ATHEROSCLEROSIS

Proceedings of the Second International Symposium

Edited by

Richard J. Jones

With 150 figures

Springer-Verlag Berlin · Heidelberg · New York 1970

Proceedings of the Second International Symposium
on Atherosclerosis
Held in Chicago, Illinois,
November 2nd-5th, 1969

Sponsored by the

1. International Society of Cardiology

Scientific Council on Atherosclerosis and Ischaemic Heart Disease

Scientific Council on Epidemiology and Prevention

2. European Atherosclerosis Group

3. American Heart Association
Council on Arteriosclerosis
Council on Cerebrovascular Disease
Council on Epidemiology

4. Chicago Heart Association

ISBN 978-3-642-48762-0 ISBN 978-3-642-48760-6 (eBook)
DOI 10.1007/978-3-642-48760-6

Softcover reprint of the hardcover 1st edition 1970

EDITORIAL COMMITTEE

RICHARD J. JONES, Chairman · LOUIS COHEN · REUBEN EISENSTEIN · GODFREY S. GETZ · GEORGE M. HASS · HUGH J. MCDONALD · RUTH PICK · ANGELO SCANU · JOHN SCHWEPPE

EXECUTIVE COMMITTEE

LOUIS N. KATZ, General Chairman
ROBERT W. WISSLER, Organizing Secretary
C. BRUCE TAYLOR, Chicago Arrangements Committee and Finance Committee
RICHARD J. JONES, Chairman of Publication Committee and Editor of Proceedings
PHILIP L. WHITE, Chicago Arrangements Committee and Chairman of Convention Services and Coordinating Committee
OGLESBY PAUL, Chairman Hospitality Committee
Mrs. R. W. WISSLER, Chairman Women's Committee
Mrs. FRANCIS KLIMLEY, Co-Chairman Women's Committee
Mrs. CORA GILLETT, Staff Representative

INTERNATIONAL PROGRAM COMMITTEE

ROBERT W. WISSLER, Chairman, Chicago, Illinois, U.S.A.
JEAN LOUIS BEAUMONT, Creteil, France
LARS A. CARLSON, Stockholm, Sweden
FREDERICK H. EPSTEIN, Ann Arbor, Michigan, U.S.A.
IVAN D. FRANTZ, JR., Minneapolis, Minnesota, U.S.A.
ROBERT H. FURMAN, Oklahoma City, Oklahoma, U.S.A.
ALAN N. HOWARD, Cambridge, England
RICHARD J. JONES, Chicago, Illinois, U.S.A.
HENRY C. MCGILL, JR., San Antonio, Texas, U.S.A.
GARDNER C. MCMILLAN, Bethesda, Maryland, U.S.A.
CLARK H. MILLIKAN, Rochester, Minnesota, U.S.A.
CONSTANTINOS J. MIRAS, Athens, Greece
MICHAEL F. OLIVER, Edinburgh, Scotland
RODOLFO PAOLETTI, Milan and Cagliari, Italy
GOTTHARD SCHETTLER, Heidelberg, Germany
DANIEL STEINBERG, San Diego, California, U.S.A.
STEWART WOLF, Oklahoma City, Oklahoma, U.S.A.

PREFACE

This is the second of a number of international symposia which will, I hope, continue to be held until atherosclerosis is no longer a major problem. The first symposium was held three years ago in Athens, Greece, under the chairmanship of Dr. Constantinos J. Miras[1], who, although he could not attend this symposium, participated actively in the deliberations of this Program Committee.

Atherosclerosis together with its sequelae constitute the most important source of morbidity and mortality in civilized countries. While a major attack is being made on the consequences, the sequelae of this disease, not enough attention is being paid to the basic cause, atherosclerosis. Yet, if the basic disease were eradicated, the major concern of this symposium, the sequelae would constitute only a minor and rare disease group.

The approach of the Program Committee was to bring together experts in the multiple disciplines which have a bearing on atherosclerosis. There is a great need for an exchange of ideas from various groups studying the basic process in many divergent ways. The hope we have is that those present (or those later studying the Proceedings) may be stimulated to attack the problem in new ways. Perhaps a breakthrough will be made or, at least, a brick or two added to build the structure, a rampart needed to defend against atherosclerosis. Better still, their contributions may help to confine it to a small area.

Conferences like this one are extremely useful in creating free interchange of views by free discussion at the formal sessions, and in the corridors, among a group of international experts of widely different backgrounds, prejudices, and viewpoints. Thus is progress achieved. Not only should these conferences continue but also the group participating in them should be expanded. We need to organize in other regions, namely in the Asian-Pacific, Latin-American, and the African areas, groups similar to those we now have in Europe and North America.

LOUIS N. KATZ
(Chairman of the Symposium)

---

[1] MIRAS, C. J., HOWARD, A., and PAOLETTI, R. (Eds.): *Progress in Biochemical Pharmacology*. Vol. 4. International Symposium on Atherosclerosis (Athens 1965). Basel: S. Karger AG. 1968.

ACKNOWLEDGEMENTS

This Symposium would not have been possible without the generous financial support of the following foundations, individuals and companies: Abbott Laboratories, American Meat Institute, American Optical Company, Ayerst Laboratories (Division of American Home Products Corporation), Albert Baer, Marion G. and S. Max Becker Jr. Foundation, Bristol Laboratories (Division of Bristol-Myers Company), Burroughs Wellcome and Company (U.S.A.) Inc., Central National Bank in Chicago, Chicago Federal Savings and Loan Association, CIBA Pharmaceutical Company (Division of CIBA Corporation), Coronary Research Foundation—Massachusetts General Hospital, CPC International Inc., Nathan Cummings, The First National Bank of Chicago, Geigy Pharmaceuticals (Division of Geigy Chemical Corporation), The Harris Foundation, Hoffman-La Roche, Inc., Albert and Mary Lasker Foundation, Lever Brothers, Eli Lilly and Company, Mead Johnson Research Center, Medtronic, Inc., Merck Sharp and Dohme Research Laboratories (Division of Merck and Company, Inc.), Arthur H. Motley—Parade Publications, National Dairy Council, National Live Stock and Meat Board, Pfizer Laboratories Division—Chas. Pfizer and Company, The Procter and Gamble Company, Psychists, Inc., Real Fresh Milk, Inc., Sandoz Pharmaceuticals (Division of Sandoz, Inc.), Schering Corporation, G. D. Searle and Company, Smith, Kline and French Laboratories, Squibb Institute for Medical Research, Standard Scientific, Statham Instruments, Inc., Sterling Drug, Inc., W. Clement and Jessie V. Stone Foundation, Travenol Laboratories, Inc. (Division Baxter Laboratories, Inc.), The Upjohn Company, Wallace Pharmaceuticals, The Wander Foundation—Dorsey Laboratories, Warner-Lambert Pharmaceutical Company, Warner-Lambert Research Institute, Wine Growers of California, Worthington Foods, Inc. and particularly the Chicago Heart Association, the American Heart Association and the National Heart Institute.

Specific support for the publication of the Proceedings has been received from Armour and Company, Armour Pharmaceutical Company, Unilever Research Laboratories—The Netherlands and the National Heart Institute, National Institutes of Health, United States Public Health Service grant No. 1 R13 HE12539-01.

Substantial guarantees against loss were also made by The Chicago Heart Association, The Council on Arteriosclerosis of The American Heart Association and The National Heart Institute of the National Institutes of Health.

The Editor is grateful for the hard-working and mutually cooperating members of the Publications Committee. Preparation of the final manuscript was accomplished with the excellent assistance of Mrs. Sylvia Bargen, Mrs. Pat Bradley and Mrs. Charlotte Greyson.

The organization of the Symposium was accomplished with grace and efficiency by Mrs. Cora Gillett and her staff assistants.

CONTENTS

V. Serum Lipoproteins

VI. Selected Papers on Lipoproteins and Atherosclerosis

VII. Regulation of Triglycerides, Including Carbohydrate-Lipid Interaction

VIII. Sterol Balance and Metabolism

IX. Selected Papers on Lipid Metabolism

X. Environmental and Host Factors in Coronary Heart Disease, Including Risk Factors: An Epidemiological View

XI. Selected Papers on Epidemiology of Atherosclerosis

XII. Nutritional Studies and Atherosclerosis

XIII. Selected Papers on Nutritional Studies

LIST OF AUTHORS

ADAMS, COLIN W. M., M.A., M.D., D.Sc., M.R.C.P., M.C. Path., Professor of Pathology, Guy's Hospital Medical School, London University, London, England

ADAMS, WRIGHT, M.D., Professor, Emeritus, Pritzker School of Medicine, Department of Medicine, University of Chicago, Chicago, Illinois, U.S.A.

AHRENS, EDWARD HAMBLIN, JR., M.D., Professor of Medicine, The Rockefeller University, New York, New York, U.S.A.

ALAUPOVIC, PETAR, Ph.D., Oklahoma Medical Research Foundation, Oklahoma City, Oklahoma, U.S.A.

ASTRUP, POUL, M.D., Professor of Clinical Chemistry, Department of Clinical Chemistry, Rigshospitalet, Copenhagen, Denmark

BAGDADE, JOHN D., M.D., Department of Medicine, University of Washington School of Medicine, Seattle, Washington, U.S.A.

BEAUMONT, JEAN-LOUIS, M.D., Professor Agregé a la Faculté de Médecine de Paris, Institut National de la Santé et de la Recherche Médicale, Hôpital Henri-Mondor, 94, Créteil, France

BERKSON, DAVID M., M.D., Chicago Health Research Foundation, Assistant Professor, Northwestern University, Chicago, Illinois, U.S.A.

BICHER, HAIM I., M.D., Ph.D., Assistant Professor, Department of Anatomy, Medical University of South Carolina, Charleston, South Carolina, U.S.A.

BIERENBAUM, MARVIN L., M.D., F.A.C.P., Atherosclerosis Research Group, St. Vincent's Hospital, Montclair, New Jersey, U.S.A.

BIERMAN, EDWIN L., B.A., M.D., Professor of Medicine, University of Washington School of Medicine and V.A. Hospital, Seattle, Washington, U.S.A.

BISS, KURT, M.D., The DeKalb Clinic, DeKalb, Illinois and The Department of Medicine, Northwestern University School of Medicine, Chicago, Illinois, U.S.A.

BJÖRKERUD, SOREN, M.D., Ph.D., Departments of Histology and Medicine I University of Goteborg, Goteborg, Sweden

BJÖRNTORP, PER, M.D., Ph.D., Assistant Professor of Experimental Medicine, First Medical Service, Sahlgren's Hospital, University of Goteborg, Goteborg, Sweden

BLACKBURN, HENRY, B.S., M.D., M.S., Professor, Lab. of Physiological Hygiene, University of Minnesota, Minneapolis, Minnesota, U.S.A.

BLATON, V., Dr. Sc., Simon Stevin Institute for Scientific Research, Brugge Belgium

BOBERG, JONAS, M.D., M.R.C. Research Fellow, King Gustaf Vth Research Institute, Department of Clinical Physiology, Karolinska Hospital, Stockholm, Sweden

BOLZANO, KLAUS, M.D., Medizinische Universitätsklinik, Innsbruck, Austria

BORN, GUSTAV VICTOR RUDOLPH, M.B., Ch.B., D. Phil., Vandervell Professor of Pharmacology, University of London and The Royal College of Surgeons of England, London, England

BOWYER, DAVID E., M.D., Post-doctoral Fellow, Department of Pathology, University of Cambridge, Cambridge, England

BOYD, G. S., M.D., Reader in Department of Biochemistry, University of Edinburgh Medical School, Edinburgh, Scotland

BRAUNSTEINER, HERBERT, M.D., Professor for Internal Medicine, Medizinische Universitätsklinik, Innsbruck, Austria

BROWN, HELEN B., Ph.D., Research Consultant, Research Division, The Cleveland Clinic, Cleveland, Ohio

BUCHWALD, HENRY, M.D., Ph.D., Assistant Professor of Surgery, Department of Surgery, University of Minnesota Medical School, Minneapolis, Minnesota, U.S.A.

CARLSON, LAR. S., M.D., Professor of Geriatrics, Chairman, Department of Geriatrics, Medical Faculty, Uppsala University, Uppsala, Sweden

CHANDLER, A. B., M.D., Professor of Pathology, Medical College of Georgia, Augusta, Georgia, U.S.A.

CHAPMAN, M. J., B.Sc., Courtauld Institute of Biochemistry, The Middlesex Hospital Medical School, London, England

CHOBANIAN, ARAM. V., M.D., Associate Professor of Medicine, Boston University School of Medicine, Boston, Massachusetts, U.S.A.

CLEMENTS, REX. S., JR., M.D., George S. Cox Medical Research Institute, Department of Medicine, University of Pennsylvania, Philadelphia, Pennsylvania, U.S.A.

COATS, D. A., Professor of Physiology, University of Melbourne, Parkville, Victoria, Australia

COHEN, LOUIS, M.D., Associate Professor, Department of Medicine, Pritzker School of Medicine, University of Chicago, Chicago, Illinois, U.S.A.

COLACO, F., M.B., B.S., Registrar, Intensive Cardiac Care Unit, K.E.M. Hospital, Bombay, India

COLLINS, F. D., Ph.D., Senior Research Fellow, Department of Biochemistry, University of Melbourne, Parkville, Victoria, Australia

CONNOR, WILLIAM E., M.D., Professor of Medicine, Director Clinical Research Center, University of Iowa College of Medicine, U. of I. Hospitals, Iowa City, Iowa, U.S.A.

CORNFIELD, JEROME, B.S., Research Professor in Biostatistics, University of Pittsburgh Graduate School of Public Health, Bethesda, Maryland, U.S.A.

CORNWELL, D. G., Ph.D., Professor and Chairman, Department of Physiological Chemistry, College of Medicine, Ohio State University, Columbus, Ohio, U.S.A.

CUMPSTON, G. N., M.R.A.C.P., Cardiologist, University of Western Australia, Perth, Australia

CURNOW, D. H., Ph.D., Professor, Clinical Biochemistry University of Western Australia, Perth, Australia

DAOUD, A. S., M.D., Professor of Pathology, Albany Medical College, Albany, New York, U.S.A.

DATEY, K. K., M.D., F.R.C.P., Professor of Medicine, Director, Department of Cardiology, G.S. Medical College, K.E.M. Hospital, Bombay, India

DAY, ALLAN, J., M.D., Professor of Physiology, Department of Physiology, University of Melbourne, Parkville, Victoria, Australia

DAY, CHARLES E., Department of Biochemistry, University of Louisville School of Medicine, Louisville, Ky, U.S.A.

DAYTON, SEYMOUR, M.D., Chief of Medical Service, Wadsworth V.A. Hospital and Professor of Medicine (UCLA School of Medicine), Los Angeles, California, U.S.A.

DE BOER, J., Ph.D., Unilever Research Laboratory, Vlaardingen, The Netherlands

DEMPSEY, MARY E., Ph.D., Associate Professor of Biochemistry, University of Minnesota, Department of Biochemistry, Minneapolis, Minnesota, U.S.A.

EGGEN, DOUGLAS A., Ph.D., Department of Pathology, Louisiana State University Medical Center, New Orleans, Louisiana, U.S.A.

EPSTEIN, FREDERICK H., M.D., Professor, Department of Epidemiology, The University of Michigan, School of Public Health, Ann Arbor, Michigan, U.S.A.

EVANS, J. GRIMLEY, M.B. (Cantab.), M.R.C.P., Research Fellow in Clinical Epidemiology, Medical Unit, Wellington Hospital, Wellington, New Zealand

FALES, HENRY, Ph.D., Head, Section on Chemistry, Molecular Disease Branch, National Heart Institute, Bethesda, Maryland, U.S.A.

FEJFAR, ZDENEK, MU Dr., D.Sc., Chief, Cardiovascular Diseases, Institute for Cardiovascular Research, World Health Organization, Geneva, Switzerland

FILO, RONALD S., M.D., Resident in Surgery, Medical School, Department of Surgery, University of Michigan, Ann Arbor, Michigan U.S.A.

FLEISCHMAN, ALAN I., Ph.D., F.A.I.C., Atherosclerosis Research Group, St. Vincent's Hospital, Montclair, New Jersey, U.S.A.

FLORENTIN, R. A., M.D., Associate Professor of Pathology, Albany Medical College, Albany, New York, U.S.A.

FRANK, CHARLES W., M.D., Associate Professor Medicine, Albert Einstein College of Medicine and Health Insurance Plan of Greater New York, New York, New York, U.S.A.

FRANTZ, IVAN D., JR., M.D., George S. Clark Research Professor, Departments of Medicine and Biochemistry, University of Minnesota, Medical School, Minneapolis, Minnesota, U.S.A.

FRANZBLAU, CARL, Ph.D., Associate Professor of Biochemistry, Boston University School of Medicine, Department of Biochemistry, Boston, Massachusetts, U.S.A.

FREDRICKSON, DONALD S., M.D., Director, Intramural Research, Chief, Molecular Disease Branch, National Heart Institute, Bethesda, Maryland, U.S.A.

FREIS, EDWARD D., M.D., Professor and Chief, Cardiovascular Research Laboratory, University Hospital, Veterans Administration Hospital, Washington, D.C., U.S.A.

FRENCH, JOHN E., K.M., D. Phil., M.C. Path., Reader in Pathology, Sir William Dunn School of Pathology, Oxford, England

FREYSCHUSS, ULLA, M.D., Research Associate, Department of Geriatrics, Uppsala University, Uppsala, Sweden

FRITZ, K. E., M.D., Department of Pathology, Albany Medical College, Albany, New York, U.S.A.

FRY, WILLIAM J., M.D., F.A.C.S., Professor and Head, Section of General Surgery, University of Michigan Medical School, Department of Surgery, Ann Arbor, Michigan, U.S.A.

FURMAN, ROBERT H., M.D., Oklahoma Medical Research Foundation, Oklahoma City, Oklahoma, U.S.A.

GEER, JACK C., M.D., Professor and Chairman, Department of Pathology, College of Medicine, The Ohio State University, Columbus, Ohio, U.S.A.

GETZ, GODFREY S., M.D., Associate Professor, Departments of Pathology and Biochemistry, University of Chicago, Chicago, Illinois, U.S.A.

GOFF, D. V., B.Sc., Biochemist, University of Western Australia, Perth, Australia

GOLDRICK, ROBERT BRIAN, M.D., F.R.A.C.P., Senior Fellow, Department of Clinical Science, The John Curtin School of Medical Research, The Australian National University, Canberra, A.C.T., Australia

GOODMAN, DEWITT, S., M.D., Professor of Medicine, Department of Medicine, Columbia University College of Physicians and Surgeons, New York, New York, U.S.A.

GOTTENBOS, J. J., Ph.D., Unilever Research Laboratory, Vlaardingen, The Netherlands

GREER, WILLIAM E., D.V.M., Director, Animal Care, Gulf South Research Institute, New Iberia, Louisiana, U.S.A.

GRESHAM, G. A., M.D., Ac.D., M.A., M.C. Pathology, Department of Pathology, University of Cambridge, Cambridge, England

GRETEN, HEINER, M.D., Medizinische Universitätsklinik, Heidelberg, Germany

GROEN, JOHANNES J., M.D., Professor, Jelcrsama Clinic, University Hospital, Department of Psychological Research, Leiden, The Netherlands

GUSTAFSON, ANDERS, M.D., Assistant Professor, First Medical Service, University of Goteborg, Goteborg, Sweden

HARMAN, DENHAM, M.D., Professor of Biochemistry and Medicine, College of Medicine, University of Nebraksa, Omaha, Nebraska, U.S.A.

HASS, GEORGE M., M.D., Professor and Chairman, Division of Pathology, University of Illinois and Presbyterian-St. Luke's Hospital, Chicago, Illinois, U.S.A.

HAUST, M. DARIA, M.D., M.Sc., Professor of Pathology, The University of Western Ontario, London, Ontario, Canada

HAVEL, RICHARD J., M.D., Professor of Medicine, Associate Director, Cardiovascular Research Institute, University of California Medical Center, San Francisco, U.S.A.

HAYTON, THOMAS, Ph.D., Atherosclerosis Research Group, St. Vincent's Hospital, Montclair, New Jersey, U.S.A.

HAZZARD, WILLIAM R., M.D., Veterans Administration Hospital, Seattle, Washington, U.S.A.

HO, KANG-JEY, M.D., Ph.D., Department of Pathology, Northwestern University, School of Medicine, The Evanston Hospital, Evanston, Illinois, U.S.A.

HOLLAND, GERALD F., Ph. D., Medical Research Laboratories, Chas. Pfizer & Co., Groton, Connecticut, U.S.A.

HOLLANDER, WILLIAM, M.D., Professor of Medicine, University Hospital, Boston University Medical Center, Boston, Massachusetts, U.S.A.

HORNSTRA, G., Research Assistant, Unilever Research Laboratory, Vlaardingen, The Netherlands

HOWARD, ALAN N., M.A., Ph.D., Department of Investigative Medicine, University of Cambridge, Cambridge, England

IMAI, H., M.D., Ph.D., Department of Pathology, Albany Medical College, Albany, New York, U.S.A.

JARMOLYCH, J., Department of Pathology, Albany Medical College, Albany, New York, U.S.A.

JARRETT, R. J., M.A., M.D., Lecturer in Medicine, Guy's Hospital Medical School, London, England

JENNINGS, ROBERT B., M.D., Professor of Pathology, Northwestern University Medical School, Chicago, Illinois, U.S.A.

JENKINS, D. J. A., B.A., Research Associate, University of Western Australia, Perth, Australia

JOHNSTONE, C. J., B.Sc., Computing Officer, University of Western Australia, Perth, Australia

JONES, RICHARD J., M.A., M.D., Associate Professor, Department of Medicine, Pritzker School of Medicine, University of Chicago, Chicago, Illinois, U.S.A.

JØRGENSEN, LEIF, M.D., Associate Professor, Assistant Director, Department of Pathology, Ulleval Hospital, University of Oslo, Oslo, Norway

KATZ, LOUIS N., M.A., M.D., D.Sc. (Honorary), Director Emeritus, Cardiovascular Research Institute, Michael Reese Hospital and Medical Center, Chicago, Illinois, U.S.A.

KEEN, HARRY, M.D., M.R.C.P., Reader in Medicine, Department of Medicine, Guy's Hospital, London, England

KEYS, ANCEL B., Ph.D., Professor and Director, Laboratory of Physiological Hygiene, University of Minnesota, Minneapolis, Minnesota, U.S.A.

KIM, D. N., M.D., Ph.D., Department of Pathology, Albany Medical College, Albany, New York, U.S.A.

KJELDSEN, KNUD, M.D., Department of Clinical Chemistry A., Rigshospitalet, Copenhagen, Denmark

KRAMSCH, DIETER M., M.D., Assistant Professor of Medicine, University Hospital, Boston University Medical Center, Boston, Massachusetts, U.S.A.

KRITCHEVSKY, DAVID, The Wistar Institute, Philadelphia, Pennsylvania, U.S.A.

LAWSON, MARGARET E., Department of Biochemistry, University of Edinburgh Medical School, Edinburgh, Scotland

LEE, K. T., M.D., Ph.D., Professor of Pathology, Albany Medical College, Albany, New York, U.S.A.

LEONARD, R. F., Research Assistant, Department of Biochemistry, University of Melbourne, Parkville, Victoria, Australia

LEVY, ROBERT I., M.D., Head, Section on Lipoproteins, Molecular Disease Branch, N.H.I., Bethesda, Maryland, U.S.A.

LEVY, ROBERT S., Ph.D., Department of Biochemistry, School of Medicine, University of Louisville, Louisville, Kentucky, U.S.A.

LEWIS, IRVING J., Department of Health, Education and Welfare, Bethesda, Maryland, U.S.A.

LILLE, ROBERT D., M.D., formerly Research Associate, Boston University School of Medicine, Lt. Commander U.S. Naval Hospital, Chelsea, Massachusetts, U.S.A.

LINDBERG, HOWARD A., M.D., Chief of Staff, Wesley Memorial Hospital, and Professor, Northwestern University School of Medicine, Chicago, Illinois, U.S.A.

LINDSTEDT, SVEN, M.D., Professor of Clinical Chemistry, Department of Clinical Chemistry, Sahlgren's Hospital, University of Gothenburg, Sweden

MARAGOUDAKIS, M. E., Ph.D., CIBA Pharmacntical Company, Research Department, Summit, New Jersey, U.S.A.

MARQUIS, NORMAN R., Ph.D., Department of Biochemistry, Mead Johnson Research Center, Evansville, Indiana, U.S.A.

MAYNARD, A. T., Senior Technician, Department of Biochemistry, University of Melbourne, Parkville, Victoria, Australia

MCGILL, HENRY C., M.D., Professor and Chairman, Department of Pathology, University of Texas, Medical School at San Antonio, San Antonio, Texas, U.S.A.

MCMILLAN, GARDINER C., M.D., National Heart Institute, Bethesda, Maryland, U.S.A.

MEDALIE, JACK H., M.B., Ch.B., Chairman and Associate Professor of Family Medicine, Tel Aviv University Medical School, Tel Aviv, Israel

MIALL, WILLIAM E., M.D., Director, Medical Research Council, Epidemiology Unit, University of the West Indies, Kingston, Jamaica

MIETTINEN, TATU A., M.D., Third Department of Medicine, University of Helsinki, Helsinki, Finland

MILLER, W. A., M.D., Chicago Health Research Foundation, Chicago, Illinois, U.S.A.

MILLS, G. L., Ph.D., Clinical Genetics Unit, Institute of Child Health, and Courtald Institute of Biochemistry, Middlesex Hospital Medical School, London, England

MOORE, RICHARD B., M.D., Instructor of Medicine, Department of Medicine, University of Minnesota Medical School, Minneapolis, Minnesota, U.S.A.

MORRIS, MANFORD D., Ph.D., Departments of Pediatrics and Biochemistry, University of Arkansas Medical Center, Little Rock, Arkansas, U.S.A.

MORRISON, ANTHONY D., M.D., George S. Cox Research Institute, University of Pennsylvania Hospital, Philadelphia, Pennsylvania, U.S.A.

MORRISON, E. S., Ph.D., Department of Pathology, Albany Medical College, Albany, New York, U.S.A.

MUSTARD, J. FRASER, M.D., Ph.D., Department of Pathology, Professor and Chairman, McMaster University, Hamilton, Ontario, Canada

NAM, S. C., M.D., Assistant Professor of Pathology, Albany Medical College, Albany, New York, U.S.A.

NEWMAN, H. A. I., Ph.D., Associate Professor, Department of Pathology, College of Medicine, Ohio State University, Columbus, Ohio, U.S.A.

NIKKILÄ, ESKO A., M.D., Third Department of Medicine, University of Helsinki, Helsinki, Finland

OLIVER, M. F., M.D., F.R.C.P., Chairman, Division of Cardiovascular Research, Royal Infirmary, and Chairman, ISC Scientific Council on Atherosclerosis and Ischemic Heart Disease, University of Edinburgh, Edinburgh, Scotland

PANGANAMALA, R. V., Ph.D., Instructor, Departments of Pathology and Physiological Chemistry, College of Medicine, Ohio State University, Columbus, Ohio, U.S.A.

PAOLETTI, RODOLFO, M.D., Professor of Pharmacology, Instituto di Farmacologia e di Terapie, University of Milan and Universita Degli Studi, Milano, Italy

PARKER, ROGER A., Ph.D., Postdoctoral Fellow, Division of Medicinal Chemistry, College of Pharmacy, The Ohio State University, Columbus, Ohio, U.S.A.

PAUL, OGLESBY, M.D., Chief of Staff, Passavant Memorial Hospital, Professor of Medicine, Northwestern University Medical School, Chicago, Illinois, U.S.A.

PEETERS, HUBERT, M.D., Lecturer, University of Louvain and Director, Simon Stevin Institute for Scientific Research, Brugge, Belgium

PEREIRA, JOSEPH N., Ph.D., Medical Research Laboratories, Charles Pfizer & Co., Groton, Connecticut, U.S.A.

PETERSON, OSLER L., M.D., Professor, Department of Preventive Medicine, Harvard Medical School, Boston, Massachusetts, U.S.A.

PINTO, IVAN J., M.D., F.R.C.P., M.R.C.P., F.A.C.C., Associate Professor of Medicine, G.S. Medical College of Bombay and K.E.M. Hospital of Bombay, Bombay, India

PORTE, DANIEL, JR., M.D., Assistant Professor, Department of Medicine, University of Washington School of Medicine, Seattle, Washington, U.S.A.

PRIOR, IAN A. M., M.D.(N.Z.), F.R.A.C.P., M.R.C.P., Director, Medical Unit, Wellington Hospital, Wellington, New Zealand

RAICHELSON, ROBERT, M.D., Atherosclerosis Research Group, St. Vincent's Hospital, Montclair, New Jersey, U.S.A.

REID, DONALD DARNLEY, M.D., D.Sc., F.R.C.P., Professor of Epidemiology, London School of Hygiene and Tropical Medicine, London, England

RITTER, MARY C., M.D., Predoctoral Fellow, Department of Biochemistry, University of Minnesota, Minneapolis, Minnesota, U.S.A.

ROBERT, LESLIE, M.D., Maitre de Recherches au CNRS, Directeur de Laboratoire de Biochimie du Tissu Conjonctif, Paris, France

ROSE, GEOFFREY, D.M., M.R.C.P., London School of Hygiene and Tropical Medicine, London, England

ROYLE, J. P., F.R.C.S., First Assistant, Department of Surgery, Austin Hospital, Parkville, Victoria, Australia

SAILER, SIGURD, M.D., Univ.-Dozent, Oberarzt der Med. Univ. Klinik, Medical Department, University of Innsbruck, Innsbruck, Austria

SANDHOFER, FRIEDRICH, M.D., Univ.-Dozent, Medical Department, University of Innsbruck, Innsbruck, Austria

SCANU, ANGELO, M.D., Associate Professor, Department of Medicine, Pritzker School of Medicine, University of Chicago, Chicago, Illinois, U.S.A.

SCHETTLER, GOTTHARD, M.D., Professor of Int. Med., Head and Chairman of the Department of Internal Medicine, President of Medical Faculties of the German Federal Republic, Heidelberg University, Heidelberg, Germany

SCHLIERF, GUENTER, M.D., Medizinische Universitätsklinik, University of Heidelberg, Heidelberg, Germany

SCOTT, R. F., B.Sc., M.D., Professor of Pathology, Albany Medical College and Albany Medical Center Hospital, Albany, New York, U.S.A.

SEIDEL, DIETRICH, M.D., Medizinische Universitätsklinik, University of Heidelberg, Heidelberg, Germany

SHAPER, A. G., M.B., M.R.C.P., M.C. Path., Research Professor in Cardiovascular Diseases, Makerere University College Medical School and W.H.O. Cardiovascular Research and Training Center, Kampala, Uganda

SHAPIRO, SAM, M.D., Health Insurance Plan of Greater New York, Albert Einstein College of Medicine, New York, New York, U.S.A.

SHORE, B., B.S., Ph.D., Division Leader, Bio-Medical Division, Lawrence Radiation Laboratory, University of California, Livermore, California, U.S.A.

SHORE, PARKHURST A., Ph.D., Professor of Pharmacology, Associate Dean, Graduate Studies, University of Texas Southwestern Medical School, Dallas, Texas, U.S.A.

SHORE, V. G., Ph.D., Biochemist, Bio-Medical Division, Lawrence Radiation Laboratory, University of California, Livermore, California, U.S.A.

Sinclair, A. J., Ph.D., Post-doctoral Fellow, University of Western Ontario, London, Ontario, Canada

Sinclair, Hugh, D.M., D.Sc., Fellow, Magdalen College, Oxford, England

Sinnett, Peter Frank, M.B., Research Fellow, National Heart Foundation of Australia, Department of Clinical Science, the John Curtin School of Medical Research, The Australian National University, Canberra, Australia

Slack, Joan, B.M., M.R.C. Clinical Genetics Unit, Institute of Child Health, London, England

Slater, Rosalind S., British Heart Foundation Unit, Department of Chemical Pathology, University of Aberdeen, Aberdeen, Scotland

Sloan, Charles, B.A., Research Associate, Department of Surgery, University of Michigan Medical School, Ann Arbor, Michigan, U.S.A.

Smith, Elspeth, B., B.A., Ph.D., Research Fellow, University of Aberdeen Medical School, Aberdeen, Scotland

Soyugenc, Rahmi, M.S., Division of Adult Healt and Aging, Chicago Board of Health, Chicago, Illinois, U.S.A.

Stamler, Jeremiah, M.D., Chief, Chicago Health Research Foundation, Northwestern University Medical School, Chicago, Illinois, U.S.A.

Stamler, Rose, M.A., Chicago Health Research Foundation, Chicago, Illinois, U.S.A.

Stein, Olga, M.D., Associate Professor of Experimental Medicine, Department of Experimental Medicine and Cancer Research, Hebrew University-Hadassah Medical School, Jerusalem, Israel

Stein, Yechezkiel, M.D., Professor of Medicine, Lipid Research Laboratory, Hebrew University-Hadassah Medical School, Jerusalem, Israel

Steinberg, Daniel, M.D., Ph.D., Professor of Medicine, Head, Division of Metabolic Disease Department of Medicine, University of California at San, Diego, La Jolla, California, U.S.A.

Stenhouse, N. S., M.Sc., Director of Medical Statistics, University of Western Australia, Perth, Australia

Stevens, E. L., R.N., Chicago Health Research Foundation, Chicago, Illinois, U.S.A.

Stossberg, Veit, M.D., Medizinische Universitätsklinik, University of Heidelberg, Heidelberg, Germany

Strong, Jack P., B.S., M.D., Professor and Chairman, Department of Pathology, Louisiana State University School of Medicine, New Orleans, Louisiana, U.S.A.

Studer, Alfred, M.D., Director, Department of Experimental Medicine, Professor of Experimental Pathology, F. Hoffmann-LaRoche & Co., Ltd, Basel, Switzerland

Summers, M., B.Sc., Biochemist, University of Western Australia, Perth, Australia

Taskinen, Marja-Riitta, Third Department of Medicine, University of Helsinki, Helsinki, Finland

TAVORMINA, PETER A., Ph.D., Department of Biochemistry, Mead Johnson Research Center, Evansville, Indiana, U.S.A.

TAYLOR, C. BRUCE, M.D., Director of Laboratories, Evanston Hospital, and Professor of Pathology, Northwestern University Medical School, Chicago, Illinois, U.S.A.

THOMAS, PETER, M.B., B.S., Senior Registrar, Intensive Cardiac Care Unit, K.E.M. Hospital, Bombay, India

THOMAS, WILBUR A., M.D., Professor and Chairman, Department of Pathology, Albany Medical College, Albany, New York, U.S.A.

THOMASSON, H. J., M.D., Consultant on Med. and Biol. Problems, Past Head of Biological Research Division, Unilever Research Laboratory, Vlaardingen, The Netherlands

THORP, J. M., B.Sc., Research Associate, Biology Department, Research Department, I.C.I. Pharmaceuticals Division, Macclesfield, Cheshire, England

TIAMSON, E., M.D., Assistant Professor of Pathology, Albany Medical College, Albany, New York, U.S.A.

TIBBLIN, GOSTA, M.D., Assistant Professor, First Medical Service, Sahlgren's Hospital, University of Goteborg, Goteborg, Sweden

TOKICK, THOMAS J., Chicago Health Research Foundation, Chicago, Illinois, U.S.A.

TURPEINEN, OSMO, M.D., Ph.D., Professor of Biochemistry, College of Veterinary Medicine, Helsinki, Finland

TYAVOKIN, V. V., Dr. Med. Sci., Chair of Hospital Therapy, Section of General Physiology, Leningrad Pediatric Medical Institute, Institute of Experimental Medicine, Academy of Medical Sciences, Leningrad, USSR

VARCO, RICHARD L., M.D., Ph.D., Professor and Chairman, Department of Surgery, University of Minnesota Medical School, Minneapolis, Minnesota, U.S.A.

VERGROESEN, A. J., M.D., Director of Biology Department, Unilever Research Laboratory, Vlaardingen, The Netherlands

VIGDAHL, ROGER L., Ph.D., Department of Biochemistry, Mead Johnson Research Center, Evansville, Indiana, U.S.A.

WAHLQUIST, MARK L., M.D., Medical Research Fellow, Department of Physiology, University of Melbourne, Parkville, Victoria, Australia

WANSTRUP, JORGEN, M.D., Associate Professor ,University Institute of Pathology, Rigshospitalet, University of Copenhagen, Copenhagen, Denmark

WATSON, PORTIA, M.S., Atherosclerosis Research Group, St. Vincent's Hospital, Montclair, New Jersey, U.S.A.

WEATHERBEE, LEE, M.D., Assistant Professor of Pathology, University of Michigan Medical School, Ann Arbor, Michigan, U.S.A.

WEINBLATT, EVE, Health Insurance Plan of Greater New York, Albert Einstein College of Medicine, New York, U.S.A.

WELBORN, T. A., M.R.C.P. (London), School of Medicine, University of Western Australia, Perth, Australia

WHITE, LAWRENCE W., M.D., Assistant Professor of Pharmacology, Established Investigator, American Heart Association, Case Western Reserve University School of Medicine, Cleveland, Ohio, U.S.A.

WHITE, PHILIP L., D. Sc., Director of The Council on Foods and Nutrition, American Medical Association, Chicago, Illinois, U.S.A.

WHYTE, HENRY MALCOLM, M.B., D. Phil., M.R.C.P., F.R.A.C.P., Professor of Clinical Science, The John Curtin School of Medical Research, The Australian National University, Canberra, Australia

WINEGRAD, ALBERT I., M.D., Department of Medicine, George S. Cox Medical Research Institute, University of Pennsylvania, Philadelphia, Pennsylvania, U.S.A.

WISSLER, ROBERT W., M.D., Professor and Chairman, Department of Pathology, Pritzker School of Medicine, University of Chicago, Chicago, Illinois, U.S.A.

WITIAK, DONALD T., Ph.D., Associate Professor Medicinal Chemistry, College of Pharmacy, The Ohio State University, Columbus, Ohio, U.S.A.

WOLF, STEWART, M.D., Professor and Chairman, Department of Medicine, University of Oklahoma Medical School, Oklahoma City, Oklahoma, U.S.A.

ZILVERSMIT, DONALD B., Ph.D., Professor, Graduate School of Nutrition and Career Investigator, A.H.A., Cornell University, Ithaca, New York, U.S.A.

KEYNOTE ADDRESS

Arteriosclerosis and its complications are the main cause of death in civilized countries. Elements of arteriosclerosis are present in all arteries, young or old, animal or human.

One cannot predict at what time the process of arteriosclerosis becomes a clinically evident disease. In spite of the impressive results of epidemiological studies of the Framingham type, it remains unclear exactly which man is going to suffer from a myocardial infarction, especially when this occurs in the absence of even one single risk factor. Why do young, lean, normolipemic, physically active, nonsmoking, normally menstruating, nondiabetic, hypotensive women sustain a myocardial infarction? I purposely have chosen an extreme example. We should study in more detail those diseases that are associated with few myocardial infarctions and slight degrees of arteriosclerosis, e.g. chronic anemias, especially pernicious anemias, cancer or leukemia. For instance among 478 obese primarily hypotensive men we did not find a case of myocardial infarction during 12 years of observation, despite the fact that 54 men were diabetics.

The systematic study of juvenile people with myocardial infarction and their relatives is a program of the International Society of Cardiology. I am glad that the Volkswagen Foundation has agreed to support a clinical institute for the study of coronary heart disease at Heidelberg University.

Germany has some peculiarities that modified the process of arteriosclerosis in a certain way. Myocardial infarctions as well as thromboembolic events were rarities toward the end of World War II and in the immediate postwar period. Similar observations had been made in other countries and after World War I. With the normalization of nutritional conditions the incidence of myocardial infarction increased markedly and in recent years has reached its highest point. Death rates from arteriosclerosis and coronary heart disease parallel the rising consumption of fat, but that is, indeed, only one factor. What is the reason for these high rates?

I would like to present some other data regarding this problem. Fig. 1 shows serum cholesterol levels of medical colleagues between 1942 and 1966. The lowest values are the result of a diet containing only about 5–10 g of fat and 10 g of animal protein and 800–1,000 total calories daily over a period of three years. Such a diet was the rule for the population in cities. Mean weight was 10–15 kg below normal. In contrast, the people living on farms held their weight at pre-war levels, had normal or high lipids and frequently developed diabetes with acidosis. In general, diabetes was rare and mild in city areas between 1943 and 1947. Since 1948, diabetes mellitus and its complications have increased considerably.

These data are in good agreement with Dr. Brown's data [247] from Albany Medical College. He showed that patients with Type IV hyperlipoproteinemia very often are obese and have pathological glucose tolerance with hyperinsulinism. One of his patients, controlled over 13 years, can be compared with our results. Abnormal glucose tolerance and hyperinsulinism are common findings in obesity. Since obesity and Type IV hyperlipoproteinemia are often correlated, weight control is a major preventive factor.

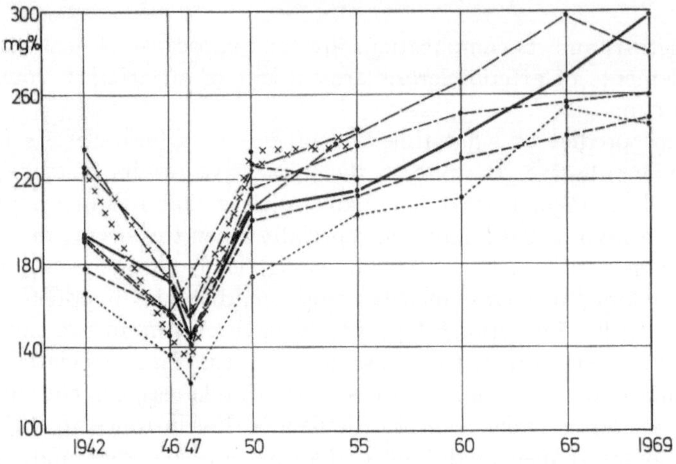

Fig. 1. Blood cholesterol in normal individuals between 1942 and 1969 (German Fed. Republ.)

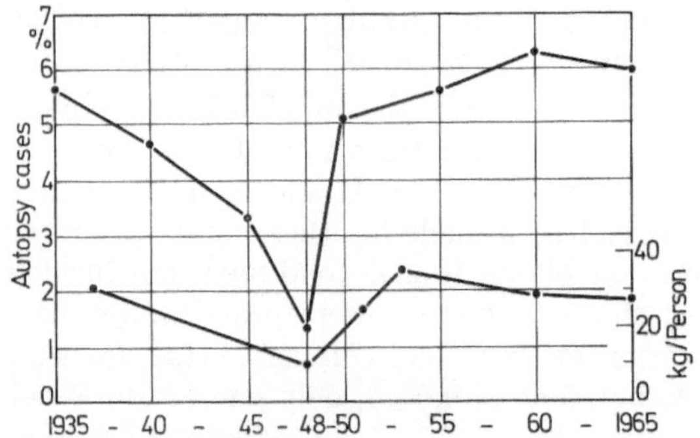

Fig. 2. Fat intake and incidence of fatal pulmonary embolism at seven hospitals[1] in the German Fed. Republ. between 1935–1965

Fig. 2 shows the incidence of pulmonary emboli according to autopsy data from Hospitals in Berlin, Frankfurt, Freiburg, Heidelberg, Marburg, Stuttgart, and Tübingen. Is arteriosclerosis a disease of thrombosis? I accept this hypothesis in most cases of arterial occlusive disease, but this must not explain the primary cause of the secondary complications. This is one of the main problems we face today.

Rokitansky's [1250] hypothesis, confirmed by findings of Duguid [408], is supported by recent data on structure, composition and function of platelets.

[1] Berlin, Frankfurt, Freiburg, Heidelberg, Marburg, Stuttgart, Tübingen.

They often agglutinate over areas of irritation of the endothelium. Platelet breakdown may increase the permeability of endothelium to plasma protein, low-density lipoprotein, and fibrinogen. Platelets also may penetrate the endothelium, especially in the presence of hemodynamic disturbances. Thus, the lipids contained in platelet cytoplasm could be liberated. Yet how does an atherosclerotic lesion, built up in this way, lead to coronary occlusion?

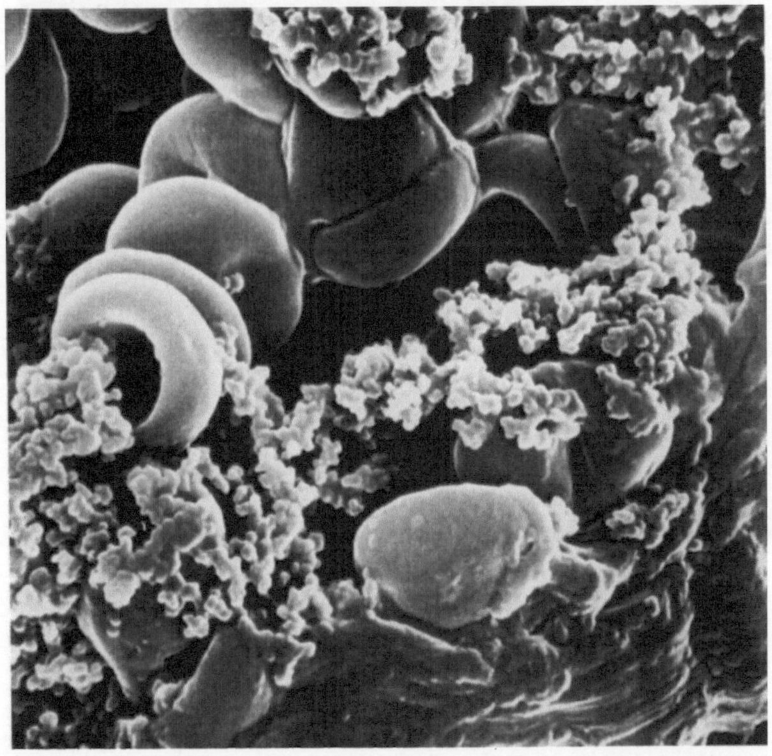

Fig. 3. Adherent aggregations of platelets and erythrocytes in a small vessel of a cheek pouch of a syrian hamster 50 minutes after intravenous administration of 300 μg/100 mg endotoxin. Magnification 5,700:1

Materials of ruptured plaques are thrombogenic. Phospholipids of the plaques contribute to tissue thromboplastic activity. Collagen could aggregate the platelets while roughened surfaces initiate clotting. Platelet stickiness, releasing factors, fibrinolytic and antifibrinolytic factors also may play a part. As a model for these processes we used the Stereoscan method. Fifty minutes after injection of endotoxin, irreversible aggregations of platelets and depositions of fibrin occur as shown in Fig. 3 (Fritsch and Urbaschek [502]). Aggregations of platelets and erythrocytes can be seen in small vessels of the cheek pouch of a Syrian hamster attached to the intimal surface. Fig. 4 shows clotted fibrin, erythrocytes and platelets. After stimulating the adventitia of the *arteria carotis* of rabbits with electrical current, platelets and the formation of fibrin aggregate 20 minutes later [504]. Twenty days later depositions of fibrin and blood cells in the intima

(Fig. 5) are found. The role of plasma lipids on platelet stickiness, as well as the influence of diet, body weight, activity, and social stress have to be examined. Pharmaco-dynamic trials offer promising results [1068, 1113, 1170].

Some clinical examples showing the importance of thrombosis especially in cases of sudden cardiac death are given herein.

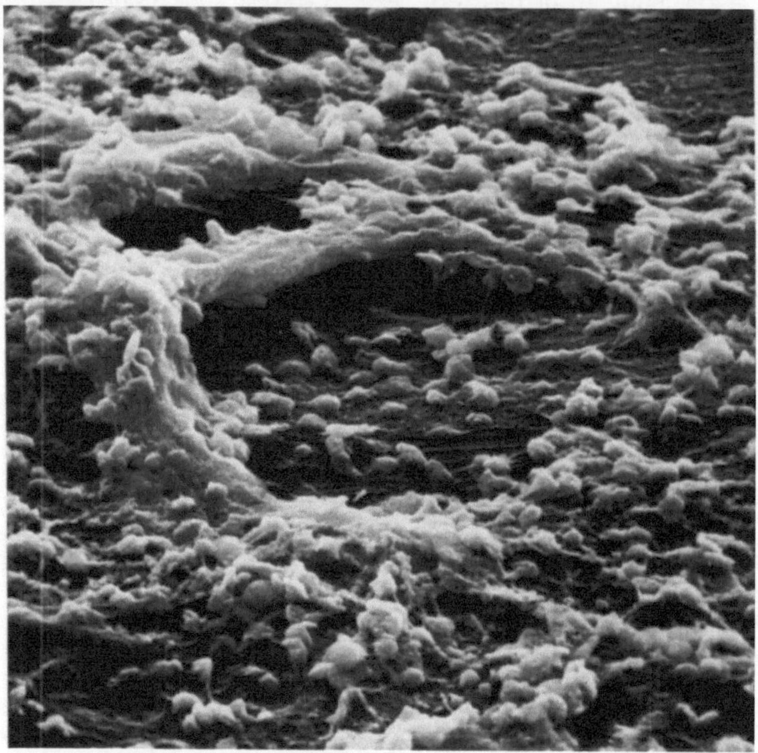

Fig. 4. Platelets and fibrin upon the intima of an arteria carotis of a rabbit 20 minutes after stimulation of the adventitia with an electrical current (170 V/1 sec). Magnification 2,000:1

Severe Coronary Artery Thrombosis in Malnourished Prisoners of War during the First Few Months after Refeeding. We saw a fair number of these patients in Germany between 1948 and 1950. Postmortem examinations revealed recent severe atherosclerotic changes, hemorrhages, and thrombosis. The vessel wall could obviously not adapt to an overnutritious diet rich in fats. Starvation might have changed the enzyme pattern and, perhaps, the composition of the ground-substance of the vessel wall. After 1950, such an exaggerated process became less frequent. It would, however, be very interesting to obtain some follow-up data on the incidence of arteriosclerosis, coronary heart disease, coronary thrombosis, etc. in people with undernutrition. To the best of my knowledge there have been no systematic studies in this area.

Severe Degrees of Atherosclerosis and Thrombosis in Young People Following a Sudden Change of Nutritional and Living Habits. We do have examples of this in men from mediterranean countries who come to work in Western Germany or Switzerland. One of these patients almost doubled his body weight from 50 kg to 95 kg within two years. He died suddenly from a myocardial infarction. At his funeral all the lean relatives stood around the grave of this prodigious man who paid a fatal tribute for his prosperous job.

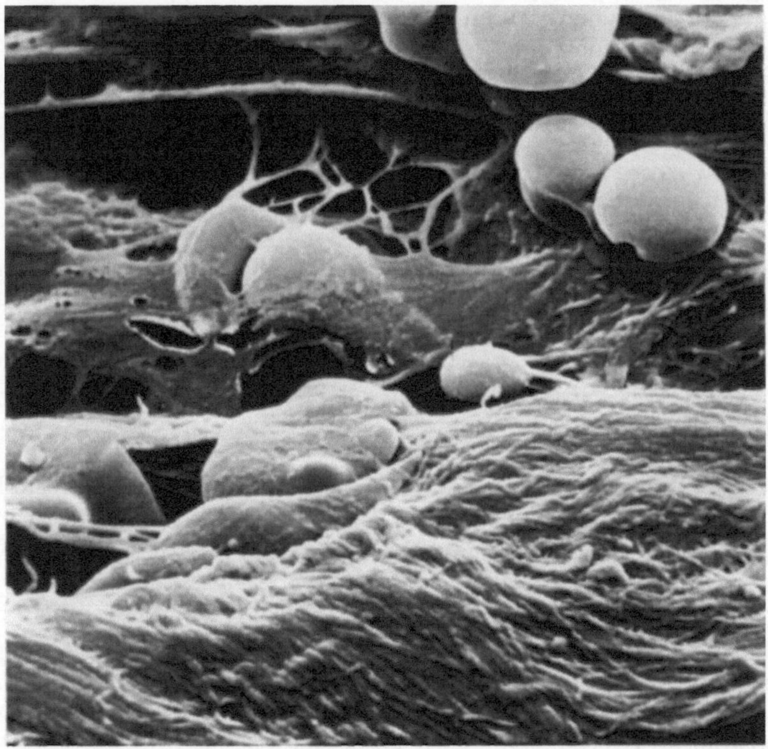

Fig. 5. Arteria carotis of a rabbit 20 days after an electrical current impulse applied to the adventitia. Fibrin and blood cells in a layer under the irritated intima. Magnification 5,500:1

Sudden Coronary Death and Acute Exacerbation of Atherosclerosis in Top Athletes at End of Their Athletic Careers. A 30-year-old bicycle champion who was the only cyclist to win the Tour de France and the Giro d'Italia in the same year abruptly stopped professional cycle-racing, considerably increased his weight, died from suicide, and demonstrated an impressive atherosclerosis.

One year after stopping active athletics a decathlon champion died with terminal thrombosis of his coronary arteries. His diet for many years contained 1 kg of meat and 10–15 eggs daily, and his body weight increased 12 kg within one year. His serum cholesterol was 450 mg-% at postmortem, but two years previously it was 195 mg-%. There was no family history of coronary disease. It seems that the abrupt change from physical training to inactivity with weight gain and rise of cholesterol are the reasons for the coronary occlusion.

There are other examples from forensic postmortem examinations. A 20-year-old man was shot after a riot. There was a severe atherosclerosis with a total occlusion of the coronary arteries. By chance we do have an absolutely normal ECG six months before his death. Further references and examples have been published earlier [1307, 1308].

Here, the importance of stress should be mentioned. Irvin H. Page states correctly that one cannot consider a successful man in a competitive society to be free of stress. Therefore, we must learn to live with stress and to prosper in spite of it. Stress alone is not sufficient to cause atherosclerosis or myocardial infarction. People in war and postwar times have lived under very stressful situations for years. Fear, needs, grief, and trouble undoubtedly cause stress. However, during these war and postwar times these people suffered from malnutrition as well as stress, particularly, but not only, in camps of all kinds. Often they had to do heavy physical work, and under these extreme situations ("Grenzsituation" according to Jaspers) men did not sustain myocardial infarctions. Hypertension, however, was not rare. Stomach and duodenal ulcers occurred under stressful conditions quite frequently, but not myocardial infarction.

I am not sure whether there are certain personality types predisposed to coronary heart disease (CHD). A careful, individual analysis of coronary patients in the Heidelberg hospitals by DeBoor did not reveal any typical psychosomatic patterns.

What are the problems we should deal with in the future? As a clinician I would like to mention a few. Epidemiology should focus not only on CHD but also on other vascular areas and should use all the available diagnostic tools. The risk factors in atherogenesis will have different weights in different vascular areas. Genetic aspects should also be more carefully studied. Some other problems are as follows. Why do people die from their first myocardial infarction with relatively small lesions in their vessels? How do necroses of the myocardium occur in the absence of a morphological defect in the coronary arteries? What is the importance of incomplete vessel occlusions for sudden cardiac death? Of special interest are myocardial infarctions, demonstrated by electrocardiograms, but with no demonstrable vascular defect. The coronary artery system has morphological peculiarities, influenced by genetics and sex, that should stimulate further studies. The influence of drugs on vascular anastomoses, on coronary flow, on myocardial nutrition and electrical phenomena are also points of great interest. There are, I believe, many promising aspects for reducing the high rates of "mankiller No. 1", arteriosclerosis.

G. SCHETTLER

Section I

PATHOGENESIS OF ATHEROSCLEROSIS

INTRODUCTION

Chairman: Robert W. Wissler

Before introducing the first panel of pathogenesis experts I want to discuss a figure (Fig. 1) which you may find helpful when considering the complex problems connected with the development of atherosclerosis. This figure attempts to present, in a simplified form, the major components of the pathogenesis of atherosclerosis starting, first of all, with the concept, now based on abundant evidence, that one of the critical factors in the development of this disease is a sustained increase in the concentration of circulating low density lipoprotein. The second point of the illustration is that platelet sticking and/or a tendency

LUMEN

1. Increase in quantity of β (LD) or α_2 (VLD) lipoproteins

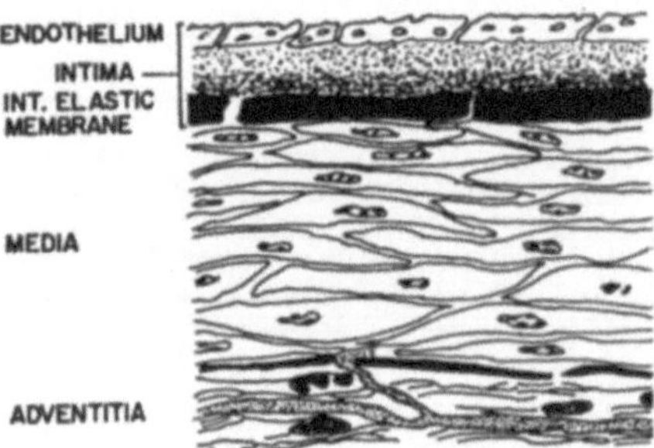

2. Increase in platelet sticking or clotting tendency
3. Increased permeability to plasma proteins due to hypertension, vasoactive amines from platelets, anoxia, toxins etc.
4. Decreased metabolism of medial cells
5. Proliferation of medial cells
6. Poorly metabolized lipoproteins accumulating in medial cells
7. Necrosis of medial cells due to accumulating lipids
8. Interruption of lymphatic drainage, vasa vasorum etc.

Fig. 1. Factors in the cellular pathogenesis of atherosclerosis. (After Gofman and Young: Atherosclerosis and its origin. Ed. by Sandler and Bourne. New York: Academic Press 1963)

toward clotting may help open the endothelium to increased migration of lipids and/or formed elements of the blood into the intima or even the media. The third line indicates that other factors such as hypertension, anoxia and various circulating toxins may also increase endothelial permeability with or without platelet sticking.

The next four lines indicate that lipoprotein molecules or some of their components, notably cholesterol and cholesteryl esters, have the capacity to produce varying reactions in medial cells whether they are located in the intima as myointimal cells or in the media. These varied reactions include altered cell metabolism; cell proliferation which can at times be very severe, so severe that it can contribute to the narrowing of the artery's lumen; lipid accumulation derived, initially at least, from the lipoproteins; and, of course, cell necrosis, which is such a very important factor in the advanced atherosclerotic lesion. Finally, the eighth point is that in rather rare instances the lipid accumulation in the wall of the artery may be accelerated because of obstruction of lymphatics in the adventitia of the arteries.

In the following presentations we will hear from four highly qualified scientists each of whom has made notable contributions to the understanding of the pathogenesis of atherosclerosis.

ARTERIAL LIPID ACCUMULATION

DAVID E. BOWYER and G. A. GRESHAM

Composition. Lipid has been recognized as a major component of most kinds of arterial lesions since the time of Virchow [1499] and questions concerning the source of the lipid and reasons for its accumulation have subsequently occupied researchers from many disciplines. The difficulty in this field for a long time was that the methods were not sufficiently sensitive for the characterization of the small amounts of lipids contained within individual lesions of different types. Consequently, analyses were often made on intima plus the underlying media. Further, it was not appreciated that lesions of different morphological types might have different lipid composition and that lipid accumulation also occurs in macroscopically undiseased intima solely with increasing age. These difficulties have been largely overcome by the use of thin-layer chromatography (TLC) for the separation of individual lipid classes, gas-liquid chromatography (GLC) for the determination of their fatty acid composition [233], and by the careful separation of intimal lesions from the underlying media and adjacent undiseased tissue.

The most significant advances have been made by the studies of Smith on human aortic tissue [1376–1379] but there are additional studies on arterial lipids of experimental animals with both spontaneous and induced atherosclerosis. The latter are important as models in the study of mechanisms of atherogenesis, e. g., various studies have employed the Rhesus monkey [1191], pigeon [1281], cholesterol fed rabbit [166, 1447, 1599], semisynthetic diet-fed rabbit [232], cockerels [194], and chickens [183].

Smith has shown for human aorta [1378] that in macroscopically undiseased intima lipid accumulates with age. The lipid in this undiseased tissue exists in two morphologically distinct forms: (1) perifibrous lipid lying along collagen and elastic fibres, and (2) lipid contained in droplets in fat-filled cells. In both kinds of lipid there is a preponderance of cholesteryl esters, and these show the most marked positive correlation with age. This is summarized from Smith's data in Table 1.

The cholesteryl esters of the two kinds of lipid are different; in the perifibrous lipid, cholesteryl linoleate accumulates, while in the fat-filled cells cholesteryl

Table 1. *Change in concentration (mg/100 mg of dry tissue) of major lipids of undiseased human aortic intima with age*

Age	PL[a]	TG[a]	Free cholesterol	Ester cholesterol	Percentage free cholesterol
20	2.5	0.5	0.8	0.2	80
80	3.2	2.5	1.9	10.0	16

[a] PL = phospholipid, TG = triglyceride.

oleate accumulates. The composition of the perifibrous lipid is very similar to that of the S_f 0–12 lipoproteins.

In a study of the lipids of the isolated intimal lesions, Smith, Slater and Chu [1379] described the lipid changes in the fatty streak (containing mainly fat-filled cells), fibrous lesions (containing collagen, without fat-filled cells), and larger lesions of both types in which there was additionally some extracellular "amorphous" lipid. In the fatty streaks, the lipid accumulation, as compared with adjacent undiseased intima, parallels the accumulation in fat-filled cells. Thus there is an increased concentration of sphingomyelin, lecithin and free cholesterol, and a large increase in cholesteryl oleate. In the fibrous plaque, the most important changes are an increase in cholesteryl linoleate and a considerable accumulation of sphingomyelin.

The highest concentration of lipid occurs in lesions having an "amorphous" component and the cholesteryl esters in this are of the same composition as those in the rest of the lesion. However, the ratio of free cholesterol to cholesteryl ester is increased. The phosphatidyl ethanolamine does not increase in amount, but there is a large increase in sphingomyelin, which in some cases accounts for 75% of the phospholipid. This is summarized in Table 2. Results of other workers are in agreement where comparable types of tissue have been analyzed [232, 516, 739, 1082].

A study of the fatty acid composition of the lecithin, sphingomyelin and triglycerides of human fatty streaks [232] showed that there were only small differences in composition compared with adjacent normal intima.

Table 2. *Percentage composition of phospholipids and percentage of free cholesterol in cellular and amorphous extracellular lipids of fatty streaks and fibrous plaques*

	LL[a]	Sph.[a]	Lec.[a]	PE[a]	Free cholesterol
Fatty streaks					
Cellular	8.7	51.2	32.7	6.2	32.7
Amorphous	11.5	65.5	20.0	2.0	46.9
Fibrous plaques					
Cellular	9.2	47.4	41.2	2.3	37.5
Amorphous	7.2	73.2	14.8	4.3	43.7

[a] LL = lysolecithin, Sph. = sphingomyelin, Lec. = lecithin and PE = phosphatidyl ethanolamine.

Mechanisms of Accumulation. Any consideration of arterial lipid accumulation must take into account the relative roles of the following possible mechanisms:

1. Deposition of blood components, either soluble lipoproteins or formed cells.
2. *In situ* synthesis.
3. Inadequate catabolism and clearance of lipid derived by step 1 or step 2.
4. Abnormal redistribution of lipid within the arterial wall during metabolism.

These questions are relevant for each lipid class. With respect to phospholipids early work showed that as a group they could be synthesized in the arterial wall and suggested that this was the major route for their accumulation [1596, 1598]. More recently studies on the incoporation of phospholipid precursors into isolated perfused arteries [232, 888], slices or cut preparations [311, 892, 1034, 1077, 1415, 1419] and homogenates [1151, 1190, 1420] showed rapid incorporation into lecithin, phosphatidyl inositol, but low rates in to phosphatidyl ethanolamine and very low rates, even in atherosclerotic lesions, into sphingomyelin. If the rates observed in these experiments are representative of those *in vivo* then *in situ* synthesis as a source of all of the sphingomyelin of the lesions must be challenged. It is known that plasma lipoproteins may cross the arterial endothelium; therefore the plasma lipoproteins could contribute to the accumulation of sphingomyelin.

With respect to the problem of cholesteryl ester accumulation it has been demonstrated that cholesterol and cholesteryl ester deposition may account for a large part of the accumulating material [1094]. Furthermore, the synthesis of the sterol nucleus occurs very slowly if at all from acetate [79]. This suggests that much cholesteryl ester may be derived by deposition. Recently, however, it has been clearly demonstrated that radioactively labelled fatty acids or fatty acids synthesized *in situ* from acetate may be incorporated into the cholesteryl esters of atheromatous lesions [5, 232, 372, 380, 888, 1092, 1514].

A greater incorporation rate of oleic acid than palmitic, stearic or linoleic acids had been demonstrated by Bowyer [232]. All of these experiments were on lesions composed primarily of fatty straks or foam cells, and the ability of these lesions to esterify cholesterol with oleic acid may explain its preponderance in that kind of lesion. It is not necessarily a unique reason for cholesteryl ester accumulation.

In any attempt to explain accumulation, account must be taken of catabolic processes. These have received little attention with respect to the arterial wall, but studies of cholesteryl ester hydrolysis [156, 375] and sphingomyelin hydrolysis suggest that catabolic processes may be the more important in controlling lipid accumulation in some cases.

Despite increasing knowledge of the chemistry and metabolism of arterial lipids, the major cause of lipid accumulation in spontaneous atherosclerosis in man is still not clear. It must be recognized that a number of mechanisms may operate either singly or synergistically.

MURAL METABOLISM

Jack C. Geer, R. V. Panganamala,
Howard A. I. Newman and David G. Cornwell

Arterial wall metabolism is a subject of considerable current interest especially with regard to changes that occur with developing lesions of atherosclerosis. A variety of methods for assaying arterial wall metabolism have been employed including enzyme localization, measurement of enzyme activity, oxygen consumption, substrate utilization, synthesis from labelled precursors, and chemical composition changes between normal arteries and those with lesions of atherosclerosis. Ultimately the pathogenesis of atherosclerosis will be detailed in metabolic terms, i.e. membrane transport, enzyme induction, energetics, synthetic activity. Present knowledge is inadequate to describe the pathogenesis of atherosclerosis in metabolic terms. The pathogenesis of atherosclerosis at this time has best been described in morphological terms, primarily gross morphology. It is generally, though by no means universally, accepted that atherosclerosis begins as proliferative lesions or fatty streaks that develop into plaques which are subject to complications of hemorrhage, ulceration, or thrombosis (complicated lesions). Whether this sequence of fatty streaks progressing to plaques and later complicated lesions accurately records the pathogenesis of atherosclerosis is of no import in the present discussion. This sequence does provide an accurate account of lesions observed with increasing age in the human and provides reference points for metabolic studies which have more meaning than "early lesions", "advanced lesions", or "severe atherosclerosis". For the present review the terms fatty streaks, fibrous plaques, and complicated lesions will be used.

Histochemical studies of normal arteries and naturally occurring and experimental atherosclerosis are numerous and recently have been reviewed by Zemplenyi [1588]. A large number of enzymes have been identified in arterial tissue [803, 1588]. The enzymes are localized primarily, if not exclusively, in the cells of the artery wall; those found in the extracellular space should be interpreted as due to diffusion until proven otherwise. In general the activity of arterial wall enzymes in the human increases up to age 40–60 years and then declines [803, 1588].

The number of reports in the literature dealing with arterial wall energetics is quite small in comparison to those dealing with morphology, diet, histochemistry, and arterial wall chemical composition. Oxygen consumption in the normal artery wall is low and does not change with age [803]. Oxygen consumption in the atherosclerotic vessel is much greater than that in the normal vessel [803, 1332, 1543]. With advancing age and/or atherosclerosis, arterial wall ATP[1] production is lower than would be predicted from the level of oxygen consumption, suggesting a defect in oxidative phosphorylation [1543]. Present

[1] Abbreviations used in this presentation include: ATP, adenosine triphosphate; CEFA, cholesteryl ester fatty acid; NADPH, nicotinamide adenine dinucleotide phosphate.

evidence indicates that about one-half of ATP production in the aorta is from glucose oxidation [803, 1332], but only about 20% of the glucose oxidized contributes to the electron transport chain producing ATP (Scott, personal communication). The substrate utilized for the remaining ATP production presently is unknown. Glucose oxidation in the aorta is primarily by glycolysis to lactic acid, and the presence of oxygen causes only a slight Pasteur effect [803, 1543]. The possibility of glucose oxidation via the hexose monophosphate pathway is of interest as the NADPH generated could drive fatty acid and sterol synthesis. Enzymes of this pathway have been demonstrated in the artery wall [803]. Metabolic studies are conflicting with regard to the amount of glucose catabolized via the hexose monophosphate pathway, varying from considerable to negligible [803, 1229]. In summary it can be said that the intermediary metabolism of the artery wall is not well understood and is in need of considerable further study.

Arterial wall composition and capacity for synthesis have been studied in regard to connective tissues and lipids. Quantitation of connective tissue mucopolysaccharides has revealed an increase in heparitin sulfate in fatty streaks [224] and no other changes [1377]. Histochemical studies showing an increase in mucopolysaccharides before lipid accumulation have not been supported by quantitative chemical studies possibly because it is the physical state rather than quantity or type of mucopolysaccharide that is responsible for the histochemical observation [224].

Lipid content and composition of human arteries has been the subject of numerous investigations since the studies of Windaus called attention to the marked increase in cholesteryl ester content associated with atherosclerosis. It is well established that arterial total lipid content increases with age, and the increase is much greater in arteries with induced or naturally occurring atherosclerosis. A distinguishing feature of atheromata is their high lipid content, primarily cholesterol. The bulk of the cholesterol found in atheromata is derived from the blood [889, 1094]. The presence of the protein moiety of serum beta lipoproteins in atheromata [776, 1573] suggests that beta lipoproteins cross the endothelium into the intima. The difference in lipid composition between the artery wall and plasma beta lipoprotein may be due to selective transport across the endothelium or selective catabolism within the artery wall. There are few studies that bear directly on the mechanism by which lipoproteins cross the endothelium and enter the arterial intima; however, there are several reports on the uptake and release of lipids by isolated cells or cells in culture [371, 376, 1263, 1514]. Most studies of arterial wall metabolism are concerned with the fate of lipoproteins after entry into the vessel wall.

As atherosclerosis progresses from the fatty streak to plaques and complicated lesions, the proportion of the arterial total lipid content made up of free cholesterol and cholesteryl esters increases markedly; phospholipids decrease; and triglycerides and free fatty acids remain essentially unchanged from the values observed in normal arteries [224, 227, 229, 740]. The rate of increase of free cholesterol with advancing atherosclerosis is considerably less than that for cholesteryl esters until well developed extensive plaques and complicated lesions are present in which the proportion of free cholesterol is greater than is observed in the early stages of atherosclerosis [1377, 1379]. The lipid composition of one segment of the arterial vasculature appears to be much like that of another except for the triglyceride content of coronary arteries which has been reported to be quite high [228]. The validity of this observation is suspect because of the technical difficulty in freeing coronary arteries from surrounding adipose tissue. Contamination of coronary artery specimens used for chemical analysis by adipose tissue fat is suggested by the reported fatty acid composition for coronary arteries which shows a high content of oleic acid [227, 229, 1330] and mimics more closely adipose tissue composition than that reported for aortic triglyceride [227, 229].

Changes in cholesterol content of the artery wall with regard to free cholesterol and cholesteryl esters have been studied in experimental animals, and the available human data is consistent with experimental results. With cholesterol feeding in the experimental animal arterial wall, free cholesterol content increases before that of cholesteryl esters; however, once cholesteryl esters begin to increase, their rate of increase is much greater than that for free cholesterol [889, 1192]. The initial high proportion of free to ester cholesterol in the artery wall could be due to selective admission or retention of the free form [889], or alternatively it may reflect hydrolysis of beta lipoprotein derived cholesteryl esters in the artery wall. The increase in cholesteryl esters may be due to esterification in the artery wall or to a decrease in activity of cholesterol esterase. Recently a lecithin-cholesterol fatty acyl transferase has been described in arterial tissue [5]. The activity of this enzyme has been found to be greater in fatty lesions than in fibrous and calcified lesions in human aorta [5]. The observed change in enzyme activity supports the possibility that cholesterol esterification in the artery wall is responsible for the change in free to ester cholesterol ratio observed in experimental lesions. Cholesterol esterase activity has been reported to decrease in experimental lesions compared to normal vessel [722, 1156] which supports the second possible reason for the observed change in free to ester cholesterol ratio in early lesions. The relative contributions of increased esterification and decreased hydrolysis to changes in free to ester cholesterol ratio observed early in the pathogenesis of fatty streaks are unknown at this time.

The increase in the ratio of free to ester cholesterol observed in plaques and complicated lesions of atherosclerosis compared to the ratio in fatty streaks may be the result of free cholesterol influx and decreased activity of the esterifying enzyme or hydrolysis of esterified cholesterol in lesions. There is rather little evidence that bears directly on either of these possibilities which, it should be mentioned, are not mutually exclusive. As stated previously lecithin-cholesterol acyl transferase activity has been reported to be less in plaques and complicated lesions than in fatty lesions [5]. This observation supports the first possibility. Cholesterol esterase activity has been observed to decrease in experimental lesions from values found in normal vessels [722, 1156]. This observation does not negate the second possibility, because the experimental lesions are comparable to human fatty streaks.

Comparison of the cholesteryl ester fatty acid (CEFA) composition of a normal human artery with fatty streaks and plaques reveals substantial differences. The CEFA composition of fatty streaks shows a significantly higher proportion of oleic and eicosatrienoic acid and lower proportion of linoleic acid than plaques or normal vessel [229, 517, 1377–1379]. The CEFA composition of normal intima and plaques is similar to that of plasma CEFA [1377]. These observations pose two questions. Why does the CEFA composition of fatty streaks differ from that of normal intima? If plaques and complicated lesions do indeed evolve from fatty streaks, why does the CEFA composition in the plaques and complicated lesions change? The observed difference in CEFA composition between normal intima and fatty streaks has been correlated with the morphological observation that most of the lipid in fatty streaks is intracellular whereas in normal intima stainable lipid when present appears to be located primarily in the extracellular space [517, 1377–1379]. The implication of this correlation is that the change in CEFA composition in fatty streaks is the result of intracellular cholesterol esterification in the artery wall reflecting cellular fatty acid synthesis, chain elongation, or availability of exogenous fatty acids. A recent study has shown incorporation of exogenous oleic acid into foam cells but not into smooth muscle cells [1514] indicating that the type of lipid containing cell present may, at least in part, determine CEFA composition. The large amount of eicosatrienoic acid found in fatty streaks in comparison to plasma is indicative of fatty acid chain elongation by aortic wall cells. The 5, 8, 11 isomer of eicosatrienoic acid is found in essential fatty acid deficiency and for this reason the identity of the isomer in fatty streaks is of interest [1377]. A trace amount of the 5,8,11 isomer has been found in human fatty streaks, but the bulk of the eicosatrienoic acid present was the 8,11,14 isomer derived from linoleic acid. Elongation and desaturation intermediates derived from oleic, linoleic, and linolenic acids have been identified in CEFA of human aorta. The acids present in highest concentration were identified as oleic, linoleic, and arachidonic [229]. A small proportion of the fatty acids are trans isomers [229].

With regard to the second question posed, why does CEFA composition change as fatty lesions become plaques? The change in CEFA composition can be correlated with intra- and extracellular localization of lipid. Plaques typically contain a large core of extracellular lipid. It has often been hypothesized that the extracellular lipid core of plaques is the result of necrosis of lipid-laden cells releasing into the extracellular space. The observed change in CEFA composition between fatty streaks and plaques and the increase in the ratio of free to ester cholesterol could be due to hydrolysis of cholesteryl esters in the extracellular space. Another possible explanation for the change in CEFA composition is influx of plasma cholesteryl esters; the CEFA composition of plaques mimics that of plasma cholesteryl esters. The questions posed by the CEFA composition of plaques and complicated lesions are much the same as those for the increase in free cholesterol to cholesteryl ester ratio in those lesions, and there is little direct evidence to support any of the possibilities. Human studies have shown that as the composition of plasma cholesteryl ester fatty acids is changed by diet the fatty acid composition of aortic cholesteryl esters in plaques and coplicated lesions changes in the same direction which indicates that the pool of cholesteryl esters in advanced lesions is not inert [181, 451].

Fatty acid synthesis by vascular tissue has been studied primarily in experimental models [721, 889, 1281, 1543, 1544]. The rate of fatty acid synthesis in vascular tissue is increased when experimentally induced lesions are present

[889, 1281]. Results of experiments with rabbits, pigeons, and subhuman primates [721, 889, 1092, 1281] are quite similar suggesting that man may react in the same way. Fatty acid synthesis takes place in the high-speed supernate: microsomal, and mitochondrial fractions of aortic cells [721]. The high-speed supernate fraction catalyzes the synthesis of palmitic and stearic acids *de novo*. The microsomal and mitochondrial fractions are involved primarily in chain elongation [721, 1542, 1544]. The increment in fatty acid synthesis in the atherosclerotic pigeon aorta is greatest for oleic acid [1281]. Isolated mitochondria from the aorta of cholesterol-fed rabbits catalyze a greater synthesis of oleic and an octadecadienoic acid hypothesized to be an 8,11 isomer than mitochondria from normal rabbit aorta [1542, 1544]. Newly synthesized and added fatty acids have been shown to be incorporated by vascular tissue primarily into phospholipids and triglycerides [889, 1419, 1514]. The rate of incorporation into cholesteryl esters is low in the normal vessel, but in the vessel with spontaneous or induced lesions, incorporation into cholesteryl esters is much greater [889, 1281, 1514]. Fatty acids derived from *de novo* synthesis or chain elongation in the aortic wall exhibit selective incorporation into phospholipids, triglycerides, and cholesteryl esters. The phospholipid fraction incorporates primarily stearic acid. The triglyceride fraction incorporates palmitic, stearic, and oleic acids. The cholesteryl ester fraction incorporates primarily oleic acid. The greatest difference in newly synthesized fatty acid incorporation between normal and atherosclerotic aorta is the increase in oleic acid incorporated into the cholesteryl ester fraction [1281]. The high proportion of oleic acid in the CEFA of human fatty streaks may be due to synthesis and increased incorporation of oleic acid into the CEFA fraction.

The phospholipid content and composition in arteries changes with the presence of atherosclerosis. The proportion of the arterial total lipid content comprised of phospholipids decreases in the atherosclerotic vessel; however, because of the increase in total lipid content in the atherosclerotic vessel, the absolute amount of phospholipid increases [224, 226, 227]. A comparison of the phospholipid composition of aortas containing predominantly fatty streaks with aortas containing predominantly plaques and complicated lesions reveals an increase in the proportion of sphingomyelin and decrease in the proportions of cephalins and lecithins in the latter [5, 224, 226, 227]. Synthesis of phospholipids by human and animal arteries as proposed by Zilversmit has been confirmed and it has been shown that in the atherosclerotic artery phospholipid synthesis is increased over that for a normal vessel [1190]. The rate of synthesis for phosphatidyl choline and phosphatidyl inositol is greater than that for sphingomyelin [376, 1190, 1514]. The accumulation of sphingomyelin in the face of a low rate of synthesis is either the result of an even slower rate of degradation or means that not all the sphingomyelin in lesions is derived from synthesis. The first possibility was suggested in a study of arterial phospholipases [1207]. There is little evidence to bear upon the second possibility. Sphingomyelin could be derived from plasma beta lipoprotein which is relatively rich in this phospholipid. Comparison of aortic sphingomyelin fatty acid [226, 227] and long chain base composition [1149] to that of other tissues including blood has shown all to be similar but not identical, thus providing no clue to the source of aorta sphingomyelin.

There are several reports that question the generally-held belief that sphingomyelin accumulation in arteries is due to the presence of atherosclerotic lesions. A recent report considers the observed increase in the proportion of aortic sphingomyelin as age-associated and not related to the presence of atherosclerotic plaques [1264]. Comparison of the phospholipid composition of human normal aorta with aorta containing fatty streaks reveals an increase in total phospholipid content with no change in the proportion contributed by sphingomyelin [224]. An increase in sphingomyelin concentration and its proportion of the total phospholipid content in plaques and complicated lesions is well established [224, 226, 1379]. The recent report stating that the increase in sphingomyelin proportion is due to age and not atherosclerosis [1264] cannot be accepted without reservation. It is difficult to believe that a normal aorta can be found in North American men 54 and 72 years of age. An age-associated increase in vascular sphingomyelin must be considered, however, as a possible contributor to the increase in sphingomyelin content and porportion reported for atherosclerotic plaques. A recent study of aging changes in the bovine species shows very little increase. In studies in which the intima is not separated from the media, the media could contribute to observed sphingomyelin content and proportion of total phospholipid; approximately 60% of medial phospholipid is sphingomyelin. With present information it is concluded that in fatty streaks the concentration of sphingomyelin increases but remains in the same proportion to the total phospholipid. In advanced lesions the concentration and proportion of sphingomyelin increase.

In the aorta of cholesterol-fed squirrel monkeys there is a correlation between increasing cholesterol concentration and certain phospholipids [1192]. With cholesterol feeding the initial rise in free cholesterol concentration is accompanied by an increase in sphingomyelin. The increase in cholesteryl esters is accompanied by an increase in phosphatidyl choline. Separate analysis of extracellular and intracellular lipids in such a model, if possible, could cast considerable light on the early reaction of the arterial wall to beta lipoprotein deposition. It would be hypothesized that the initial rise in free cholesterol and sphingomyelin results from extracellular deposition of plasma beta lipoprotein, and the later observed increase in cholesteryl esters and phosphatidyl choline is the result of intracellular cholesterol esterification and phospholipid synthesis. Sphingomyelin has been localized histochemically in the extracellular space, and it also has been localized in the microsomal fraction of cells [1192].

The relative contribution of cholesterol synthesis by the artery wall to cholesterol accumulation is an unsettled question. It has been established experimentally that sterol synthesis occurs in the artery wall, and that the synthesis is enhanced when atherosclerosis is present [889, 1282, 1543]. Only a small percentage of the sterol synthesized is cholesterol. The principal product of synthesis according to one group is the sterol precursor squalene [889] and according to another investigator is cholestanol [1282]. With present information it appears that only a very small amount of the cholesterol in fatty streaks or plaques could be derived from synthesis by cells of the artery wall.

Of the lesser components of the arterial total lipid content there are a few reports concerned with cerebrosides and plasmalogens. Cerebrosides comprise a larger proportion of the total lipid content of fatty streaks than that of normal vessel or plaques [477]. The similarity of aortic and plasma cerebroside fatty acids has prompted the suggestion that aortic cerebrosides originate from the plasma [477]. Plasmalogens in the human aorta decrease in concentration with advancing lesions of atherosclerosis [998]. The alk-1-enyl composition of plasmalogens from human aorta, plasma, and erythrocytes differ [1148] suggesting that those in the aorta are not derived from the plasma. The role, if any, that cerebrosides and plasmalogens play in the pathogenesis of atherosclerosis remains to be determined.

In summary, our present knowledge of the metabolism of the arterial wall and the pathogenesis of atherosclerosis consists essentially of a series of more or less isolated bits of information as outlined here. The relationship of these bits to the origin and development of atherosclerosis or even to each other is too vaguely understood to justify speculation at this time. The plethora of data does, however, raise two questions in regard to their comparability which are of immediate importance for future work. The first question is that of terminology: present lack of uniformity, and variation in exactness of definition makes it very difficult to determine whether, and to what degree, any two reports are comparable. The second is whether any two investigators have indeed assayed the same material, e.g. exactly how much media was included in a supposedly pure intimal sample.

INJURY AND REPAIR IN THE PATHOGENESIS OF ATHEROSCLEROTIC LESIONS*

M. Daria Haust

The numerous theories concerned with the etiology and pathogenesis of atherosclerosis attest to the fact that none can account for all the features of this arteriopathy. Observations in man and experimental animals, however, lend some support to each theory, and it becomes apparent that the various factors implicated in atherogenesis are not mutually exclusive of each other; rather, they all may fit into a certain sequence of events (or alternative events) that culminate in the genesis and progression of atherosclerotic lesions. In terms of general pathology all the various factors implicated represent forms of injurious elements, and what is observed as a lesion is the morphological representation of a reaction of the vascular wall (specifically intima) to these and an attempt at repair and restoration of functional and structural integrity. Peculiarities of function, structure, nutrition and internal "circulation" of large (elastic) and medium-size

* The work herein has been supported by grants-in-aid MT-1037 from the Medical Research Council of Canada and T. 3–11 from The Ontario Heart Foundation, Toronto, Canada.

(muscular) arteries [8, 598], i.e. those involved in atherosclerosis, are all responsible for the uniqueness of this reaction and of the repair tissue which, in turn, is an important factor in the progression of atherosclerotic lesions.

The intima of normal arteries, like the cardiac valves and the cornea, is not vascularized, and with the exception of the outer part of the elastic arteries, the media also lacks capillaries. Blood pressures in the arterial lumina are at all times high and capillaries from vasa vasorum, supplied with blood under low pressure, would collapse if present in the inner layers of the arteries. The same applies to the lymphatics in which the pressure is even lower and the walls thinner than those of the blood capillaries. Lymphatic capillaries normally drain that part of tissue fluid not returned to blood capillaries, and keep tissue fluids free from substances that escape from blood capillaries in normal, but particularly damaged, tissues. In the absence of lymphatic capillaries, the arterial wall may be unable to rid itself of such substances as readily as other tissues. If, alternatively, blood capillaries connecting with the arterial lumen were created to supply the inner arterial wall, their thin walls exposed to the high blood pressure, would rupture and the ensuing intramural hemorrhage would cause structural damage and functional impairment of the arterial wall. Nevertheless, this high pressure is the instrumental force in the entry of nutrients from the blood into intima, because it creates pressure and diffusion gradients across the arterial wall, a "milking" action of systolic stretch and diastolic recoil facilitating the transmural passage of the nutrients and metabolites, and the ultimate entry of the latter into the adventitial blood capillaries and lymphatic channels. Evidence is forthcoming from animal experiments and studies on the human postmortem material that under normal conditions plasma proteins enter the intima from the lumen. It was shown that labelled albumin and lipoproteins injected into the circulation of dogs entered the aortic wall readily [413]. In man, small quantities of albumin and lipoproteins can be demonstrated by fluorescent antibody techniques in normal aortic intimas of all ages; fibrinogen does not enter the aortic wall under normal conditions [636]. In the process of filtration and diffusion, the intimal and medial acid mucopolysaccharide-rich ground substance plays an important role. It acts as a sponge taking up the substances entering the wall, thus facilitating the constant change of volume of the arterial wall with pulsation. This change of volume in turn promotes the movement of substances and fluids across the wall. All these mechanisms operate satisfactorily under the conditions of homeostasis, and normally, the clearing of substances is in equilibrium with the influx from the lumen. However, the fine balance of the many factors relating either to the circulation or to the arterial wall can be upset by a multitude of causes. Focal intimal accumulations of local metabolites and substances derived from blood result from such an "upset".

The peculiarities of arterial structure and function would be a curiosity only, were it not for the fact that in addition to the difficulty in maintaining homeostasis, they are also responsible for the limited capacity of the wall to "handle" abnormal circumstances. Even under optimal normal conditions there is an inherent tendency for the native tissues to degenerate prematurely because of the constant tension under which they operate, and the difficulty in maintaining the quality and circulation of tissue fluids bathing the intercellular substances. The diffuse intimal thickening that increases with age further adds to difficulties in nutrition and clearing of the arterial wall of various substances [1048].

Following injury the preceding problems become much more exaggerated. The arterial local defense mechanisms are hampered by the absence of blood and lymphatic capillaries in the intima and media, and by lack of "rest", a factor important in promoting the healing phase. The nature of the injurious agent, duration of exposure to it, the status of the host, as well as the mural reaction, will determine—as elsewhere in the body—the initial local manifestations, the nature and success of repair, and the ultimate outcome of the entire process.

Many factors have been shown experimentally to be injurious to the endothelium and intima, and to produce lesions resembling in some or most aspects those of human atherosclerosis. These factors include physical, chemical, metabolic and biological forms of injury. Innumerable experiments were carried out utilizing various microorganisms and their toxins; electric stimulation; ionizing irradiation; heat; cold; direct trauma; forces applied to the body as a whole such as rapid deceleration, negative and positive G-forces, and mechanical vibration; neurovascular disturbances; hypo-, and hypervitaminotic states, manipulation of endocrine organs or their active principles; enzymes; conditions of stress; changes in hemodynamics; quantitative and qualitative alterations of normal plasma components either by dietary means, administration of drugs or other means; generally altered metabolic states; numerous chemicals and poisons; various hypoxic states; and others. Detailed reviews on these experimental data are available in the older and more recent literature [406, 724, 1043, 1238, 1453].

It is important to stress, however, that the experimentations with the various forms of injury seldom result in production of lesions limited to the intima only, because in most instances there were some accompanying changes in the other arterial coats. Moreover, some lesions so produced are diffuse rather than focal. Nevertheless, much has been learned in general terms from these experiments regarding the nature of arterial reaction to adverse conditions, and the ability of the wall to repair and regenerate. This knowledge is useful in assessing the role of injury to the arterial wall in the pathogenesis of atherosclerosis.

Judging from the type of tissue reaction in response to injury in atherosclerosis, the injury cannot be very severe, but rather subtle. Were the injury severe the manifestations would be evident not only in the intima but in all arterial layers, and necrosis as well as cellular exudates would dominate the reaction, all features not characteristic of atherosclerosis. It is conceivable that the susceptibility of the endothelium and the intima to injurious factors of rather low intensity exceeds that of other tissues because of the arterial peculiarities (see the preceeding), and stimuli considered to be within physiological range elsewhere, may have adverse effects upon the intima. Some injurious factors are involved in the initiation of atherosclerotic lesions, others are responsible for the progression of the latter, and thus reference is often made to initiating and aggravating factors. These are not always separable, and one form of injury may be influential at both levels. With relevance to human atherosclerosis the various injurious factors may be conveniently grouped together as either related to hemodynamics, to blood components (including normal constituents and elements in transit), or to the arterial wall itself.

The inception of the process leading to atherosclerosis may proceed in one of two ways (Fig. 1), regardless of the nature and derivation of the injurious agent [396, 1261]. When the latter resides in the lumen, i.e. all the blood factors and some of the hemodynamic factors, it may injure the endothelium severely enough to abolish the active control mechanism of filtration (permeability) with consequent indiscriminate (in composition and/or amount) influx of blood constituents into

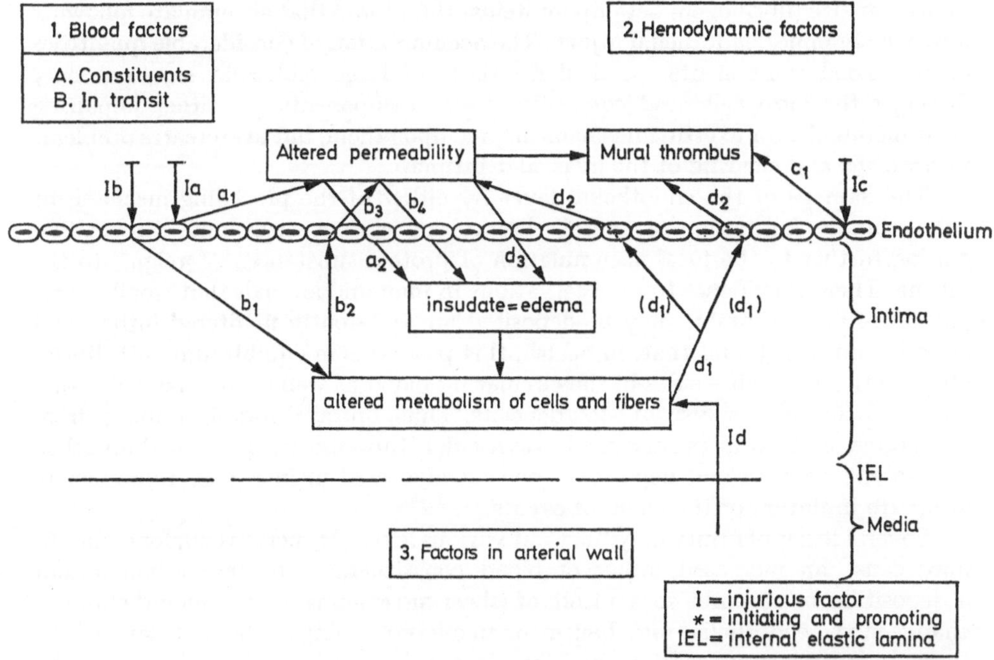

Fig. 1. Injury and repair in the pathogenesis of atherosclerosis. Injurious factors and their mode of action. Injurious factors (*Ia*), derived from the lumen (either blood or hymodynamic factors) may act upon endothelium whose differential permeability becomes altered (a_1) and this results in insudation of blood constituents into the intima (a_2); the insudate may alter the metabolism of intimal cells and fibers aggravating the local conditions. Alternatively, injurious factors (*Ib*) derived from the lumen (either blood or hymodynamic factors) may "pass" through the endothelium without affecting it, but alter the metabolism of intimal cells and/or fibers (b_1); this in turn affects the integrity of endothelial cells (b_2), followed by altered permeability (b_3), and insudation (b_4). Other factors derived from the lumen (*Ic*) may precipitate mural thrombosis (c_1). Factors derived from the wall itself (*Id*) and characterized by an altered metabolism of the vascular cells and fibers will influence the endothelial integrity via the latter (d_1); mural thrombus and/or altered permeability (d_2) and insudation (d_3) follow

the intima. Alternatively, the injurious agent may traverse through the endothelial lining without damaging it sufficiently to induce the previous chain of events, and acts instead upon the subendothelial intimal tissues directly. The damaged intimal elements will affect secondarily, possibly through their altered metabolites, the integrity of endothelium; again, this will be followed by indiscriminate permeability and the preceding sequence of events. The injurious factors may reside *a priori* in the vessel wall itself, as is no doubt the case in some inherited connective tissue disorders, and thus alter metabolism of the wall; or they may be certain hemodynamic factors exerting their influence through changes of the intimal components, rather than via alterations of endothelium. The amount and nature of substances entering the intima reflect the degree of endothelial damage. Severe injury will result in the passage from the blood of substances with larger molecular size (fibrinogen, beta lipoproteins) than those that accumulate following a relatively minor endothelial injury. The accumulation of considerable quantities of the blood components, particularly those of large molecular size, not only damages the local cells and connective tissue components, by either impairing their metabolism or exerting mechanical force upon them, but also creates problems in drainage and clearing of the avascular intima.

The damage of the endothelial layer by either of the preceding mechanisms will promote formation of mural thrombi of various sizes and composition adding further to the focal accumulation of protein substances "foreign" to the intima. There is evidence from observations in man and animals that small, mural platelets-fibrin thrombi, may be deposited on apparently unaltered intima and endothelium [519], and that, in health, this process is in equilibrium with fibrinolytic activity which resides in the circulating blood as well as arterial wall itself, and is responsible for lysis of such deposits. Thus, mural thrombi, resulting from the action of factors promoting intravascular thrombosis, or from diminished fibrinolytic activity and deposited upon an unaltered intima, may represent an alternate initiation of the chain of events.

Several forms of injury may "act" at various levels. Hypertension, for example, may cause an increased influx of blood constituents into the intima and/or a deposition of thrombi as a result of (sheering) trauma to the endothelium, a change in the endothelial metabolism, or an overstretching of the vascular surface, thus exposing larger areas to the blood (increased permeability). Alternatively, it may contribute to the build-up of the lesion by causing minute ruptures (by overstretching the wall) in the internal elastic lamina [632] with subsequent reactive proliferation of intimal fibrous tissue. Hypertension may be acting, on the other hand, through all these various mechanisms. Blood lipids are often cited as factors involved at several levels. High concentration of plasma lipids, especially those of certain types, may create *per se* an abnormal milieu for arterial endothelium, causing injury to the latter with consequent insudation and/or mural thrombosis; high concentration in plasma may be reflected in high content of these lipids in the intimal (insudative) lesions with difficulties of removal. Moreover, certain plasma lipids are considered to promote thrombosis and thus atherosclerosis, either by altering the fibrinolytic systems, or by influencing the platelets [1072]. Nicotine may be injurious by acting either directly upon the endothelium, or by influencing the neurovascular function, or both.

It is known from observations in man that atherosclerosis affects some arteries with predilection, and even in a given artery, it localizes more in one than another segment. This pattern was reproduced in animals, with various forms of injury showing a predilection for different sites. Moreover, it was convincingly shown in experimental animals that the components of the arterial wall differ in their susceptibility to various forms of injury. Elastic fibers, for example, when suitably exposed to irradiation are damaged, and the changes are similar to those observed in aging. Fragmentation of elastic tissue may follow direct but slight trauma, whereas other vascular components do not show apparent changes. All cellular elements are destroyed by heat or cold, but the elastic framework, although altered, remains intact. Endothelium is the component most sensitive to ionizing radiation, while the connective tissues are rather resistant to it, and the smooth muscle cells occupy the midposition on this scale [1453].

Following the local manifestation of injury (either in the form of intra-intimal edema, i.e. insudate, thrombus deposition, or both), there will be an attempt at repair by the vessel wall. The mobilization of the arterial defense mechanisms depends in large measure upon the structural and metabolic state of the wall. Any atherosclerotic lesion may be viewed as an outcome of defensive and offensive forces operating at a given arterial segment in a given time interval.

Minute injuries to the endothelium and/or intima may be followed by a *restitutio ad integrum* analogous to that observed in the regeneration and healing by first intention in the skin. Thus, the small amount of probably serous edema that accumulates in a focal intimal area following injury may only separate but not damage the local tissues and be reabsorbed into the adventitial circulation entirely because it contains only small molecular, readily diffusible substances (albumin). Thus, a completely normal structure and function is restored. However, this complete restitution is seldom, if ever, achieved in arteries. It is more probable, that some of this albumin-containing intimal edema remains unabsorbed; organization of this proteinaceous fluid by native cells results in a slight increase in local connective tissues. Serofibrinous insudates into the intima and those containing large pools of beta, or prebeta lipoproteins follow more severe injury, and present problems to repairing forces. Fibrinogen and the large lipid complexes contained in such insudates precipitate in the intima (fibrinogen being converted to fibrin) because their large molecular size does not render them amenable to reabsorption. Fibrin, if in moderate quantities, can be organized and thus contributes to local increase in connective tissue; the same applies to the apoproteins which are believed to originate in tissues from the lipoprotein complexes that enter in the insudate. The lipid component of these complexes, however, must be phagocytized by local cells, or those entering the area for this purpose, if it is to disappear.

The arterial forces of repair must not only dispose of substances that "intrude" into the intima, but also replace the native intimal tissues that were damaged either mechanically or by altered metabolism as a result of the massive serofibrinous insudate. The intima's ability to regenerate its tissues is remarkable. Moreover, the process of organization of exogenous proteins and that of regeneration of damaged native tissue components are both "molded" into formation of connective tissues adapted to the local needs. It is avascular, like normal intima, and the cells, collagen, and elastic fibers are not distributed haphazardly, as in the case of the conventional granulation tissue, but rather, all are arranged in a layer-like fashion parallel to the lumen (Fig. 2), and blend imperceptibly with the components of adjoining normal intima. This can be interpreted as an attempt at physiological adjustment of a pathological process simulating the normal intima. An interesting biological phenomenon of functional adaptation is observed in such areas of repair. The cells responsible for organization and elaboration of all connective tissue elements are not fibroblasts, but smooth muscle cells proliferating in the intimal loci of repair (Fig. 3) [638]. These cells provide, in addition, a contractile element needed in a thickened collagenous area, and this need may be a priori the reason for their presence in these lesions [641].

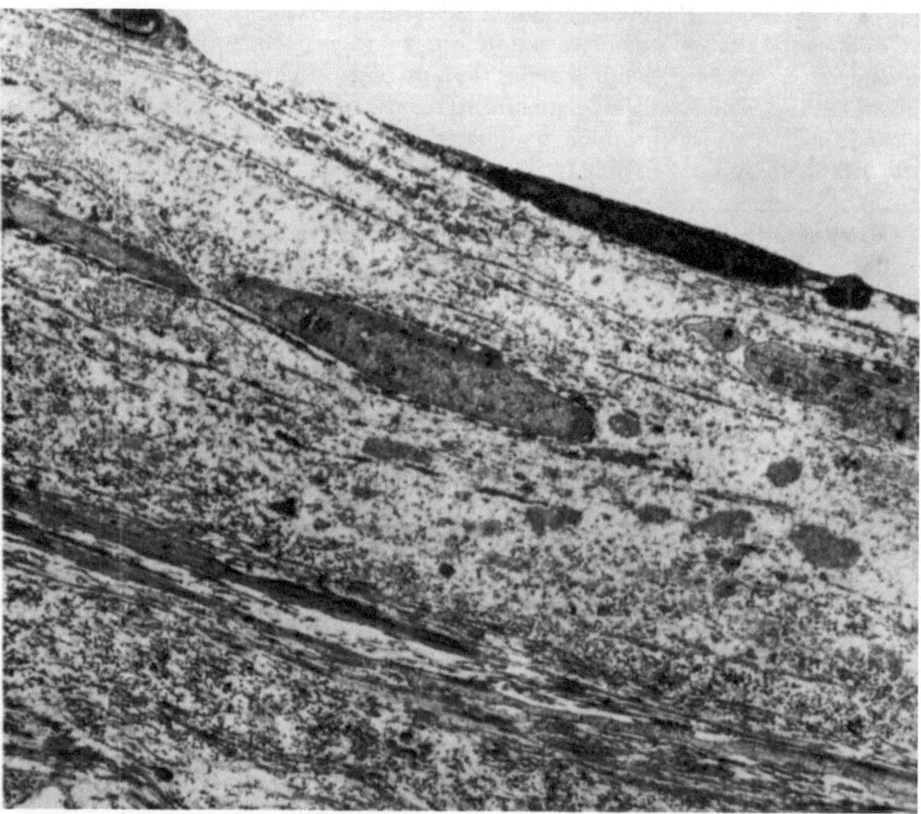

Fig. 2. Electron micrograph of a luminal area of a white atherosclerotic plaque removed at necropsy from a human aorta. The subendothelial components (cells and fibers) are all arranged in layers parallel to the lumen. Tissues were fixed in glutaraldehyde, post-fixed in osmic acid, embedded in Epon-812 and thin sections stained with uranyl acetate and lead citrate. ×5,500

Small mural thrombi may be either lysed or organized. The arterial wall determines, perhaps even more than does the fibrinolytic system of the blood, whether a mural thrombus deposited upon its surface will be lysed or will remain and be organized. Astrup [71, 72] reviewed the subject of thromboplastic and fibrinolytic properties of normal and atherosclerotic arteries; the latter have less fibrinolytic activity than the former. Evidence supporting the view that substances released from the arterial wall may be important in the break-up of mural thrombi is forthcoming from the observations that fewer thrombi precipitate on porous vascular than on nonporous synthetic grafts [618], the latter being more accessible to "permeation" by enzymes or enzyme-activators important in the dissolution of thrombi. When small thrombi are organized the resulting connective tissues assume features similar to, or indistinguishable from, those described. Mural thrombi of larger size are usually organized by two concomitantly operating processes: the superficial (luminal) layers of the thrombus are replaced by the avascular type of granulation tissue, whereas the capillaries and fibroblasts containing an orthodox type of granulation tissue develop at the base of the thrombus [640]. When the two processes meet the organization is completed, and the resulting lesion is the characteristic white pearly fibrous plaque. Often,

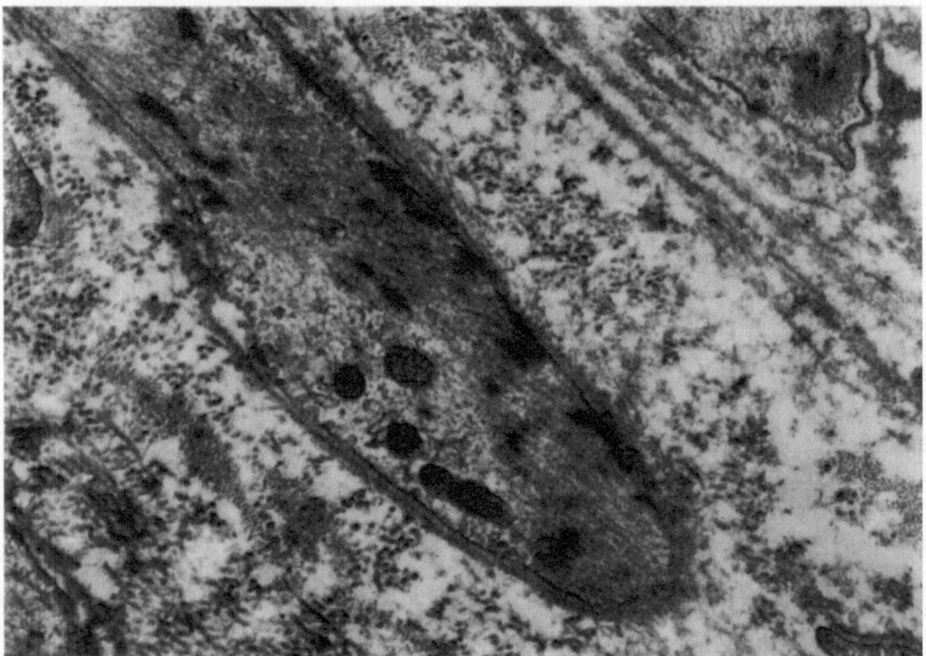

Fig. 3. Higher magnification of a subendothelial area similar to that seen in Fig. 2. Smooth muscle cells in all stages of maturation are the only cells observed. They are closely associated with the numerous fibrils and fibers proliferating in the extracellular space. ×27,500

layers of "younger" connective tissues are observed in the luminal aspects of such plaques. They represent insudation into the substances of the latter with subsequent organization.

The avascular reparative connective tissue fulfills its role of structural and functional adaptation only when it develops in small quantities. Since an intimal area of repair is susceptible to subsequent repeated injuries, this will in time result in considerable local accumulation of the avascular tissue composed of layers, each representing an episode of injury, and each composed of connective tissues of different stages of maturation. Accumulated avascular connective tissues, no matter how much structurally similar to normal intima, are liable to degenerative changes secondary to local hypoxia (insufficient diffusion of nutrients from lumen). In addition, substances traversing the wall from the lumen become arrested and precipitate in such areas more readily, adding further to local metabolic difficulties and degenerative changes which in turn stimulate the process of repair and further accumulation of connective tissue.

The successful completion of the arterial repair process depends upon numerous local and general factors. The content and amount of the intimal edema is important, and some reference to these has been made previously. When the lipids entering the intima cannot be phagocytized and carried away by macrophages, they remain in the area giving rise to a lipid pool. In addition, high content of lipids may influence greatly the quality of the repair tissue; in hypercholesterolemic rabbits repair of injured vascular wall by regeneration of the intima is markedly delayed and altered. Fibroblasts rather than smooth muscle cells are present, but only in small numbers. There is also paucity of regenerating elastic elements, and premature hyaline degeneration of collagen fibers [789]. When the intimal forces of repair are not sufficient to organize all the *in loco* arrested and precipitated proteins derived from blood, they remain in the area and in time degenerate and contribute to the lipid pool of the lesion. The same applies to the organization of a large mural thrombus when either or both of the two types of granulation tissues (avascular from the lumen, orthodox from the base) fail to develop adequately and to meet, leaving unorganized and subsequently degenerating remnants of the thrombus. The resulting pool of lipid material is the hallmark of atheroma [1029]. Unorganized masses of proteins also stimulate proliferation of capillaries from the lumen. The high blood pressure to which these are exposed makes them liable to rupture, and the ensuing hemorrhages into the plaque further add to local difficulties [1157].

Other factors may influence the efficacy of the repair process such as: the age and sex, deficiencies of vitamin C, pyridoxine and choline, hypervitaminosis D, adrenal cortical hormones, and many others. Most of these act by either directly or indirectly influencing the development and the integrity of connective tissues.

It may be stated in conclusion that the tissues of intimal repair, so ingeniously designed for adaptation of structure and function of injured arteries, ultimately contribute to progression of atherosclerosis.

THROMBOSIS AND ATHEROGENESIS

A. STUDER

The significance of thrombosis in atherogenesis is herein presented. Interest will therefore be focused upon the earliest stages of arteriosclerosis with consequent exclusion of thrombotic complications encountered as a secondary pathological feature in sclerotically altered vessel walls.

There exists conclusive evidence for the presence of fibrin deposits within arteriosclerotic human arteries. Haust et al. [639, 642] by the fluorescent antibody technique have demonstrated fibrin in white plaques at all stages of development. These findings were confirmed for man by Kao and Wissler [776], Woolf and Carstairs [1570], and for Holstein-Frisien cows by Likar et al. [872]. It would appear legitimate to infer from this a relationship between thrombosis and arteriosclerosis. Nevertheless the origin of the intramural fibrin still remains to be determined. In particular it is not clear whether it is incorporated into the vessel wall as such, or whether it enters the wall in the form of fibrinogen and is transformed into fibrin only within the wall.

Consideration should first be given to the hypothesis of Duguid [410] which claims that fibrin is produced by coagulation in the lumen, deposited on the intima, endothelialized, and finally incorporated into the vessel wall. Many authors have attempted to support Duguid's hypothesis by the demonstration of alterations in the vessel wall after intravascular injection of fibrin clots [60, 299]. By this method fibrin clots were obviously incorporated into the organism as foreign bodies. There was organization of emboli, formation of lipid foam-cells, recanalization, and incorporation of the remaining emboli. There would thus exist a morphological correlation with arteriosclerosis. However, it is hardly conceivable that arteriosclerosis is a consequence of constantly recurring and relatively massive emboli [1435].

Remember that experimental injection of fibrin clots is a drastic measure and does not correspond to physiological conditions. Physiological conditions are approached somewhat more closely by inducing endogenous fibrin formation. This is achieved by intravenous administration of minute amounts of thrombin, but fibrin layers on the intima are rarely detected in rabbits and not at all in rats. Fibrin incorporated into the vessel wall was rarely observed, despite inhibition of fibrinolysis by treatment with epsilonaminocaproic acid. In fact, the fibrin formed is found to disappear almost completely within hours in rats and within days in rabbits [394, 1437–1439]. Hence experiments with intravascularly injected or endogenously produced fibrin in animals do not lead to a satisfactory understanding of the presence of fibrin in the human vessel wall.

Under normal conditions fibrinogen perfuses the arterial intima from the lumen. Its pattern of distribution is comparable to that of other plasma proteins such as lipoproteins, albumins, and gammaglobulins demonstrated intramurally. Increased infusion of fibrinogen appears to disturb the metabolism of the intima, and this in turn may lead to retention of fibrinogen [190].

There is, in fact, evidence against the encrustation theory. By means of the fluorescent antibody technique, material in fatty streaks has been shown to react with fibrinogen antibodies. Geer [514, 515] concluded from his studies on fatty deposits in human and baboon aortas, that these consist of precipitated blood lipoproteins. Recently Wissler (personal communication) documented platelet antigen near the center of early aggregates. Conversely, he detected hardly any evidence of fibrin on the surface of the developing lesion and little evidence of its being incorporated into a developing lesion until the latter is far advanced. Wissler concluded from these findings that fibrin may be formed from fibrinogen as it moves through the wall of the artery.

In any case plasma deposits in the intima are important as a source of lipids [514, 515]. In experiments with rabbits and pigs Packham et al. [1141] showed that protein accumulations are focal and that the sites at which they occur are associated with the presence of small mural thrombi. These observations suggest that the vascular endothelium undergoes changes that promote localized insudation of plasma proteins and that blood platelets probably play a role in this process. Their possible participation in increasing endothelial permeability may be direct (mechanical) or indirect.

A primary endothelial lesion may occur by stretching of the wall due to raised blood pressure [414] or circulatory disturbances [1141]. In such a primary lesion subendothelial collagen is exposed, and this is known to induce aggregation of platelets [230, 729]. In addition, it can be demonstrated that platelets will adhere to the denuded basement membrane [103]. Whether the presence of collagen is required in the basement lamina for this reaction is not known. Also unanswered is the question as to whether platelets can adhere to intact endothelium, even though some authors [519, 737, 1290] insist that they have observed platelets on unaltered endothelium. The possibility has to be considered that there may be minute submicroscopical changes in the vessel wall which are not demonstrable by present-day methods [65, 1046]. French [493] has pointed out that in some instances platelets adherent to apparently normal endothelium were associated with nearby breaks in the endothelial continuity.

The injury to the endothelium may also be initiated by platelet aggregates. These form in the bloodstream under conditions of disturbed flow when platelets collide with each other, with other formed elements such as leukocytes or erythrocytes, or directly with the arterial wall, thereby releasing factors which cause their adherence and aggregation. Apart from this mechanical process, aggregation of platelets can be initiated by a variety of intravascular "biochemical" stimuli such as trypsin, serotonin, epinephrine and norepinephrine, long-chain saturated fatty acids, uric acid crystals, antigen-antibody complexes, gammaglobulin-coated surfaces as well as bacteria and viruses (for review see Mustard et al. [1069], Marcus [924]) although, the concept of a primary immunologically-induced injury of platelets by endotoxins has recently been challenged [1057]. All these stimuli including collagen seem to cause the platelets to swell, form pseudopods, and release ADP, the most potent nucleotide responsible for platelet adherence. The ADP released is thought to derive from ATP stored in the platelets [203]. The ATP is broken down to ADP by the contractile protein thrombosthenin located in platelet granules and on the membrane [149]. Both thrombin and ADP have been observed to initiate a contractile wave in the platelets [1545]. Recently endothelial cells have been demonstrated to contain a contractile protein similar to, if not identical with, platelet thrombosthenin and smooth muscle actomyosin [128, 129]. It remains to be determined whether there exists a connection between the different contractile systems. This view of ATP-derived ADP has been contested, at least for collagen- and thrombin-induced ADP release and it was proposed that these two agents liberate preformed platelet ADP [630, 701].

Apart from ADP, platelets release a substance that increases endothelial permeability. Contrary to previously held views, it can now be regarded as established that ADP itself also initiates a release of platelet contents [1140].

Among the factors released, histamine and serotonin have been identified and shown to cause gaps which appear between endothelial cells [905, 1265]. The endothelium is induced to contract. In regions of high pressure this contraction does not lead to a narrowing of the lumen but to a tearing apart of endothelial cells. Majno and Leventhal [904] have pointed out that endothelium and smooth muscle are structurally and biologically related, and thus it is not surprising that the endothelium should react to substances known to cause contraction of smooth muscle. There is evidence that apart from histamine and serotonin a third factor is mainly involved in increasing vascular permeability [1140].

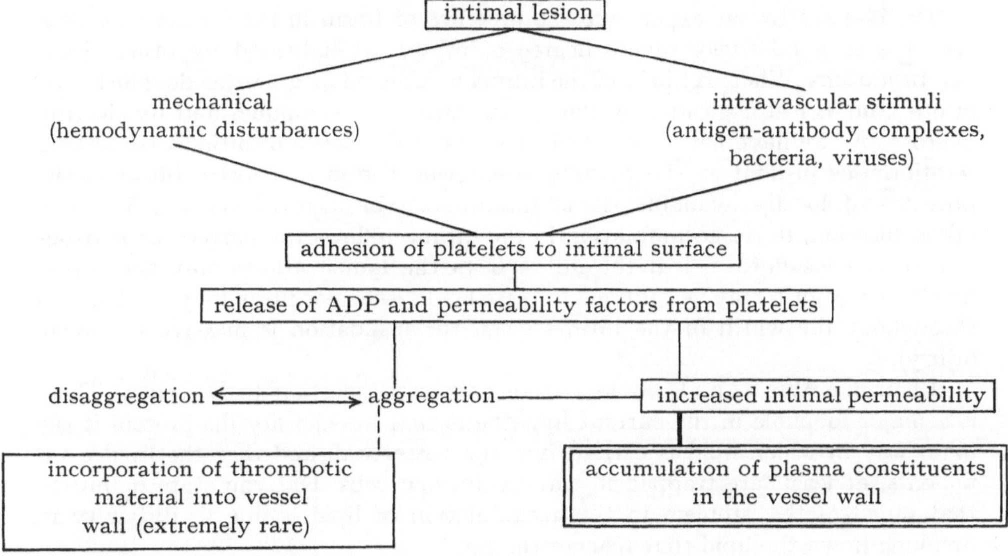

Fig. 1

During degranulation of platelets due to phagocytosis there is release of enzymes such as acid phosphatase [702, 1004, 1181], beta glucuronidase [702, 1004, 1181), cathepsin [1181], and arylsulphatase [1181]. It was concluded from this that some of the platelet granules released are lysosomes [925, 1248]. Polymorphonuclear leukocytes have long been known to release permeability factors, some of which are lysosomal enzymes: these cause damage to cells [544, 688, 1047]. These observations led Packham et al. [1140] to examine whether platelet lysosomal enzymes had a comparable injurious effect. After ultracentrifugation of homogenized platelets in a sucrose gradient, it became evident that platelet membranes and granules do, indeed, show permeability factor activity. In another experiment Mustard et al. [1069] demonstrated that after incubation of cell cultures with platelet lysosomal enzymes the cells show extensive vacuolization and become disrupted.

As the damaging effect of platelet aggregates upon the endothelium has been established and as increased permeability of the endothelium leads to intensified infiltration and deposition of plasma proteins in the vessel wall, the participation of platelet aggregation in atherogenesis—though not exclusive—must be regarded as probable. The schema in Fig. 1 outlines the various mechanisms reviewed.

PANEL DISCUSSION ON PATHOGENESIS OF ATHEROSCLEROSIS

Chairman WISSLER: I would like to begin the panel discussion by asking Dr. Haust, where does fibrin deposit in the vessel wall, and especially where is it located in the early lesions? Is it associated with platelets? It appears from Dr. Studer's presentation and your own that fibrin does enter the artery wall. In our experience it enters the pre-existing media as fibrinogen, and, then, often fibrin forms in between the smooth muscle cells.

Dr. HAUST: In our experience the presence of fibrin in the intima was associated with a relatively severe degree of injury, as indicated by other tissue manifestations. Whereas fibrin in the intima of affected arteries was demonstrated in our studies histologically, by fluorescent antibody techniques and by electron microscopy, we have never observed platelets in the depth of intimas containing serofibrinous insudates. The fibrinogen entering the intima forms fibrin in the presence of locally available tissue thromboplastins. To answer Dr. Wissler's other question, fibrin accumulation in the intima follows the pattern of distribution of the insudate, i.e., if the influx from the lumen affects only the superficial layers, fibrin may be confined to these layers, whereas fibrin may be observed throughout the width of the intima when the insudation is massive (= severe injury).

Chairman WISSLER: I would like to address a question to Dr. Geer. There is a major loophole in the current hypothesis that low-density lipoprotein is the main way in which lipid is carried into the vessel wall and that the lipid components, at least, are trapped in the myointimal cells. Did you state definitely that much of the problem in the accumulation of lipid is due to difficulty in breaking down the lipid that reaches the cell?

Dr. GEER: I think the problem is in the inability to degrade or remove portions of the plasma lipoprotein from the intima, most notably cholesterol. There is no evidence that the artery wall can degrade cholesterol, and thus accumulation must be due to an inability to transport it out of the artery wall. The same situation may apply for the sphingomyelin; however, the artery wall can degrade sphingomyelin to a limited degree.

Dr. BOWYER: It seems to me that we have to take into account the biochemical balance between the reactions of synthesis and catabolism. We should remember that this balance is not the same in the smooth muscle and the foam cell. We should consider the possibility of different kinds of biochemical mechanisms of lipid accumulation associated with the two cell types.

Chairman WISSLER: Do you think two cell types occur in man?

Dr. BOWYER: From a biochemical standpoint, yes.

Dr. POLLOCK: I am convinced that all the cells in the arterial wall are capable of storing lipids; certain cells are more capable than others. Now, I would like to refer to some unpublished observations concerning trauma and atherogenesis. If an aortic ring segment is placed into a diffusion chamber which is implanted subcutaneously, and the host animal is fed cholesterol, foam cell plaques develop only in previously traumatized tissue. If the aortic ring has been cut, intimal cushions develop on the shoulders of the cut. This observation suggests that only three factors were essential for atherogenesis in this experiment: (1) a susceptible arterial segment, (2) trauma, and (3) hypercholesterolemia. The last two factors need not be in this sequence. I realize, of course, that these experimental observations are not necessarily applicable to human atherogenesis.

Dr. GOTLIEB (Chicago, Illinois): Dr. Haust, when does an "injury" or a stressful situation in an artery become an injury, i.e., what is the minimum threshold where it might be operative in atherogenesis? Can this be defined?

Dr. HAUST: I wish we knew the threshold for injury in the intima. It is conceivable that whatever may be a normal stimulus, i.e., within physiological range for other tissues, may represent an injury to either endothelium or intima because of the very peculiar functional and nutritional conditions in which endothelium and intima find themselves. There is, furthermore, no rest period allowing proper and complete regeneration and repair as is the case in some other tissues. Judging from the kind of tissue response to the injury leading to atherosclerosis in the vessel wall, this injury cannot be very intense, for we observe neither intense cellular exudate nor much necrosis. There is some necrosis seen in the course of atherosclerosis, but this is a late and secondary phenonemon.

Dr. SMITH: This is a comment rather than a question, but I hope it will evoke some response from the panel.

In examining the maturation of lesions, from what we think are early stages to what we think are late stages, we have found a difference in behavior between primarily fatty streak lesions and primarily fibrous lesions. In what we consider are fatty streak type lesions, we start with an early stage in which all the lipid is within the cells, and we progress to a stage where there is a thin cap containing fat-filled cells overlying a typical atheroma. In our fibrous series we start with what perhaps is just intimal hyperplasia, suffused with peri-fibrous type lipid, and end up with a thick collagenous cap overlying a typical atheroma.

Now, as the fatty streak type lesion progresses from earliest to latest stage, there is no, or very little, increase in its total lipid content on a dry weight basis, but as the fibrous type lesions progress, there is a tenfold increase in its lipid content on a dry weight basis. Therefore it seems that in fatty streak type lesions the atheromatous center may be formed by disintegration of the pre-existing fat-filled cells, whereas in the fibrous type lesion we are getting a tremendous inflow of plasma type lipid.

Dr. GEER: I think the very basic question you are asking here is: Is the fatty streak the precursor of the plaque?

Section II

THE REACTIONS OF THE ARTERIAL WALL

LOCAL FACTORS IN ATHEROGENESIS: AN INTRODUCTION*

C. W. M. Adams

The mechanism of atherogenesis is complex; it is the summation of factors acting on the arterial wall from the blood and of those that result from changes in the arterial wall itself. Clearly, many exogenous and endogenous factors are interrelated, but this introduction is primarily aimed at surveying local pathogenic factors in the arterial wall itself.

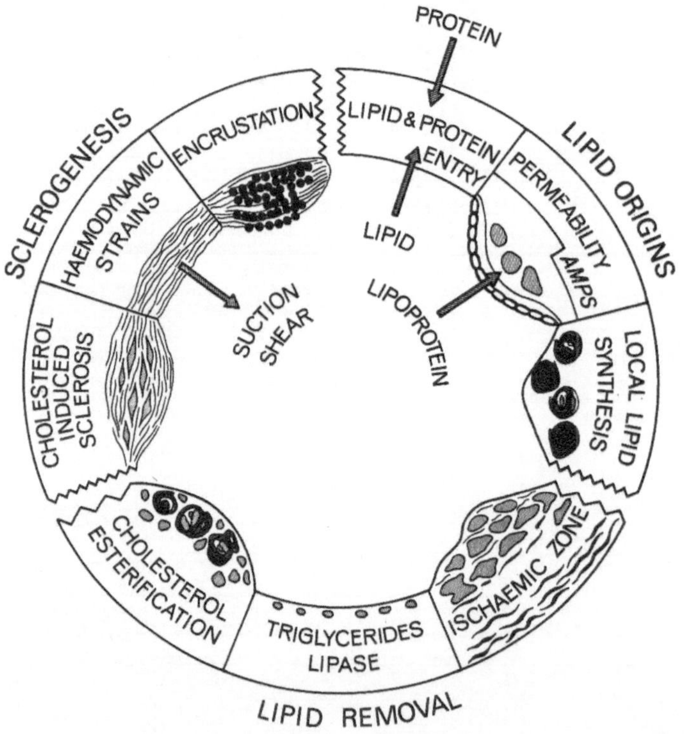

Fig. 1. Local atherogenic mechanisms

An important characteristic of human atherosclerosis is that the lesions comprise two major elements: (a) lipid deposition (athero), and (b) fibrotic organization (sclerosis). Both these features must be taken into account in hypotheses concerned with the pathogenesis of atherosclerosis.

* Various aspects of the work reported herein have been supported by the British Heart Foundation, The Tobacco Research Council, Messrs. Natterman Inc. (Köln), Chas. Pfizer Ltd. (Sandwich) and the U.S. Public Health Service.

In this survey of local factors, three aspects will be discussed: the cause of sclerosis, the origin of the lipids, and disordered lipid removal (see Fig. 1).

THE CAUSE OF SCLEROSIS

Three mechanisms have been advanced to explain the fibrosis in atherosclerotic lesions.

Encrustation. Platelet and fibrin encrustation [411], with resulting fibrous organization of the denatured protein is an attractive explanation for the sclerosis; it has received support from the histoimmunological [1572] and ultrastructural [643] identification of fibrin in the lesions. However, this mechanism does not account for the large amounts of lipid in the plaque, nor would it seem that such encrustations are of frequent occurrence. The stratified appearance of coronary atherosclerosis [1129] is frequently cited as evidence of previous thrombotic episodes with subsequent organization. Nevertheless these "geological layers" can only strictly be interpreted as evidence of the episodic nature of the disease: such episodes could be due to events other than mural thrombosis and fibrin encrustation.

Hemodynamic Stress. The nature of the mural strains caused by the stress of pulsatile blood flow have been reviewed by Macdonald [949]. The most important of these appears to be longitudinal shearing stress in which the tunica intima and inner arterial wall tend to be pushed forward over the relatively tethered outer arterial wall. This generalized shearing stress is supplemented at curves and constrictions in the arterial tree by suction pressure which pulls inwardly on the arterial wall [1459]. These strains might reasonably be expected to evoke a proliferative response from the connective tissue of the inner arterial wall, particularly at the potentially weak intimomedial junction, to repair or anticipate structural damage.

Benign essential hypertension provokes proliferative changes in all layers of certain smaller arteries (hypertensive arteriosclerosis). In the larger arteries that are involved in atherosclerosis, hypertension might be expected to exaggerate the various strains previously enumerated and, thus, to increase connective tissue proliferation in the tunica intima.

Lipids. Free cholesterol and its more saturated esters induce proliferative changes and fibrosis when implanted subcutaneously [3, 1390]. These sclerotic changes are reduced or absent when the sterol is dispersed by phospholipid added to the implant [19], or when the sterol is dispersed in lipoprotein. In view of the large amount of relatively saturated esterified cholesterol in an atherosclerotic lesion, it is not unreasonable to regard sterol-induced organization as the major sclerogenic factor in atherosclerosis, particularly with regard to the fibrous cap that overlies the "fatty atheroma".

THE ORIGIN OF THE LIPIDS

Plasma Lipoprotein Entry. In the filtration theory, low density lipoprotein is considered to enter the arterial wall from the lumen; and, due to the instability of its molecular structure, it is thought to shed its lipids during passage through the inner arterial wall [1144]. This concept was supported by immuno-electrophoretic identification of lipoprotein within the inner arterial wall [524], and, subsequently, by histoimmunological studies [776, 1521, 1525]. However, the filtration theory of lipoprotein was compromised when it was shown that the influx ratio of free/ester cholesterol into the arterial wall *in vivo* [1094] and *in vitro* [628] does not correspond to the concentration ratio of these lipids in plasma lipoproteins: more free cholesterol enters than ester, even though low density lipoprotein contains more ester than the free sterol. Our own preliminary studies in the cholesterol-fed rabbit indicate that only in severe atheroma does the entry of the ester rise to similar values to that of the free sterol.

Cholesterol appears mainly to enter the arterial wall from the lumen, as judged by autoradiographic and quantitative histochemical studies [17, 18, 22].

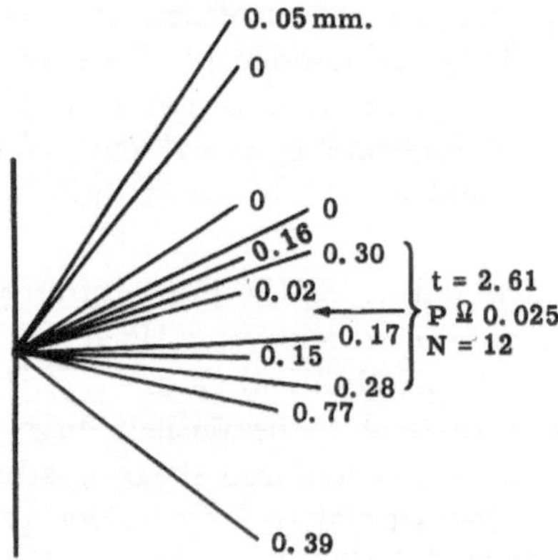

Fig. 2. Calculated slopes for entry gradients of ^{125}I radioactivity adjusted to a common left-hand point. The abscissae represent progression of multiple layers (6–10) from the inner intima (left) to the outer intima (right). The figures refer to maximum plaque thickness (mm) in the immediately adjacent aortic specimen

Nevertheless, globulins and albumin labelled with ^{125}I seem to enter the normal or mildly atheromatous rabbit aorta mainly from the outer or adventitial surface [22]. However, as such cholesterol-induced atheroma become more severe the entry gradient of (^{125}I)-albumin across the rabbit aorta reverses, so that more enters from the inner surface of the vessel (Fig. 2; unpublished data). This reversal of plasma protein entry in severe atheroma is attributed to increased permeability of the endothelium or subendothelial tissues in the diseased vascular wall, with resulting leakage of plasma proteins from the lumen. In a recent study in man, lipoprotein peptide usually appeared to enter the adult arterial wall from the lumen [1325]. However, in a six year old boy more lipoprotein entered the outer arterial wall than the inner. Possibly, only in youth is the human arterial wall sufficiently "normal" to be comparable with the normal rabbit aorta in respect to protein entry. Clearly more quantitative data about the extent and location of lipoprotein in the normal and diseased vascular wall are required. Moreover, information is required about the fate and distribution in the arterial wall of lipoprotein labelled in both the protein and cholesterol moieties. Such an experiment would convincingly show whether or not cholesterol enters the normal endothelium and intima in company with lipoprotein.

Arterial Permeability. Little is known about how macromolecules enter and traverse vascular endothelium [493]. Likewise, the role of disordered ground substance in atherogenesis has been little explored. Changes in the hydration of mucopolysaccharides and of acid mucopolysaccharide-protein binding could well alter the pore size and thus permeability of the ground substance in the *tunica intima* [1050]. Much remains to be explored in this field and little concrete evidence is available about arterial permeability.

Arterial Lipid Synthesis. Most workers are agreed that the human arterial wall has little capacity to synthesize sterols, although some species appear to have greater capability in this respect than others. The arterial wall has a marked capacity for synthesizing phospholipid and to a lesser extent triglyceride. Arterial lipid synthesis will be discussed in the next paper by Zilversmit.

DISORDERED LIPID REMOVAL

Triglycerides. An important feature of the lipids that accumulate in atherosclerosis is that the triglyceride concentration is rather trivial. The predominant lipid is cholesterol (ester > free), while phospholipid occupies an intermediate position. The relative absence of triglyceride from the lesions could be ascribed to the action of the arterial wall lipase (tributyrin lipase). The activity of this enzyme declines in the aging rat aorta [1590] and human aorta [16]. Nevertheless, when activity in the latter study was referred to surface area rather than wet weight or protein, as much enzyme was present in a unit segment of an old aorta as in a young aorta. It follows that a segment of the human arterial wall would have the same capacity to catabolize triglyceride entering from the lumen in old age as in youth.

Cholesterol Transport and Mural Hypoxia. It is not clear how cholesterol is transported across the arterial wall. As the influx ratio of free/ester cholesterol into the arterial wall does not correspond to the ratio of these lipids in plasma (see above), it is highly unlikely that plasma lipoprotein is the transport vehicle for cholesterol in and across the normal arterial wall. Although lipoprotein presumably leaks into the damaged atherosclerotic arterial wall (see above), some other vehicle must be involved in transmural transport in the normal vessels. From available evidence the only plausible vehicles are phospholipid-cholesterol micelles and lipoprotein endogenously synthesized within the arterial wall. Both such transport vehicles (phospholipid and protein) require energy for their synthesis. It can, therefore, be inferred that impairment of energy production in the aging arterial wall would cause diminished production of these lipotrophic transport vehicles.

Qualitative and quantitative histochemical evidence shows that enzymes concerned with arterial aerobic energy production decline in the middle and inner-middle parts of the human tunica media with advancing age (Fig. 3) [13, 15, 18, 1589]. The impaired metabolism of the middle media probably results from the progressive nonatherosclerotic intimal thickening that proceeds in many human arteries throughout life (unpublished data). Such diffuse intimal thickening may possibly result from hemodynamic stresses (see above). As the tunica intima thickens, the diffusion pathway of oxygen and similar small molecules from the

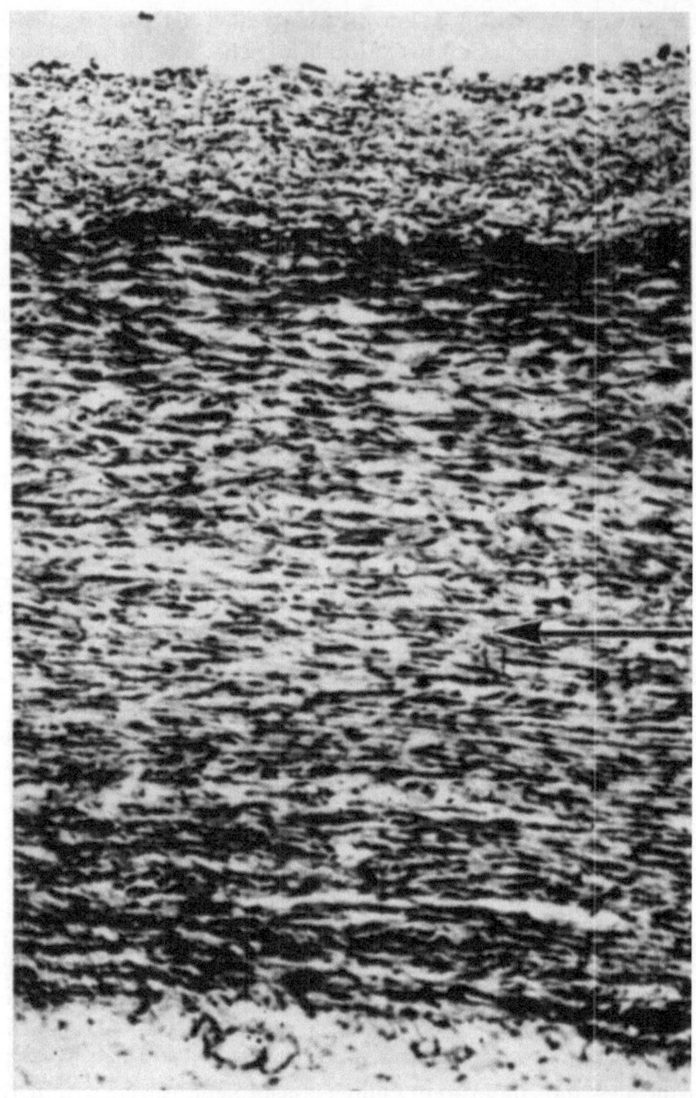

Fig. 3. Decreased NADH-tetrazolium reductase (Coenzyme I reductase) activity in the smooth muscle fibres of the middle media (arrow) in the aorta of a woman aged 52 years. Intima at top, Nitroblue tetrazolium, ×92. (Reproduced with permission from the Journal of Atherosclerosis Research)

lumen to the mid-media [804] would become overextended and, hence, the mid-media would suffer hypoxia. Small arteries are nourished by direct permeation from the lumen; but, at a critical mural thickness, the outer part of the vessel is nourished from *vasa vasorum* in the tunica adventitia [13, 1566, 1567]. For this reason the middle and, subsequently, the inner parts of the human aortic media suffer hypoxic damage with advancing age; the outer media retains normal enzymic activity as it is nourished by the *vasa vasorum*.

Hypoxia of the middle and inner parts of the tunica media would result in diminished energy production by the smooth muscle fibers in this zone and, hence, the synthesis of phospholipid and protein would locally decline. If these lipotrophic agents are required for the transport of cholesterol out of the arterial wall, their diminished synthesis would lead to the accumulation of cholesterol within the innermost zones of the vessel. Thus lipid would be deposited predominantly in the tunica intima, as is seen in the typical atherosclerotic lesion.

Cholesterol Esterification. As stated cholesterol is highly sclerogenic when injected subcutaneously. In a study of the relative sclerogenic properties of

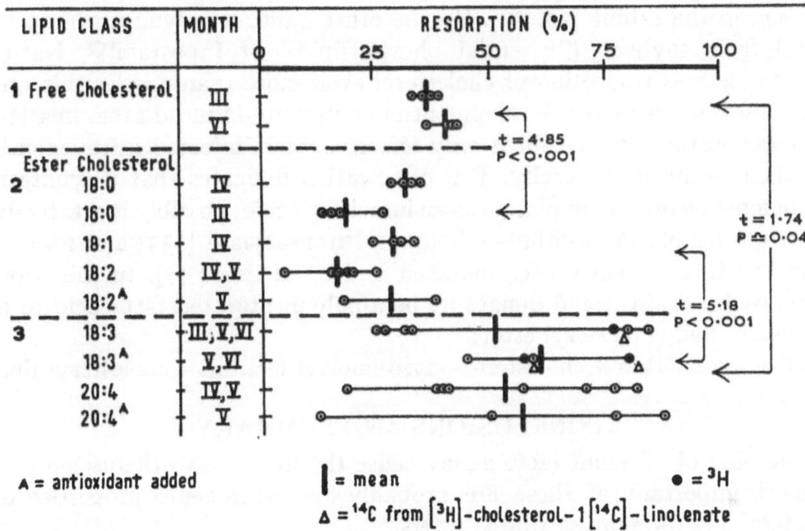

Fig. 4. Resorption rates of free and esterified (^{3}H)-cholesterol from 3-week subcutaneous implants in the rat. (Reproduced with permission from the Journal of Atherosclerosis Research)

cholesterol and its esters [3], we found that these lipids could be ranked in the order (most→least sclerogenic) as follows:

monounsaturated esters > free cholesterol > saturated esters > linoleate (18:2) > linolenate (18:3) > arachidonate (20:4).

If results from subcutaneous implants can be extrapolated to the connective tissues of the arterial wall, it can be inferred that the more polyunsaturated cholesteryl esters are less atherogenic and would cause less damage than the free sterol and its more saturated esters. Studies on the resorption speeds of labelled cholesterol and its esters from subcutaneous implants indicate that free cholesterol is resorbed more rapidly than saturated monoene and diene esters, but usually more slowly than triene and tetraene esters (Fig. 4) [4]. Although Rothblat et al. [1262] showed that cholesterol is mainly transported into cultured cells in free form and not as ester, our results suggest that the triene and tetraene cholesteryl esters are usually more readily mobilized from tissues than the free sterol. Nevertheless, the transcellular and intracellular mechanisms for cholesterol transport remain a problem that requires proper elucidation.

Our studies indicate that the formation of highly polyunsaturated cholesteryl esters might be beneficial in atherosclerotic lesions. Cholesterol esterification increases during severe atherosclerosis [5, 888, 1156]. However, the fatty acid pattern of the cholesteryl esters in the plaques provides no information about the role of polyunsaturated esters. If these esters are rapidly turned over (mobilized) their levels would remain low.

The phospholipids that are synthesized within the arterial wall (see Zilversmit, this volume) may play a surface-active role in dispersing cholesteryl esters. However, although relatively saturated egg lecithin accelerates the resorption of subcutaneously implanted cholesterol, it fails to ameliorate cholesterol-induced atheroma in the rabbit [14, 20]. On the other hand, a polyunsaturated lecithin derived from soybean ("essential phospholipid" of Lipostabil®, Natterman, Köln) accelerates resorption of cholesterol even more than egg lecithin and also practically suppresses the development of cholesterol-induced atheroma [14, 20]. This polyunsaturated lecithin is only effective when injected intravenously and fails when administered orally. This observation indicates that polyunsaturated lecithin must be present in plasma as an intact molecule; possibly it acts by forming a substrate for plasma lecithin→cholesterol transacylase [534] and for a related enzyme that has recently been detected in arterial tissue [5]. In this way polyunsaturated lecithin would donate its beta-polyunsaturated fatty acid to form a polyunsaturated cholesteryl ester:

Dilinoleyl lecithin + cholesterol→lyso-linoleyl lecithin + cholesteryl linoleate.

CONCLUSIONS AND SUMMARY

A number of different factors may cause the fibrosis in atherosclerotic lesion the most important of these are probably the sclerogenic properties of free cholesterol and its more saturated esters.

Cholesterol does not seem to enter the normal arterial wall by direct filtration of plasma lipoprotein through the endothelium but, when the vessel wall is already diseased, plasma protein appears to leak directly into the lesion. Phospholipid and some triglyceride are actively synthesized within the arterial wall.

Triglycerides do not accumulate to any great extent in atherosclerotic lesions, possibly because they are metabolized by the arterial wall lipase. By contrast, cholesterol cannot be significantly degraded by the arterial wall and presumably can only be removed by certain lipotrophic vehicles, such as phospholipid and protein. The metabolic impairment of the middle and inner tunica media of senescent human arteries would result in locally reduced synthesis of such lipotrophic agents and, hence, would promote the accumulation of cholesterol in the inner arterial wall.

Implantation studies indicate that polyunsaturated cholesteryl esters produce less tissue reaction and fibrosis than the free sterol and its more saturated esters. Thus, it would be advantageous to the arterial wall to form polyunsaturated cholesteryl esters, by the action of either cholesteryl ester synthetase or lecithin→cholesterol transacylase. Implantation studies with labelled cholesteryl esters show that Δ_3 and Δ_4 cholesteryl esters are usually mobilized more rapidly from tissues than free cholesterol, which in turn is more rapidly mobilized than its saturated, Δ_1 and Δ_2 esters. The form and vehicles in which cholesterol is transported out of cells and tissues is a problem that requires further investigation.

METABOLISM OF ARTERIAL LIPIDS*

D. B. ZILVERSMIT

It is, of course, well known that various lipids accumulate in the arterial wall during the early stages of atherogenesis. Although cholesteryl ester and free cholesterol are quantitatively the most important lipid fractions that accumulate, several phospholipids, particularly sphingomyelin and phosphatidyl choline, also greatly increase in concentration in atheromatous aortas.

In the present discussion data which elucidate the process of lipid accumulation and the balance of lipid influx and lipid release in arteries developing atherosclerosis will be reviewed. In addition, phospholipid biosynthesis in the normal and atheromatous arterial wall will be discussed. Space limitations do not allow

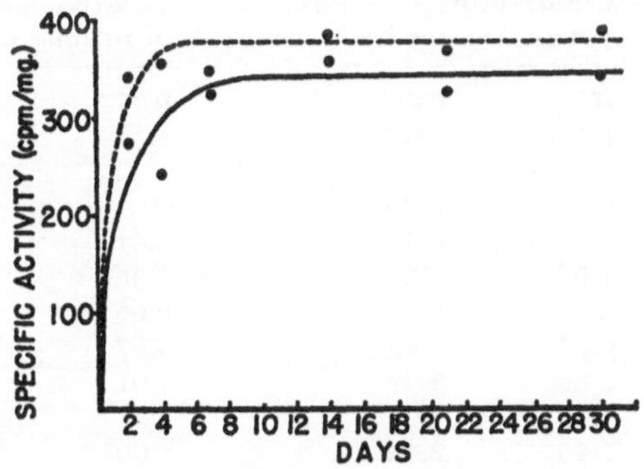

Fig. 1. Specific activities of free (—) and esterified (- - -) cholesterol with time in the plasma of a rabbit fed a 1% cholesterol-^{14}C diet for 30 days. (From Newman and Zilversmit [1094])

a comprehensive review of the literature, and most of the experimental work presented here was performed in the author's laboratory.

It is well known that, in the cholesterol-fed rabbit, serum cholesterol may reach concentrations up to 3 g or 4 g/100 ml. Although it is reasonable to assume that the cholesterol which accumulates in various tissues of these rabbits (liver, skin, artery) is derived directly from blood cholesterol, no quantitative information on this point was available before the use of labeled cholesterol. Newman and Zilversmit [1094] made use of the theorem that if the cholesterol of the arterial wall is entirely derived from plasma, and if the specific activity of plasma cholesterol is held constant during the growth of the cholesterol containing lesion, then the specific activity of cholesterol in the atheromatous lesion is equal to the specific activity of serum cholesterol. These conditions are found to hold

* The work herein has been supported in part by funds provided by Public Health Service Research Grants HE 2181 and HE 10933 from the National Heart Institute, United States Public Health Service and in part by funds provided through the State University of New York. The author wishes to thank L. Barry Hughes for excellent technical assistance.

approximately during the development of atheromatous lesions in rabbits fed a diet containing 1% labeled cholesterol for 21 to 87 days [1094]. Fig. 1 depicts the course of serum free and esterified cholesterol specific activities in a rabbit fed 1% cholesterol-^{14}C for a period of 30 days. At the end of the dietary periods the animals were sacrificed and the specific activities of free and esterified cholesterol in the intima-media portions of the entire aorta in the thorax were divided by those of plasma. In Table 1 relative specific activities close to unity signify the absence of appreciable cholesterol biosynthesis by the arterial wall of animals in which atherogenesis proceeds rapidly, i.e. in animals exhibiting a striking increase in arterial cholesterol content above basal levels. This conclusion is

Table 1. *Cholesterol contents and relative specific activities of aortic intima after prolonged cholesterol-4-^{14}C feeding*[a]

Cholesterol-^{14}C in diet	Cholesterol per intima-media[b]		Relative specific activity of intimal cholesterol[c]	
days	free (mg)	esterified (mg)	free	ester
0	0.32	0.06	—	—
21	0.40	0.17	0.41	0.19
21	1.06	1.38	1.36	1.19
21	0.56	0.23	0.66	0.43
21	0.74	0.43	0.67	0.83
25	2.80	2.97	1.01	0.89
30	1.21	2.95	1.25	1.00
43	1.40	2.48	1.00	0.92
87	4.40	8.20	1.09	0.94

[a] Data from Newman and Zilversmit [1094].
[b] Intima-media from total thoracic portion of aorta (see text).
[c] Relative specific activity equals specific activity of intima-media cholesterol fraction divided by average specific activity of corresponding plasma fraction.

strengthened by the very low incorporation of acetate-^{14}C into the cholesterol of atheromatous aortas as compared to that incorporated into the fatty acid portion of the cholesteryl ester [380, 1092].

The foregoing experiments strongly suggest that cholesterol accumulating in the atherosclerotic plaque is derived from circulating lipoproteins in plasma. The rather low relative specific activities of cholesterol in the arteries with low cholesterol content suggest that isotopic exchange of plasma and arterial cholesterol does not proceed as rapidly in near-normal arteries as in arteries in which atherogenesis is full blown. This, as well as other evidence summarized elsewhere [1594], has led to the hypothesis that atherogenesis appears to be a consequence of, or at least proceeds in parallel with, an increased permeability of the arterial wall towards cholesterol or cholesterol-containing lipoproteins. The increased permeability may be a direct consequence of the high cholesterol concentration in blood plasma, or it may be related to degradation products of cholesterol such as bile acids, or to other lipid or nonlipid substances present in the blood of cholesterol-fed animals.

The foregoing experiments were not designed to yield information about the rate at which plasma cholesterol enters atherosclerotic plaques at different stages of their development. To measure this rate one must carry out experiments in which the influx of labeled plasma cholesterol into the arterial wall is measured relatively early after isotope dosage so that little or no return of label from artery to bloodstream occurs. We tried to accomplish this by feeding animals a high cholesterol diet until sizable lesions had developed and then switching them for a very short period to a diet containing labeled cholesterol. Some results are shown in Table 2. These rabbits were maintained on 1% cholesterol diets for 15, 30 or 60 days. During the last two days of the dietary period the animals received the same amount of cholesterol but now the cholesterol was labeled

Table 2. *Comparison of cholesterol influx and retention by aortic intimas at different stages of atheromatosis*[a]

Days on 1% cholesterol diet	Intimal cholesterol content[b]		Cholesterol influx[b]		Cholesterol retention[b]	
	free (mg)	ester (mg)	free (μg/day)	ester (μg/day)	free (μg/day)	ester (μg/day)
15	0.49	0.14	56	67	14.2	7.2
30	0.88	0.47	122	109	25.3	18.2
60	2.73	4.72	406	240	70.4	101.0

[a] Data from Newman and Zilversmit [1094]. Mean values for three or four animals per group.

[b] Per total thoracic portion of aorta.

with ^{14}C. By dividing the average specific activity of plasma cholesterol into the total cholesterol-^{14}C of the thoracic aorta, at the end of the experiment a value approximately twice the cholesterol influx per day was obtained. Several interesting conclusions can be drawn from the data in Table 2. The accumulation of free and esterified cholesterol in the arterial wall starts out slowly and proceeds to gather speed as the lesions become larger. Up to 90 days after the beginning of the cholesterol diet both free and esterified cholesterol content of the artery increase exponentially [1094, 1095]. It is clear from Table 2 that the influx of free and esterified cholesterol also increases steadily as the degree of atherosclerosis, as measured by cholesterol content of the artery, increases. It is also of interest to compare the rate of cholesterol influx with the rate of cholesterol retention by the arterial wall. The rate of cholesterol retention was calculated from the rate of increase in chemically determined arterial cholesterol at different stages of atherogenesis. Table 2 shows that the cholesterol influx exceeds cholesterol retention by a factor of 2 or 3. This means that turnover of free and esterified cholesterol is taking place in the atheromatous plaque. Apparently a removal mechanism exists, presumably an efflux of cholesterol back into the bloodstream and this efflux also appears to increase with the duration of cholesterol feeding. All these observations are compatible with the hypothesis that during atherogenesis the permeability of the arterial wall to cholesterol gradually increases. This increase does not appear to be related to aging because even in newborn rabbits on a high cholesterol intake, arterial cholesterol accumulated rapidly (unpublished observations).

Another interesting observation was made, namely, that free cholesterol appears to penetrate the arterial wall relatively faster than cholesteryl ester [1094, 1096]. The concentration of cholesteryl ester in plasma exceeds that of free cholesterol by a factor of 3. If cholesterol entered the artery as part of a lipoprotein complex one would expect that the mass of free and esterified cholesterol entering per unit of time would also differ by a factor of 3. The failure to find such a relationship as well as the previously mentioned finding that cholesterol accumulates exponentially in the arterial wall appear to rule out a simple filtration process as the primary mechanism by which cholesterol accumulates in the arterial wall. Other studies by ourselves [1096] as well as by Dayton and Hashimoto [382] have shown that the uptake of free and esterified cholesterol by the artery does not depend on metabolic activity of the artery. The studies of Jensen [747], on the other hand, appear to show that the rate of glycolysis is related to the rate of cholesterol influx. Jensen believes that in the normal artery plasma cholesteryl ester may be rapidly bound to the endothelial cell but fails to penetrate deeper, while free cholesterol may be able to reach the deeper layers of the artery. Our own studies on the esterification of labeled precursors of cholesteryl ester in the arterial wall suggest that the permeability of the arterial wall to serum cholesterol is less than that to serum unesterified fatty acids [1092]. In a typical experiment, aortic strips from cholesterol-fed rabbits were incubated with serum which contained lipoproteins labeled with free cholesterol (^{3}H) and albumin labeled with free fatty acids (^{14}C). After 6 hours of incubation about 0.006% of added ^{3}H and 0.13% of added ^{14}C were found in the arterial cholesteryl ester, a twentyfold difference. Although an interpretation of these results is difficult because of the unknown extent of isotope dilution of labeled lipids by the exchangeable cholesterol and fatty acids in the intima-media of the arterial wall, the results are consistent with the hypothesis that serum free fatty acids can penetrate to the esterifying sites in the intima-media more rapidly than the serum-free cholesterol. Relatively rapid conversion of serum fatty acids to esterified cholesterol in the normal arterial wall has also been demonstrated by Stein and Stein [1419]. Day and Wahlqvist [378] studied the uptake of labeled oleic acid by cholesteryl ester and other lipids in atheromatous lesions of rabbits while Wahlqvist, Day and Tume [1514] performed similar studies on human arteries. In the latter two studies, both radiochemical and radioautographic methods were employed.

Attention will now be placed on some other lipids in the arterial wall, namely the phospholipids. Although the phospholipids do not increase to the same extent as the cholesterol and cholesteryl ester, their accumulation is by no means minor. In the human lesion, particularly the sphingomyelin appears to increase [13] whereas in the rapidly induced atheromatous lesion of the rabbit, both lecithin and sphingomyelin increase 4 or 5 fold [946]. Studies undertaken with radioactive phosphate [1356, 1598] and radioactive acetate [1093] have shown that the source of this phospholipid is primarily synthesis *in situ*. This synthesis of phospholipids, which also takes place in human atheromas [1597], might serve to solubilize cholesterol deposits in the arterial wall [1598]. More recently, this hypothesis has been amplified by numerous studies undertaken in the laboratory of Professor Adams [13]. Notwithstanding the attractiveness of this hypothesis, there does not appear to be any direct evidence that the *in situ* synthesis of phospholipids has a beneficial effect in retarding the development of the atherosclerotic lesions.

Recently attention has been focused on the phospholipids of the arterial wall in an effort to localize the type of cell primarily responsible for the accelerated phospholipid synthesis. In one such study, atheromatous aortas were subjected to partial digestion with collagenase and elastase, and foam cells were isolated from these arteries [376]. Although it was evident that the isolated foam cells contained only about 2% of the total lipid of the atheromatous lesions, these cells appeared to play a significant role in the total biosynthesis that was observed

Table 3. *Phospholipid-^{32}P of foam cells, supernatant and residue of atheromatous rabbit aortas incubated with ^{32}P phosphate* [a]

	Phospholipid-^{32}P percentage	Lipid P μg	Specific activity cpm/μg
Foam cells	11.3 ± 0.8	12.3 ± 0.9	2,660 ± 162
Supernatant	48.2 ± 2.2	420 ± 55	350 ± 24
Residue	40.4 ± 3.1	341 ± 38	360 ± 9

[a] Day, Newman and Zilversmit [376]. Three aortas were incubated with ^{32}P for four hours. Values are mean ± S.E. The values reported as "foam cells" include cells and their wash fluid.

in atheromatous aorta. For example, in one experiment shown in Table 3, atheromatous aortas were incubated with a buffer containing radioactive phosphate for four hours and foam cells were separated from a milky looking "supernatant" fraction (probably mostly extracellular material) and a residual mass (probably mostly undigested material). The specific activity of the phospholipids in the cells was about eight times as high as that of the phospholipids in the supernatant or residue. It is not known whether the labeled phospholipid in the "supernatant" may represent, at least in part, the contents of cells disrupted during the isolation procedure.

One line of evidence that such may well be the case may be seen in the results of a recent experiment (shown in Table 4, unpublished observations). After a four-hour incubation of an atheromatous rabbit aorta with ^{32}P-phosphate, foam cells were isolated from the intima-media preparation. Phospholipid-^{32}P in individual phospholipid fractions was determined in "foam cells", "supernatant" and "residue". Table 4 shows that the specific activity of phospholipids in foam cells were five to seven times as high as in the other fractions. Yet the distribution of ^{32}P of individual phospholipid fractions in the three tissue fractions was practically identical. Although this finding does not prove that all labeled phospholipids were derived from the same source, the finding is compatible with the idea that all labeled lipids are formed in one site, i.e. the foam cell.

Although one cannot conclude from these results that phospholipid synthesis takes place primarily in the foam cell of the lesion, one can conclude that most

Table 4. *Distribution of individual ³²P-phospholipids in atheromatous rabbit aorta fractions* [a]

	PL^{32}P per arterial fraction [b]					PLP	spec. act. [c]
	PE	PI	PC	Sp	Ly		
Whole artery	4.6	29	63	0.9	1.4	100	100
Foam cells	4.1	21	70	1.2	0.7	2	518
Supernatant	5.4	28	63	1.0	1.9	38	107
Residue	4.2	31	62	0.9	1.2	60	82

[a] Intima-media after two hours incubation with ^{32}P-phosphate.
[b] Expressed as percentage of total PL^{32}P in each fraction.
[c] Expressed as percentage of whole artery.
Abbreviations: PE = phosphatidyl ethanolamine; PI = phosphatidyl inositol; PC = phosphatidyl choline; Sp = sphingomyelin; Ly = lysolecithin.

Table 5. *Distribution of phospholipid ³²P in layers of pig aorta*

	Tissue wt g	P incorporated [a]	PE	PI	PC	Sp	Ly	PI/PC
Endothelium [b]	—	0.005	24.0	17	43	0.4	3.4	0.4
Media 1	0.26	5.3	1.3	59	39	0.4	0.4	1.5
Media 2	0.42	1.8	1.2	64	33	0.4	0.4	1.9
Media 3	0.53	0.2	2.4	55	40	0.5	0.4	1.4
Media 4	0.51	0.5	2.4	53	42	0.6	0.3	1.3
Media 5	0.64	3.5	6.6	51	39	0.5	0.4	1.3

[a] mμ moles P/incorporated into phospholipid per gram of tissue in four hours; endothelium calculated per whole sample. Figures in columns 3–7 are percentages of total PL^{32}P in each layer. Column 8 gives ratio of ^{32}P in PI and PC for each layer.
[b] Endothelium derived from same area as slices of media. Numbers after media refer to slices from lumen surface to adventitia. For abbreviations see Table 4.

of the phospholipid in the atheromatous aorta is metabolically much less active than that present in these cells. It is even possible that most of the phospholipid, and possibly other lipid present in the lesion, is metabolically inert. Such lipid deposits might well be the beginning of necrotic areas which are commonly seen in advanced human lesions but are rarely observed in experimentally induced lesions in rabbit aortas [1562].

Comparisons between the phospholipid synthesis in foam cells and that in normal rabbit arteries revealed that in the normal artery the phosphatidyl inositol, which represents chemically only a very small fraction of the total phospholipid, exhibits by far the highest ^{32}P content [1077, 1091]. Since the normal artery exhibits a phospholipid synthesis pattern which differs markedly from that of the atheromatous aorta we became interested in localizing the sites of phospholipid synthesis in the normal artery. Several studies were performed in both rabbit and pig aortas. The intimal cell layer was removed with a frozen glass plate and thin layers of the intima-media were peeled off in succession. In one such experiment (unpublished observations) shown in Table 5 it is shown that the relatively high synthesis of phosphatidyl inositol from ^{32}P precursors is not localized in the endothelial cell but instead seems to take place in the media which is, of course, the locus of smooth muscle cells. Parker et al. [1151] have suggested that smooth muscle cells in the artery evolve into foam cells, rich in cytoplasmic organelles, and that the increased phospholipid synthesis in the atheromatous aorta is linked to the additional requirement for membrane phospholipids. However, if the normal smooth muscle cell synthesizes primarily phosphatidyl inositol, and if it is true that the foam cell synthesizes primarily phosphatidyl choline, one of two possibilities appear to exist: (1) the foam cell is derived from the smooth muscle cell but the uptake of cholesterol transforms the metabolic pattern of the cell from one that incorporates ^{32}P primarily into phosphatidyl choline, or (2) most foam cells in the atheromatous lesion of the rabbit are not primarily derived from smooth muscle cells but from other cell types, e.g., circulating macrophages. Apparently, macrophages have a similar phospholipid synthesis pattern to that found in foam cells [373]. Day and Wahlqvist [378] conclude from their work on the conversion of various lipid precursors to esterified products by medial and intimal portions of normal and atherosclerotic rabbit aortas that the lipid metabolism of foam cells differs considerably from that of the differentiated cells in the media. It appears likely that further biochemical studies may add a new dimension to the study of foam cells, a study which so far has been the exclusive domain of the microscopist.

SUMMARY

The studies cited here, and others not quoted, indicate that in aortic lesions of rabbits fed high cholesterol diets, cholesterol and cholesteryl ester appear to accumulate at rapidly increasing rates and are derived primarily from the circulating blood. The kinetic studies of lipid influx, accumulation, and biosynthesis, do not support the hypothesis that the accumulation of lipid in the atheroma is governed primarily by a process of simple filtration and retention of intact lipoproteins. They do suggest, however, that in the cholesterol-fed animal there is a gradual increase in the permeability of the arterial wall which promotes the influx and retention of serum lipoprotein cholesterol.

The phospholipids, which accumulate in the arterial wall, appear to be derived primarily from local synthesis; and it is evident that the foam cells play an important role in the total biosynthetic mechanism. The pattern of phospholipid synthesis in the foam cells is quite different from that observed in normal smooth muscle cells. This raises the question as to whether the foam cell is derived from a cell type different from the smooth muscle cell, or whether the uptake of cholesterol is capable of modifying the phospholipid synthesizing pattern of the smooth muscle or multipotential cell.

THE LIPOPROTEINS OF THE LESIONS*

ELSPETH B. SMITH and ROSALIND S. SLATER

Lipid in the arterial intima occurs in at least two distinct morphological and chemical forms, fine extracellular droplets with a chemical composition closely resembling the S_f 0–20 lipoprotein (LP) of plasma, and larger intracellular lipid droplets with a bizarre and highly characteristic cholesteryl ester fatty acid pattern suggesting synthesis *in situ* [1378]. In aging normal intima and in fibrous thickenings and plaques the accumulating lipid appears to be of the former type whereas in fatty streaks and flecks and, at least in part, in raised fatty plaques it appears to be of the latter type [1379]. More precise information on the relationship between infiltration of plasma lipoprotein and the accumulation of these different types of lipid is urgently required.

There is no doubt that plasma low density lipoprotein (LDLP) is present in the arterial wall. It has been demonstrated in extracts by immuno-electrophoresis [1133, 1475] and in the wall itself by several workers using immuno-fluorescent microscopy. Unfortunately there are rather marked differences in the details of their findings. Thus Knieriem, Kao and Wissler [812] considered that virtually all the plasma LDLP was intracellular in all types of lesion whereas Walton and Williamson [1521] found it to be virtually all extracellular. In fatty streaks (not very precisely defined) Haust [636] and Woolf and Pilkington [1573] found diffuse extracellular fluorescence, and some focal fluorescence which might be intracellular, whereas Walton and Williamson did not find fluorescence within fat-filled cells. Both latter authors found strong, diffuse fluorescence in small fibrous thickenings in which all the lipid seemed to be extracellular. The findings of Walton and Williamson seem to be closely in line with the chemical-morphological data from our laboratory [1378, 1379].

Unfortunately neither immuno-electrophoresis nor immuno-fluorescence are readily quantified, and the interpretation of studies on the amount of LDLP entering the arterial wall using lipoprotein with labelled cholesterol has been rendered uncertain by the recent work of Newman and Zilversmit [1096] and Hashimoto and Dayton [628]. They have demonstrated that labelled cholesterol in plasma lipoproteins is incorporated into arterial lipids even after inhibition with KCN or boiling the artery; this is also true for the reverse exchange. From the data presented by Newman and Zilversmit it appears that the counts taken up are dependent on the arterial cholesterol level rather than the amount of plasma LP. Hashimoto and Dayton interpret this independence of enzymic mechanisms as a physico-chemical exchange. This would be comparable with the exchange which occurs between red cells and lipoproteins [66, 593] and other membrane systems, such as mitochondria, and lipoproteins [559]. This exchange

* The work herein was wholly financed by the British Heart Foundation, to whom the authors are most grateful. Thanks are also extended to Professor S. C. Frazer for provision of laboratory facilities.

probably accounts for the complete equilibration between subcellular fractions and injected labelled cholesterol and for the constant specific activities, found in dog aortas by Hollander and Kramsch [695] and Hollander et al. [696].

Another approach to quantification has been homogenization of arterial tissue and fractionation of the extract by ultracentrifugation under the conditions used for plasma lipoproteins [604, 696]. This provides a convenient method for measurement, but the nature of the material which is found in the various fractions is open to considerable doubt. It is known from the field of oil seed technology that homogenization of lipid/protein mixtures produces a range of stable lipid/protein aggregates [1380], and these show ultracentrifugal flotation characteristics comparable to plasma lipoproteins (personal observation). The mixture of lipids and proteins found in arterial intima would seem to be ideally suited to the formation of nonspecific aggregates of this nature. Slater and Smith [1375] found a high extraction of cholesterol but a very low activity of immunologically intact plasma S_f 0–20 LP in homogenates of aortic intima. The amount of plasma LDLP in arterial extracts can be determined by a quantitative immunological assay, but for the lipid material which is not accounted for by plasma LP it is difficult to see how to differentiate between lipoproteins specifically synthesized in the lesions and nonspecific lipid/protein aggregates of the same density.

In this laboratory we are using the quantitative immuno-plate method of Fahey and McKelvey [447] to measure the amount of plasma LDLP in the ultracentrifugal S_f 0–20 LP fraction of extracts made from scissor-minced human aortic intima, and some of our findings follow.

METHODS USED FOR EXTRACTION OF PLASMA LDLP OF INTIMA AND ITS IMMUNOLOGICAL DETERMINATION

Human aortas were obtained within 24 hours of death, the intimal surface wiped and blotted with saline-moistened filter paper, and homogeneous areas of normal or mildly atherosclerotic intima selected and stripped, taking samples for histological control, as described previously [1378].

Extraction and preparation of lipoprotein. Various methods have been tried: (a) homogenization in a standard glass tissue grinder; (b) extraction of slices 10 μ or 20 μ thick prepared in a cryostat; and (c) scissor-mincing in saline. Maximum immunological activity is obtained by method c (see Table 1), and the following standard procedure has been adopted.

The tissue is weighed into a small glass weighing pot, 2 ml 0.9% NaCl solution added, and the tissue chopped with fine scissors. The extract is then carefully pipetted off, and the procedure repeated four times giving a total of 10 ml extract. This is separated into $S_f > 20$ and S_f 0–20 LP fractions by preparative ultracentrifugation, the fractions dialyzed, concentrated against polyethylene glycol and adjusted to 1 ml for immuno-assay and cholesterol estimation.

Immuno-assay. The immunoplate method of Fahey and McKelvey [447] is used; goat antihuman LDLP serum is incorporated in the gel, and human serum S_f 0–20 LP used as standard. The cholesterol content of the standard is measured, and the calibration curve constructed as ring diameter against S_f 0–20 cholesterol.

Ten µl aliquots of the intimal LP fractions are used for immuno-assay and suitable aliquots for determination of total cholesterol in the S_f 0–20 fraction. The threshold for reliable immuno-assay is about 0.1 mg S_f 0–20 cholesterol in 1 ml, and results from samples with less than this amount have been rejected. No immunological activity has been obtained in intimal $S_f > 20$ fractions.

Definition of terms. The residual tissue is extracted with solvent for determination of residual tissue cholesterol, then dried and weighed, and all concentrations are in terms of mg/100 mg of this extracted dry tissue. The components measured are defined in the following way: *S_f 0–20 cholesterol:* total cholesterol in the ultracentrifugal S_f 0–20 fraction; *immuno-beta-cholesterol:* calculated cholesterol content of the immunologically determined plasma LP in the S_f 0–20 fraction; and *total cholesterol:* sum of the cholesterol in the S_f 0–20, $S_f > 20$ and residual tissue fractions.

RESULTS: LIPOPROTEINS EXTRACTED FROM NORMAL INTIMA AND EARLY LESIONS

Effect of Method of Extraction on Fractions Recovered from normal Intima. The method of extraction is of such vital importance that the results of preliminary studies, in which samples of normal intima were divided into two parts and extracted in different ways, are given in Table 1. In the first pair of samples where

Table 1. *Effect of extraction method on lipid components extracted from intima*

Age and sex	Treatment of sample	Cholesterol mg/100 mg dry tissue		Percentage immuno-beta cholesterol in S_f 0–20 fraction	Percentage total tissue cholesterol extracted
		immuno-beta	S_f 0–20		
59, F.	Homogenized	0.18	2.11	8.5	35.4
	Cryostat slices (20 µ)	0.40	1.25	32.0	20.5
55, M.	Cryostat slices (10 µ)	0.13	0.50	26.0	22.1
	Cryostat slices (20 µ)	0.17	0.44	38.8	14.8
50, F.	Cryostat slices (10 µ)	0.07	0.34	20.4	22.5
	Scissor-minced	0.17	0.24	70.8	12.4

a homogenate is compared with 20 µ cryostat slices the homogenate contained almost twice as much S_f 0–20 LP cholesterol and less than half as much immuno-beta cholesterol as the slices. Throughout the series of experiments the mildest manipulations have given the lowest extraction of immunologically inert lipids, and the highest immunological activity.

It appears that homogenization: (1) produces a large amount of material in the S_f 0–20 and $S_f > 20$ fractions which does not have the immunological properties

Table 2. *Effect on immunological activity of homogenization of intima and of plasma S_f 0–20 LP*

Treatment of sample[a]	Mg immuno-beta cholesterol in 1.5 ml extract	Percentage inactivation
Scissor-minced	0.789	
Homogenized	0.265	66.0
Minced residue homogenized	0	
Scissor-minced after addition of 0.15 ml plasma S_f 0–20 LP	0.912	
Homogenized after addition of 0.15 ml plasma S_f 0–20 LP	0.324	72.0
0.15 ml plasma S_f 0–20 LP[b]	0.182	
0.15 ml plasma S_f 0–20 LP homogenized alone	0	100
0.15 ml plasma S_f 0–20 LP homogenized with minced residue	0.052	71.4

[a] In all cases intima was divided into four parts, each of which was extracted with 10 ml saline and the extract was concentrated to 1.5 ml.

[b] Volume made up to 10 ml. then concentrated to 1.5 ml.

Table 3. *Cholesterol fractions and intimal thickness of normal intima in different age groups*

Age group	Number	Cholesterol mg/100 mg dry tissue				Thickness of intima, in μ
		immuno-beta	S_f 0–20	S_f >20	total	
12–33[a] av. 24	9	—	0.105 ± 0.060	0.078 ± 0.047	2.79 ± 1.95	61 ± 38
20–39	8	0.289 ± 0.154	0.537 ± 0.269	0.107 ± 0.062	3.48 ± 1.74	69 ± 29
40–49	23	0.380 ± 0.240	0.536 ± 0.335	0.112 ± 0.066	4.55 ± 1.68	166 ± 44
50–59	29	0.429 ± 0.304	0.612 ± 0.417	0.144 ± 0.138	5.63 ± 2.10	179 ± 40
60–69	19	0.412 ± 0.221	0.662 ± 0.397	0.274 ± 0.233	6.70 ± 1.74	193 ± 47

[a] S_f 0–20 cholesterol values were below the level permitting reliable immunoassay.

of plasma lipoprotein, and (2) causes actual loss of immunological activity. This latter observation is confirmed in the experiment recorded in Table 2.

Amount of Immuno-beta Cholesterol in Normal Intima. The results obtained in 88 samples of intima which were both macroscopically and microscopically normal are summarized in Table 3. No sex differences were detected and the series contains equal numbers of men and women. In 9 out of the 17 subjects under the age of 40 the concentration of S_f 0–20 cholesterol was below 0.1 mg/ml which is the threshold for reliable immunological assay. The other parameters for these samples are shown at the top of the table, but they are not included in subsequent correlations. The significance of this group with very low S_f 0–20 LP levels is not understood.

Table 4. *Correlation coefficients for relationship of cholesterol fractions with age, and with intimal thickness*[a]

	Age		Thickness	
	r	p	r	p
Immuno-beta-cholesterol	0.086	>0.1	0.370	<0.001
S_f 0–20 cholesterol	0.189	>0.1	0.364	<0.001
Total cholesterol	0.469	<0.001	0.372	<0.001

[a] The group of aortas not assayed immunologically is excluded from these calculations.

All the extracted fractions show a wide scatter within each age group, and when the anomalous low group is excluded there is no significant correlation with age; by contrast, total cholesterol is significantly correlated with age. It can be seen in Table 3 that there is a progressive increase in intimal thickness with age, and in Table 4 a comparison is made of the correlation coefficients between lipid parameters and age and lipid parameters and intimal thickness. Immuno-beta and S_f 0–20 cholesterol are more highly correlated with thickness than with

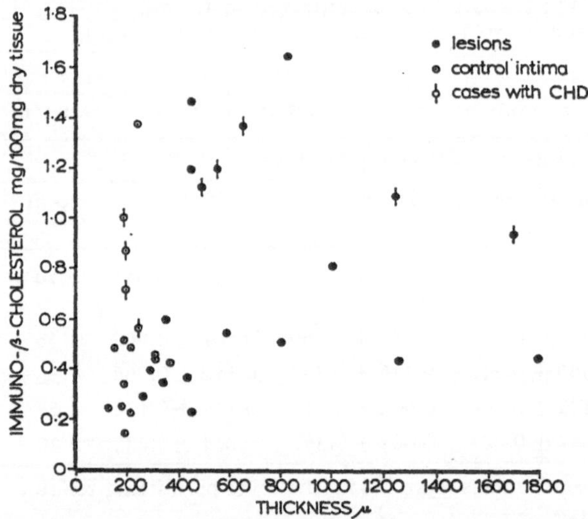

Fig. 1. The relationship between immuno-beta cholesterol and intimal thickness in fibrous lesions and controls from the same aortae. Samples from cases with CHD are marked with a bar

age, but total cholesterol is more highly correlated with age than with thickness, as was found previously [1378].

Immuno-beta Cholesterol in Early Atherosclerotic Lesions. Early lesions were selected macroscopically in two classes, raised fibrous plaques, nodules or ridges, and fatty streaks or flecks. A control sample of macroscopically normal intima was taken from the nearest possible site in the same aorta. The lesions were finally classified from the histological sections, and only early lesions of clearly defined type were included: (a) fibrous thickenings with intact perifibrous lipid and no

Table 5. *Comparison of cholesterol fractions and intimal thickness in fibrous lesions with immuno-beta cholesterol levels above and below 0.65 mg/100 mg dry tissue*

Immuno-beta cholesterol	Number	Average age	Cholesterol, mg/100 mg dry tissue			Percentage immuno-β cholesterol in S_f 0–20 fraction	Thickness of intima, in μ
		age	immuno-beta	S_f 0–20	total		
Above 0.65	9	49	1.214	2.457	7.23	49.5	820
Below 0.65	6	53	0.415	0.975	7.15	42.5	890
Difference			$p=0.001$	$p=0.001$	$p>0.1$	$p>0.1$	$p>0.1$

fat-filled cells; and (b) fatty streaks or flecks with the lipid within fat-filled cells which show no sign of disintegration.

a) *Fibrous Lesions.* In Fig. 1 the immuno-beta cholesterol is plotted against intimal thickness for fibrous lesions and their control samples. It can be seen that immuno-beta cholesterol is generally higher in the lesions than in the controls; it does not, however, increase progressively with thickness but seems to be highest in a group of medium lesions between 400 μ and 900 μ maximun thickness. There seems to be a slight division at about 0.65 mg immuno-beta cholesterol/100 mg dry tissue, and in Table 5 the cholesterol fractions in lesions above and below this level are compared. There is no significant difference between the two groups in thickness, total cholesterol content, or percentage of immuno-beta cholesterol in the S_f 0–20 fraction. The difference lies in the amount of S_f 0–20 extracted. We have been unable to find any consistent morphological differences between these two groups of fibrous lesions.

b) *Fatty Streaks and Flecks (Lipid Mainly in Fat-Filled Cells).* Very surprisingly, in fatty streaks containing numerous and confluent fat-filled cells the immuno-beta cholesterol is *lower* than the control samples; this is found in spite of higher S_f 0–20 and very much higher total cholesterol in lesions than in controls (Table 6). In addition to the low levels of immuno-beta cholesterol in lesions containing fat-filled cells the levels in the controls for these lesions also appear to be low. This is examined in the lower half of Table 6 where the controls for the 15 fat-filled cell lesions are compared with all other samples of normal intima in the same age range. In the lesion controls immuno-beta cholesterol and S_f 0–20 cholesterol are significantly lower although total cholesterol is higher. It thus appears that fat-filled cells are associated with low levels of immuno-beta cholesterol both in their immediate vicinity and in the surrounding normal intima.

Immuno-beta Cholesterol in Aortic Intima in Relation to Coronary Heart Disease (CHD). In the autopsy material collected there were 33 aortas from cases with CHD, and of these 19 could not be used because they were totally involved with gross atherosclerosis. The 14 aortas with minimum involvement had high levels of immuno-beta cholesterol, and in Table 7 samples from the cases with CHD (all men) are compared with men in the same age group with all other conditions excluding hypertension and cerebro-vascular accidents. In 8 out of the 14 cases with CHD macroscopically normal intima was found to be ridgy and irregular on microscopic examination; this condition was found in 7 out of the 28 controls (difference in incidence of borderline significance, $p=0.04$). In these rather

Table 6. *Comparison between lipid fractions in lesions containing numerous fat-filled cells and adjacent normal intima, and between these normal controls and normal intima from all other aortas in same age group*

	Number of samples	Cholesterol, mg/100 mg dry tissue		
		immuno-beta	S_f 0–20	total
Fat-filled cell lesions				
Lesion	15	0.148	0.517	15.25
Control		0.236	0.381	6.28
Difference		$p = 0.01$	$p = 0.02$	$p = 0.001$
Normal intima				
Controls from above	15	0.236	0.381	6.28
Other normals	54	0.470	0.668	5.36
Difference		$p = 0.001$	$p = 0.001$	$p = 0.005$

Table 7. *Comparison of immuno-beta cholesterol and total cholesterol in samples of intima from men with CHD and all other men in the same age group (excluding hypertension and cerebrovascular accidents)*

	Normal intima	Irregular intima	Fibrous lesions
CHD			
Number of samples	6	8	5
Immuno-beta cholesterol, mg/100 mg dry tissue	0.730	0.990	1.158
Total cholesterol, mg/100 mg dry tissue	6.20	4.80	7.47
Thickness of intima, μ	226	244	926
Other conditions			
Number of samples	21	7	10
Immuno-beta cholesterol mg/100 mg dry tissue	0.383	0.613	0.753
Total cholesterol, mg/100 mg dry tissue	5.53	4.18	7.06
Thickness of intima, μ	176	291	804
Difference in immuno-beta cholesterol	$p = 0.01$	$p = 0.1$	$p = 0.002$
Difference in total cholesterol	$p > 0.1$	$p > 0.1$	$p > 0.1$

heterogeneous samples the immuno-beta cholesterol levels showed a wide scatter, and the difference is not significant, but in normal intima and in fibrous lesions the immuno-beta cholesterol is significantly higher in cases with CHD, although there is no difference in total cholesterol content.

SUMMARY AND CONCLUSIONS

This study has demonstrated four salient points

1. In attempts to measure the amounts of plasma lipoprotein in the intima the method of extraction is of primary importance. The immunological integrity of the lipoprotein is easily destroyed and a large amount of material can be extracted which lacks the immunological properties of plasma lipoprotein although its ultracentrifugal behavior is similar.

2. The immuno-beta cholesterol is substantially raised (about threefold, compared with normal intima in the same age range) in about half the early fibrous lesions which have been examined, but in the remainder it is not significantly increased. The high levels of immuno-beta cholesterol are associated with a high extraction of S_f 0–20 LP, while total cholesterol is the same in both groups. In the high group, immunologically intact plasma S_f 0–20 LP accounts for about 17% of the total cholesterol of the lesion. We have been unable to recognize any consistent morphological differences in the two groups.

3. In fatty streaks and flecks containing numerous fat-filled cells the immuno-beta cholesterol is significantly *lower* than in adjacent normal intima, and this control intima is in turn significantly lower than all other samples of normal intima in the same age range. Thus fat-filled cells seem to be associated with low levels of immuno-beta cholesterol both in their immediate vicinity and in the surrounding tissue.

4. In samples of normal intima and of fibrous lesions from men with CHD the immuno-beta cholesterol is significantly higher than in men with other conditions in the same age group, although total cholesterol is unchanged.

The significance of these findings is not clear. No correlation has been found between immuno-beta cholesterol and total tissue cholesterol, thus the presence of a large amount of plasma lipoprotein in the intima is not necessarily associated with increased lipid deposition. The low levels found in association with fat-filled cells is most suprising; possible explanations might be phagocytosis and destruction of immunological properties within the cell, or some form of disruptive action at the cell surface. The strikingly different CEFA composition of plasma S_f 0–20 LP and fat-filled cells [1378] is difficult to reconcile with wholesale phagocytosis, whereas Robertson's studies on intimal cells in tissue culture [1239, 1240] tend to support the latter idea, and also suggest that there may be some association between fat-filled cells and anoxia.

In the cases with CHD the most obvious explanation of the high levels of immuno-beta cholesterol would be high serum cholesterol levels. Unfortunately serum cholesterol was available in only 6 out of our 88 cases, and only one of these had CHD, so that this association cannot be tested.

In spite of these uncertainties the association shown by the level of immunologically intact plasma lipoprotein with CHD and different types of lesion seems to be highly relevant to the understanding of the atherogenic process.

REACTIONS OF ENDOTHELIAL AND SMOOTH MUSCLE CELLS IN THE ATHEROSCLEROTIC LESION

R. F. Scott, J. Jarmolych, K. E. Fritz, H. Imai, D. N. Kim and E. S. Morrison

The chief reactions of smooth muscle cells and endothelial cells in atherosclerosis can be summarized under four headings: (1) multiplication, (2) dedifferentiation, (3) accumulation of lipid, and (4) cell degeneration and death. Each of these reactions in both human and experimental lesions will be discussed in turn and then some additional specific metabolic reactions of these cells in atherosclerosis will be covered briefly. At the end of the presentation an attempt will

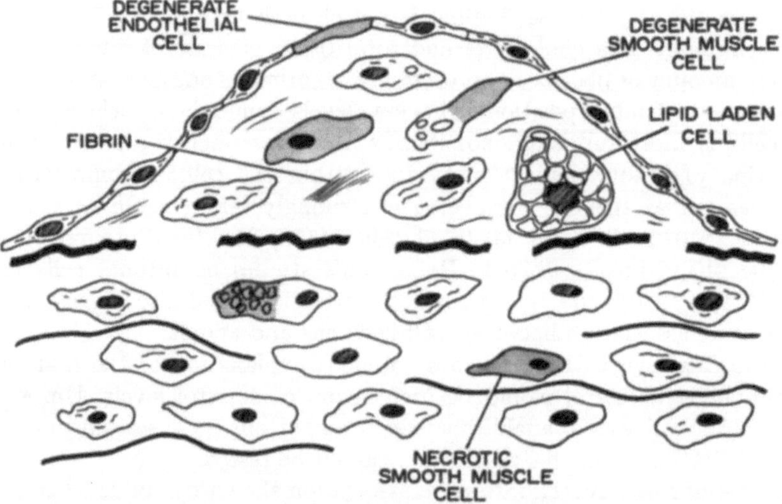

Fig. 1. This figure illustrates the proliferative atherosclerotic lesion, which is visible on gross examination. The proliferative lesion is characterized by an accumulation of cells within the intimal space. All of the cells that can be identified with certainty appear to be smooth muscle cells, although some are so laden with lipid that it is not possible to determine what kind of cells they are. Some of the increased intimal smooth muscle cells in experimental lesions induced in swine and monkeys display individual cell death or degeneration while the remaining ones display morphologic evidence of increased metabolic activity and varying stages of maturation. Mucopolysaccharides and small elastic fibers are present, as well as collagen. Masses of fibrin are seen in some lesions. The endothelial cells overlying the proliferative lesion display occasional individual cell degeneration or death, while the remaining endothelial cells appear more metabolically active than endothelial cells in stockfed swine. The internal elastic lamina beneath the proliferative lesion is often difficult to identify with certainty, since large parts of it may be missing. For this reason it is often not possible to demarcate the area of the upper media from that of the proliferative lesion in the intimal space [1332]

be made to relate these reactions to each other and to the pathogenesis of atherosclerosis.

The grossly visible atherosclerotic lesions in both human and in experimental animals can be divided into two phases: the initial proliferative phase and the later atheromatous phase [468, 1332, 1462]. The proliferative phase is illustrated in Fig. 1. Most of the reactions of endothelial cells and smooth muscle cells in human atherosclerosis have been described in the proliferative lesion. The lesion in humans is slow in developing (requiring years) compared to the rapidly developing proliferative lesion in cholesterol-fed swine, which can be induced in four to six weeks. Because of the rapidity of the development of the animal lesion, cell reactions are better studied in the experimental animal. The cells within experimental lesions, at least in swine and monkeys, are the same type as are seen in the human atherosclerotic lesion. Additional experimental models such as cell culture and organ culture have also been used to study the reactions of smooth muscle cells, and some observations from organ culture experiments will be included in the presentation.

REACTION I: MULTIPLICATION

The human proliferative atherosclerotic lesion is composed of an accumulation of cells within the intimal space. Haust [637] and Geer [514] demonstrated some years ago that the cells composing this lesion are largely smooth muscle cells covered by an intact endothelial surface. The human lesion, as judged morphologically, is composed of mature cells displaying varying amounts of metabolic activity. Because of its slow speed of development, the human lesion does not lend itself well to studies regarding proliferation of its cellular elements. Studies of experimental lesions morphologically similar to the human lesion, however, do provide direct evidence of smooth muscle cell multiplication within the lesion.

Swine fed hypercholesterolemic diets develop within four to six weeks proliferative atherosclerotic lesions in the aorta [468]. These lesions are composed, like the human lesion, predominantly of smooth muscle cells. In swine the smooth muscle cells morphologically show more metabolic activity than do the cells in comparable human lesions, presumably because of the rapidity with which the lesions develop. Evidence that these smooth muscle cells are actively proliferating within the intimal space more rapidly than in other sites in the arterial wall is provided by two studies. In one study tritiated thymidine was injected into the swine before they were killed. The labeling index of tritiated thymidine in the nucleus of cells within the proliferative lesion as measured by autoradiography was considerably greater than thymidine uptake into normal aortic wall [1462]. Increased DNA synthesis within the proliferative lesion as compared to normal artery wall was also demonstrated by biochemical methods [1462]. In another study in swine it was found that the number of mitotic figures within the proliferative lesion were significantly higher than in either adjacent area without visible lesions in hypercholesterolemic diet-fed swine, or in the aortas of stock-fed swine (personal communication). These studies suggest that, at least in the swine lesion produced by a hypercholesterolemic diet, the mass of smooth muscle cells in the intimal space which actually constitute the lesion arise by multiplication *in situ*. An older study of McMillan and Duff [959] and recent studies of McMillan and Stary [960], and Sparagen [1393] provide similar data regarding rabbit atherosclerosis. The findings do not exclude the possibility, of course, that at least initially some of the cells in the lesion are derived from the circulating blood above or from the media beneath the lesion.

The same type of study using tritiated thymidine *in vivo* that demonstrated increased smooth muscle cell DNA synthesis within the proliferative atherosclerotic lesion also showed greater DNA synthesis of endothelial cells covering the lesion, compared to endothelial cells in normal aorta [1462]. Despite the increased rate of endothelial cell DNA synthesis, there is no obvious accumulation of endothelial cells within the lesions, suggesting that endothelial cells have a relatively rapid rate of turnover.

Studies of smooth muscle cell multiplication using medial explants have shown that the increased smooth muscle cell multiplication which occurs in hypercholesterolemic swine is not a transient reaction which disappears rapidly with the removal of the stimulus to multiplication. Strips of medial aortic tissue were removed from swine fed a hypercholesterolemic diet and from swine on a stock diet. Both were grown in a medium containing normocholesterolemic serum. At both four and nine days after the explant was made and after several changes of the nutrient media, DNA synthesis was still considerably higher in the explant of smooth muscle cells taken from the hypercholesterolemic swine (unpublished data, A. S. Daoud) than in explants from control animals. This study suggests at least three possibilities: (1) It may be that despite the lapsed time of nine days, and multiple changes of nutrient media, the substance or substances that originally stimulated smooth muscle cell multiplication in the hypercholesterolemic swine were still present in the explanted tissue. (2) The control mechanisms of smooth muscle cells within the aorta of the hypercholesterolemic swine are permanently changed, and the cells continue to proliferate more rapidly regardless of the nutrient media they are grown in. (3) These cells are not permanently changed and the substance or substances originally inducing the excessive proliferation are no longer present in the explant but that the process of increased cell proliferation, once started, takes a considerable time to reverse itself to normal levels.

REACTION II: DEDIFFERENTIATION AND DIFFERENTIATION

The fact that smooth muscle cells under certain circumstances are capable of fairly vigorous multiplication led to the question of whether or not they dedifferentiated before undergoing mitoses. In the early human lesion Geer found, among the easily identifiable smooth muscle cells, stellate star-shaped cells [514]. On the basis of their morphologic characteristics he suggested that these stellate cells may have been either cells differentiating into smooth muscle cells or smooth muscle cells dedifferentiating. He did not however observe any mitotic figures in the lesions he studied, although an occasional mitotic figure has been found in the human proliferative lesion (Haust).

In the rapidly produced proliferative lesions in swine [363] and monkeys [1328] fed hypercholesterolemic diets, what appears to be dedifferentiation of smooth muscle cells has been observed. There appears to be transition from mature smooth muscle cells to three morphologically different types of cells; in some instances features suggesting transition from one cell type to another were observed. The three cell types have been called modified smooth muscle cells, fibroblast-like cells, and primitive cells. The mitotic figures observed in these types of lesions occur in modified smooth muscle cells, i.e., in a smooth

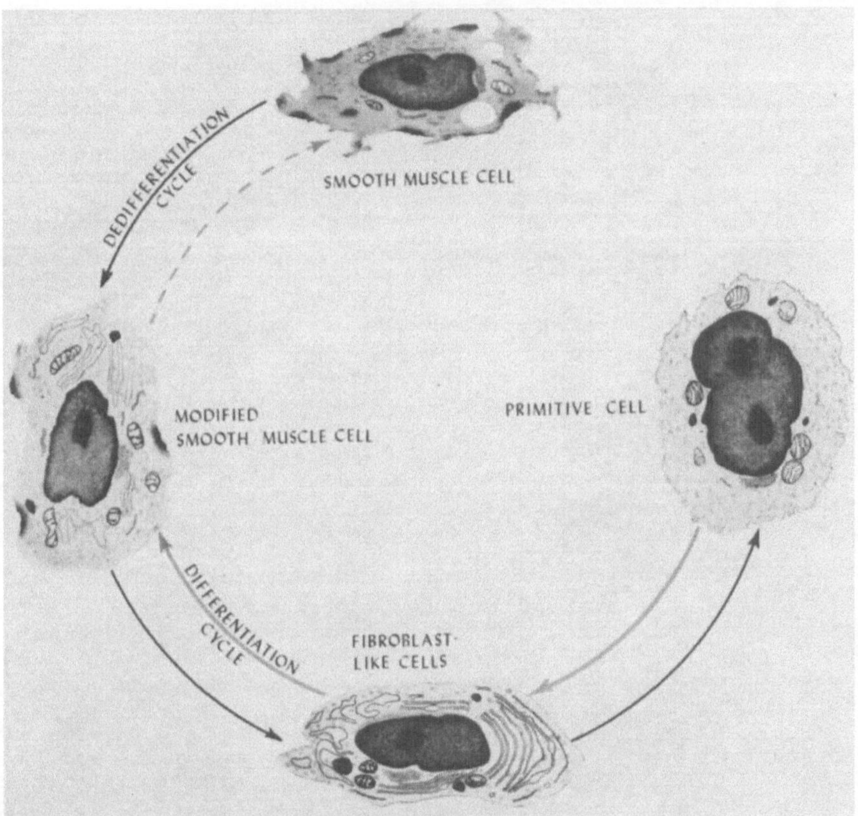

Fig. 2. Schematic drawing illustrating the stage of dedifferentiation seen in organ culture from medial tissue

muscle cell which appears at least partially dedifferentiated, having few if any myofilaments within its cytoplasm.

Studies of cultured strips of aortic media from swine have also demonstrated apparent dedifferentiation and differentiation of smooth muscle cells. When examined by electron microscopy, smooth muscle cells within the strip of media gradually show progressive loss of myofilaments and dense bodies with an increase in the numbers of organelles. By the fourth day most cells contain few if any myofilaments and resemble fibroblasts or primitive cells. By the fourth day an outgrowth of cells from the medial explant appears. These cells at first exhibit few features identifying them as smooth muscle cells. Gradually thereafter the cells in the peripherv differentiate toward smooth muscle cells and by the 21st day

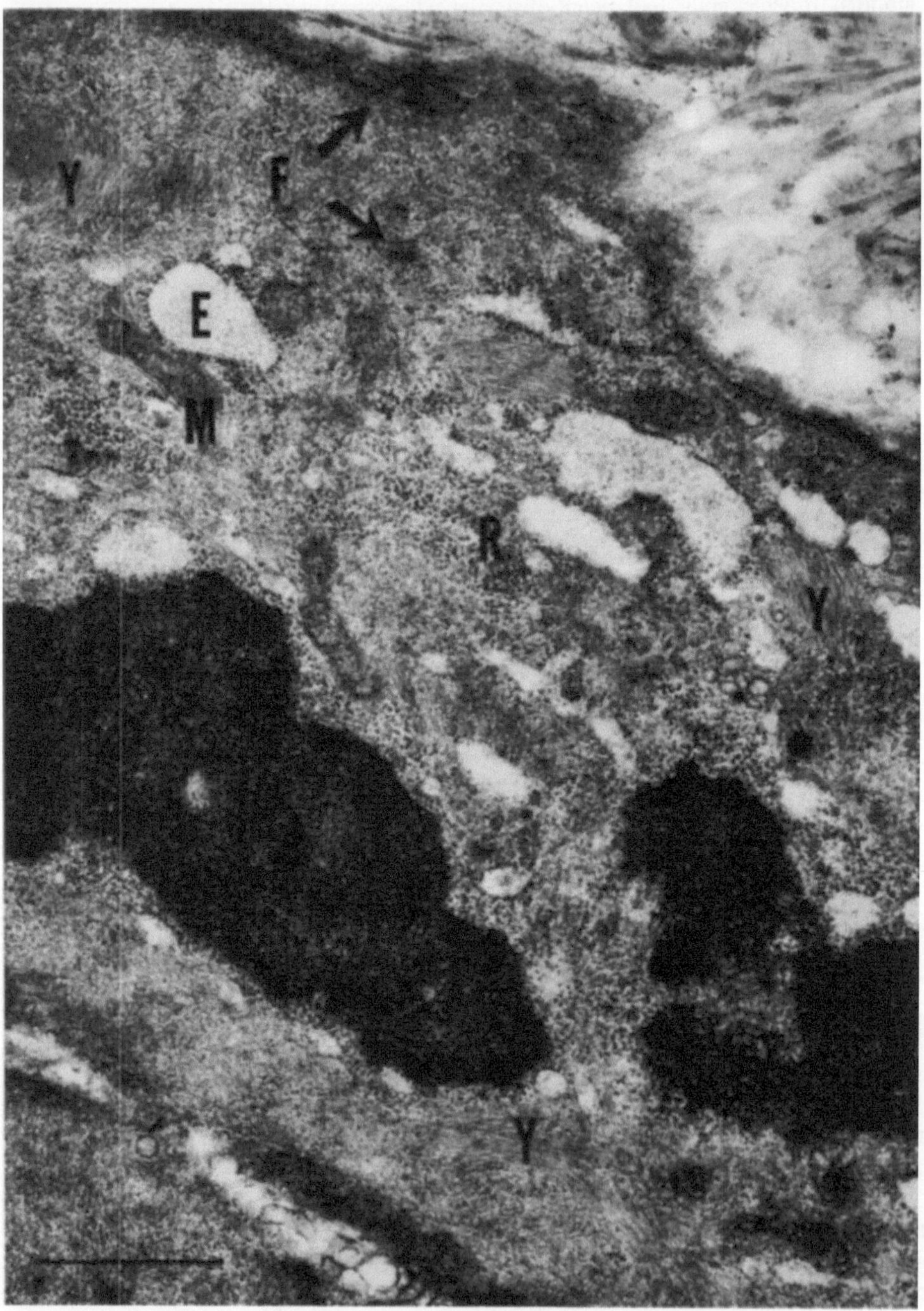

Fig. 3. Myofilaments (*Y*) in this dividing aortic medial smooth muscle cell of a control swine are seen in small bundles oriented irregularly instead of in a uniform longitudinal pattern. Accordingly, fusiform densities (*F*) are also irregular in orientation. The ones with arrow are nearly perpendicular to each other. Ribosomes (*R*), mitochondria (*M*) and slightly distended granular ER (*E*) are marked

almost all the cells contain varying numbers of myofilaments, and a few can be classified as mature smooth muscle cells. From the seventh day onward, these proliferating cells begin to synthesize first mucopolysaccharides, and later (13–21 day) elastic tissue and collagen (see Fig. 2) [745].

That smooth muscle cell multiplication and mitoses can occur in other than dedifferentiated smooth muscle cells has been shown by studies of grossly normal aorta both in swine fed hypercholesterolemic diets for three days and in swine fed stock diets [470]. In this study, significantly more mitotic figures were found in the aortas of the hypercholesterolemic group. In both dietary groups, however, the mitoses were found in apparently differentiated smooth muscle cells (Fig. 3). The findings suggest that it is not necessarily a special group of aortic cells which are capable of multiplying; almost any mature smooth muscle cell has the potential to divide, even without first undergoing dedifferentiation.

While the evidence available points to the conclusion that smooth muscle cells are capable of dedifferentiation and that, in the proliferative lesion at any rate, mitoses in smooth muscle cells are more frequent in these partially dedifferentiated cells, other possibilities exist. There may be within the proliferating lesion totipotential stem cells which are the original source of the smooth muscle cells, or it is possible that the smooth muscle cells are derived initially from other cell types, such as the endothelial cell, through a process of metaplasia.

REACTION III: ACCUMULATION OF LIPID

The type of lipid within the atherosclerotic lesion, its location within the lesion, and its origin will no doubt receive a thorough discussion at this symposium. We would like to touch on only one point about lipids: the distribution of lipid within the cells of the lesion. In the very early, barely visible, human and animal atherosclerotic lesion the lipid, seen by electron microscopy, is both intracellular and extracellular [514]. In most grossly visible lesions in both humans [1327] and animals [1328] however, the lipid appears to be chiefly intracellular in location. It appears to lie within the cytoplasm in droplet form, at times enclosed by a membrane. By electron microscopy it is difficult to tell if the intracellular membranes of the smooth muscle cells either contain or are associated with the excess lipid within the cell. This point may be of considerable importance. If the excess intracellular lipid is either bound to or an integral part of cell membranes, the altered chemical composition of the membrane may be reflected in both altered morphology and function of the membrane. The distribution of labeled cholesterol within the normal arterial smooth muscle cells of the dog and monkey has been studied by cell fractionation. In these normal smooth muscle cells cholesterol incorporation was greatest in the microsomal fraction, with lesser amounts in the nuclear debris, mitochondrial and supernatant fractions [695]. No fractionation studies appear to have been done of the distribution of lipids in smooth muscle cells in an atherosclerotic lesion. Fractionation studies done of hepatic cells containing large amounts of cholesterol, however, show that the majority of the greatly increased amounts of cholesterol remains within cell sap, and only a small proportion of it is associated with intracellular membranes [1042].

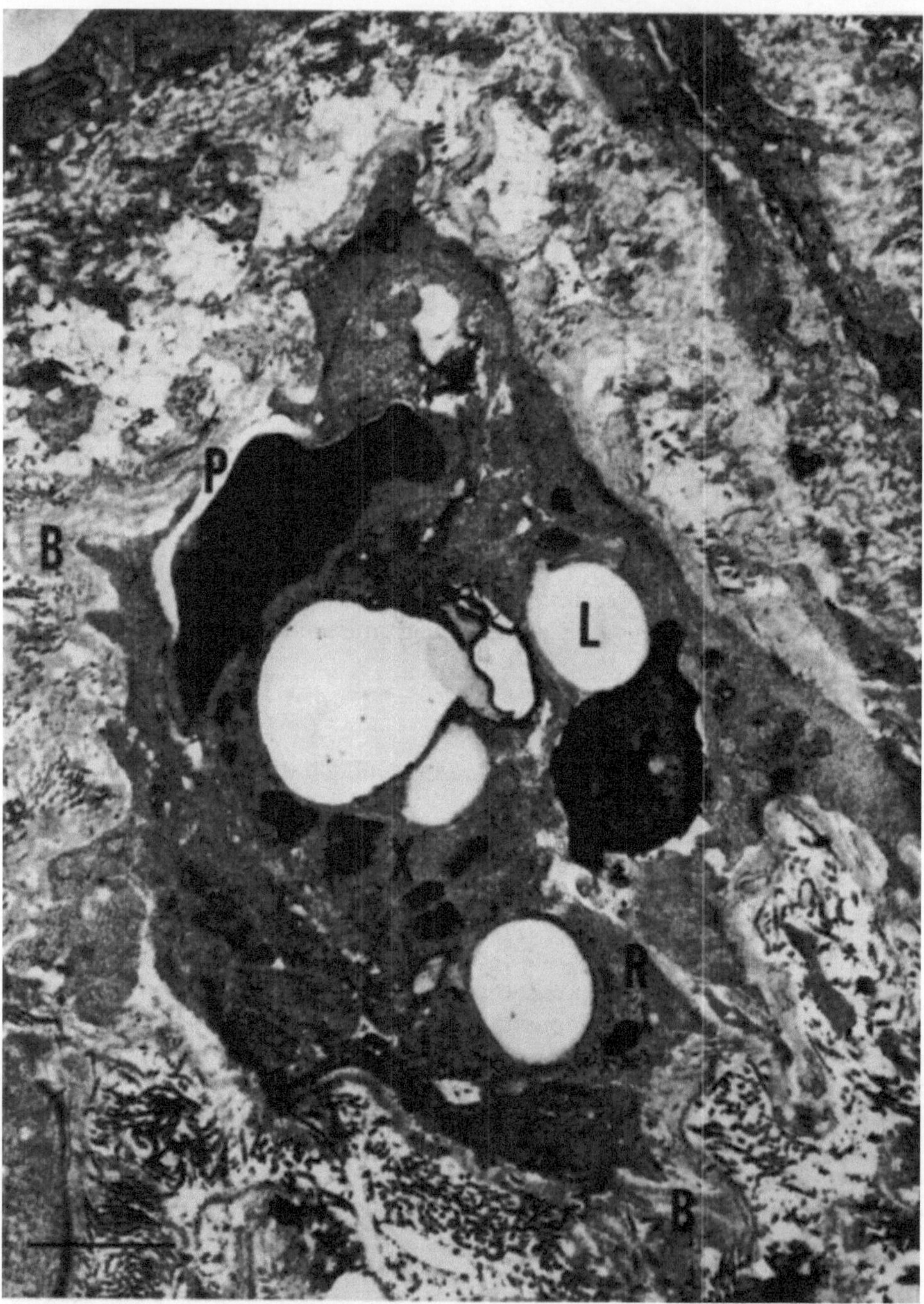

Fig. 4. Intimal lesion illustrating pyknosis (*P*) and karyorrhexis (*X*) in a predominantly proliferative lesion in a pig. Note the apparent lack of discontinuity or other distortions attributable to undesirable artefacts in the area. Neutral lipids are usually dissolved out completely or demonstrable only as a narrow, homogeneous gray zone lining vacuoles (*L*). Extremely dense, amorphous material is consistent with pyknotic and fragmented nuclear debris as seen in light microscopy. The aggregate of cell debris is

REACTION IV: DEGENERATION AND NECROSIS

Cytoplasmic degeneration in proliferative human lesions has not been searched for systematically. Available reports of electron microscopy studies understandably stress the description of well preserved cells and not degeneration. In experimental lesions, however, definite evidence of isolated smooth muscle cell and endothelial cell degeneration and death (Fig. 4) is seen fairly frequently in the rapidly developing experimental proliferative lesion in swine [363, 736]. The degeneration manifests itself by swollen, fractured mitochondria and more dramatically by the presence of dense irregular cytoplasmic bodies and ghost bodies.

SELECTED METABOLIC REACTIONS

The metabolic reactions of endothelial and smooth muscle cells with reference to lipid metabolism have already been dealt with by other speakers. Therefore, the following remarks will be confined to the metabolic reaction of smooth muscle cells to aspects of carbohydrate metabolism and the supply of adenosine triphosphate (ATP) in the aortic wall. Studies of the isolated proliferative lesions in high cholesterol diet-fed swine have shown that per milligram of DNA there is a higher rate of respiration in the proliferative lesion than in adjacent intima-media of grossly normal areas of aortic wall. The rate of respiration in the apparently normal wall in these hypercholesterolemic diet-fed swine however was significantly higher than in the aortic wall of stock-fed swine, suggesting that metabolic changes in smooth muscle cells occur before evidence of grossly visible proliferation is present. The rate of glycolysis was not significantly different in the lesion from adjacent normal areas of aorta from the hypercholesterolemic swine or stock-fed swine. It appears that if extra ATP is required by a developing proliferative lesion, it is derived from oxidative phosphorylation and not glycolysis [1332]. In a study using rabbits, however, it has been suggested that in the visible atherosclerotic lesion in this animal there is uncoupling of oxidative phosphorylation [1542]. If this result can be confirmed in other animals, it would mean that despite increased tissue respiration in the proliferative lesion, there is no increased ATP production via oxidative phosphorylation. Studies utilizing glucose labeled in the C1 and C6 position in human atherosclerotic lesions and in arteries from experimental animals have suggested that glucose contributes very little to oxidative phosphorylation; the majority of it appears to be converted to lactic acid [873]. Similar studies show that the amount of glucose used by the pentose shunt pathway is relatively small compared to that utilized for glycolysis [1229].

Studies of arterial wall carbohydrate metabolism led to the statement for many years that up to 50% of the ATP available to the artery wall is derived from glycolysis, with the remaining 50% being produced by oxidative phosphorylation. It has been therefore presumed that the smooth muscle cells of

surrounded by a narrow rim of apparently viable smooth muscle cells (*S*) which also have increased basement membrane materials (*B*). E: endothelium with relatively wide cytoplasm at the cell junction (arrow). Their nexi are characteristically end-to-end unlike in smooth muscle the artery wall derive at least one half of their ATP requirements utilizing an anaerobic system. That this may not be the case is shown by recent experiments using intima-media strips from normal swine aorta when the tissue was not precooled to 4° before respiration measurements were made. The cooling of smooth muscle cells of the arterial wall before measuring tissue respiration and glycolysis apparently decreases irreversibly both the rate of tissue respiration and of glycolysis. The decrease is not equal in each case however, respiration being decreased fivefold while glycolysis is only decreased by 50%. If the normal artery is kept at 37° before glycolysis and tissue respiration is measured, only 40% of the ATP appears to be derived from glycolysis, and 60% from oxidative phosphorylation, assuming complete coupling (Scott, unpublished data). Since most of the published studies of carbohydrate metabolism of smooth muscle cells in the normal wall and atherosclerotic lesion have been done using pre-cooled tissue, it is possible that some of the results may have to be reinterpreted.

COMMENT

Within the last four years it has become more apparent than ever that the smooth muscle cells and endothelial cells are not inactive cellular elements but are capable of exhibiting a fairly wide range of reactions during the development of atherosclerosis. Considerable work remains to be done to elucidate more details covering both the morphologic and, especially, the metabolic reactions of these cells, but enough is known about them to formulate some hypotheses concerning the relationships of these reactions and their bearing on atherosclerosis. One of the older theories concerning the relations of these reactions of endothelial and smooth muscle cells is that degeneration and necrosis, with or without visible lipid accumulation, is the primary change, and that multiplication of cells with accompanying dedifferentiation is a secondary phenomenon. In other words, atherosclerosis is basically a process of damage to smooth muscle and endothelial cells, with consequent repair manifested by proliferation. Another possibility is that the first cell reaction in the artery wall in atherosclerosis is not necrosis but excessive proliferation of smooth muscle cells, with or without dedifferentiation. The necrotic and degenerating smooth muscle cells develop as a consequence of the abnormal proliferation. The evidence for and against these theories will be presented later in the symposium by Dr. W. A. Thomas in his discussion of plasma lipids and experimental atherosclerosis.

THE MACROMOLECULAR MATRIX OF THE ARTERIAL WALL: COLLAGEN, ELASTIN, MUCOPOLYSACCHARIDES*

L. Robert

The arterial wall can be assimilated to a specialized connective tissue characterized by its cellular and fibrillar elements. The fibrous stroma contains several different types of macromolecules, such as collagen, elastin and glycoproteins. They are synthesized *in situ* by the cells of the vessel wall. The distribution of these macromolecules is different in the intimal, medial, and adventitial layers and changes with age and in atherosclerosis. Some of the most important results obtained during the last years on the composition and metabolism of these macromolecules will be summarized herein.

ELASTIN

A soluble precursor of elastin (tropoelastin) was isolated from the aorta of pigs raised on a copper-deficient diet [1291]. It has a molecular weight of 67,000 and an amino acid composition similar to elastin, except for the presence of much higher amounts of lysine (Table 1). These lysine residues are known to be involved in crosslinking of the proelastin molecules during fibrillogenesis (Fig. 1) [220, 1155]. Dityrosine crosslinks were also described in some elastin preparations [784]. The crosslinked tropoelastin, submitted to the mechanical traction of the pulsing arterial wall, undergoes conformational changes resulting in the fibrous, branching structures seen under the microscope.

One of the key enzymes involved in these crosslinking reactions is a copper and pyridoxal-phosphate containing amine-oxidase. This probably explains the inhibition of crosslink formation in the presence of lathyrogenic agents as β-aminoproprionitrile as well as in the copper-deficient pig aortas and explains their frequent aneurysm formation and rupture [292, 1155]. Polymeric elastin forms a three-dimensional crosslinked fibrous network intimately entwined with collagen, proteoglycans and structural glycoproteins. Drastic methods have to be used to purify elastin and to free it from all other "contaminants". Therefore, the usual criteria of purity cannot be easily applied to such preparations. Elastin obtained by a variety of methods shows a relative constancy of amino acid composition; however significant variation in certain amino acids can be observed. Chemical and immunological studies lead to the conclusion that fibrous elastin as prepared by the usual methods is not homogeneous but contains variable amounts of structural glycoproteins which are associated with it in its native state (Table 2). A great deal of information on the structure of elastin could

* The following abbreviations are used herein: SGP: structural glycoprotein; Glc: glucose; Gal: galactose; UDP: uridindiphosphate; Hypro: hydroxyproline; OHLys: hydroxylysine; MPS: mucopolysaccharide and AMP: acid mucopolysaccharide.

Table 1. *Amino acid composition of some macromolecules of the arterial wall*[a]

Amino acid	Tropo-elastin[b]	Fibrous elastin[c]	Collagen[d]		Structural glycoproteins[e]	
			normal	athero-scler;	water soluble fraction	insoluble fraction
Aspartic	2.9	8.8	6.31	6.24	67.0	97.3
OH Proline	11.2	14.5	12.82	11.38	0	0
Threonine	13.8	7.4	1.91	1.87	35.0	58.0
Serine	9.4	8.1	2.66	2.35	37.0	61.0
Glutamine	18.3	20.9	11.67	11.34	100.0	100.0
Proline	108.7	93.8	10.64	11.07	79.0	56.5
Glycine	333.7	328.9	28.00	25.77	200.0	95.3
Alanine	218.1	233.3	8.43	7.89	165.0	827.2
Cystine (1/2)	0.0	0.0	—	—	90.0	80.5
Valine	120.6	124.9	2.58	2.54	1.0	28.5
Methionine	0.0	1.7	1.24	1.22	0.5	0.7
Ileucine	18.8	19.6	1.54	1.64	31.2	47.2
Leucine	46.2	57.4	3.93	4.09	73.0	82.0
Tyrosine	15.6	16.9	0.97	1.13	17.2	30.3
Phenylalanine	27.9	32.3	2.13	2.18	27.3	33.5
Isodesmosine (1/4)	0.0	8.1	—	—	—	—
Desmosine (1/4)	0.0	8.3	—	—	—	—
Lysine	47.5	7.6	4.61	4.26	35.0	61.3
Histidine	0.0	1.1	1.09	1.09	12.0	23.5
Arginine	7.1	6.6	8.29	7.95	28.0	49.2
Hydroxylysine	—	—	1.05	1.25	1.3	±

[a] Results given as residues per 1,000 residues unless otherwise indicated.
[b] From copper deficient pig aorta [1291].
[c] From normal pig aorta [1291].
[d] From rabbits, results as a percentage [476].
[e] Unpublished data.

Table 2. *Composition of the carbohydrate portion of some macromolecules isolated from the aorta*

Substance analysed	Percentage of dry weight	
	hexose	hexosamine
TCA-extract, rich in polymeric		
collagen (pig aorta)[a]	1.9[d], 2.7[e]	1.3[d], 3.0[e]
elastin (human aorta)[b]	1.0–1.7	0.42
SGP (pig aorta)[c]	2.1	2.9
SGP (sheep aorta)[c]	3.1	2.8
SGP (horse aorta)[c]	2.9	2.3

[a] From Moczar, Robert (unpublished data).
[b] Elastin prepared by NaOH-extraction (45 min, 100°).
[c] Purified, urea-soluble fraction.
[d] 1st TCA-extract, OH-pro content 15%.
[e] 2d and 3d TCA-extract, OH-pro content 16% and 10.8% respectively.

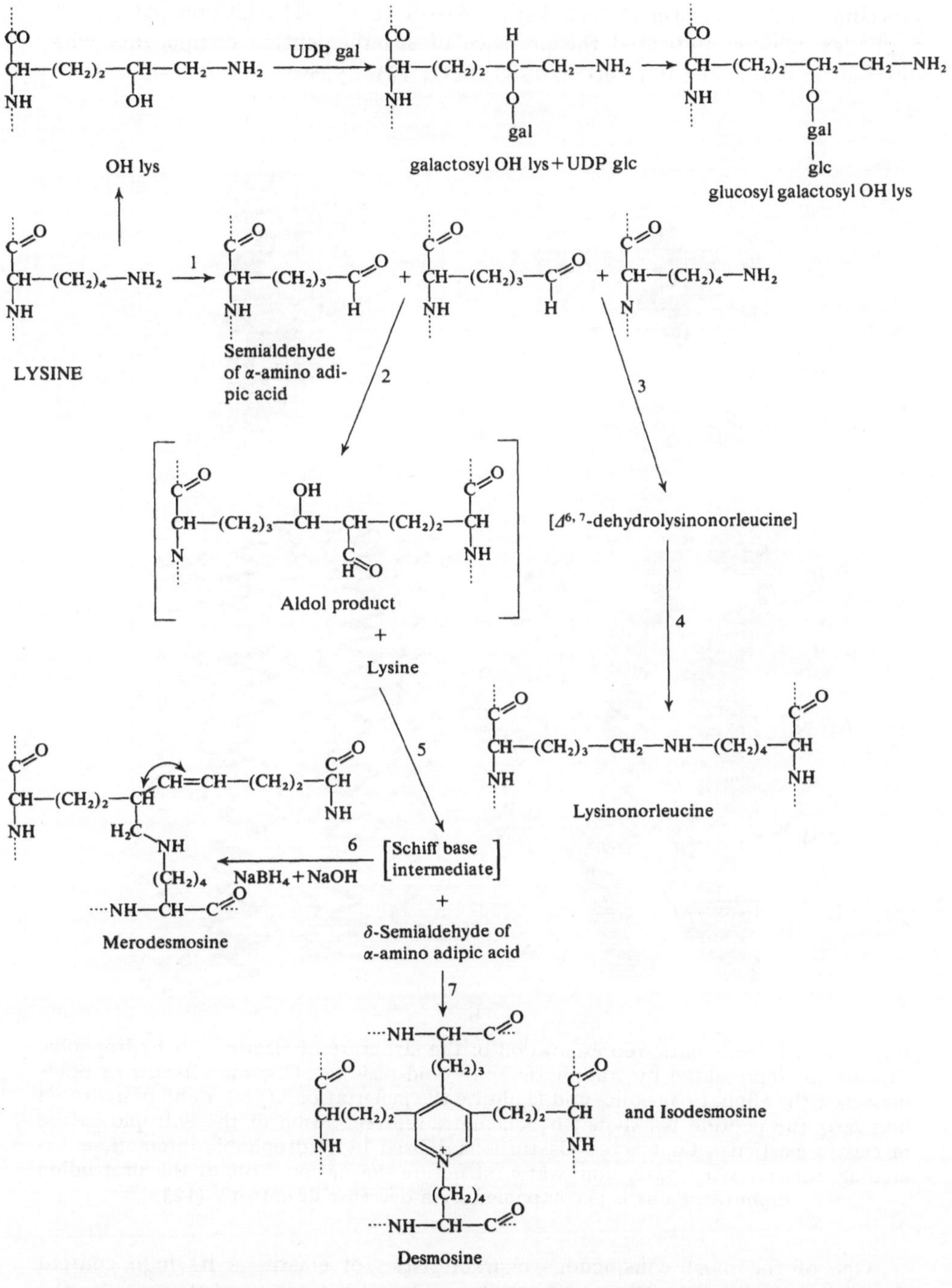

UDP gal

OH lys

galactosyl OH lys + UDP glc

glucosyl galactosyl OH lys

LYSINE

Semialdehyde of α-amino adipic acid

[$\Delta^{6,7}$-dehydrolysinonorleucine]

Aldol product

+

Lysine

Lysinonorleucine

[Schiff base intermediate]

+

δ-Semialdehyde of α-amino adipic acid

$NaBH_4 + NaOH$

Merodesmosine

and Isodesmosine

Desmosine

Fig. 1. Crosslink formation in collagen and elastin from lysine (2d and 3d row) Hydroxylation of lysine and glycosylation of hydroxylysine in collagen (first row) (Modified after Bornstein [220])

be obtained by preparing water-soluble derivatives using controlled degradation procedures (alpha-elastin [1155], kappa-elastin [819]). The elution pattern on Sephadex columns indicated the presence of several peptide components with different amino acid compositions [788, 1232, 1233, 1259].

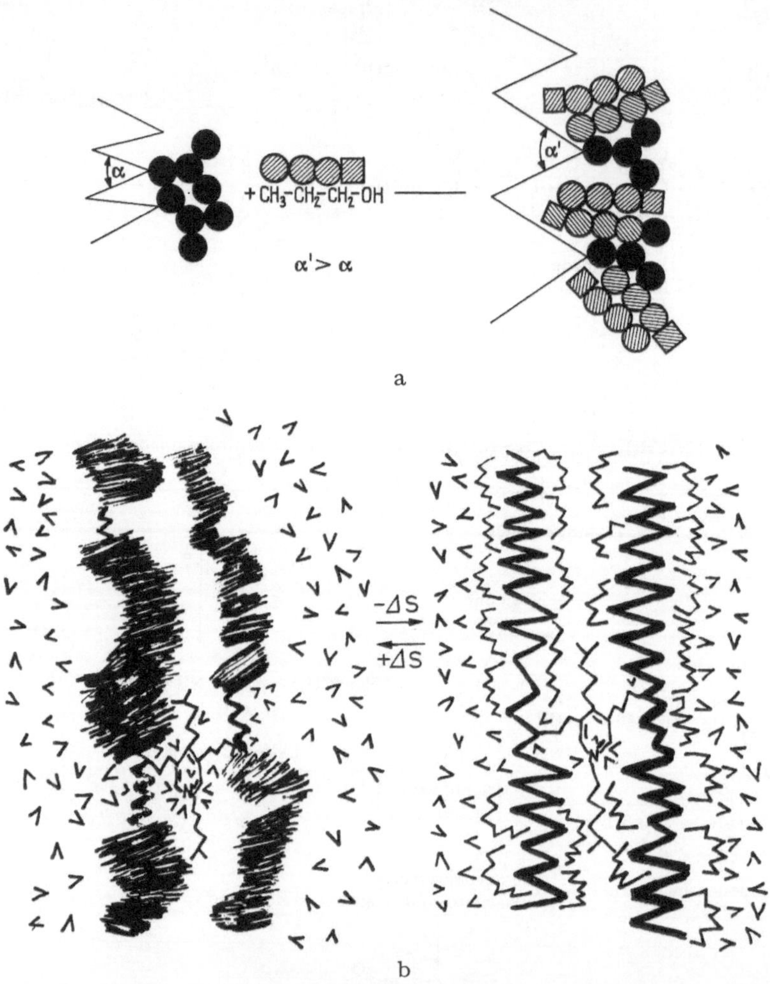

Fig. 2a and b. Schematic representation of the structure of elastin. a A hydrophobic "region" is represented by 2 aliphatic aminoacid residues. Organic solvents or lipids dissociate the aliphatic residues and facilitate the penetration of water and of hydrated ions near the peptide backbone; b Schematic representation of the entropic nature of elastin elasticity. Contracted elastin is stabilised by hydrophobic interactions excluding water. After extension water structure formation around the protruding aliphatic chains is accompanied by a decrease of entropy [1235]

One of the most conspicuous characteristics of elastin is its high content of apolar amino acids. This explains, in part at least, some of the peculiarities of its tertiary and quaternary structure, such as the high proportion of alpha-helices [549] and coacervation when the cold aqueous solution of alpha- or kappa-elastin is heated to temperatures over 25° C, as well as the strong hydrophobic interactions in elastin. These strong hydrophobic interactions may explain the resistance of elastin to acid or alkali in aqueous media and the rapid hydrolysis of peptide bonds in the presence of organic solvents. This "solubilization-promoting efficiency" of organic solvents depends on their composition and steric structure [819, 1235]. The rupture of hydrophobic interactions by organic solvents can lead to a partial "unfolding" of the peptide structure, forcing hidden peptide chains to come in close contact with the aqueous solvent (Fig. 2).

The entropy-factor of the elasticity of elastin can be explained by this behavior. The chains of extended elastin will return "spontaneously" to their contracted conformation re-establishing maximal hydrophobic interactions. This contraction is accompanied by an increase of entropy because of the disorganization of water structure built up around the exposed hydrophobic residues during extension [1235]. Fig. 2 shows schematically this behavior. The strong affinity of elastin for lipids can also be explained by the same principle. The extended hydrophobic structures, resistant to water, appear permeable to lipidic substances which can play the same role as the aliphatic chains of alcohols (Fig. 2a). Such molecules can be "dissolved" in the hydrophobic regions and will "stack" between the apolar residues of elastin. This finding probably explains the strong complex forming capacity of elastin with lipids and lipoproteins and may play a predominant role in the lipid deposition in the arterial wall [1235].

The slow degradation of elastic fibers was recognized as one of the early signs of the pathological alteration of the vessel wall. Several authors found evidence in favor of the existence of an elastolytic enzyme in blood plasma [595, 886]. A protease is present in blood platelets attacking elastin at pH 8.0—8.6 and is liberated from platelets during their aggregation on collagen or by ADP [1231]. This mechanism of enzyme liberation would enable the platelets to "inject" this "elastase" into small denuded portions of the arterial wall during their adhesion, even in the absence of permanent thrombus formation.

The very sensitive method of determination of elastase action with ^{125}I or ^{131}I-labelled elastin showed that chymotrypsin in high concentrations attacked elastin, as did several other proteases [1233]. This attack may be directed primarily against the structural glycoprotein component of elastic fibers and may explain their partial "solubilization" by such enzymes in accordance with morphological observation on the *in vivo* degradation of elastic fibers, showing first a fragmentation followed by a slow degradation and not a sudden lysis of elastin.

COLLAGEN

The synthesis of collagen can be readily studied by measuring the incorporation of labelled proline in collagen-hydroxyproline. Besides collagen (12% to 13%) and elastin ($\leq$1.5%) no other proteins of connective tissue are known to contain significant amounts of this amino acid. The amino acid composition of aortic-collagen is shown in Table 1. A crucial step in collagen biosynthesis is the hydroxylation of proline and lysine, required for the assembly and secretion of completed tropocollagen molecules [553].

An important reaction taking place after the peptide chains leave the polysomes is the glycosylation of some of the hydroxylysine side chains of collagen by two specific transferases. The first will transfer galactose from UDP-galactose to the delta-hydroxyl-group of hydroxylysine (OH-Lys) (Fig. 1); the second enzyme then transfers glucose from UDP-glucose to only some of the hydroxylysyl-galactose units formed (Fig. 1). The ratio of OH-Lys-Gal to OH-Lys-Gal-Glu to total OH-Lys is an important tissue-specific molecular parameter of collagen morphology [564, 1236]. Aortic collagen is characterized by a OH-Lys-Gal to OH-Lys-Gal-Glu ratio of about unity, by the total hexose content of about 6.6% for the whole stroma, 1.9 to 2.7% for TCA-extractable collagen and by a OH-Lys-content of about 1.0%. The hydroxylysine content seems to increase in the atherosclerotic aorta to about 1.25% [476, 1017] (see Tables 1 and 2).

Tissue specificity of collagen metabolism is first reflected in the great variation in collagen content of different tissues. Recent and precise determinations carried out by Frey [497] on rabbit aorta gave a total hydroxyproline content of 1.04 μMol/g of fresh tissue, as compared to 0.07 μMol/g for liver and 1.39 μMol/g for skin. Gerber, Gerber and Altman [522] have shown that the turnover time of polymeric collagen varies from tissue to tissue between 30 and 300 days. Biosynthesis appears fastest in the skin, followed by aorta and by the tendon [775]. The turnover rate decreases from skin to tendon to aorta. These results would suggest a more important degradation of freshly synthesized tropocollagen in aorta than in tendon. Recent studies by Frey [497] indicate a rapid incorporation, *in vitro*, of ^{14}C-proline into soluble and insoluble aortic collagen. Total incorporation and specific activity in aortic-soluble collagen was much lower than in liver or skin. This would indicate a strong dilution of freshly synthesized aortic tropocollagen in a slowly degrading pool. Similar remarks can be made on the incorporation in polymeric collagen, the low specific activities do not permit, however, a detailed comparison of these tissues. The degradation of polymeric collagen is probably initiated by specific tissue collagenases. Some of these enzymes appear to be of lysosomal origin, as are also the cathepsins which can attack collagen at acid pH [105].

Another facet of collagen tissue specificity is the ratio of hydroxylated proline to total proline [220, 1176], hydroxylysine to total lysine [275] and glycosylated hydroxylysine to total hydroxylysine [1236]. Frey [497] found a value of 0.82 μMol of hydroxyproline per μMol of proline for rabbit aorta, as compared to 1.19 for liver and 0.75 for skin collagen. It appears after his results that the degree of hydroxylation of proline might be a factor in determining the metabolic fate of tropocollagen, strongly hydroxylated molecules are more likely to be degraded than those having an intermediary degree of hydroxylation. These rapidly degraded tropocollagen molecules may be at the origin of the collagen-like substance present in blood serum [497].

ACID MUCOPOLYSACCHARIDES AND PROTEOGLYCANS

Proteoglycans are complex molecules containing several high molecular-weight glycosaminoglycan chains covalently linked to the serine or threonine residues of the core proteins through a special sequence containing xylose and galactose [844, 1171, 1247]. Little is as yet known of the core protein. It appears however, that it may be a glycoprotein having a composition similar to that found for "noncollagen proteins" of several connective tissues and for some structural glycoproteins. It also appears from recent studies that hybrid molecules can exist containing several different kinds of polysaccharide chains (chondroitin-4-sulfate, chondroitin-6-sulfate, keratan-sulfate, or dermatan-sulfate) linked to the same core protein. Such a hybrid proteoglycan was recently isolated from aorta by Buddecke [263], containing chondroitin-4-sulfate and dermatan-sulfate in a ratio of about 3 to 1. Table 3 shows the main polysaccharides extracted and characterized from aorta as well as their relative contribution to the total mucopolysaccharide content determined in normal tissue [512] and Table 4 shows the total MPS, collagen and lipid content in normal human aorta, and

Table 3. *Distribution of total acid mucopolysaccharides of adult rabbit and rat aorta between the four main molecular species. Determined by CPC-cellulose chromatography (c) and by cellogel electrophoresis (e) from Picard et al.* [512, 1172]

MPS	Percentage of total MPS			
	rabbit		rat	
	c	e	c	e
Hyaluronate	37	40	11.5	12
Heparan sulfate	27	26	35	31
Dermatan sulfate	17	15.5	40	41
Chondroitin 4 and 6 sulfate	19	18.5	13.5	16

in atheromatous plaques of increasing severity. Detailed characterization of the purified mucopolysaccharides showed the presence of hyaluronic acid, chondroitin-4 and 6-sulfate, dermatan-sulfate and heparitin-sulfate [1172]. The concentration of the individual acid mucopolysaccharides changes independently with age and pathological conditions. Their evolution is different in the intimal layers, rich in acid mucopolysacharide, and in the medial and adventitial layers [832]. Total acid mucopolysaccharide tends to increase with age up to 20–25 years and decrease later. Chondroitin-4-sulfate, however, increases steadily up to at least 40 years. A significant increase in total acid mucopolysaccharide together with an increase in collagen was observed only in the fatty streak type of lesions [1377]. In fibrous plaques the acid mucopolysaccharides are decreased and collagen is increased. This change is even more conspicuous in calcified plaques where the total acid mucopolysaccharide is severely decreased and collagen accounts for more than 60% of total proteins (Table 4). Individual acid mucopolysaccharides again behave differently; hyaluronic acid does not change or decreases. Chondroitin-sulfate, heparitin-sulfate, and mainly intimal dermatan-sulfate increase moderately with increasing involvement of the aortic wall and decrease then after 30% to 40% of involvement. Chemical determinations do not confirm the very strong increase of acid mucopolysaccharides suggested by the increase of metachromasia in aging and pathological arterial wall. Histochemical studies on arterial glycoproteins were recently reviewed by Velican and Velican [1496]. Relative compositional changes were noted also in dissecting aneurysms of Marfan's syndrome [916] and were interpreted as a relative increase of chondroitin-6-sulfate. Similar increase in metachromasia was often noticed in conditions leading to weakening of aorta and eventually to aneurysm formation (lathyrogenic agents, copper deficiency, mucopolysaccharidoses, idiopathic dissecting aneurysm). An increase of the dermatan-sulfate/chondroitin-sulfate ratio accompanies generally the degradation of elastic fibers.

The physiological and pathological role of aortic proteoglycans may well be related to the "excluded volume" effect [844]. The accumulation of β lipoprotein in the arterial wall may be due partly to such physicochemical effects [741] partly to specific complex formation with certain AMP's [164] or with specific antibodies (Beaumont, see this volume). The thermoanalytical method renders possible a direct *in situ* determination on normal and atherosclerotic aortas, giving qualitative and quantitative indication of the AMP's and of their state of association with lipoproteins [163]. As a result of treatment with poly-

Table 4. *Mucopolysaccharide, collagen and total lipid content of normal and pathological human aortas (from E.B. Smith* [1377]*). Results are expressed as percentage of total protein*

	Normal[a]	Fatty streaks	Fibrous plaques	Calcified plaques
Collagen[b]	24.8	26.3	41.0	60.7
MPS[c]	2.62	3.02	2.47	1.21
Lipids	9.80	30.6	47.3	109.0

[a] Individuals of 11 to 75 years.

[b] Calculated with an OH-proline-content of 12%.

[c] Calculated from uronic acid + hexosamine value taking their sum as 74% of total MPS.

unsaturated phosphatidyl choline, thermogravimetric analysis indicated a return to normal of aortic mucopolysaccharides [165].

Recent experiments suggest an increased incorporation of ^{35}S in mucopolysaccharides of atherosclerotic aorta [263, 635, 1173]. The regulation of their turnover depends not only on the synthetic processes [1173] but also on the degradative enzymes [264]. Dermatan-sulfate and heparitin-sulfate generally show a high rate of incorporation of $^{35}SO^4$ and a slower incorporation is found in chondroitin-sulfate. The same relationship is obtained with other markers such as ^{14}C-glucose. Aortic dermatan-sulfate appears to turn over much faster than skin dermatan-sulfate ($t^1/_2$ of 5–7 days as compared to 40 days in skin). The identification of UDP-Nac-galactosamine-sulfate-^{35}S in aorta may be of importance for the understanding of the synthetic processes of mucopolysaccharides in this organ [1172, 1173].

GLYCOPROTEINS

Several investigators have noticed the presence of glycoproteins in aorta which did not appear to be related to serum glycoproteins or to acid mucopolysaccharides. Some of these substances were purified and characterized [96, 137, 1017]. In chicken aorta, they were shown to increase with age as mucopolysaccharides and elastin decrease [509]. Aorta exhaustively extracted with aqueous buffer solutions such as 1 M $CaCl_2$ still contained appreciable amounts of glycoproteins. Sialic acid determinations performed on such fibrous stroma preparations gave results of the order of 100 to 400 μg/100 mg of dry tissue [1236]. These glycoproteins were isolated by extracting with 8M urea. Table 1 gives the amino acid composition of this "structural glycoprotein" (SGP) preparation from pig aorta and Table 2 gives its hexose and hexosamine content. Its amino acid composition was similar to that of the structural glycoproteins isolated from other connective tissues. Detailed investigations of the glycopeptides isolated from the purified SGP showed a similar composition to those isolated from pronase digests of native aorta. The molecular weight of purified glycopeptides was from 2,500 t0 4,000, they contained galactose, glucose, N-acetylglucosamine, mannose, fucose, and sialic acid in varying ratios. At least seven different glycopeptides were isolated from one Sephadex peak by high voltage electrophoresis,

Table 5. *Specific activity of subfractions of the polymeric stroma of rabbit aorta incubated with ^{14}C-lysine (5 μC) for four hours at 37°. Extraction and fractionation of the fibrous stroma by the method described* [1237]. *Results of unpublished data*

	No.	Specific activity cpm/mg prot. (average ± σ)		
		TCA-extract[a]	urea extract[b]	KOH-ethanol-extract[c]
Rabbits treated with Freund's adjuvant only	4	393 ± 212	6810	631 ± 381
Rabbits immunised with SGP-fraction of human aorta in Freund's adjuvant	3	538 ± 90	4870	1,773 ± 942
Rabbits fed a cholesterol-rich diet	3	393 ± 160	4860	591 ± 317

[a] Contains mainly the polymeric collagen.
[b] SGP-fraction.
[c] Elastin fraction.

having regularly increasing sialic acid/fucose ratios from 2.2 for the slowest migrating fraction to 6.7 for the fastest migrating glycopeptide, and suggesting a pronounced microheterogeneity for the carbohydrate chains of aortic SGP. Thin layer fingerprinting of the partial hydrolysates of glycopeptides isolated from aortas of several species showed slightly different patterns suggesting a species specificity for the glycans of SGP [1016, 1017].

Aortas incubated *in vitro* with ^{14}C-lysine or proline incorporate these amino acids in the macromolecules of the fibrous stroma. This incorporation is strongest in the structural glycoprotein fraction and least strong in the polymeric elastin fraction, collagen being in between (Table 5). These results confirm those obtained with other connective tissues such as cornea and tendon, showing that structural glycoproteins have an active metabolism and a significantly higher turnover than the fibrous proteins to which they are linked. The implication of this finding for the tissue specificity of fibrillogenesis has already been discussed.

CONCLUSIONS

Recent investigations clearly indicate the close adaptation of the macromolecular composition of the fibrous stroma of the arterial wall to anatomical, physiological, and mechanical circumstances [607]. The previously cited data confirm and extend this conception and reveal the extreme complexity of the regulatory processes which determine the local evolution of the relative concentrations of each individual macromolecule. Among the four major proteoglycanes, elastin, collagen and structural glycoproteins, one can estimate at least ten such macromolecules. As they all show structural and conformational microheterogeneity, the number of such regulatory processes must be high indeed. Most of the important recent advances concern the structure and composition of elastin and glycoproteins. The regulation of the crosslinking processes of elastin and collagen, whether intra- or intermolecular, appear to play a key role in the regulation of the mechanical properties of the vessel wall. The metabolic disturbances of atherosclerosis possibly manifest themselves by interfering with these regulatory processes. The immunochemical properties of the macromolecular components of the vessel wall may be of as much importance in the pathological increase of catabolic processes as in the disruption of the elastic membranes. Experiments undertaken in several laboratories along the lines here outlined will eventually lead to a detailed molecular description of the normal and pathological vessel wall.

Discussion Following Papers by Dr. Adams and Dr. Zilversmit

Dr. Y. Stein: I would like to confine my remarks to one major phospholipid component which accumulates in the normal human artery with age, i.e., sphingomyelin. If one plots the phospholipid accumulation in the histologically normal human ascending aorta, male or female, one can see that total phospholipid accumulates with age, expressed either per gram wet weight, per unit DNA, or per the number of cells in the artery. The main phospholipid components which comprise 90–95% of the total phospholipids of the aorta are sphingomyelin, phosphatidyl ethanolamine, lecithin, phosphatidyl inositol, and phosphatidyl serine. The only marked rise is in sphingomyelin, while lecithin, phosphatidyl ethanolamine and phosphatidyl inositol show a very small rise.

Recently the phospholipases of several mammalian aortas (rabbit, rat, dog and human) have been determined by quantitative assay procedures. The hydrolysis of lecithin and phosphatidyl ethanolamine rises very markedly with age when expressed per unit of DNA. In contrast, the hydrolysis of sphingomyelin decreases with age. We believe that the study of phospholipases in normal and pathological aortas may shed some light on the mechanism of accumulation of specific phospholipids.

Dr. Walton: I want to focus attention on a tissue other than the aorta itself, because there is another site which provides almost a natural control. I refer to the cardiac valve.

Almost any pathologist knows that one frequently sees lipid accumulation in the mitral valve as a flat area near the margin of the valve or as rounded accumulations nearer to the aortic valve. It is only the anterior mitral cusp that is ever involved. The aortic valve is also involved, but the valves on the right side of the heart never show this kind of lipid accumulation. When one looks at such a valve, one finds that the lipid is almost entirely peri-fibrous, to use Dr. Smith's phrase, and it is confined to about one-half to two-thirds of the valve and never extends through the full thickness. Lipid seems to be distributed from the ventricular surface halfway through the valve.

When looking for immunofluorescence with a specific anti beta lipoprotein antiserum, one can see that there is a very good correspondence between distribution of the lipoprotein by this method and of lipid as shown by the lipid stain. The antiserum is directed against the protein portion of the low density (Beta) lipoprotein. The good correspondence, therefore, suggests that the whole of the molecule is present.

As time goes on one sees fibrosis, and the thickening of the intimal surface in the ventricle will give the appearance of an arterial plaque. It is notable that the valve has no muscularis. Also, there is a kind of natural control in that the valves on the right- and left-hand sides of the heart are virtually identical as far as acid mucopolysaccharides, and so on, are concerned. Yet, it is only the valves on the left side of the heart and not the ones on the right which become involved. This rather suggests, particularly from the distribution, that the lipoprotein is being forced actively into the substance of the valve, and this is perhaps further borne out by the fact that these lesions increase with hypertension.

Dr. Wissler: Prof. Adams suggested that Dr. Zilversmit's data with labelled lipids localizing in the aorta should be interpreted as evidence against serum lipoproteins as a primary source of the lipid in the aorta. I wonder if Dr. Zilversmit interprets his data similarly?

Dr. Zilversmit: It could, indeed, mean this. The fact is that labelled free cholesterol goes in faster than esterified cholesterol, i.e., relative to the ratio of free to esterified cholesterol in serum. This observation can be interpreted as entry of free and esterified cholesterol, independent of protein.

However, there is an alternate explanation. It could be that the lipoprotein goes in as a unit, and that over and above this there is an exchange reaction of serum free cholesterol with free cholesterol in the arterial wall.

I would like to comment on Dr. Walton's remarks. He touched on the same point. I don't understand how the presence of beta lipoprotein shows that the lipoprotein enters intact, or at least that this is an important process. If one tests for albumin or high density lipoprotein, I would guess that these proteins would also be found in the lesion or in the heart valves discussed previously. I wonder if anyone has any comment on the validity of the use of the immunofluorescent technique as evidence for the specific uptake of intact beta lipoprotein.

Dr. Walton: We have used antisera specific for albumin, high density lipoprotein, low density lipoprotein, gamma globulins, fibrinogen, and alpha-2 globulin. We were able to demonstrate only beta lipoprotein present in any significant amount.

Dr. Wissler: This has been our experience also. We have used the same controls in our fluorescent microscopy studies. We do them on unfixed tissues, and under these conditions the predominant serum protein we find is low-density lipoprotein in all the lesions we have studied. Occasionally we find small clumps of interstitial fibrin but they are not related to lipid localization.

Dr. Chobanian: Dr. Zilversmit, you indicated that cholesterol synthesis may contribute to cholesterol present in the normal intima but probably had little role in the atherosclerotic tissue. In these studies, following 21 days of cholesterol feeding, you observed differences in cholesterol specific activity between the arterial wall and plasma. Did you observe any pathological changes at this early stage?

Dr. ZILVERSMIT: We have not looked at these arteries with histological techniques but grossly you cannot see any lesions.

Dr. GOTTLEIB: Can we interpret lipid influx on a biophysical basis of molecular porosity rather than a biochemical basis and enzymatic transport into the endothelium?

Dr. ZILVERSMIT: I think this is possible.

Discussion Following Dr. E. Smith's Paper

Dr. ADAMS: Dr. Smith, can you explain your results on different cholesterol and lipoprotein levels in terms of differential metabolism? Perhaps, the protein is broken down quickly while the sterol stays intact.

Dr. SMITH: I frankly don't know how to explain my results, either in relation to peri-fibrous lipid accumulation or in relation to fat-filled cells. I always objected to the term "lipophage" as implying that such cells were phagocytozing lipoproteins. However, they seem to be associated with low levels of intact plasma lipoprotein in the intima, so perhaps they are really doing something of this sort.

How to explain the relationship between the still insoluble lipoprotein which is presumably what we are extracting, and the insoluble lipid which perhaps is being stained by immunofluorescence, and is presumably not coming out, I don't quite understand.

Dr. INSULL: We have been interested in determining whether or not the human arterial fatty streaks can be divided into physical compartments that we can analyze separately. We have used the polarizing microscope to view isolated fat droplets of the type Dr. Smith showed. These are dichroic under polarized light, with Maltese crosses and two colors in them. Some of the droplets are not birefringent and are barely seen.

In a study with Dr. Dieter Lang, who worked with us in Professor Schettler's department, we analyzed the chemical composition of the droplets and observed that the lipids of these droplets consisted of 95% cholesteryl esters, 2% free cholesterol, 1% phospholipid and 2% triglyceride. In other words, they were essentially pure cholesteryl ester. These esters had the fatty acid composition almost identical with that which Dr. Smith showed.

I think this unusual lipid composition indicates that there is a highly selective mechanism operating to synthesize these droplets. They are also selective in terms of structure, because a large portion of these droplets are liquid crystals under polarized light as well as having a unique chemical composition.

The lipid composition does not resemble that of the conventional lipoproteins. Therefore the question comes: Is there selection of specific lipids at the interface between the droplet and the cytoplasm of the cell or between the cell membrane, and the extracellular space?

Dr. ADAMS: Dr. Weller, in London, showed that fractions that contain a great deal of these liquid crystal structures, showing this particular type of Maltese cross anisotropism, contain more free cholesterol and phospholipid than cholesteryl ester. Dr. Weller made the point that it is the isotropic droplets which contain cholesteryl ester. Is this in complete divergence with your conclusions?

Dr. INSULL: We do not observe a difference in lipid composition with the proportion of anisotropy. I cannot explain the difference between Dr. Weller's results and ours.

Dr. LAZZARINI ROBERTSON, JR.: We have studied the transport of low density lipoprotein (LDL) fractions across the cell surface of primate arterial intimal cells. Using *in vitro* or *in vivo* labeling of the protein moiety with ^{131}I and the lipid with ^{14}C or ^{3}H cholesterol, we found that splitting of the LDL occurred in the presence of ATP, resulting in faster incorporation of labeled sterol than of the carrier protein into the cell cytoplasm (*Wistar Inst. Symposium*, ed. G. H. Rothblat and D. Kritchevsky [Monograph No. 6, 1967] 115–128).

The question as to how lipoproteins get across endothelial and subendothelial cells and eventually across the arterial wall as a whole is not the only one. Are mechanisms for LDL transport and available preferential storage of lipids seen in vascular cells (and eventually across the arterial wall) based in general on the identification of the protein moieties of lipoproteins by their ultracentrifugal or electrophoretic characteristics or by using immunologic or isotopic labels? If the carrier protein partially remains on the cell surface while the lipid enters the cell, it is possible that part of this extracellular protein may subsequently be mobilized across the arterial wall and eventually removed through the vasa vasora. This would result in a net increase of intracellular lipids (particularly those that cannot be catabolized such as cholesterol and its esters) in cells of the intima and inner media without concurrent elevations of carrier protein content. I believe that some of Dr. Smith's very interesting experimental findings could be explained on this basis.

Dr. KRITCHEVSKY: I would like to mention some data obtained by Dr. George Rothblat on the uptake of cholesterol by cells grown in tissue culture.

Using delipidized serum to which cholesterol was added, it has been found that the further addition of phospholipid to this medium actually inhibits the influx of cholesterol into the cell. If the cells are prelabeled and then incubated in a medium with a cholesterol-phospholipid ratio resembling that of beta lipoprotein, very little of the cholesterol emerges. If the medium contains a ratio similar to alpha lipoprotein, then cholesterol emerges from the cell.

In addition to the other factors under consideration there is a gradient against which the cholesterol comes out of the cell, and the gradient is in favor of cholesterol leaving the cell if beta lipoprotein in the medium is low.

Dr. DAY: I would like to refer to some recent work (Campbell, Fidge, and Day, unpublished data) we have done with ^{131}I-labeled lipoprotein, in which it is possible to label both the lipid and the protein moiety. In cholesterol-fed rabbits, we have investigated the entry of both the protein and the lipid moiety *in vitro*; and have found that a considerably larger amount of lipid than protein enters the intima.

Dr. SMITH: I suppose that as long as we have not been able to demonstrate rapid synthesis of the sterol in the cells, they must be getting it from the lipoprotein. None of the studies in lesions of which I am aware have clearly demonstrated a rate of synthesis that could account for the large amounts of cholesterol which accumulate. On the other hand, most of these studies have been done on cholesterol-fed animals. Perhaps feedback mechanisms may be inhibiting cholesterol synthesis, whereas in naturally-occurring atherosclerosis synthesis might be occurring.

Discussion Following Papers by Dr. R. Foster Scott and Dr. Robert

Dr. ADAMS: Dr. Robert, could it be that this lipid binding by elastic tissue explains the fact that biochemists find no lipid in elastic tissue, whereas histochemists for a long while have been reporting lipid associated with vascular elastic fibers?

Dr. ROBERT: It is difficult to answer this interesting question, because the studies I have discussed are *in vitro* investigations, and naturally they are only indirectly related to what histochemists see. Recent studies from our laboratory have demonstrated the presence of "bound lipids" in elastic tissue; K-elastin, prepared by ethanolic KOH degradation of fibrous elastin, was fractionated on Sephadex columns; the tail fraction was shown to contain a lipo-peptide, rich in fatty acids. Another lipid-rich fraction can be isolated from elastic tissue after extraction of polymeric collagen by hot trichloroacetic acid, by extracting the residue with 8M urea. This urea extract contains, together with some elastin and with the structural glycoprotein fraction, some neutral lipids and phospholipids. These "bound lipids" of the arterial wall might well be those seen by the histochemists.

Dr. WISSLER: Mrs. Rose Jones, who very recently joined our laboratory, has been employing labelled antibodies in various proteins to establish by electron microscopy whether these proteins enter the artery cells and, if so, where they are localized within the cells. The method of labelling the antibodies is based upon the horseradish peroxidase method pioneered by Prof. Morris Karnovsky and adapted to this purpose by Prof. Barry Pierce of the University of Colorado. I wish to demonstrate the use of peroxidase-labelled antibody to low density lipoprotein on the aortic tissue of a monkey, fed an average American diet for two years. From these preliminary observations we believe that this kind of immune histochemistry at the electron microscope level does indeed tend to support the earlier immunofluorescent data and that we do find the low-density lipoprotein antigen in the medial cell. Usually the label is present near lipid droplets. As a test for specificity, we could not find evidence of labelling when the block of aorta was treated first with unlabeled antibodies, a similar technique one uses as a control for fluorescent microscopy. We conclude that we have preliminary evidence that the low density lipoprotein is indeed in the artery's medial cell and often near the lipid droplets.

Dr. MORRISON: I was particularly interested in Dr. Robert's studies on elastin. We also found lipid associated biochemically with normal elastin, especially cholesteryl ester with elastin from the cat.

Dr. BJORKERUD: I agree with Dr. Scott in his conclusion that atherosclerosis is a disturbance of a proliferative repair reaction. We have reached the same conclusion from studies of a repair reaction characterized by proliferation without accumulation of lipids induced in the rabbit aorta by superficial, longitudinal mechanical trauma. This lesion is temporary and leads to restoration of the wall architecture [170]. A repair reaction characterized by proliferation, tissue damage, accumulation of lipids, which is not regressive, i.e. an atherosclerotic lesion, can be induced by transverse mechanical trauma [169]. Therefore, it is feasible to differentiate the normal repair reaction from the disturbed one. One further point of interest is that artery segments with normal repair reactions do not have increased permeability to albumin tagged with Evans blue, while segments with disturbed repair reaction have an increased permeability.

Dr. GERÖ: Recently we found evidence, by the use of a thermoanalytical method, mentioned by Dr. Robert, for the identification of complexes in the atherosclerotic intima of beta lipoprotein (LP) and mucopolysaccharide (MPS). In the first part of these experiments *in vitro* studies were performed by the use of a series of MPS-preparations (GAG, according to the new chemical nomenclature), among them MPS mixtures isolated from aortic intimas.

A peak was found at about 240° on the thermal decomposition curves characteristic for the protein-bound structural MPS-s. This peak diminished to an inflexion, or even disappeared, when the aortic MPS-s were precipitated by the addition of beta-LP and converted into a complex consisting of MPS-s and beta-LP. The typical MPS peak at 240° became visible again after the dissociation of the complex by the extraction of the lipids with organic solvents.

These experiments were extended, and we studied the thermal decomposition of biological materials, e.g. aortic tissue samples obtained from human subjects and experimental animals. The characteristic MPS peak at 240° was detectable on the decomposition curves of young, healthy aortic intimas, indicating the presence of the normal structural MPS-s. On the curves of the atherosclerotic samples a significant decrease, in some cases even a lack, of this maximum could be established; presumably indicating the formation of MPS-beta-LP complexes. In the delipidated atherosclerotic intimal tissue the characteristic MPS peak reappeared again as a result of the dissociation of the complexes and so the derivatogram became similar to that of the healthy aortas.

Dr. KRUT: Earlier, Dr. Zilversmit raised a point with respect to the alteration in permeability of atheromatous lesions. We have found evidence that this does occur for cholesterol by tracing labeled cholesterol in the atheromatous arterial wall. It occurs also with albumin. This does not appear to be a function of the size of the lesion, since an increased rate of ingress of albumin is seen whenever a lesion is present, regardless of its size. Access is directly from the luminal surface in these vessels.

The other point I might mention is with respect to the transport of the beta lipoprotein. If one labels a lipoprotein with cholesterol and labels beta globulin relative to globulin and injects these simultaneously, one finds that the globulin as well as the cholesterol gains access to existing lesions at an increased rate. But the rate at which the globulin traverses the vessel wall, both at the site of a lesion and over normal vessel wall, is greater than the rate at which cholesterol traverses the vessel wall.

This suggests that the transport of cholesterol into the normal or atheromatous vessel wall does not require that it be transferred as part of a lipoprotein complex derived from plasma.

Dr. WALTON: If one examines an experimental lesion in the cholesterol-fed rabbit, by treatment with sheep anti-rabbit beta lipoprotein, one can see quite a lot of beta lipoprotein there. One can also see that the fluorescent antibody is not evenly distributed, that there are apparently black holes in among the bright green fluorescence. The corresponding lipid stain shows that the black holes for the most part correspond to the position of intracellular lipid. One can actually do this on precisely the same section, so that although this is not quantitative it is highly discriminatory.

This would suggest that if the material inside the lipid-laden cell is, in fact, beta lipoprotein which has been phagocytozed, it probably has had the protein moiety detached from it, since the antiserum is directed against the protein moiety. Alternatively, the lipid inside these cells may come from quite a different source.

Dr. SMITH: I would like to make a comment about the cholesteryl esters in cells other than those in the aortic intima. I have examined fat-filled cells in xanthomatous lesions, and the fat-filled cells in the adrenal cortex, which are producing steroids. In the xanthomas one finds exactly the same pattern as in the aorta with the very high cholesteryl ester containing high oleic and low linoleic acids.

Again, in the adrenal cells, one also finds this same pattern. Therefore, it rather looks as though this pattern is in some way typical of cells which are accumulating large amounts of lipid. This is also, I think, in line with some work done on cholesteryl esters produced in gut; they were preferentially esterified with oleic acid. It looks as if cells esterify cholesterol with a high proportion of oleic acid, and the liver is, perhaps, producing lipoprotein with a fatty acid composition which is rather unique.

Dr. INSULL: We have recently had an opportunity to compare the cholesteryl ester fatty acid composition in the fatty streaks and fibrous plaques of two human populations that have quite different fatty acid sources, namely, Japanese and American men.

There were distinctive differences between the fatty acid proportions in the esters of fatty streaks and in the esters of fibrous plaques, but there was no difference between the two population groups. This seemed to indicate that the fatty streak lesions have a specific fatty acid pattern and the fibrous plaques another specific, but different, fatty acid pattern. The index acid that is of most interest here is the linoleic which in fatty streak esters was about 15%, but in the fibrous plaque esters it was 30% to 35%, quite a significant difference.

Dr. BEAUMONT: The homogenization seems harmful to the extraction of lipoprotein from the arterial wall. Do you know why, Dr. Smith?

Dr. SMITH: We have done some experiments with homogenizing beta lipoprotein itself, and this completely destroyed the immunological activity. We then tried homogenizing it with some previously extracted arterial tissue residue present, and this gave a small measure of protection. My original idea was that beta lipoprotein was perhaps getting stuck onto larger lipid particles in the artery wall homogenate, and then perhaps it was too large to diffuse into the gel. I think from these later experiments of homogenizing lipoprotein alone that it must somehow be mechanical disruption of the lipoprotein; but as to where the apoprotein goes, I have no suggestions.

Section III

THROMBOSIS AND ATHEROSCLEROSIS

INTRODUCTION TO THE PLATELET AND THE ARTERY*

J. F. Mustard

It is now well established that platelets play a part in the development of arterial lesions and the complications arising from them [493, 1062]. Platelets may be involved in the mechanisms causing focal areas of vessel injury where the early changes of the vessel wall occur [1141]; they are involved in the formation of mural thrombi which can become organized and contribute to vessel wall thickening [493, 1062]; they are involved in the formation of thrombi which occlude arteries [1062]; they are involved in the formation of intravascular platelet aggregates which can disrupt the microcirculation and lead to tissue injury and organ dysfunction [758, 759]. Most of these events will be described in more detail in later presentations. Our understanding of the role of the platelets in these reactions has been greatly advanced by the recently acquired knowledge of platelet aggregation and the release reaction of platelets.

Platelet aggregation. Platelet aggregation is caused by adenosine diphosphate (ADP) [508], thrombin [571], collagen [711], antigen-antibody complexes [1049], gamma-globulin coated surfaces [1064], epinephrine [1011], serotonin [1011], endotoxin [390], bacteria [1140, 1361], and viruses [748]. Most of these stimuli are thought to cause platelet aggregation by inducing the release of platelet ADP [629], although the reaction of platelets with endotoxin and some of the reactions involving gamma globulin may occur through the process of immune adherence [668, 1396]. For some of the aggregating stimuli such as bacteria and viruses, the mechanism through which they act has not been established.

The effect of ADP on platelets can be divided into four stages for the purposes of description: (1) an initial change in shape which consists of swelling, centralization of granules, and the formation of pseudopods; (2) the adherence of these altered platelets to each other; (3) the deaggregation of the platelets; and (4) restoration of the deaggregated platelets to their original shape and sensitivity to ADP. The initial effect of ADP on platelets is independent of calcium and magnesium [1373]. It is very difficult to inhibit this ADP-induced shape change completely. The second stage of platelet aggregation requires calcium and is inhibited by chelating agents such as citrate, EDTA and EGTA [213]. This stage is also inhibited by ATP, 2-methyl thio AMP [982], AMP [1136], 2-chloroadenosine [206], adenosine [206], the pyrimido-pyrimidine compounds [429], prostaglandin E_1 (PGE_1) [810], and a number of other compounds. *In vitro*,

* The following abreviations are used herein: EDTA = Ethylene diamine tetraacetate; EGTA = Ethylene glycol diaminoethyl tetra-acetate; ATP = Adenosine triphosphate; AMP = Adenosine monophosphate; ADP = Adenosine diphosphate and PGE_1 = Prostaglandin E_1.

PGE_1 has been shown to be the most potent inhibitor of ADP-induced aggregation [428, 1526]. However, its mechanism of action has not been established. Platelet deaggregation requires magnesium and metabolic energy [799] and does not depend on the removal of ADP [1136, 1267]. Very little is known about the requirements for the restoration of the deaggregated platelets to their original state.

It is apparent from this description that ADP-induced platelet aggregation is a reversible process. It has been proposed, however, that high concentrations of ADP can induce irreversible aggregates by causing the release of platelet ADP [899, 1004]. Although this is a reasonable interpretation of data from some *in vitro* studies, the evidence is not conclusive. Platelets deaggregate in the presence of concentrations of ADP adequate to cause aggregation [1136, 1267]. Evidence from a number of *in vivo* experiments indicates that ADP-induced aggregates, even when induced by massive doses of ADP, are reversible and that these platelets quickly return to the circulation and subsequently have a normal life span [211, 759, 1070]; and, finally, the surfaces of the containers in which platelet aggregation is studied *in vitro* can become coated with plasma proteins and cause the release of platelet constituents [1137]. Although it is questionable whether ADP can cause irreversible platelet aggregation, there are factors which can potentiate ADP-induced aggregation; these include epinephrine [1005] and serotonin [101]. Two important aspects of platelet aggregation *in vivo* are: (1) the source of the ADP, and (2) the factors which stabilize the platelet mass.

The Platelet Release Reaction. Thrombin, collagen, antigen-antibody complexes, gamma-globulin coated surfaces, some bacteria and some viruses cause the release of platelet constituents as well as platelet aggregation [1140]. Among the constituents released are the nucleotides ATP and ADP, serotonin, potassium, epinephrine, histamine, and some lysosomal enzymes [261, 365, 703].

The release of nucleotides and serotonin is very similar to the release or secretion of storage granule contents from other cells such as the adrenal medulla. This process has been called stimulus-secretion coupling by Douglas [399]. Metabolic energy and external divalent cations are required for the release of constituents following stimulation [399, 703].

The release of ADP, serotonin, and epinephrine from the platelets is important in causing more platelets to adhere to those which have already clumped. It seems likely that these compounds are the messengers which alter the platelets in the flowing blood so that they become adhesive and stick to each other.

Among the substances released from platelets exposed to release-inducing stimuli are some which increase vessel permeability [1063, 1066, 1140]. In addition to histamine and serotonin, there is a factor (or factors) with a molecular weight of between 10,000 and 20,000 which increases vessel permeability and causes contraction of smooth muscle. One component of this material may be similar to the cationic protein which is released from leukocyte granules [743] and causes the release of histamine from mast cells. In addition to these substances, platelets also release lysosomal enzymes which can cause tissue injury [365, 703, 1004]. It is possible that when platelets interact with the vessel wall they may increase the permeability of the endothelium and thus contribute to the localized accumulation of protein and lipoprotein in the wall of arteries [1141]. The factors released from platelets may also be important in the vasculitis which has been observed to develop in association with platelet aggregation [727].

The release of platelet constituents is inhibited by a number of compounds. Some of the inhibitors of ADP-induced aggregation also inhibit the release reaction. These include ATP, AMP, adenosine, PGE_1, methyl xanthines, and the pyrimido-pyrimidine compounds [703]. There are also some compounds which do not block ADP-induced aggregation but inhibit the release reaction; these include the imipramine class of compounds [1006] and the nonsteroidal anti-inflammatory and related drugs [443, 1114, 1139, 1142, 1530] (sulphinpyrazone, phenylbutazone, acetyl salicylic acid, sodium salicylate and indomethacin). Many of these compounds have been demonstrated to inhibit the formation of hemostatic plugs in response to vessel injury [443, 1142], the formation of thrombi in injured small vessels [215], and the formation of deposits in extracorporeal shunts [442, 443]. Dipyridamole (persantin), sulphinpyrazone, and acetyl salicylic acid inhibit platelet aggregation in man, and dipyridamole has been shown to reduce the incidence of thromboembolic complications in patients with artificial cardiac valves [1441]. The two classes of compounds which appear to be most promising in the management of thrombo-embolic disease are the pyrimido-pyrimidine compounds and the nonsteroidal anti-inflammatory drugs. When one takes into consideration dosage requirements, toxicity, and efficacy in man, the most useful compounds seem to be dipyridamole, sulphinpyrazone and acetyl salicylic acid.

Platelets and Blood Coagulation. Although the initial platelet aggregation which occurs in response to injury to the blood involves mechanisms which are independent of blood coagulation, the mass is unstable unless there is adequate fibrin formation around the platelet aggregate [1067]. Morphological evidence indicates that in the initial stages, blood coagulation is largely localized around the platelets [715, 760]. There are several reasons for this. When platelets are aggregated by ADP, the platelet phospholipid or phospho-lipoprotein becomes available for the clotting reaction. This phospholipid material is important in the interactions of factor IX with factor VIII and of factor V with factor X [665, 666]. The effect of the phospholipid is to cause a marked acceleration of the clotting reaction which leads to thrombin formation at a rate that is greater than the rate at which thrombin can be neutralized by antithrombin. Since many of the clotting factors are adsorbed on the platelet surface [1076], the circumstances are ideal for a localized acceleration of the clotting reaction when the platelet phospholipid is exposed.

As well as causing the formation of fibrin from fibrinogen, thrombin also causes further platelet aggregation by inducing the release of platelet ADP.

When fibrin formation is impaired, the platelet mass which forms in response to vessel injury is unstable, and fragments frequently break off [689, 1067]. Usually during the initial stage a new mass forms to replace the lost sections. Thus it has been found that with heparin therapy the platelet masses which form in response to vessel injury embolize more frequently than they do in control animals [505]. When platelet aggregates containing fibrin are induced in the microcirculation by the intravenous infusion of thrombin, the platelet aggregates do not immediately break up as they do with an ADP infusion [1070,

1071]. After several hours, however, the aggregates do break up and many of the platelets return to the circulation. In these circumstances it appears that the fibrin around the platelets is lysed by the intense fibrinolytic activity in the microcirculation.

Thus, even thrombin-induced aggregates are unstable *in vivo* unless the fibrin component is maintained.

When a platelet mass persists it is gradually transformed to a mass of fibrin [343, 760]. This subsequently becomes organized into an endothelium-covered intimal thickening rich in smooth muscle cells, collagen, and elastic tissue. In some circumstances this organized thrombus may include lipid-rich foam cells which represent macrophages that have phagocytized platelets and platelet debris [603].

It has also been suggested that slight injury to the vessel wall can initiate thrombus formation through the coagulation mechanism [65]. Such injury is thought to increase the permeability of the endothelium to plasma proteins, leading to the activation of factor XII of the coagulation mechanism as the plasma proteins come in contact with the collagen. Some of the thrombin which is formed diffuses out to the vessel lumen and causes fibrin formation and platelet aggregation on the endothelium. There is some experimental evidence which supports this concept. Fibrin in which the thrombin has been neutralized does not readily adhere to platelets or cause platelet aggregation [714]. However, if this fibrin is exposed to circulating blood, a platelet aggregate will form on the surface of the fibrin that is exposed to the blood [714]. It appears that the mechanism involves the generation of thrombin on the surface of the fibrin, with fresh fibrin formation and platelet aggregation.

SUMMARY

Platelets may be involved in the development of vascular disease and its complications through a variety of mechanisms. The stimuli which can induce platelet aggregation range from vessel wall stimuli such as collagen, to intravascular stimuli such as antigen-antibody complexes, viruses, and bacteria. These platelet aggregates can initiate mural thrombi, occlusive thrombi, and transient disturbances of the microcirculation with resulting tissue injury and organ dysfunction. They can also induce vascular injury and increased vessel permeability, and may be in part responsible for the localization of lipid deposits in the vessel wall. In view of our knowledge of the mechanisms involved in platelet aggregation, it is now possible to introduce new methods for the prevention of thromboembolic disease with drugs already available, such as dipyridamole, sulphinpyrazone, and acetyl salicylic acid.

FORMATION AND FATE OF A THROMBUS

John E. French*

The events which occur during the formation of a thrombus and its subsequent fate can to some extent be deduced from the histological study of natural thrombi as they occur in man. However, the thrombi seen postmortem, or even the fresher specimens obtained from surgical material, may have been present *in situ* for days or weeks before they are examined and have undergone degenerative changes which obscure their early features. Most of the detailed morphological information about the early stages of thrombus formation has, therefore, been obtained from studies on experimental animals, where events can be observed directly in living preparations, or in which a thrombus can be fixed at chosen intervals for histological examination.

Many experiments of this type, carried out since the end of the last century, have led to the concept of thrombus formation as a fairly ordered sequence of events [495, 1184]. In most experimental models, thrombosis begins with a local accumulation of platelets, some of which are attached to the vessel wall; more platelets then aggregate at the site to form a predominantly platelet mass which may give rise to multiple small emboli or continue to build up until it impedes blood flow. When the latter occurs, platelets at the periphery of the mass undergo morphological changes, the so-called viscous metamorphosis, leucocytes adhere to them, and polymerised fibrin is seen in significant amounts for the first time. Mural thrombi may not advance beyond this stage, but if the lumen is completely occluded coagulation extends into the stagnant column of blood and may add considerably to the total bulk. Further changes occur with the passage of time; there is an increase in the proportion of fibrin to platelet material and in the number of leucocytes to be followed by autolytic and degenerative changes and eventual organization of any unresolved material that remains.

While these events can be considered as distinct stages in thrombus growth their relative contribution varies in different situations depending, for example, on the type, size, and configuration of the vessel in which the thrombus is formed and on the local conditions of blood flow. Moreover, when a growing thrombus has reached a particular stage it does not necessarily progress to the next and, in the initial stages at least, each step is potentially reversible.

The main features of thrombus formation as outlined have been recognised for many years, and the more recent morphological studies have not resulted in any major changes in interpretation; but, by the use of improved techniques for viewing living preparations and by electron microscopy, it is now possible to depict the events more clearly and to fill in some of the points of detail. Thus, there is a continuing consolidation of the structural basis on which a detailed explanation of thrombosis in physiological and biochemical terms needs to be built. An account will be given here of some of the new developments; a more comprehensive review of studies on the fine structure of experimental thrombi has recently been published [494].

* Deceased May 15, 1970.

INITIAL STAGES

The induction of thrombosis in experimental animals usually involves some form of injury to the vessel wall. Under these circumstances the first stage in thrombus formation, as detectable by direct microscopy, is the accumulation of platelets in the lumen of the vessel at the injured site. This appears to be explained by the retention of platelets which are brought by the blood flow into contact with the injured wall or with other platelets that have already become adherent. No mechanism has been proposed whereby platelets could be specifically attracted to a site of injury, although presumably if the circulating platelets possessed increased adhesiveness it is more likely that they would be retained.

ADHESION OF PLATELETS TO THE WALL

The fact that platelets do not normally adhere to the endothelial surface of blood vessels has led to attempts to construct artificial surfaces with similar properties [752] but the precise physico-chemical properties that would be required to explain this effect are not understood. Earlier suggestions that the endothelial surface is covered by an adsorbed layer of protein have not been supported by observations with the electron microscope. However, the demonstration by use of the dye ruthenium red that endothelial cells have a surface coating rich in polysaccharide material [894] could possibly have a bearing on this point. Endothelial cells probably have a role in the reversal of the early stages of thrombosis since they contain enzymes which can break down adenosine diphosphate [923] and also an activator of the fibrinolytic system [1202], but it seems doubtful that these properties would be concerned in the prevention of adhesion to a normal surface.

Intact endothelium can develop a property, so far unexplained, of stickiness to leucocytes [563], but observations on living vessels do not suggest that platelets respond to this change in the same way. Degenerate or vacuolated endothelial cells have been observed in injured vessels, but adherence of platelets at these sites does not apparently occur until the cells desquamate; nor do platelets adhere readily to injured endothelial cells *in vitro* [1478]. Accumulation of platelets has been described at sites of minimal injury in veins when there is neither destruction nor complete separation of endothelial cells, but in this case it has been proposed that local activation of the coagulation mechanism at the surface of the injured cell, rather than platelet adhesion, is the primary event [65].

In most of the procedures used to induce thrombosis there is an actual destruction of endothelial cells which allows platelets to make contact with the exposed subendothelial tissue. Thus in experimental arterial thrombi one usually finds that the endothelium is missing completely from the sites where the thrombus is attached. In veins, visible platelet accumulation can be induced by much milder forms of injury and the loss of endothelial continuity may be less extreme. Nevertheless, exposed subendothelial tissue is commonly present even though with minimal injury this may occupy no more than the gap between two separated endothelial cells [64, 493].

The components of the wall which may be exposed when the endothelium is lost consist of the collagen and elastic fibers of the subendothelial space, the intimal ground substance and, depending on the degree of injury, the endothelial basement membrane or the inner surface of the internal elastic lamina. Platelets are known to adhere to extravascular collagen fibers during the formation of a haemostatic plug and to collagen fibres inserted as a suture into the lumen of an artery [760]. Moreover, studies on the properties of platelets *in vitro* have indicated that platelets will adhere readily to collagen, but not to elastin [1388] and that mucopolysaccharides prepared from the ground substance of the aorta do not themselves cause platelet aggregation [1051]. A specific interaction between collagen and the platelet membrane is suggested by the very close approximation (100–200 Å) of the two surfaces when in contact and by the apparent breaks observed in the platelet membrane under these conditions [440, 714]. On the basis of these observations it is reasonable to suppose that exposed collagen fibers may be the major stimulus for platelet adhesion during thrombus formation.

Electron microscopy of transverse sections of some injured vessels has shown typical collagen fibers at the sites where platelets are adherent. In other vessels, however, the platelet membrane appears to follow closely the contours of the inner surface of the internal elastic lamina or to be separated from it only by a zone of carbohydrate-rich material, as indicated by positive staining with ruthenium red (Sheppard and French, unpublished data). In mildly injured veins a very close approximation has been observed between the platelet surface and the endothelial basement membrane. This spacing is similar to that seen when platelets are in contact with collagen fibers, but in this case no collagen could be identified mophologically [103]. These findings keep open the possibility that platelets adhere to components in the wall other than collagen and that elastin or ground substance may have different properties in their native state from those observed with isolated materials *in vitro*.

In arteries, thrombosis may develop no further than the stage of platelet adhesion if the flow remains rapid and linear. When the endothelium is removed from the mid-abdominal aorta of a rabbit by passing a roughened probe into the lumen, it can be seen from *en face* preparations that only single platelets, or small platelet clumps, are scattered over the surface of the denuded area [1185]. Under these circumstances it is possible to view the adherent platelets by scanning as well as by transmission electron microscopy [1350]. The platelets are spread over the surface in a manner which is strikingly similar to that observed by the same technique when platelets adhere to glass [1303]. They show elongated cytoplasmic projections, some of which are branched, and may be completely flattened or show a central hump, presumably where the granules are concentrated (Fig. 1). It is still not clear, however, whether the platelets are clinging specifically to the network of fibers or more generally to the inner surface of the elastic lamina. Scanning electron microscopy has also been used by Frost and Hess [503] to illustrate the early and later stages of thrombus formation in arteries of the rabbit at sites of injury by heat or cold.

AGGREGATION OF PLATELETS

When the conditions for further growth of the thrombus are favorable, more platelets adhere to those already attached to the wall, and a chain reaction is set in motion which builds up a mass consisting almost entirely of platelets [207].

A local release of adenosine diphosphate (ADP), either from platelets which have adhered to the wall and to other platelets, or from damaged tissue in the wall itself, is thought to be the effector mechanism; certain morphological features of the platelet mass are consistent with this view.

The adherent platelets at the base of the thrombus show, in addition to the pseudopodia already mentioned, structural changes which indicate swelling and loss of granules. These changes are similar to those observed in other situations

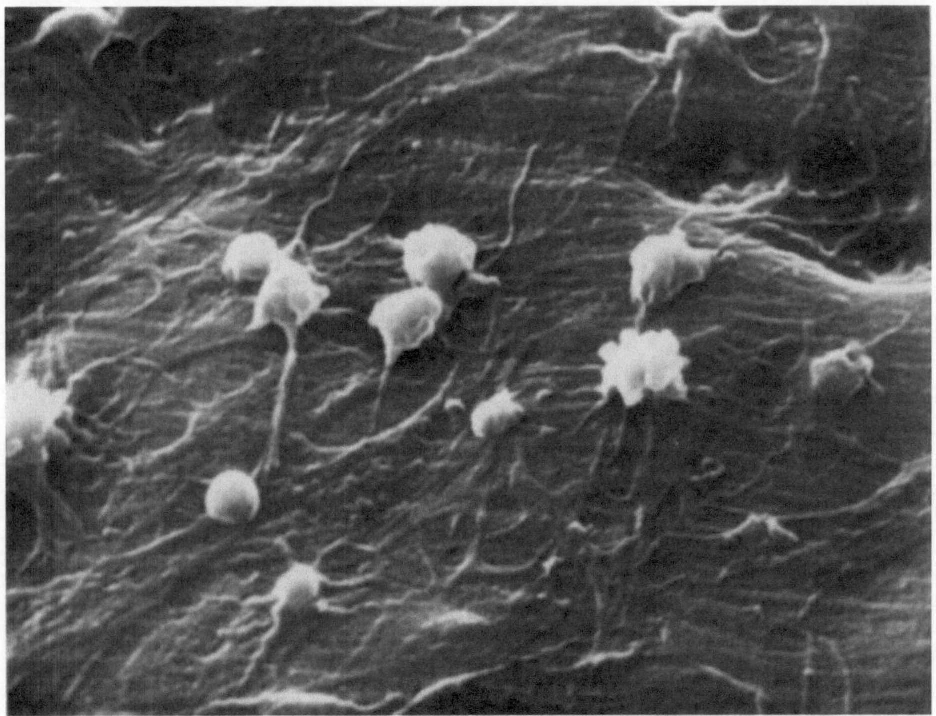

Fig. 1. Platelets adherent to the inner surface of the abdominal aorta in a rabbit at a site where endothelium had been removed. Micrograph taken on a Cambridge Mark II A Stereoscan scanning microscope. Reproduced by permission of the Cambridge Scientific Instrument Company. ×7,500

where platelets in contact with collagen fibers are known to release ADP [714, 1436]. In transverse section, the platelet mass shows a very characteristic mosaic pattern. The individual platelets have, in general, retained their internal structure, but they show some variation in density and irregularities in their surface contours which indicate swelling and pseudopod formations; they are very tightly packed together, but their surface membranes appear intact and are separated from each other by a fairly regular spacing of about 200 Å. Usually no fibrin can be detected within the platelet mass at this stage, and in this and other respects it resembles the aggregates which can be induced by ADP both *in vitro* and *in vivo* [710, 1078].

With standard methods of electron microscopy no material has been clearly identified in the space between the adjacent platelet membranes in this compact structure and, as with the gap of similar dimensions which can be seen between the plasma membranes of other types of cell in contact, its nature is not fully understood. Regularly arranged threads or filaments have been described bridging the gap in platelet aggregates induced by addition of ADP to blood *in vitro*, and it has been suggested that these filaments could represent extracellular material, possibly fibrinogen [713]. Recent evidence indicates that platelets have a surface coating of material rich in carbohydrate which can be shown by staining procedures

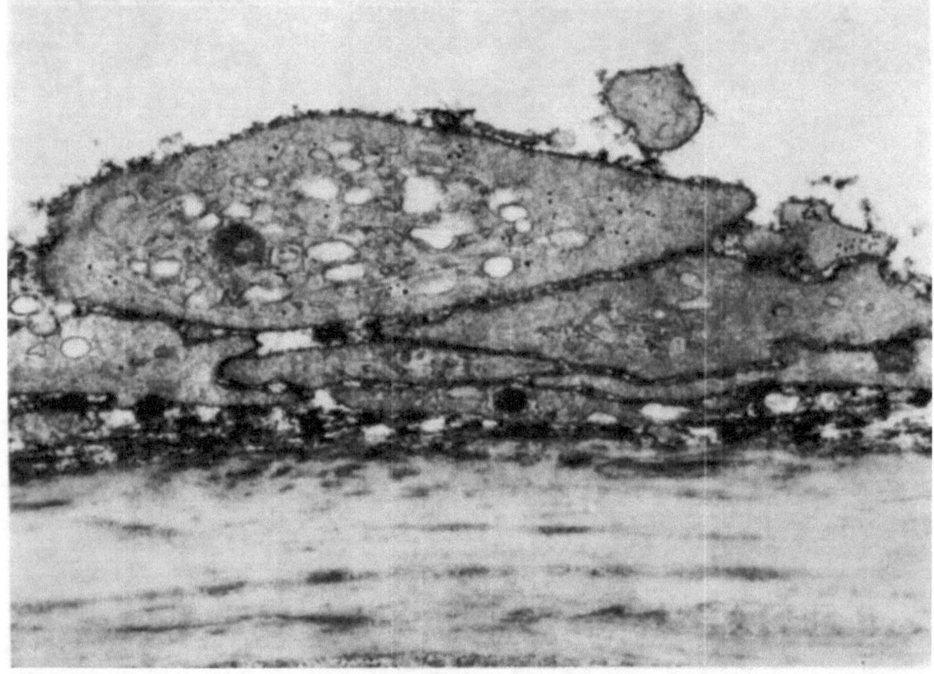

Fig. 2. A group of platelets on the exposed surface of the internal elastic lamina of the aorta in a rabbit. Material on and between the platelet membranes and between the platelets and the internal elastic lamina is stained with ruthenium red. Electron micrograph. ×34,000

that are more or less specific for carbohydrate complexes [133, 494]. It seems possible, therefore, that the gap is more apparent than real and that glycoproteins on the surface of the platelet membranes are the major components of this so-called space (Fig. 2).

Without the added support of fibrin, the platelet mass at this stage is inherently unstable so that small or larger fragments may be detached from it and swept away by the bloodstream. Under appropriate conditions, this platelet embolism followed by regrowth of the mass may occur repeatedly at fairly regular intervals over quite long periods and provides a means of assessing, more or less quantitatively, in experimental animals the effectiveness of drugs or changes in the blood which influence platelet behavior [61, 705]. The phenomenon has its clinical counterpart in the formation of platelet emboli from mural thrombi in the carotid arteries and their subsequent lodgement in vessels of the retina or brain [587].

When observed in the living circulation it usually appears that the mass is disrupted mechanically if it grows to such a size that it can no longer withstand the force of the blood flow. However, since platelet aggregates induced by ADP *in vitro* may also come apart again after an interval [212], it is possible that a similar chemical mechanism, involving breakdown of ADP by phosphatases in the blood or vessel wall, is operating *in vivo* at this stage.

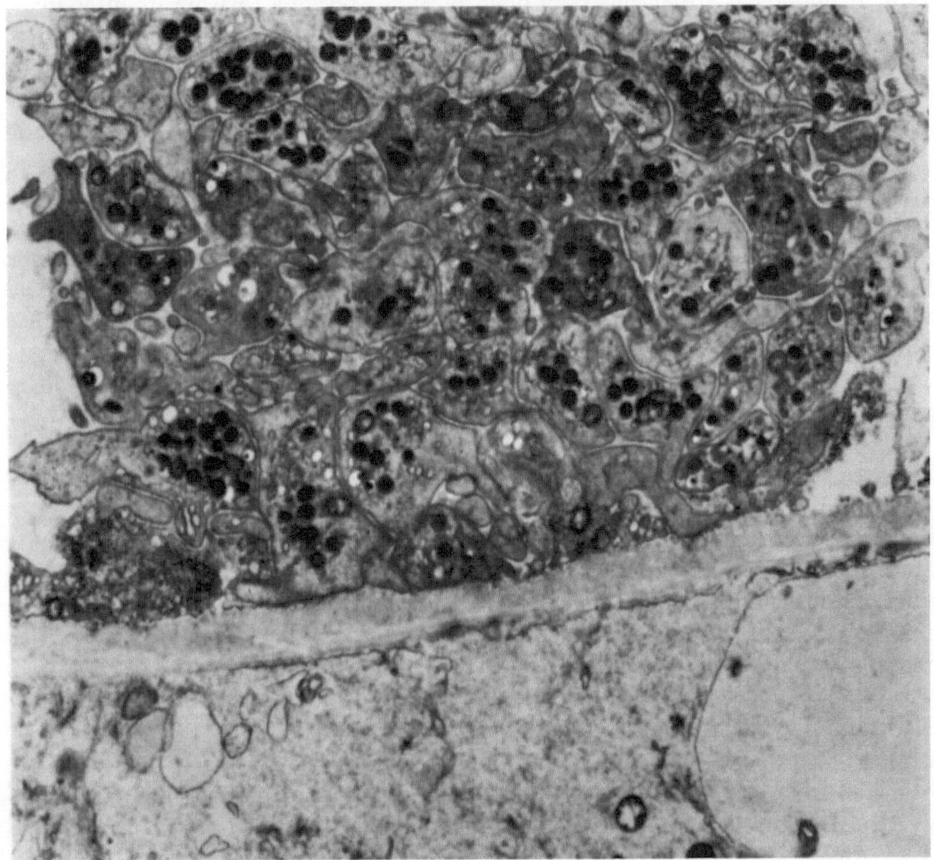

Fig. 3. A mass of platelets at a site of mechanical injury in a cerebral artery in a rabbit. The size of the mass had been increased by external application of ADP. Electron micrograph. ×14,000

The size and configuration of the platelet mass which forms will depend on a number of local factors. While rapid flow will tend to wash it away, slowing of flow or whirling or eddying currents in the stream will make more platelets accessible to it. The extent of platelet aggregation may also be augmented when chemical mediators are released locally from damaged tissue in the vessel wall. The application of ADP to the surface of moderately injured arteries, or infusion of ADP into their lumen, will cause visible aggregates to form under circumstances in which they cannot otherwise be seen by direct microscopy [704, 1388]. Electron microscopy of such vessels indicates that the effect of ADP is to make platelets aggregate with those already attached to the wall rather than to initiate the adhesion of platelets to the injured area (Fig. 3)—(Sheppard, Honour and French, unpublished data).

STABILIZATION OF PLATELET THROMBI

Under conditions where the platelet mass can grow to sufficient size to impede flow, it undergoes either generally or in plasma "pockets" within its interstices, a series of changes beginning at the free edges which serve to increase its stability. The platelets become swollen with bulbous outward projections so that the aggregates come to be surrounded by a fringe of relatively translucent nongranular bodies. Concurrently, fibrin makes its appearance as a network of fine strands around the nongranular bodies; this network extends inwards for a short distance from the edge but it does not, at this stage, penetrate the central parts of the mass. It is usually considered that thrombin has now been activated around the edges of the mass since platelet-fibrin aggregates with similar structural features are formed *in vitro* when thrombin is added to platelet-rich plasma [710], or *in vivo* when thrombin is infused intravascularly [1495]. At this stage, leucocytes which had not taken part in the earlier development begin to adhere around the edges of the platelet mass, apparently attaching specifically to the nongranular bodies rather than to intact platelets.

In some experimental thrombi an accumulation of fresh platelets has been observed external to the zone of nongranular bodies and fibrin formation in an earlier deposit, which suggests that the stabilized mass can still continue to grow in an episodic manner [391, 760]. Indeed, it is not clear why all mural thrombi should not continue to grow at this stage since thrombin, no less than ADP, is a potent stimulus to platelet aggregation. One possible explanation suggested by studies *in vitro* is that fibrin, once it has become stabilized on the surface of the mass, may no longer provide a surface to which platelets will adhere [714]. On the other hand it appears that the platelet-fibrin thrombus is potentially reversible. Mustard, Jorgensen, Hovig, Glynn and Rowsell [1065] found that, although infusion of thrombin in swine causes a fall in the platelet count and the formation of platelet-fibrin thrombi in small vessels, these microthrombi gradually break up over a period of two hours, and the platelets are returned to the circulation. This effect can probably be attributed to a local activation of the fibrinolytic mechanism. Application of streptokinase to freshly formed hemostatic plugs causes the plugs to break up with renewed bleeding through them [689]. Streptokinase has also been shown to disperse small thrombi in injured veins, leaving the injured area covered only by one to three layers of adherent platelets [936]. It is suggested that fibrinolysis could represent a regulatory mechanism in the early development of a thrombus determining whether, in a particular instance, a surface deposit of platelets and fibrin will break up or persist to undergo further growth or organization.

The growth of a thrombus, until it occludes or nearly occludes the lumen of a vessel, brings about a change in the relative contribution of platelets and fibrin. With cessation of flow fresh platelets are no longer brought to the site, while activated clotting factors are no longer diluted and washed away. The conditions are therefore favorable for coagulation to spread into the stagnating column of blood on either side of the obstruction. It has been pointed out that this wider extension of the clotting process may occur before the circulation has been brought entirely to a halt. Thus, the coagulation part of a thrombus may show, in contrast to a clot formed *in vitro*, an arrangement of fibrin in coarse bands or membranes. This streamline pattern of the fibrin suggests that it may begin to form along the contact surfaces of laminae of flow in the sluggish stream [755].

When the growth of a mural or occluding thrombus has come to a halt, further alterations begin to occur in the platelets and in the distribution of fibrin and leucocytes. Within a few hours the platelets within the aggregates become less densely packed and show an increasing degree of degeneration of internal structure, but they can still be recognized by electron microscopy from the persistence of their boundary membranes. In contrast to the appearance in fresh thrombi, fibrin can now be identified in the wider spaces between the membranes of the platelet remnants, and at the edges of the aggregates the fibrin in its original position forms coarser strands. Thus with the passage of time there is an apparent fibrinous transformation in the parts of the thrombus formerly occupied by platelet material [391, 760].

In addition to the leucocytes which are incorporated in the thrombus as it grows, others invade it later from the surrounding blood and vessel wall. Granulocytes rapidly show degenerative changes and by release of their lytic enzymes aid in the gradual digestion of the mass. Macrophages derived from blood monocytes, which are incorporated or migrate into the thrombus, are able to ingest red cells and platelets and through this process may be transformed into highly vacuolated foam cells [760, 1183, 1424]. Following the initial increase in fibrin, there is a progressive loss at this later stage, presumably as a result of fibrinolytic activity. Since the loss is most marked where the thrombus is in contact with circulating blood, it appears that the plasma system is the more active, but zones of lysis are also observed around incorporated leucocytes, particularly the macrophages [760]. During the course of these events the thrombus shrinks so that mural thrombi become more compact, while occluding thrombi may develop clefts or be drawn away from the wall at points at which they are not firmly adherent.

At the time when a thrombus is undergoing partial resolution, reactive changes begin in the vessel wall with the gradual transformation of the residual mass into organized connective tissue. Endothelium covers the free surface of mural deposits and comes to line the clefts or fissures in an occluding mass. It has been established that endothelium can divide mitotically, and growth of preformed endothelial cells from the free edges probably plays an important part in providing this new lining [493]. However, since the layer of cells forms rapidly under some circumstances, it has been proposed that the new endothelium is derived from cells in the circulating blood [760, 1424, 1569]. This point has not been finally established, but it has been shown that blood monocytes can spread out on the free surfaces to form at least a temporary surface or pseudoendothelium [746]. In any event it is not known whether a new cellular lining can form rapidly enough to be an important factor in limiting further growth of a thrombus at this stage.

The cells which penetrate the substance of the thrombus during organization have, in contrast to the fibroblasts in healing tissue at other sites, the morphological features of vascular smooth muscle. Since these cells have apparently the ability to synthesize both collagen and elastic fibers, the mass is eventually transformed into tissue which is rich in these fibers and cells though there may be, in addition, a variable amount of residual extracellular debris and, as pointed out, macrophages or foam cells [760]. Organized occluding thrombi may obliterate the lumen of a vessel permanently or be traversed by new blood channels which can take a variety of forms [1323]. Mural thrombi are incorporated into the wall with the formation of intimal plaques which in arteries may reproduce many of the features of the atherosclerotic lesion [1569].

THROMBOSIS AND THE DEVELOPMENT OF ATHEROSCLEROTIC LESIONS

A. B. Chandler

Thrombosis as a factor in the pathogenesis of the localized lesions of atherosclerosis was recognized by Rokitansky [1251] over a century ago. He maintained that localized thickening, atheromatous change, and calcification of the arterial wall are due to the repeated deposition of blood elements on the lining membrane of the vascular wall and the deposit's subsequent metamorphosis and degeneration. This hypothesis was not generally accepted at the time. The main objection was that the lesion of atherosclerosis is in the intima not on the surface and, therefore, could not be due to a surface deposit [891]. This seemingly important objection turned out to be unfounded when it was shown that endothelium can grow over a thrombus and incorporate it into the vascular wall.

With the exception of occasional brief reports [922, 1591], Rokitansky's hypothesis was disregarded for many years. Mallory [911], in his Harvey lecture of 1912, considered elevated plaques of fibrous tissue on the intimal surface of the aorta usually, perhaps always, to be formed by the organization of thrombi. Mallory also remarked on the endotheliozation of thrombi stating that the lining endothelial cells quickly cover over the surface of any fibrin within the lumen. He pointed out that fibrin, when not lysed, is a strong stimulus to the proliferation of fibroblasts and likened the process to the formation of thick plates of fibrous tissue on the surface of the spleen following acute infections. As Rokitansky had previously observed, Mallory noted that plaques are often stratified; the connective tissue, replacing two or more layers of fibrin formed at different times, could be recognized like the layers marking the annual growth of a tree.

A more detailed investigation of the role of thrombosis in atherosclerosis was made by Clark, Graef and Chasis [313]. They studied atherosclerotic lesions in the aorta and coronary arteries and concluded that the hyalinized bands of "fibrinoid" in plaques are thrombotic in nature. A gradual transition from masses that were clearly mural surface deposits to those covered by endothelium and collagenous tissue was observed. In agreement with Mallory and Rokitansky, they also found a progressive increase in the size of plaques as the result of repeated deposits of fibrin. Even though the hyalin bands in plaques were considered to be largely remnants of fibrin, the term "fibrinoid" was retained because the possibility of the occurrence of other blood elements could not be eliminated. These observations were confirmed and extended by Duguid [408].

Thrombic Constituents in Plaques. The hyalin fibrinoid material in plaques was thought by Duguid [408] to represent patches of unorganized fibrin. Lesions of this sort were considered the essential link in the chain of evidence which connects atherosclerosis with thrombosis. Further evidence of fibrin in atherosclerotic plaques was obtained by the use of immunofluorescent techniques [1572] and by electron microscopy [643, 858]. However, the presence of fibrin in a plaque is not conclusive evidence of its thrombotic origin, because fibrinogen could get to the site by filtration across the endothelium or by hemorrhage and then be converted to fibrin.

Blood platelets, which are a major constituent of arterial thrombi, also have been detected in plaques by immunofluorescent techniques [1570]. Platelets are a more reliable indicator of thrombus than fibrin. Although platelets might reach a lesion by hemorrhage, they are not as apt to penetrate endothelium as fibrinogen. Nevertheless, identification alone of elements from the blood in a plaque is of less significance than the morphological studies that trace the transition of a thrombus to a plaque.

Reaction of the Vessel Wall. Duguid [408] emphasized that the origin of a plaque from a thrombus may be obscured. As a thrombus is covered by new endothelium, the underlying endothelium disappears and is replaced by the invasion of connective tissue from the intima which obliterates the original line of demarcation. Crawford and Levene [343] showed in their study that thrombi are organized by ingrowth of the overlying endothelial cells as well as by connective tissue from the intima. This explains why thrombotic material often becomes encased by connective tissue and further obscured.

A prominent feature of organizing thrombi is a smooth muscle cell capable of synthesizing collagen [640, 1032]. These modified smooth muscle cells are usually more numerous than fibroblasts in organizing thrombi [641]. They are often present in the connective tissue of the intima of arteries [42] where they can invade the base of an attached thrombus. The recent demonstration of actomyosin [128], and of myofibrils [1199] in endothelial cells strongly supports the idea that the smooth muscle cells organizing a thrombus can also be derived from endothelium [42, 641].

Small mural thrombi are organized by an avascular process [409, 640, 654] whereas larger thrombi tend to become vascularized [518]. Capillaries sprout off the newly grown overlying endothelium to provide a direct blood supply from the lumen [343, 518, 1032]. They also grow through the wall from vasa vasorum and penetrate the thrombus at its base and sides [518, 1032]. Geiringer [518] considers luminal vascularization the hallmark of an organized thrombus. Capillaries growing into a thrombus have fibrinolytic activity [1472] and thus contribute to the resolution of a thrombus as it organizes. Even though these vessels may atrophy in time, some usually remain. Hemorrhage from these vessels can enlarge the plaque and further encroach on the lumen [1032].

Little is known about the rate of growth of endothelium over thrombi. Crawford's [340] study of healing arterial needle puncture wounds would indicate that endothelial regeneration is fairly slow. Hemostatic plugs in the puncture wounds are covered by endothelium in six to eight days. Variations in the rate of endotheliozation relative to that of thrombolysis could be a significant factor in determining the amount of thrombus incorporated into the arterial wall [368]. Rapid covering of a thrombus by endothelium could inhibit thrombolysis and thus contribute to the growth of the plaque.

Occlusive Thrombi and Thrombo-emboli. Occlusive as well as mural thrombi can become incorporated into the intima of arteries as atherosclerotic plaques [408] Occlusive thrombi may retract before endotheliozation is complete and in that

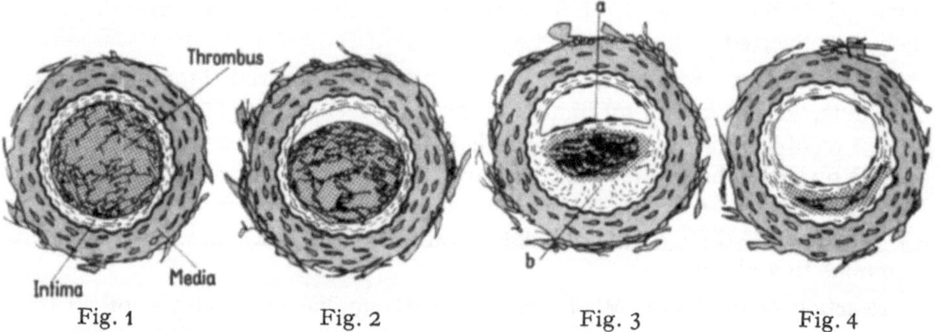

Fig. 1 Fig. 2 Fig. 3 Fig. 4

Figs. 1—4. An occlusive thrombus (Fig. 1) may retract eccentrically to form a single channel (Fig. 2) as it organizes and becomes covered by endothelium (Fig. 3). organization takes place from the overlying newly grown endothelium (Fig. 3, a) and from the preexisting intima (Fig. 3, b) to encase in fibrous tissue the residual thrombus which may undergo fatty degeneration, thus producing an atherosclerotic lesion (Fig. 4). By permission of Professor J. B. Duguid [410] and the publisher

way become mural or parietal in position (Figs. 1–4). Several investigators, studying the pathogenesis of pulmonary hypertension due to thrombo-emboli, have suggested that plaques in the pulmonary arteries are formed by the organization of retracted emboli [94, 135, 295]. Barnard [94] reviewed the subject and reported the conversion of thrombo-emboli to plaques in one case. The conversion of thrombo-emboli to plaques is important evidence of the thrombotic origin of atherosclerosis because such emboli sometimes lodge in normal arteries[1].

Sources of Lipid. Crawford and Levene [343] observed that when two zones of organization fail to meet, the remnants of the thrombus may undergo regressive changes to grumous fatty debris. According to Duguid [408] fatty degeneration occurs most often in red thrombi composed of tightly packed blood corpuscles and little fibrin. Among the cellular elements of blood in thrombi, platelets are a major source of lipid. Foam cells characteristic of those in atherosclerotic plaques can be derived from monocytes that have phagocytized lipid-rich platelets

1 In this regard it should be noted that atherosclerotic plaques, derived from thrombi in arterial prostheses form, in the absence of a true arterial wall [1471].

in thrombi [300]. Plasma, of course, is also a constituent of thrombi and may vary considerably in amount according to the type of thrombus. Lipoproteins of plasma have been identified in recent and organizing thrombi [1574] and their presence in definitive atherosclerotic plaques is well established [776].

Another source of lipid is from hemorrhage into a vascularized thrombus. Morgan [1032] points out that repeated small hemorrhages could lead to the accumulation of large amounts of lipid, especially cholesterol which is so resistant to absorption. He compares the process to the formation of a cholesteatoma following hemorrhage into a nodular goitre.

Frequency of Lesions. At present there seems to be general agreement that recurrent thrombosis is a major factor in the growth of atherosclerotic lesions from an early stage [492]. However, it is not established how often thrombosis initiates the atherosclerotic process on a normal arterial wall. Duguid [409] found microthrombi in varying stages of organization in 15 of 50 aortas in autopsy material from cases ranging in age from 3 to 73 years. The thrombi often were found near the mouths of branches, one of the sites where atherosclerosis begins. In some instances the thrombi had formed on an apparently healthy arterial wall. He suggests that such a high frequency of these lesions indicates that thrombosis is a common cause of intimal thickening. Movat, Haust and More [1046] reported similar observations. Heard [654] and Crawford and Levene [343] also found a high prevalence of aortic thrombi, but none was observed on an entirely normal vessel wall.

EXPERIMENTAL STUDIES

Duguid's work in the 1940's prompted several experimental studies. Much of the work was at first concerned with the study of the fate of fibrin clots and whole blood clots, not thrombi [617, 655]. When clots are injected into the circulation of rabbits as emboli that lodge in pulmonary arteries, fibrous intimal plaques form as a result of incorporation of the emboli into the arterial wall. Even though the emboli are occlusive they subsequently retract to become eccentric while undergoing the process of conversion to plaques. This point is of interest because it bears out similar observations in man. It would seem from these experiments that red blood cells in the clots are not a significant source of lipid. Plaques derived from clots contain little fat even though the animals may have been made hyperlipemic [670, 1464].

Fibrofatty Thrombotic Plaques. In a subsequent study in the rabbit, Hand and Chandler [603] used platelet-rich thrombi rather than clots as emboli. Typical fibrofatty atherosclerotic plaques containing abundant foam cells and foci of calcification formed in as short a period as three weeks. No dietary manipulations to produce hyperlipemia were employed. Organization of the retracted thromboemboli occurs both from the overlying new endothelium and the intima in the same way that Crawford and Levene [343] describe in aortic thrombi.

The major source of lipid in these plaques is thought to be platelets which are rich in lipids including cholesterol. Platelets are phagocytized by monocytes in the thrombi and disintegrate into lipid droplets, thus converting the monocytes or macrophages into foam cells characteristic of those in an atherosclerotic plaque. Nonphagocytized platelets often become calcified, possibly because of their high lipid content.

In electron microscopy studies of plaques derived from experimental platelet thrombi, Still [1424] and Casley-Smith et al. [294] found miniature cholesterol clefts in foam cells by 30 days. Fatty plaques in man contain a variety of lipids including cholesterol which is largely esterified [223, 225]. Although most cholesterol in platelets is not esterified [374, 943], Day and Gould-Hurst have shown by their experiments that macrophages can esterify ingested cholesterol [314].

Other Sources of Lipid. Red blood cells are a potential source of lipid in thrombotic plaques [95] but platelets contain considerably more lipid than red blood cells [93] and, as already noted, whole blood clot-emboli do not form fatty plaques. Degenerated and phagocytized granulocytes may contribute some lipid [294, 1424]. Friedman and Byers [500] have demonstrated that another source of lipid in thrombotic plaques is by way of diffusion of plasma from highly permeable new capillaries within an organizing thrombus.

Variable Composition of Plaques and Thrombi. Atherosclerotic lesions may be atheromatous and contain much lipid or sclerotic scars composed largely of fibrous tissue. Many forms exist between these extremes. Thrombi also vary considerably in composition. Mixed white and red thrombi form plaques that contain some foam cells [457], but not in such quantity as in plaques derived from platelet-rich or white thrombi [603]. These experiments indicate that the composition of the thrombus may influence the kind of plaque that forms. Arterial thrombi characteristically contain numerous platelets, but wide variations in composition occur. This is one reason atherosclerotic lesions may differ from each other.

Thrombi also may change in composition over a period of time. In a study of experimentally-induced mural thrombi in the carotid artery of the pig, Jörgensen and his associates [760] found that almost pure platelet thrombi form at first but over a period of time fibrin replaces many of the platelets before a plaque begins to take shape. Aortic mural thrombi, though retaining some platelets, undergo a similar transformation to compressed fibrinous remnants before incorporation into the arterial wall [1569, 1571]. These thrombi are mural, not occlusive, and the plaques that form are largely fibromuscular. Occlusive platelet-rich thrombi, however, retain their platelets and do not accumulate fibrin while undergoing transformation to fibrofatty plaques [603]. Thus, the type of thrombus, whether mural or occlusive, also may influence the composition of the plaque that eventually forms.

Topography. The topography of atherosclerosis in the pig is similar to that in man. In a study of coronary arteries and the aorta in the pig, microthrombi were found at sites of predilection for the development of atherosclerosis [519]. The thrombi had formed about branches and bifurcations on apparently normal endothelium and in some instances were undergoing incorporation into the intima.

Mustard [1061] found that thrombi develop in a similar pattern in experimental arteriovenous shunts made of plastic in the form of arterial branches and bifurcations. The formation and distribution of thrombi in these shunts illustrate the influence of hemodynamic forces and arterial configurations in the pathogenesis of thrombosis. Thrombi regularly form in the shunts about the branches and bifurcations at the same sites where atherosclerosis begins in arteries.

DIETARY AND PLASMA LIPIDS

Dietary and plasma lipids may be important in the thrombotic origin of atherosclerosis for several reasons. Both arterial and venous thrombosis are associated with high fat diets and hyperlipemia in man [131]. Diets rich in fat, especially saturated fat, cause thrombosis in animals [717, 1463] and increase an animal's susceptibility to experimentally-induced thrombosis [1107, 1109, 1220]. The thrombogenic effect of these diets is thought to be related to alterations in the quantity and the quality of plasma lipids. Hyperlipemia seems to be a double-edged sword, because thrombolysis is inhibited in this condition thereby increasing the stability of a thrombus once it has formed [961].

Ardlie and Schwartz [60] studied the effect of dietary-induced hyperlipemia and hypercholesterolemia on the fate of platelet-rich pulmonary thromboemboli in the rabbit. Thrombolysis was inhibited and the resultant plaques contained greater amounts of lipid and calcium than those in normocholesterolemic animals. They suggested that lipid-rich plasma trapped within the emboli is an important source of the enhanced lipid content of the plaques.

SUMMARY

The concept that some atherosclerotic lesions are thrombi altered by degeneration and organization is based on anatomical studies that trace the incorporation of thrombi into the walls of arteries. Both occlusive and mural thrombi can be incorporated into the intima by endotheliozation and undergo metamorphosis to atherosclerotic plaques. Occlusive thrombi become plaques by retracting to a mural or parietal position before they are covered by endothelium. In the later stages of metamorphosis, degeneration and organization of a thrombus may be so advanced the thrombotic origin of a plaque is obscured.

Thrombosis can account for the local character and the varied composition of atherosclerotic lesions. Both cellular and extracellular components of a thrombus influence the kind of plaque that forms. Fibrin seems to be important in stimulating fibrosis; and cellular elements, especially platelets, are a major source of lipids. Plasma lipids also contribute to the fat content of thrombi.

A prominent feature of organizing thrombi is a smooth muscle cell with fibrogenic properties. Small mural thrombi are organized by an avascular process, whereas larger thrombi are apt to become vascularized. Hemorrhage into a vascularized thrombus enlarges it and leads to the accumulation of lipid from the extravasated blood.

It is not known at present how often thrombosis initiates the atherosclerotic process; however, the growth of lesions from an early stage in their development frequently can be attributed to recurrent thrombosis. Multiple episodes of thrombosis form layers that progressively enlarge the plaques.

THROMBOSIS AND THE COMPLICATIONS OF ATHEROSCLEROSIS

LEIF JØRGENSEN

Atherosclerotic lesions are frequently associated with mural fibrin thrombi [1032]. This observation has led to the hypothesis that atherosclerotic plaques are the result of the incorporation and organization of such thrombi. Since fibrin masses on the intimal surface most likely are derived from plateled thrombi [755, 760] the presence of mural fibrin thrombi indicates that platelet thrombosis is frequent in arteries. In recent studies, small platelet thrombi have in fact been a common finding in the aorta of several species [1141]. The sites of predilection for these platelet thrombi are those where the earliest atherosclerotic lesions develop; these sites correspond to areas of disturbed flow [1058]. Thus, it is reasonable to assume that platelet thrombosis goes on in the arteries continuously or intermittently. Probably, it is partly counterbalanced by disaggregation of the platelets and by fibrinolysis.

Compared with this small-scale thrombosis, the formation of large, clinically significant thrombi in association with atherosclerotic plaques must be a rare event. Nevertheless, thrombosis as a complication of atherosclerosis is generally considered to be one of the most important causes of tissue ischemia and infarction. The prevalence of coronary thrombi in patients with recent myocardial infarction is somewhere between 37% and 91% according to autopsy studies from the last decade (Table). In other organs, it is more difficult to indicate how many infarcts are associated with thrombi on atherosclerotic plaques. This is mainly due to the problem of differentiating between locally formed thrombi and arrested emboli. The latter are much more frequent outside the heart than in the coronary arteries. In a Norwegian autopsy population, it is reasonable to expect that 45% to 50% of all large, recent cerebral infarcts are caused by thrombi on atherosclerotic plaques [761].

Table. *Percentage of cases with observed arterial thrombi among patients with recent myocardial or cerebral infarction according to some autopsy reports from last decade*

Authors	Percentage of cases with arterial thrombi
Myocardial Infarction	
Spain and Bradess [1391]	37–54[a]
Ehrlich and Shinohara [423]	50
Jørgensen et al. [757]	61
Sinapius [1364]	80
Harland and Holburn [610]	91
Cerebral Infarction	
Jørgensen and Torvik [761]	Approx. 45–50

[a] Patients surviving 1–24 hours: 37%; patients surviving more than 24 hours: 54%.

Why does the thrombotic process sometimes accelerate from a minute mural lesion to a significant obstruction or complete occlusion of the lumen? Several local and general factors are possibly involved, such as: (1) acute intimal edema; (2) hemorrhage into the atherosclerotic plaque; (3) rupture of intimal collagen fibres; (4) hemodynamic disturbances; and (5) increased systemic tendency to thrombosis.

Several authors have noted a localized intimal edema in association with arterial thrombi [969, 1032, 1351]. On the assumption that the edema is acutely formed, it has been considered an important pathogenetic factor in many instances of coronary thrombosis, particularly in younger persons [969]. However, platelets may release factors which increase vessel permeability and platelet aggregates may damage the vessel wall [728, 758, 759]. Therefore, any edema present underneath a thrombus may well be secondary to the thrombus.

The frequency of hemorrhage into the atherosclerotic plaque underneath the thrombus has been repeatedly stressed [1032]. The bleeding may be due to rupture of small vessels within the plaque [1032], or to a break in the intimal lining [302, 327, 501]. In the latter case, the bleeding usually takes place into soft, necrotic masses. However, the importance of intimal hemorrhage for the initiation of thrombosis should not be overestimated. Hemorrhages from vasa vasorum are frequent, even without obstructing thrombosis [1527]. Smaller hemorrhages from intimal vessels in association with thrombi may well be incidental or perhaps caused by the thrombosis. Morgan [1032] maintains that only the larger hemorrhages are capable of initiating thrombosis. Among the larger hematomas, Jørgensen et al. [759] found that only those due to rupture of necrotic plaques were associated with thrombi. In such cases, the thrombus is probably not caused by the hemorrhage directly, but the rupture of the necrotic plaque may be looked upon as a common cause of both the hemorrhage and the thrombus [302, 327, 501].

At present, rupture of the innermost layer of atherosclerotic plaques is considered the most important precipitating cause of arterial thrombosis [302, 327, 501]. Particularly characteristic is rupture of the layer covering soft necrotic material leading to discharge of necrotic debris into the arterial lumen [302, 327, 501] or, as already mentioned, to bleeding into the plaque. The rupture results in exposure of collagen to the flowing blood; this is a strong stimulus for platelet reactions [714]. Furthermore, the sudden changes in the volume of the ruptured plaque, the discharge of material into the lumen, and the presence of a flap of partly detached intima must create alterations in the flow pattern and, thus, favor platelet thrombosis [302]. On the other hand, the observation of a thrombus covering a fissure in the intima does not necessarily indicate that the break is the primary event, and thrombosis is the secondary. In smaller vessels, platelet aggregation may secondarily cause rupture of the inner vascular lining [unpublished data]. The possibility that platelet aggregation may create similar lesions in larger arteries should not be overlooked. However, it cannot be doubted that an intimal rupture, particularly over necrotic material, markedly accelerates the thrombotic process.

There is no unanimous agreement, however, that most arterial thrombi are related to rupture of necrotic plaques. Both Fischer [459] and Jørgensen et al.

[unpublished data] could clearly separate coronary thrombi into those associated with rupture of a necrotic plaque and those unattended by such a lesion. The latter type comprised two-thirds and one-half, respectively, of all thrombi. Thrombi not associated with rupture of a plaque were apt to occur independent of underlying intimal necrosis or hemorrhage [459] and they were possibly more preventable by anticoagulant therapy [unpublished data]. Thrombi on ruptured necrotic plaques were particularly frequent in men with evidence of hypertension and in patients with prolonged survival after the first attack of angina pectoris

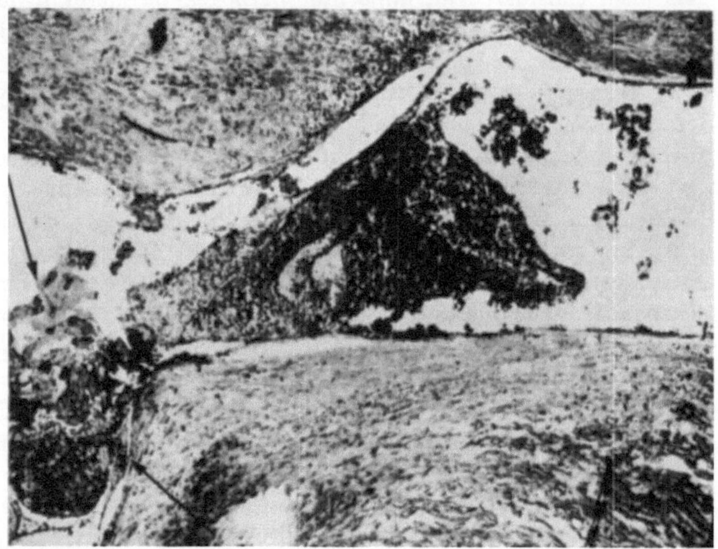

Fig. 1. Longitudinal section through a stenotic part of the descending branch of left coronary artery with a mixed platelet and coagulation thrombus. The patient, an 83 year old woman, died within a few hours of acute myocardial infarction. The blood flow has been from right to left. At the lower "lip" of the stenosis, just at the beginning of the expansion, there is a platelet aggregate (between the arrows). The platelet masses appear gray; the black strands within the aggregate are fibrin membranes. At the stenosis, upstream to the platelet aggregate, there is an occluding coagulation part composed of red blood cells (black) and fibrin membranes (black). The latter components appear as curved lines, probably reflecting the flow pattern during the formation of the coagulation part in retarded flow [757]. There is no rupture of necrotic plaque. Phosphotungstic acid-hematoxylin. ×32

[unpublished data]. These distinctive features of the two types of thrombi make it likely that their pathogenesis is different.

One important pathogenetic factor in thrombosis not related to rupture of a necrotic plaque is the hemodynamic disturbances, turbulence and eddies created by the atherosclerotic stenoses [1230]. The significance of flow disturbances in the a initiation of thrombosis is well known [714, 755, 1058]. A narrowing of the lumen will introduce focal points of high velocity gradients which favor platelet aggregation [395]. A high shearing stress may also cause erythrocyte damage [1089], followed by release of adenosine diphosphate [619] and platelet aggregation. In experimental thrombosis, the site of predilection of the initial deposit has been within the stenosis or at the beginning of the poststenotic luminal expansion [755]. Human arterial thrombi not associated with rupture of a necrotic plaque may have a similar location (Fig. 1). In these cases, one need not assume that the platelet reactions are initiated by changes in the underlying intima since, in areas of disturbed flow, thrombi may form irrespective of the character of the exposed surface [714, 1058]. Destruction of endothelium, if present, may well be secondary to the massing of platelets [758].

Hemodynamic disturbances are presumably present all the time in atherosclerotic arteries. In fact, some arterial thrombi have obviously been under formation for an extended period of time (Fig. 2). However, large arterial thrombi

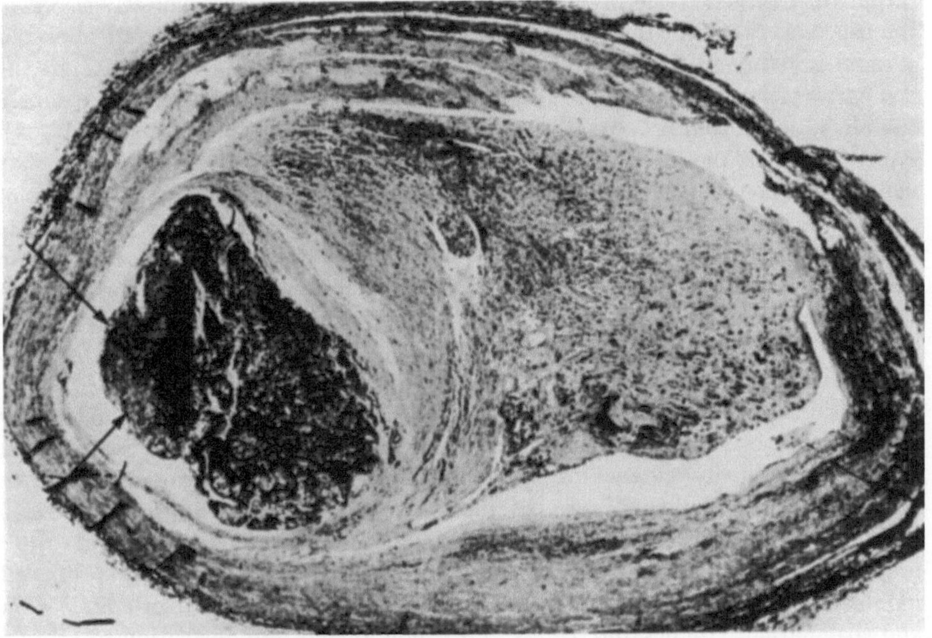

Fig. 2. Transverse section through the proximal part of the left internal carotid artery with a layered thrombus. The patient, a 72 year old man, got a right-sided hemiparesis and drowsiness nearly 5 months before death. Later, the symptoms varied somewhat until he became comatous shortly before death. The thrombus is composed of a large organized part to the right, a smaller fibrin-rich part to the middle left (black), and a recent platelet part to the extreme left (at the arrows). There is no rupture of necrotic plaque. Martius yellow-scarlet red-soluble blue. ×15

may also arise within an apparently short time (Fig. 1). If the hemodynamic disturbances are of importance, why does the thrombosis take place at the time it does? In order to explain this, one has to assume that additional thrombogenic factors come into play. Theoretically, they could be related to either the local vascular bed or a systemic factor.

A local precipitating factor could be sudden alterations of flow in smaller vessels of the arterial territory. Spain and Bradess [1391] stressed the fact that the prevalence of coronary thrombi found at autopsy increases with time of survival after the onset of the acute myocardial disease. They explained this by assuming that the thrombi generally developed as a result of diminished flow in the coronary arteries rather than being the cause of the myocardial disease. However, Spain and Bradess [1391] did not recognize the frequent occurrence of thrombi related to ruptured necrotic plaques. The lower frequency of coronary thrombi in the group dying immediately can be largely accounted for by assuming that it takes more than a few minutes for a sizeable thrombus to form secondary to the rupture, which itself produces lethal myocardial ischemia.

Several authors have compared the length of the clinical history with the apparent "histological age" of the coronary occlusion and the myocardial infarct [423, 1364]. In some cases it appeared that the occluding thrombus has followed rather than preceded the myocardial necrosis. Again, this observation has led to the conclusion that the thrombus is secondary to reduction of flow in the infarcted arterial territory [423]. However, this conclusion is probably only valid for the last part which has completed the occlusion; older parts, representing the previously stenotic mural thrombus, are at least of the duration of the clinical history [1364]. Based on experimental flow studies, Müller and Otto [1056] suggested that vasoconstriction or platelet aggregates in small vessels could alter the pattern of flow in the main artery and induce occluding thrombosis. In a study of thrombus formation in stenotic arterial grafts, Eiken [424] showed that a decrease in the peripheral flow induced by injection of noradrenaline resulted in a considerable shortening of the graft occlusion time. Altogether, it seems likely that an obstruction to the peripheral flow may accelerate the thrombotic process, but it is hardly the sole cause.

Acceleration of a local arterial thrombosis can probably also take place under the influence of a systemic factor. Of particular importance perhaps are catecholamines suddenly released into the blood. In animals, these hormones stimulate coagulation [1135] and promote thrombosis [1351]. In man, the catecholamines potentiate platelet aggregation [947] and coagulation [1518]. Connor et al. [321] found that, in rabbits, pituitary extract or adrenocorticotrophin (ACTH) produced mobilization of free fatty acids and, thereby, stimulation of platelet aggregation and coagulation. Hughes and Tonks [728] showed that administration to rabbits of sodium phosphate combined with a steroid (2α-methyl-9α-chlorocortisol acetate) caused platelet aggregation in myocardial and lung vessels. In man, the possible importance of pituitary and adrenocortical hormones in the acceleration of arterial thrombosis remains to be clarified.

According to Born and Philp [219], alimentary lipemia increases the tendency to platelet aggregation in the microcirculation of the rat. In man, there is evidence that coagulation is stimulated by alimentary lipemia [404], but the results of studies on platelet function during alimentary lipemia have been controversial [404, 709]. However, when given over a limited period, a diet rich in dairy or saturated fat is clearly thrombogenic [605].

Reports of the acute effects of one or a few cigarettes on platelet function have not been consistent [540, 1351]. However, the "thrombus formation time" in a Chandler loop is shortened [433]. The long-term effect of smoking may be more important than the acute effect [540].

In recent years the serious question has been raised as to whether oral contraceptives increase the incidence of arterial thrombosis in women of child-bearing age. Blood coagulability has been increased [421], but the epidemiological evidence of an association between the medication and arterial thrombosis is still somewhat equivocal [738].

At present, the significance of systemic factors in the formation of local thrombi in atherosclerotic arteries can only be a matter of conjecture. More exact knowledge is desired because, if systemic factors do play a role, and if they can be influenced by simple measures, prevention of thrombosis as a complication to atherosclerosis may be possible.

In arterial thrombosis, the effect of the thrombus on the tissue supplied by the artery varies considerably. An occluding thrombus does not necessarily lead

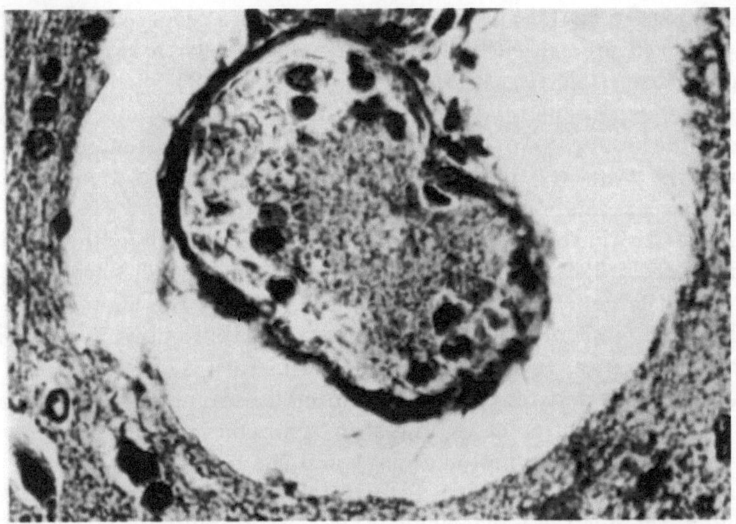

Fig. 3. An intracerebral artery in a case of thrombosis of the internal carotid artery. The lumen is nearly filled by a platelet aggregate which may have been detached from the carotid thrombus. Hematoxylin-eosin. $\times$ 560

to extensive infarction. The occurrence, size, and localization of infarcts depend on the available collateral circulation [762, 1474]. If the thrombus gives rise to only a moderate stenosis the blood supply would theoretically be sufficient even without calling upon anastomoses. In the carotid artery, a detectable reduction of flow and pressure does not occur before the lumen is reduced by 80–90% [238]. According to Robbins and Bentov [1230] a stenosis of an artery will be without effect until its resistance reaches a higher level than the peripheral resistance of the arteriolar and capillary bed.

A complicating factor in a mural arterial thrombosis is the embolization of platelet aggregates from the thrombus to the peripheral arterial bed. Platelet aggregates in peripheral arteries were observed at autopsy downstream to arterial thrombi both in cases of myocardial [756] and cerebral infarction [762, 1474] (Fig. 3). Clinically, the passing of platelet aggregates in to the cerebral microcirculation has been particularly associated with transient ischemic cerebral attacks. Passage of microemboli in the retinal arterioles has been observed during transient visual loss [587]. Experimentally, Denny-Brown and Meyer [389] observed passage of microemboli in the leptomeningeal vessels of monkeys. The emboli lodged temporarily in small arteries. This was accompanied by transient sludging of red blood cells, stasis, and local hypoxia. Honour and Russell [705] showed that microemboli from experimental platelet thrombi in arteries of rabbits tended to take a stereotyped course into the same small branches. This is probably explained by a strictly laminar flow. If microemboli in man also tend to pass down the same vessel each time, one may account for the fact that the symptoms at each of the repeated cerebral attacks are often the same.

Although particularly frequent in cases of intermittent or recurring symptoms, microembolism probably occurs in all clinical types of cerebral infarction [762, 1474]. Gunning et al. [587] suggested that the transient ocular and cerebral ischemic attacks were caused by friable microemboli, whereas less friable emboli might cause irreversible tissue damage. However, even transient platelet aggregation in the microcirculation may be enough to cause infarction in the heart [759] and in the kidneys [756]. Meyer et al. [978] showed that more severe damage to the cerebral tissue was produced by widespread embolization of small particles than by mere ligation of the artery.

In cases of carotid thrombosis, two general patterns of circulatory disturbance may be discerned [1474]. In some patients, the clinical course is brief and stormy, the infarcts are large, and the thrombus occludes both the main artery and the collaterals of the circle of Willis. In these cases, the thrombus itself is obviously of decisive importance. In other patients, the history is prolonged, the infarcts are less extensive and patchy, and the thrombus may still be nonoccluding at autopsy. Among the latter cases, there are probably patients in whom microembolism determines the symptomatology and the brain lesion.

Similar patterns of circulatory disturbance may also occur in the heart. On the one hand, there is the large, single infarct associated with a thrombus which is often occlusive; on the other, there are multiple, small infarcts with or without demonstrable coronary thrombosis [423]. The histological appearance of many of the thrombi may suggest a protracted development [1364]. As already mentioned it often appears as if only a nonoccluding thrombus has been present at the clinical onset of the infarction [1364]. In cases of sudden death, stenotic mural thrombi are more frequent than occluding thrombi [1364]; in small myocardial arteries platelet aggregates may be encountered, even when death is instantaneous [Haerem, personal communication].

Thus, there is evidence that an arterial thrombus may give rise to clinical symptoms and tissue damage both by obstruction of the main lumen and by showering of platelet aggregates to the peripheral arterial bed. In the brain, these showers may give rise to transient ischemic attacks; in the heart, they may be responsible for some cases of sudden death. Gunning et al. [587] suggested that microembolism may even give rise to some instances of "coronary insufficiency", but they did not present any direct evidence for this.

When affecting the kidneys, microembolism may play a particularly important role. According to Moore and Mersereau [1028], multiple, repeated emboli from mural thrombi in the aorta of rabbits upstream to the renal arteries may produce cortical infarcts, scars with atrophy of the nephrons, increased granularity of the juxtaglomerular cells, and hypertension. Similar effects may even be produced by only one episode of transient platelet aggregation in the renal microcirculation of rabbits [756]. The renal lesions produced in these experiments are remarkably similar to those of human kidneys in cases of primary hypertension [1028]. The question arises whether microembolism from mural atherosclerotic thrombi in the aorta may be a cause of nephrosclerosis and hypertension in man [756, 1028].

In all autopsy series of ischemic disease there remain a number of cases with tissue infarction without demonstrable thrombosis [423, 762, 1364]. The atherosclerosis of the supplying arteries is usually just as severe in these cases as in those where a thrombus is found [unpublished data, 762]. There are several explanations for the infarcts with apparently open arteries. One is that the thrombus has been overlooked, but that can hardly account for all the cases. A form of thrombosis may be involved after all. In myocardial ischemia, platelet aggregates were found in smaller arteries with equal frequency whether a coronary thrombus could be demonstrated or not, while in a consecutive autopsy series, platelet aggregates in the myocardial arteries were definitely less frequent [756, 757]. From the available evidence in studies of both brain and heart [756, 762] it seems unlikely that all arterial platelet aggregates found at autopsy are secondary to ischemia. In a case of apparently open arteries, peripheral platelet aggregates could derive from an unstable upstream thrombus not present at the moment of death. At a site of disturbed flow, due, for instance, to atherosclerosis, platelet aggregation could occur within the lumen without attachment of the aggregates to the vessel wall [755]. At a site of vascular damage, platelet masses may form repeatedly and dislodge completely each time [705]. At present, all that can be said about the role of such unstable thrombi is that they are a potential cause of tissue ischemia and should be the subject of further investigation.

SUMMARY AND CONCLUSIONS

A small-scale thrombosis is probably going on in arteries continuously or intermittently. At times, the thrombotic process accelerates and gains clinical significance. Larger thrombi in association with atherosclerotic plaques are one of the most important causes of tissue ischemia and infarction.

There are two main mechanisms by which larger thrombi form in atherosclerotic arteries: one is by rupture of a necrotic plaque followed by bleeding into the plaque or discharge of necrotic debris into the lumen; the other is disturbance of laminar flow at stenoses. The latter mechanism may be potentiated by obstruction to flow in the peripheral arterial bed. Thrombosis is also favored by systemic factors, such as release of catecholamines into the blood or use of a diet rich in saturated fat.

An arterial thrombus may give rise to clinical symptoms and tissue damage both by occluding the lumen and by a showering of platelet aggregates into the peripheral arterial bed. In the brain, these showers may give rise to transient ischemic cerebral attacks. In the heart, they may be responsible for some of the cases of sudden death. Experimentally, platelet aggregation in the microcirculation may alone cause infarction.

Microembolism from atherosclerotic thrombi in the thoracic aorta may give rise to nephrosclerosis and hypertension.

Even in cases of infarction with no demonstrable thrombus in proximal arteries, platelet aggregates may be found in peripheral arteries within and near the ischemic tissue. It is suggested that some of the aggregates could represent microemboli from an unstable upstream thrombus not closely connected with the vessel wall and not present at the moment of death.

Discussion Following Dr. Jørgensen's Paper

Dr. Born: Earlier in the symposium, evidence has been given showing that the lesions of atherosclerosis, and also the deposition of thrombotic material in large arteries, tend to begin around the openings of branches. That this localization may be due to blood flow properties, is an old hypothesis. Recently, I suggested to Dr. Helen Payling-Wright that these properties might also affect the endothelium and that such an effect might show itself in a higher rate of replacement of endothelial cells around the openings of branches than elsewhere. Dr. Payling-Wright has, indeed, demonstrated such a difference; experiments were as follows:

Apparently normal guinea-pigs weighing 300/400 g received tritiated thymidine (0.1 mc/100 g) 24 and 16 hours before being killed. Sheets of endothelial cells suitable for autoradiography were made by stripping away all other layers from rapidly frozen, partially fixed aortas. Slides prepared from the aortas were exposed autoradiographically for six weeks before developing and staining. With this technique we have established that the proportion of cells showing mitosis is higher around the mouths of branches leaving the aorta than in areas remote from branches. The ratio is about 1.7 to 1 and almost constant in different animals in which the absolute proportions of platelet cells varies considerably. These observations suggest that endothelial cells exposed to the effects associated with blood flow turbulence are replaced more frequently than endothelial cells not so exposed. This may have implications as regards both lipid infiltration into the arterial wall and deposition of platelets and other material from the lumen.

Dr. Robert: There was some question this afternoon about whether platelets adhere to anything other than collagen. We have recently purified elastin from the aorta and ligamenta nuchae by eight different methods, but none of these purified elastins made platelets more adherent.

Dr. Engelberg: Is there any evidence that platelet aggregation per se, without the intervention of fibrin formation to build up the thrombus, can form a clinically significant occlusive thrombus?

Dr. French: A situation in which platelet aggregates without fibrin have clinical significance is seen in the platelet emboli which arise from mural thrombi in the carotid arteries and go to the retina or the brain.

Dr. Chandler: I think Dr. Engelberg was also referring to the possibility of their formation entirely in the blood stream as well. There is evidence in hemolytic reactions, for example, that thrombi can form from aggregation of the platelets within the bloodstream, if not on the vessel wall. Some have fibrin, some don't.

Dr. JØRGENSEN: We heard from Dr. French that the platelets stick to collagen. We have shown that the platelets may also adhere to a damaged endothelial cell. The peripheral membrane of the endothelial cell is absent. The platelets are in close contact with the internal cellular structures, including the altered nucleus.

Dr. ROBERT: Dr. Rafelson with Dr. Boyce proposed a theory for platelet aggregation in terms of actomyosin hybridization. As epithelial cells also contain some actomyosin-like protein in their cell membrane, platelets could adhere to them. Dr. Jørgensen's observation might be considered as a direct confirmation of their theory.

Dr. BICHER: It has been known for a long time that the formed elements of the blood aggregate in thrombosis. From the discussion here, it appears that only the platelets are involved. I wonder if the red cells shouldn't be considered too as part of this series of events.

The following evidence must be considered: first, red cell aggregation has been described with many of the same conditions under which platelet aggregation is increased. Secondly, there are a number of publications that prove that platelet adhesiveness in PRP is much less than in whole blood. Thirdly, there is no doubt that the red cell can provide the adenosine diphosphate that can induce platelet aggregation. Fourthly, there is no doubt that the red cell is part of the final thrombus. Finally, changes in the physical behavior of red cells affect the ability of the blood to oxygenate tissue, and this should undoubtedly be considered in the origin of the endothelial lesion.

Dr. FRENCH: There may be situations where damaged red cells by releasing ADP affect platelet aggregation. In small blood vessels, increased permeability, which occurs in inflammation, for example, may lead to compaction of red cells and actual blockage of the lumen.

Dr. JØRGENSEN: The red blood cells may have an important role as a source of ADP. The red cells may be damaged by mechanical trauma and then release ADP. This may initiate platelet aggregation.

Another aspect is that the red blood cells may adhere to collagen. We have evidence that a thrombus formed on collagen may contain more red cells than a thrombus formed in another way.

Dr. WISSLER: There is one other way in which the platelet may be active in the atherogenic process. For a number of years now we have been observing with immunofluorescence little clumps of fibrin quite deep in the wall of arteries, particularly aortas and coronary arteries. These are located interstitially, i.e. in between the medial cells, and we have always been puzzled as to why fibrin should be there.

About four years ago one of our graduate students, Dr. Gorden Stottznar, began to use the ferritin label as an immunohistochemical method. He found that there are, indeed, not only clumps of fibrin deep in the wall of arteries, but frequently there are little areas of platelet antigen associated with the fibrin. Since Mrs. Rose Jones has joined us, we have begun to study some of the aortas from Rhesus monkeys fed table-prepared, average American diets, and one electronmicrograph that Mrs. Jones has taken shows that, very deep in the thickened intima, there is evidence of a degenerating platelet. Around it are strands that we believe to be fibrin. We believe that this is not a part of organization of a thrombus but that this platelet has made its way into the intact vessel and that little clumps of fibrin have been formed around it.

Dr. SCHWARTZ: We did some studies on the organization and fate of artificial pulmonary thromboemboli in which we found that the phagocytosis of red cells was not essential in the development of lipid-laden plaques.

A second point concerns the possibility that the phagocytosis of platelets may not be the only source of lipid in the resultant lesions. Phagocytosis of the debris derived from degeneration of the extensive leucocytic infiltrate which is seen only in the organization of platelet-rich thrombi may be another possibly important source of lipid.

Finally, a question: Can the qualitative composition of the lipid that is derived from the phagocytosis of the formed elements, particularly platelets, really account for the qualitative composition of the lipid in the organizing thrombus, particularly since the platelet lipid consists predominantly of phospholipid, with some free cholesterol and little or no cholesteryl ester?

Dr. MUSTARD: I would like to comment on Dr. Wissler's point. Whether one considers his lesion a thrombus depends on the definition of thrombosis. If one platelet sticks to the vessel wall mass, that to me is a thrombus. Therefore, no matter what is done afterwards, it was a thrombus.

Dr. WISSLER: I would like to have platelets with fibrin and trapped red cells on the surface first. I think that individual platelets may well be getting into the wall of the vessel and may be responsible for some of the interstitial accumulation of fibrin there!

Dr. STAMLER: I think we are getting close to a central issue which has been before us since Duguid wrote. I put it squarely to Dr. Chandler.

For years we have seen Dr. Duguid's schematic. We have heard about the embolic experiments in the lungs of animals, and we have seen advanced atherosclerotic plaques in coronary arteries with superimposed thrombosis. This modern basis for the old Rokitansky hypothesis of encrustation has been before us for years, yet there is no new evidence, by the advocates of the Duguid hypothesis, from man or experimental animals, to support the idea of early plaque formation by encrustation with endothelialization. I would like Dr. Chandler to say if I am right or wrong, that there is practically no solid evidence, certainly nothing new in recent years, for the Duguid hypothesis on early atherogenesis.

Dr. CHANDLER: If by early atherosclerotic lesions we mean small then we must know the incidence of microthrombi in the walls of arteries. In fact there is little data on this point and the four or five reports are discussed in my paper. Furthermore, the problem is not as simple as finding microthrombi. Not only can a small intimal lesion produce a thrombus, but the thrombus itself can lead to further injury of the vessel.

Dr. MUSTARD: Dr. Stamler has asked a very fundamental question. Because of the shortness of time I would like to use the chairman's prerogative in an attempt to reply to his challenge. I think there is little doubt that the organization of mural thrombi contributes to the development of atherosclerosis particularly in the later stages of the process. Dr. Chandler has presented a very clear account of this process. This process, however, may only be important in the development of stenotic lesions which lead ultimately to either rupture or occlusion of the vessel at critical points. I would agree that it is difficult to conceive of the organization of mural thrombi as playing an important part in the development of the earlier changes in the vessel wall. In addition, I think it would be wrong to infer that thrombosis is the only change which is occurring in the later stages of the process. Thus, thrombosis is probably only a component of the process, albeit an important one.

With respect to the earlier changes which occur in the vessel wall, I think we should keep in mind the nature of the environment in which these changes are occurring. There is a vessel wall, flowing blood with disturbed flow patterns around vessel orifices and branches, and the constituents of the blood. In injury to the microcirculation both the polymorphonuclear leukocyte and platelet release factors which increase vessel permeability. In addition, it is known that activation of plasma proteins can generate factors such as kinins which increase vessel permeability. It is possible that the interaction of constituents of the blood, in particular the formed elements with the vessel wall, could in larger vessels cause focal areas of injury with increased endothelial permeability. As I tried to demonstrate in my introductory remarks, if one examines the accumulation of protein in the intima of the vessels of normal healthy animals one finds that the pattern of protein accumulation is focal. Prime sites for the accumulation of protein are around vessel orifices and right-angle branches. Histological examination of the sites shows that there is intimal edema, with formed elements on the surface of the endothelium, and in some cases polymorphonuclear leukocytes in the intima. Examination of tissues from regions in which protein does not accumulate to such an extent shows much less change and, indeed, very little intimal thickening and only the occasional red blood cell on the surface of the vessels. Fry has proposed that these areas of focal injury are caused by hemodynamic factors. In our own studies and in his studies there is clear-cut evidence from electron microscopic examination of endothelial injury. Although Fry's explanation for the endothelial injury could be correct, it is also possible that the formed elements themselves have caused the alterations in the endothelium. Even if the formed elements are not the primary factors causing increased vessel permeability their accumulation at these sites in response to the injury would surely influence the process. Surely alterations in the endothelium associated with increased permeability could be an important factor in lipoprotein accumulation at these sites. I think the evidence discussed gives a fairly clear indication that the accumulation of beta lipoprotein in the intima could cause tissue proliferation.

You may not consider the accumulation of a few platelets and leukocytes on the endothelial surface as a thrombus, but I would point out that it is the same process as is involved in the more florid thrombus which we usually associate with pathological conditions. Thus, in considering the thrombogenic theory in the development of atherosclerosis, I believe one has to extend one's point of view to consider more subtle changes, formed element interactions with the vessel wall and their effects on increasing vessel permeability. These changes themselves are probably unimportant unless there are other factors which modify the process. I think it is reasonable to speculate that one of the factors which modifies this process is the accumulation of abnormal lipoprotein complexes which are difficult to metabolize. Furthermore the lipid accumulation may itself alter the vessel wall causing further formed element interactions with it. Thus, in reply to your question, it is my opinion that you cannot separate this form of a thrombogenic theory from the other theories and that they are interrelated. It is time that we considered them as a whole rather than as separate units.

Dr. E. Smith: In answer to Dr. Schwartz, the table shows a comparison of the lipid in platelets with the lipid in intimal fat streaks. The cholesterol in the

Table. *Lipids in platelets and intimal fatty streaks (mg/100 mg dry tissue)*

	Platelets	Fatty streaks	Fat-filled cells only
Total cholesterol	3.07	24.4	87.8
Phospholipid	13.8	5.8	23.5

platelets is very low in concentration compared with the cholesterol in the fatty streaks, and there is, in fact, virtually no esterified cholesterol. The phospholipid is two to three times higher than that in the fatty streak. In this fatty streak material, in fact, approximately one-third of the sample is occupied by fat-filled cells. If one then estimates the actual amount of lipid within the fat-filled cells, which is in the last column, the difference in lipids is quite phenomenal. The fat-filled cell would have to ingest about 30 times its own weight of platelets in order to produce enough cholesterol, and it would then have nearly 400 mg of phospholipid to get rid of in order to reach the measured composition of lipid. I think it is a very a complicated hypothesis in terms of lipid content.

It is possible that the platelet will make the cell start doing something else, but I don't think it can really supply the lipid in the lesion.

Section IV

SELECTED PAPERS ON PATHOGENESIS OF ATHEROSCLEROSIS, INCLUDING THROMBOSIS

THE EFFECTS OF EXPOSURE TO CARBON MONOXIDE, HYPOXIA AND HYPEROXIA ON THE DEVELOPMENT OF EXPERIMENTAL ATHEROMATOSIS IN RABBITS

Poul Astrup, Knud Kjeldsen and John Wanstrup

A number of epidemiological and clinical studies have recently shown a considerable increase in incidence of occlusive arterial diseases in smokers, most conspicuously among young individuals. A central role of tobacco smoking in the development of arteriosclerotic cardiovascular disorders has long been suspected, but the basic pathogenetic mechanisms responsible for such an atherogenic effect of tobacco smoke remains to be elucidated. For several years attention was focused on the action of nicotine and other alkaloids on the cardiovascular system; but it is important to stress that it has never been possible through the action of such substances to produce lesions in the vasculature which can be confidently accepted as atherosclerotic in nature.

Astrup [68] and Astrup et al. [69] in studies dealing with various cardiovascular disorders called attention to yet another component of tobacco smoke, i.e. carbon monoxide. It was demonstrated that carboxyhemoglobin concentrations from 10–15 and even 20% were not uncommon in heavy smokers, and it was hypothesized that a carbon monoxide-induced tissue hypoxia might be an important factor in the acceleration of cardiovascular disorders of the arteriosclerotic type.

Since then a number of experiments have been performed in an attempt to confirm and elucidate an accelerating effect of carbon monoxide-induced hypoxic states on the degenerative cardiovascular changes of arteriosclerotic type. The present paper is a concentrate of our experimental findings and investigations on the involved biological mechanisms. The results are discussed with special relation to present understanding of basic pathogenetic mechanisms in atherogenesis.

MATERIALS AND EXPERIMENTAL PROCEDURES

The experimental model chosen was a well-known, easily reproducible, classical one, i.e. the cholesterol-fed rabbit. The animals were obtained from the same source and inbred, and initial weights were between 2,500–3,000 g.

By using gas-mixing pumps it was possible to mix atmospheric air with calculated amounts of carbon monoxide, nitrogen and oxygen. These gas mixtures were led through airtight chambers containing cages with the rabbits.

The following experiments were carried out:

A. Cholesterol-fed rabbits were exposed to a carbon monoxide-containing atmosphere for 10 weeks, causing an average carboxyhemoglobin concentration of 15–20% [70].

B. Cholesterol-fed rabbits were exposed to an oxygen-deficient atmosphere (10% oxygen) for eight weeks [809].

C. Cholesterol-fed rabbits were exposed to an oxygen-enriched atmosphere (28% oxygen) for 10 weeks [807].

D. Rabbits fed a normal diet were exposed to a carbon monoxide-containing atmosphere for 13 weeks, causing an average carboxyhemoglobin concentration of 11% [1522].

Control groups were treated in exactly the same way as the experimental groups, but were breathing atmospheric air. To omit the influence of individual differences in the response of serum cholesterol to cholesterol feeding, the animals after two weeks were divided into two groups (experimental and control) each having approximately the same average rise in serum cholesterol.

After the experimental period the animals were killed, macroscopic and microscopic autopsy was performed. Special emphasis was laid upon the changes in the hearts and aortas. Furthermore the content of cholesterol, phospholipids, and triglycerides in the aortic tissue was determined.

RESULTS

As shown in the table the analyses of the aortic tissue cholesterol content showed highly characteristic and significantly different values in the experimental groups compared to those of controls. It will be seen that tissue cholesterol in the carbon monoxide-exposed animals was 2.5 times greater than in controls;

Table. *Mean of total cholesterol content of aortic tissue (mg/100 g wet weight)*

	Test number		
	I	II	III
Experimental group ($N=12$)	1774	1399	303
Control group ($N=12$)	703	412	596
Significance	$p<0.001$	$p<0.001$	$p<0.001$

I. Cholesterol feeding and moderate carbon monoxide exposure for ten weeks.
II. Cholesterol feeding and hypoxia (10% O_2 in N_2) for eight weeks.
III. Cholesterol feeding and hyperoxia (28% O_2 in N_2) for ten weeks.

in the hypoxic animals this difference in cholesterol deposition was even more pronounced. Similarly the triglycerides in the aortic tissue were significantly increased in the carbon monoxide-exposed and hypoxic animals, while the phospholipids showed only minimal and nonsignificant changes compared to the controls. On the other hand hyperoxia seems to prevent lipid tissue deposition since the aortic cholesterol content in the hyperoxic group was only half of that in the control group.

Macroscopically it was easy to discern between experimental and control animals, as the former showed far more pronounced changes both in degree

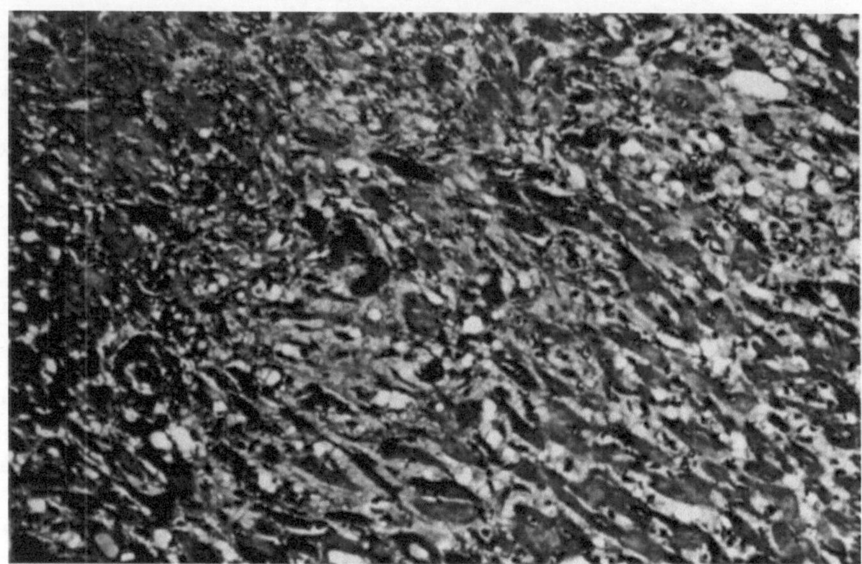

Fig. 1. Myocardium from hypoxic cholesterol-fed rabbit. Pronounced interstitial lipid infiltration is present, causing severe degeneration of the myocardial fibrils. H-E stain ×140

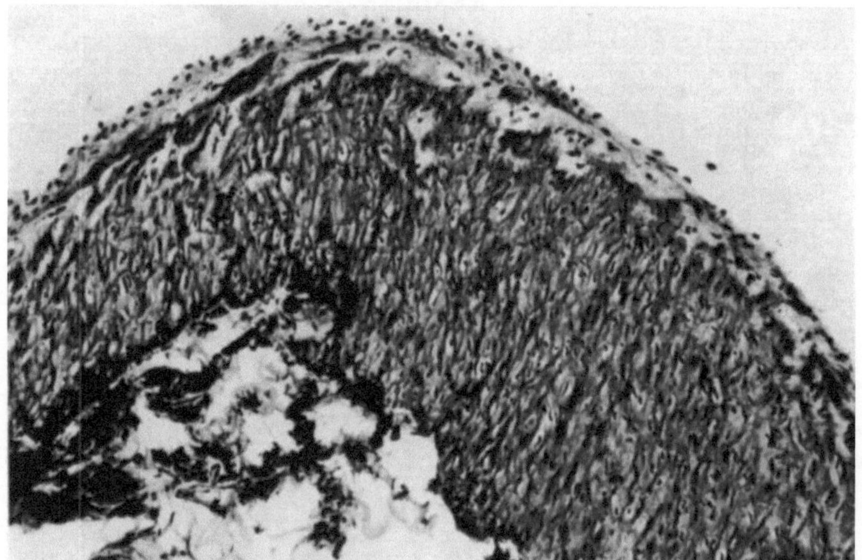

Fig. 2. Aorta from CO-exposed rabbit on a normal diet. Marked intimal-subintimal edema, splitting of the luminal architecture and prominent endothelial cell proliferation are seen. H-E stain ×140

and extent. Microscopy fully confirmed this macroscopic impression. Especially in the hypoxic group a deep "transmural" lipid infiltration of the vascular wall was a conspicuous feature, causing a prominent interstitial "xanthomatosis" in the perivascular structures, e.g. the myocardium (Fig. 1). This "transmural" lipid vascular deposition was in clear contrast to what was seen in the control groups, where the elastic membranes represented at least a relative resistance. In the experiments dealing with rabbits on a normal diet and exposed to small concentrations of carbon monoxide (average 11% carboxyhemoglobin) for 13 weeks, it was possible to demonstrate multifocal vascular damage of the early arteriosclerotic type. These were localized to the intima-subintima zone and characterized by focal edema, reactive fibrosis, and a variety of accompanying degenerative changes and prominent endothelial cell proliferation (Fig. 2).

Other relevant autopsy findings included the frequent occurrence of exudate in the serous cavities (peritoneum, pericardium and pleura), especially in the carbon monoxide-exposed groups. Apart from quantitative differences the changes in the carbon monoxide exposed and the hypoxic groups were identical.

COMMENTS

The biological mechanisms involved in the hypoxic production of vessel injuries are uncertain, but some interesting observations should be mentioned. The frequent presence of abnormal amounts of fluid with relatively high protein concentrations (2–3 g/100 ml) in the serous cavities in many of the carbon monoxide-exposed animals [70, 1522] suggested an increased permeability of the endo- and mesothelial membranes caused by carbon monoxide. Also the localized edematous areas in the aorta, comparable to the well-known valvular and subendocardial edema, probably reflected a disturbance in the transport of fluid across the arterial wall. The findings of an increased vascular permeability for albumin [1362] in human subjects after moderate carbon monoxide and hypoxic exposures suggested that the edema may originate in permeability changes. It should also be stressed that exposure of human individuals to carbon monoxide and to hypoxia is followed by a significant decrease of plasma volume and accumulation of fluid in various tissues. This has been demonstrated at high altitude by other investigators and by Asmussen and Knudsen [67] during carbon monoxide exposure. This decrease in plasma volume is explained by an increased vascular permeability to high molecular substances. The transmural and perivascular accumulation of lipid in our experimental animals also indicates an increased permeability through the vascular membranes. This is also supported by the findings of Robertson [1240] who exposed intimal cells cultivated *in vitro* to decreasing concentrations of oxygen in the surrounding medium, down to 1%, and found increases of six to seven times the uptake of cholesterol, while the synthesis of fatty acids decreased considerably.

The disturbances in enzymatic activities causing the permeability changes of the vessel walls seem to effect the same oxygen-demanding systems during exposure to carbon monoxide as well as to hypoxia, since the lesions are qualitatively similar. The underlying mechanisms of these permeability changes and their significance under physiological and pathological circumstances need further clarification. As the carbon monoxide-exposed rabbits had carboxyhemoglobin values which are not uncommon in heavy smokers, we feel that it is not unreasonable to assume that carbon monoxide in tobacco smoke might be a major factor in the increased morbidity and mortality rates from arteriosclerotic cardiovascular diseases found in smokers.

LOCALIZATION OF LIPID SYNTHESIS BY FOAM CELLS IN ATHEROMATOUS LESIONS*

ALLAN J. DAY and MARK L. WAHLQVIST**

The development of the atherosclerotic lesion is characterized by the accumulation in the intima of increasing amounts of lipid, in particular, of cholesteryl ester and of phospholipid. The origin of this lipid and its role in the pathogenesis of atherosclerosis, however, is still the subject of intensive investigation in various laboratories. Much of the phospholipid and possibly the fatty acid in experimental and human atherosclerotic lesions arises by synthesis *in situ* [1093, 1592]. The cholesterol, on the other hand, appears to originate from the serum by infiltration [162]. In early lesions most of the lipid is present in the foam cells scattered throughout the intima, and the suggestion has been made that these foam cells contribute to the synthesis of lipid in the atherosclerotic arterial wall. This possibility has been investigated in our laboratory, initially using normal macrophages as a model system [371] and more recently, using either foam cells isolated from atherosclerotic lesions or atherosclerotic arteries incubated *in vitro* with ^{14}C-labeled oleic acid. Foam cells isolated from experimental atherosclerotic lesions take up and incorporate ^{32}P-labeled phosphate, ^{14}C-labeled acetate, and ^{14}C-labeled oleic acid into phospholipid and cholesteryl ester [376, 377, 380]. Autoradiographic studies published recently have demonstrated that the fatty acid which is incorporated into phospholipid and cholesteryl ester in the atherosclerotic arterial wall is localized to intimal foam cells [378, 1514].

Herein the question of phospholipid synthesis in the atherosclerotic artery is investigated and data presented indicating that most of such synthesis is localized to the foam cells.

METHODS

Atherosclerotic aortas obtained from rabbits fed 1% cholesterol and 3% peanut oil in the diet for one to four months were used. Human arteries were obtained at surgery or from renal transplant donors. The arteries were incubated *in vitro* in 50:50 Hank's solution: rabbit/human serum containing either ^{14}C-labeled choline or ^{3}H-labeled oleic acid. Following incubation and suitable washing and fixing, portions of the intima were extracted for radioassay and separated into lipid components. The remainder was sectioned and examined by autoradiography using Kodak AR10 stripping film.

---

* Data presented herein is derived from Day and Wahlqvist [379] and Wahlqvist and Day [1513], and is published with the permission of Academic Press.

** This work was supported by grants from the National Heart Foundation of Australia, National Health and Medical Research Council of Australia and U.S.P.H.S Grant No. R05-TW00318. Technical assistance by Mrs. G. M. Neill, Misses J. Dare and A. Lawrence is also gratefully acknowledged.

RESULTS AND DISCUSSION

Experimental Rabbit Atherosclerosis. Up to 11.3% of the ^{14}C-labeled choline present in the medium was taken up by the atherosclerotic rabbit intima and incorporated into phospholipid. Incorporation of the choline into phospholipid in the intima was linear over the four hour period studied and separation of individual phospholipids by thin layer chromatography indicated that most of the choline (80–90% of the total) had been incorporated into lecithin with lesser amounts into the other choline containing phospholipids, sphingomyelin (1.2–5% of the total) and lysolecithin (6.4–13.4% of the total).

In order to confirm that most of the ^{14}C-labeled choline in the artery was present as lipid, radioassay of the protein precipitate and of the Folch wash

Table 1. *Grain counts (No. grains/100 μ^2)* [a] *in autoradiographs prepared from rabbit aortas incubated in vitro with ^{14}C-labeled choline*

Period rabbit cholesterol fed (months)	Incubation time (hours)	Intima		Media
		foam cells	extracellular	
1	4	8.3	5.4	6.2
2	4	8.3	4.5	3.2
3	4	10.7	6.7	9.9
3	1	6.5	1.1	2.0
3	3	11.3	4.6	5.9
3	4	9.6	3.2	5.4
4	0.25	7.3	2.2	14.5
4	0.5	5.9	1.9	7.3

[a] At least 6,000 μ^2 assessed for each feature.

was carried out. Following the standard fixation and washing procedures used, it was found that 94–98% of the ^{14}C-labeled choline present in the artery was present in the lipid extract, so that localization of ^{14}C by autoradiography was indicative of localization of phospholipid synthesis. Autoradiographs indicated that while some of the ^{14}C-labeled phospholipid synthesized was scattered throughout the arterial wall, most of it appeared in the foam cells. Grain counts (Table 1) showing this localization give a quantitative picture of these observations.

When ^{3}H-labeled oleic acid was incubated with atherosclerotic rabbit aortas, most of the oleic acid taken up was incorporated into phospholipid and cholesteryl ester as has been previously shown [378]. Following extraction of the sections with cold acetone most of the ^{3}H-labeled lipid, with the exception of the phospholipid, was removed, so that in the sections presented for autoradiography 88.9% of the ^{3}H was present as phospholipid. This ^{3}H-labeled phospholipid was present almost entirely in foam cells (Fig. 1) so that it can be concluded that the incorporation of ^{3}H-labeled oleic acid into phospholipid which takes place in the atherosclerotic arterial wall occurs predominantly in the foam cells.

Human Atherosclerosis. Similar findings were observed in human fatty streak lesions. ^{14}C-labeled choline was taken up and incorporated primarily into lecithin

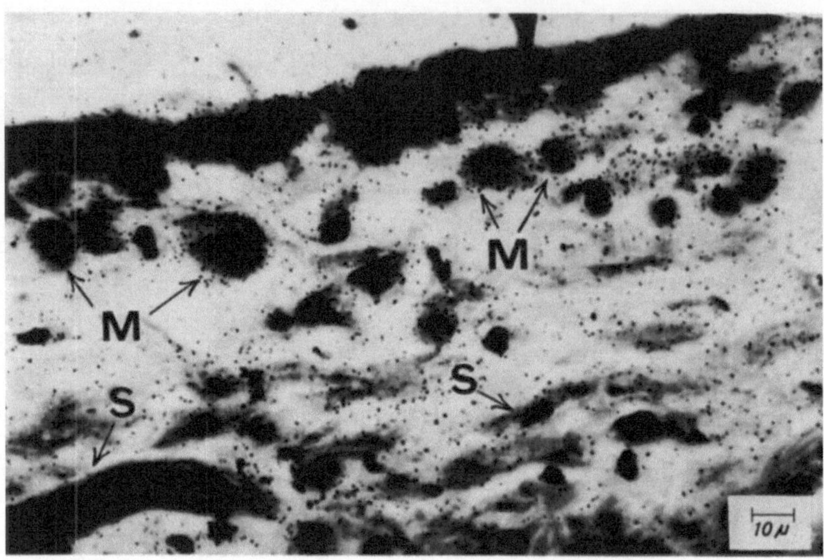

Fig. 1. Autoradiograph of a rabbit atherosclerotic lesion incubated with ^{3}H-oleic acid followed by acetone extraction of the sections. There is localization to superficial round mononuclears (*M*) with little label in spindle-shaped cells (*S*). Hematoxylin and Sudan IV

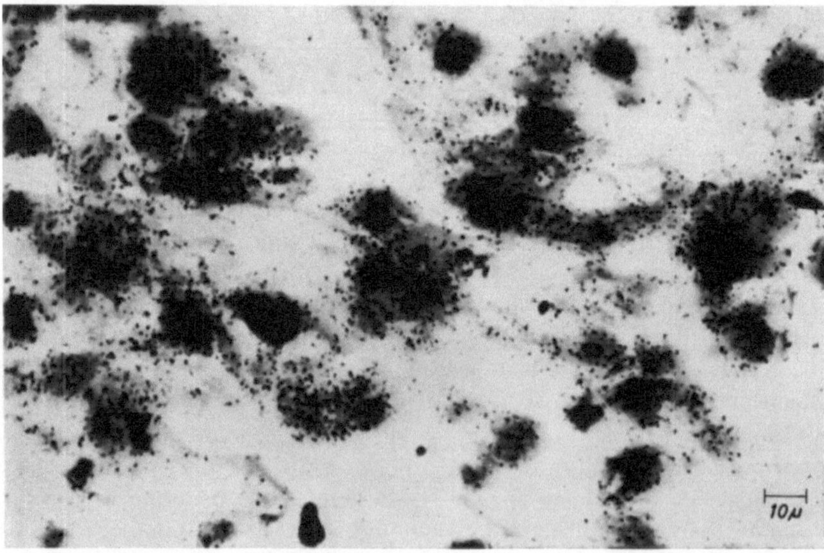

Fig. 2. Autoradiograph of a human atherosclerotic lesion incubated with ^{14}C-choline. Hematoxylin and Sudan IV

by the intimal lesions. Autoradiography showed clear localization of such incorporation to the foam cells of the atherosclerotic lesions (Fig. 2). Quantitative assessment by grain counting indicated that the localization was rather more clear cut than was the case with the rabbit lesions (Table 2). When ^{14}C-labeled oleic acid was used as a precursor followed by acetone extraction of the sections prepared, incorporation of the fatty acid into phospholipid could be observed by autoradiography as a foam cell phenomenon.

Table 2. *Grain counts (No. grains/100 μ^2) in autoradiographs prepared from human atherosclerotic lesions incubated with ^{14}C-labeled choline*[a]

Lesion	Intima				Media
	foam cells	non-sudanophilic round mononuclears	spindle-shaped cells	extra-cellular	
Complicated	14.8	1.5	0.3	0.2	0.1
Fatty streak	14.1	3.0	1.6	2.0	1.6

[a] 6,000 μ^2 counted.

It can be concluded, therefore, that in both human and rabbit atherosclerotic lesions the incorporation of precursors into phospholipid *in vitro* takes place predominantly in the foam cells present. Clearly then, synthesis and metabolism of lipid by these cells influences the composition and development of the atherosclerotic lesion.

THE ROLE OF ARTERIAL ELASTIN IN THE LIPID ACCUMULATION IN HUMAN ATHEROSCLEROTIC ARTERIES

DIETER M. KRAMSCH, WILLIAM HOLLANDER and CARL FRANZBLAU

Accumulation of stainable lipids on structurally altered intimo-medial elastic membranes appears to be one of the earliest manifestations of atherosclerosis [21, 639, 1378]. The present study was undertaken to correlate structural and metabolic changes of arterial elastic membranes in atherosclerotic arteries.

METHODS

Radioautography of arteries was performed according to the method of Kramsch et al. [821] two to four months after intravenous injection of ^3H-cholesterol into moribund humans. Elastin from intimal layers of normal and atherosclerotic aortas (containing some medial elastic membranes) was purified according to the method of Lansing et al. [841], and analyzed for its amino acid and lipid composition. Purified and defatted arterial elastin was incubated with

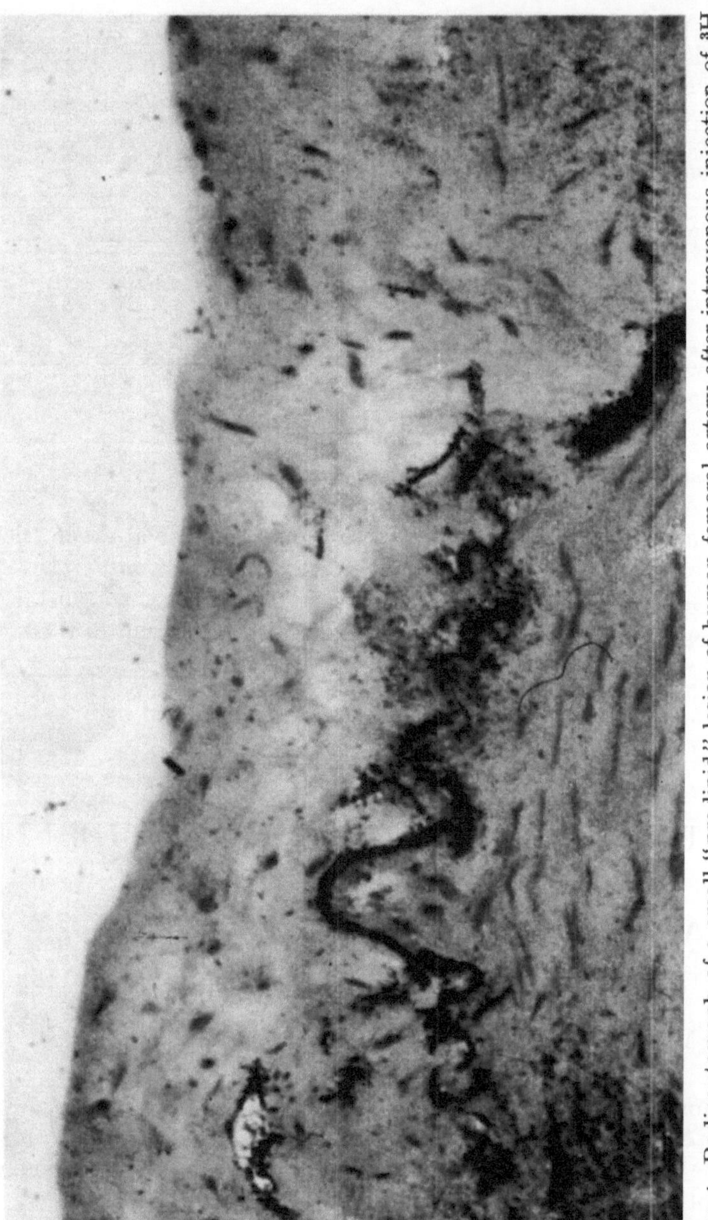

Fig. 1. Radioautograph of a small "pre-lipid" lesion of human femoral artery after intravenous injection of ^{3}H-cholesterol. The black bands represent dense accumulations of ^{3}H-cholesterol on the unstained internal elastic membrane which is split and fragmented. Relatively little cholesterol radioactivity is present, diffusely scattered, in the cellular layers of the thickened intima and in the media. No stainable lipids were detectable in Oil Red 0-stained serial sections from this lesion. Hematoxylin eosin, exposure three weeks, $\times 600$

lipoprotein fractions of normal and hyperlipoproteinemic human serum as well as with lipoproteins extracted from human arteries.

RESULTS

The radioautographs revealed accumulations of cholesterol radioactivity in foam cells and on the fragmented elastic membranes of atherosclerotic plaques.

In advanced plaques no cholesterol radioactivity was found in the amorphous center of the plaque but ^{3}H-cholesterol accumulated on the fragmented elastic membranes at the base and on both sides of the lesion. Dense accumulations of ^{3}H-cholesterol on fragmented internal elastic membranes but not in the cellular

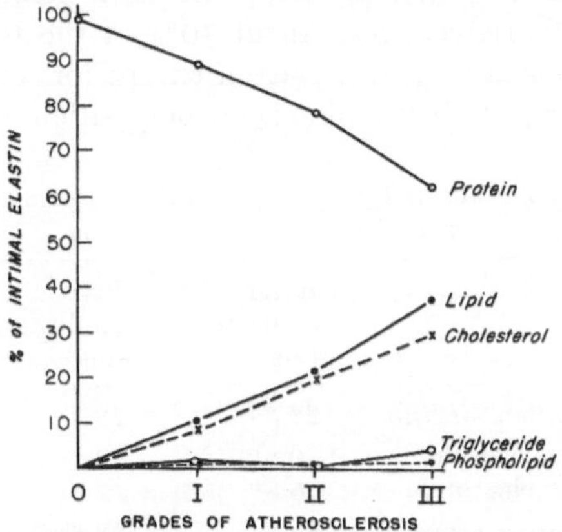

Fig. 2. Protein and lipid composition of plaque elastin from human aortic plaques with increasing severity of atherosclerosis. Grade 0 = intima with no atherosclerotic lesions; Grade I = fatty streaks and pinpoint lesions; Grade II = large confluent plaques; Grade III = severe calcified and ulcerated plaques

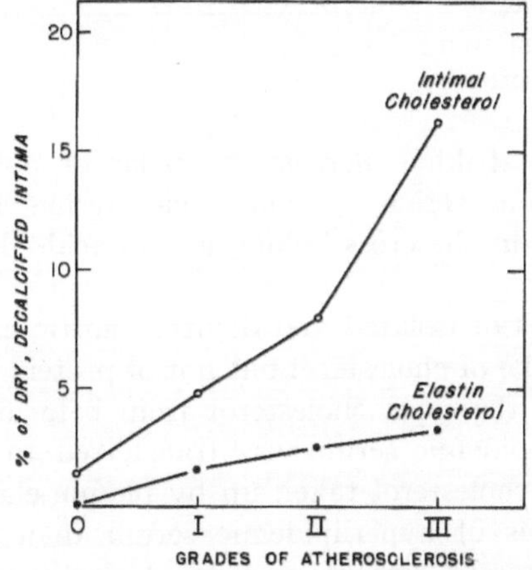

Fig. 3. Total intimal cholesterol content as compared to intimal elastin cholesterol content in human aortic plaques with increasing severity of atherosclerotic as a percentage of dry, calcium-free tissue. Grades of atherosclerosis as in Fig. 2

intima also occurred in small so-called prelipid lesions, i.e., in the absence of stainable lipids (Fig. 1).

Radiochemical analysis of purified arterial elastin revealed that the uptake of intravenously injected ^{3}H-cholesterol by plaque elastin was twice as high as that by normal elastin. Arterial elastin appeared to be a protein-lipid complex containing normally 98% protein and 1 to 2% lipid. The protein and lipid composition of plaque elastin was altered as compared to normal elastin. With increasing severity of atherosclerosis, the lipid moiety increased, and the protein moiety decreased (Fig. 2). In severe plaques the elastin contained about 37% lipid and 63% protein. The lipid increase in plaque elastin was mainly due to large increases in cholesterol, especially ester cholesterol, with minor increases in phospholipids and triglycerides. About 30% of the total intimal cholesterol of plaques was contained in plaque elastin, except for severe plaques with large amorphous centers (Fig. 3). The amino acid composition of plaque elastin protein

Table. *Lipid uptake by normal and plaque elastin incubated with lipoprotein fractions of hyperlipidemic human serum*

		Ester cholesterol (mg)	Free cholesterol (mg)	Phospholipids (mg)	Triglycerides (mg)
	Incubation medium	*22.5*[a]	*12.4*	*9.4*	*43.1*
$d < 1.006$	Normal elastin	0.8[b]	0.1	0.5	1.3
	Plaque elastin	16.8[b]	2.7	2.7	9.1
	Incubation medium	*20.3*	*8.5*	*16.6*	*8.4*
d 1.006–1.063	Normal elastin	2.8	0.2	4.2	1.1
	Plaque elastin	14.8	2.1	4.2	2.7
	Incubation medium	*5.3*	*0.8*	*13.8*	*2.5*
d 1.063–1.210	Normal elastin	0	0	0.2	0
	Plaque elastin	0	0	0.8	0

[a] Incubation medium 10 ml.
[b] Per 50 mg elastin protein.

also was altered with striking increases in polar or polar acting amino acids (aspartic acid, threonine, serine, glutamic acid, lysine, histidine and arginine) and marked decreases in the cross-linking amino acids desmosine, isodesmosine and lysinonorleucine.

In vitro incubations of isolated and defatted aortic elastin with serum lipoproteins revealed uptake of cholesterol but not of protein by plaque elastin. After 24 hours over 75% of the ester cholesterol from beta and prebeta lipoproteins of normal and hyperlipidemic serum was transferred to plaque elastin (Table). The amounts of ester cholesterol taken up by plaque elastin were greater from low density lipoproteins of hyperlipidemic serum than from those of normal serum. The ester cholesterol uptake by normal elastin was much less than by plaque elastin. Only minor amounts of free cholesterol, phospholipids and triglycerides were transferred to both, normal and plaque elastin. Similar lipid transfers to elastin occurred from arterial lipoproteins. The transferred cholesterol was not removed by subsequent incubation with serum apolipoproteins ($alpha_1$, beta and prebeta) or trypsin. No cholesterol transfer occurred from $alpha_1$-lipoproteins or chylomicrons.

CONCLUSION

In conclusion, the deposition of lipid in elastin of fragmented intimal elastic membranes accounts, at least in part, for the accumulation of lipid in the plaque. The prerequisite for lipid accumulation in plaque elastin appears to be an altered amino acid composition of the elastin protein in the plaque. The mechanism involved in the accumulation of lipid in plaque elastin appears to be an interaction of the altered elastin protein with serum or arterial low density lipoproteins. The amount of lipid incorporated into diseased elastin appears to be dependent on the concentration of the low and very low density lipoproteins. The binding of lipid to diseased elastin appears to be firm and may be irreversible.

DEMONSTRATION OF THE POLYOL PATHWAY IN THE AORTIC WALL*

Anthony D. Morrison, Rex S. Clements, Jr., and Albert I. Winegrad

The presence of the polyol pathway in a tissue in which the intracellular transport of glucose is not rate limiting provides the basis of a pathological mechanism that has been implicated in the development of cataracts in diabetes mellitus and galactosemia [800, 1178]. Polyol: NADP oxidoreductase (E.C. 1.1.1.21) catalyses the reduction of a number of aldose sugars to their respective polyol derivatives; this reaction is essentially irreversible in mammalian tissues [674].

$$\text{Glucose} + \text{NADPH} + \text{H}^+ \rightleftharpoons \text{Sorbitol} + \text{NADP}^+$$

Polyol: NADP oxidoreductase

$$\text{Sorbitol} + \text{NAD}^+ \rightleftharpoons \text{Fructose} + \text{NADH} + \text{H}^+$$

L-iditol: NAD oxidoreductase

Polyol: NADP oxidoreductase has high Km's for glucose and galactose whose polyol derivatives (sorbitol and dulcitol) accumulate within the lens in diabetes and galactosemia. The intracellular accumulation of these polyols is accompanied by an increased water content of the lens, a decreased ability to maintain normal intracellular Na^+ and K^+ concentrations, a defect in the active transport of amino acids, and a decreased intracellular concentration of free myoinositol [333, 800, 1178]. These effects have been attributed to the osmotic consequences of polyol accumulation since these compounds cross cell membranes slowly; however, Horecker [707] has speculated that the diversion of NADPH to polyol formation may also play a role. We have previously observed that rabbit aortic intima and media are freely permeable to glucose [1558]. The presence of the polyol pathway in the aortic wall would, therefore, provide a mechanism by

* This work was supported in part by grants from the USPHS, AM 04722, AM 05556, GM 06405 and the Heart Association of Southeastern Pennsylvania. The authors thank Mrs. J. Moffatt, Mrs. M. A. Fletcher and Mrs. Joan Feuer for expert assistance; Dr. Floyd Kupiecki of the Upjohn Co. for samples of prostaglandins E_1, E_2, and $F_{1\alpha}$ and Dr. Albert J. Plummer of the Ciba Co. for samples of Val-5-Hypertensin II.

which elevated plasma glucose levels could result in increased sorbitol formation with consequences similar to those described in the lens. Neutralized perchloric acid extracts of whole rabbit thoracic aorta were found to contain 13.7 ± 0.7 nmoles of sorbitol per g, a concentration five to six times that present in normal rabbit plasma. This suggested that sorbitol was either synthesized or actively concentrated in the aortic wall. Using an *in vitro* preparation, which is comprised of tubular sections of intima and media only from rabbit thoracic aorta [1558], we observed a progressive increase in aortic sorbitol concentration with increasing medium glucose concentration (Fig. 1). In experiments, using paired samples from the same rabbit aorta, the sorbitol content increased 14.1 ± 2.5 nmoles/g

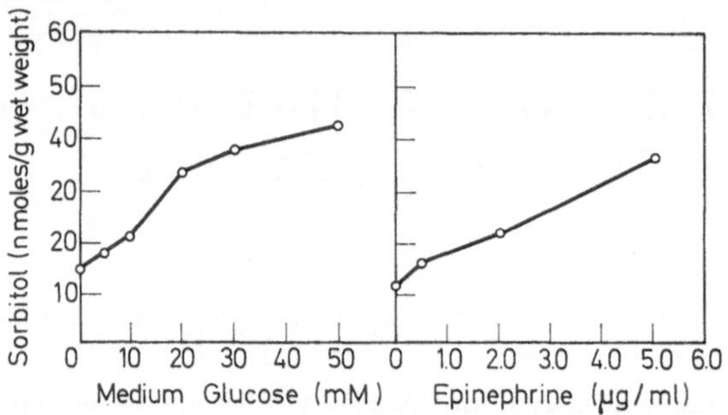

Fig. 1. Pooled aortic samples from 6 rabbits incubated in Krebs-HCO_3 buffer pH 7.4, gas phase 5% CO_2 in air. Left: Samples incubated for 2 hours. Right: Medium glucose concentration 5 mM, samples preincubated for 30 minutes, then transferred to fresh medium containing glucose (5 mM) and epinephrine, and incubated for 30 minutes. [From Clements, R. S., Jr. et al.: Science **166**, 1007–1008 (21. November 1969), Copyright 1969 by the American Association for the Advancement of Science.]

when the medium glucose concentration was increased from 5 to 50 mM. Thus, the ambient glucose concentration appears to regulate the sorbitol content of the aortic wall.

The enzymatic capacity for sorbitol synthesis from glucose in the aortic wall has also been established by the isolation and partial purification of polyol: NADP oxidoreductase from human and rabbit aorta [314]. As shown in the table these enzymes catalyze the reduction of a wide range of aldoses. They have less than 10% of their activity when NADH is substituted for NADPH. Their pH optima are in the range of 6.2; they are activated by sulfate ion and inhibited by chloride ion. L-gulonate: NADP oxidoreductase was also isolated from human and rabbit aorta; this enzyme similarly catalyzes the reduction of a wide range of aldoses, however, the Km's glucose for the human and rabbit aortic enzymes are of the order of 2 M, and it is probable that this enzyme functions primarily in the reduction of D-glucuronate to L-gulonate in the uronic acid pathway.

In the course of these experiments we observed that the sorbitol content of the aortic wall could be acutely altered by the addition of a number of hormonal and pharmacological agents *in vitro*. This provides the first evidence that the activity of the polyol pathway is regulated by factors other than substrate concentration. As shown in Fig. 1 epinephrine (0.5 to 5 μg/ml) increased the sorbitol content of the aortic wall during a 30-minute incubation in media

Table

Substrate	Rabbit polyol: NADP oxidoreductase		Human polyol: NADP oxidoreductase	
	K_m (mM)	relative V_{max}	K_m (mM)	relative V_{max}
D-Glyceraldehyde	0.13	100	0.05	100
D-Erythrose	0.23	54	0.08	74
D-Ribose	20	29	11	43
D-Xylose	15.4	23	14	62
D-Glucuronate	37	77	20	44
D-Glucuronolactone	6	44	7.2	111
D-Glucose	56	23	100	33
D-Galactose	290	22	39	24
NADPH	0.006		0.007	

Activity was assayed spectrophotometrically at 340 mμ in 1.0 ml of potassium phosphate buffer (67 mM) pH 6.2 containing NADPH (0.1 mM) at 30° C. The K_m NADPH was determined in the same system using D-xylose (0.3 M) as substrate.

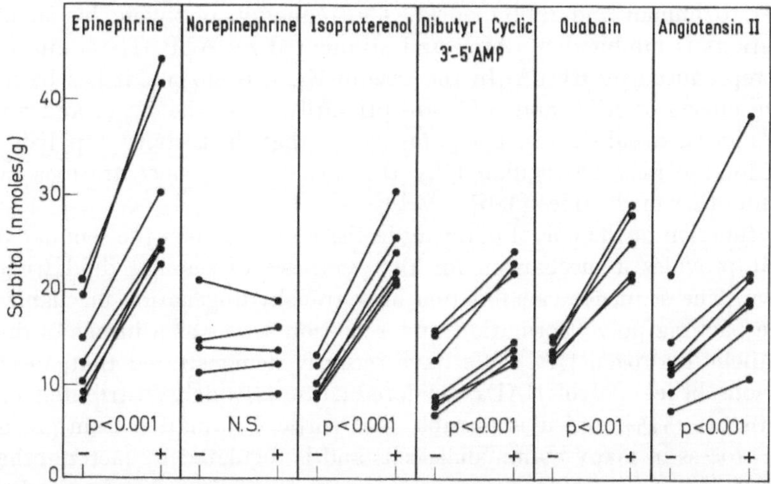

Fig. 2. Paired samples of rabbit thoracic aorta pre-incubated in Krebs-HCO_3 buffer pH 7.4, gas phase 5% CO_2 in air, glucose (5 mM) for 30 minutes; samples transferred to fresh medium and one of each pair incubated as a control (−) and the other with the agent indicated (+) for 30 minutes except in experiments with ouabain (1 hr.) and angiotensin II (2 hrs.). Concentrations added were, L-epinephrine and L-norepinephrine, 2 μg/ml; DL-isoproterenol, 4 μg/ml; dibutyryl cyclic 3′, 5′ AMP, 10^{-4} M; ouabain, 10^{-5} M; angiotensin II, 1 μg/ml. [From Clements, R. S., Jr. et al.: Science **166**, 1007–1008 (21. November 1969), Copyright 1969 by the American Association for the Advancement of Science.]

containing a constant glucose concentration. Norepinephrine (2 μg/ml) had no effect *in vitro*, but isoproterenol *in vitro* also produced significant increases in aortic sorbitol content (Fig. 2). The effects of epinephrine and isoproterenol could be reproduced by the addition of dibutyryl-cyclic 3′,5′ AMP *in vitro* (Fig. 2). Ouabain and angiotensin II added *in vitro* also increased the aortic sorbitol concentration (Fig. 2). Prostaglandins E_1, E_2, and $F_{1\alpha}$ (1 μg/ml) were also tried in this system; however, they did not increase the aortic sorbitol content, nor did they inhibit the response to epinephrine. When aortic samples were incubated in Krebs-bicarbonate buffer containing 5 mM glucose the addition of glyceryl trinitrate (2.6×10^{-4} M) caused a 30% reduction in the aortic sorbitol concentration. (Mean $\Delta = -3.0 \pm 0.4$ nmoles/g $N = 8$.)

The mechanisms by which these hormones and pharmacological agents produce their effects have not been fully elucidated. The aorta lacks glucose-6-phosphatase activity [1581], and it is, therefore, unlikely that phosphorylase activation acutely alters the intracellular free glucose concentration. The effect of epinephrine can be demonstrated in the absence of oxygen and is accompanied by increased lactate production. The ouabain effect, however, occurs without a significant increase in lactate production.

The demonstration of these acute hormonals effects caused us to re-examine the evidence that the activity of polyol:NADP oxidoreductase is regulated primarily by substrate concentration. Polyol:NADP oxidoreductase was isolated and partially purified from rabbit lens, pancreas, and sciatic nerve [316] in addition to human and rabbit aorta. The reduction of xylose by all of these preparations is inhibited by ADP and stimulated by ATP. These effects could not be reproduced by EDTA. In the case of the lens enzyme it has been shown that the effects of ADP and ATP are primarily upon the V_{max}, and not upon the K_m's for these substrates. The data suggest that the activity of polyol:NADP oxidoreductase may be regulated by the intracellular concentrations of ATP, ADP and other nucleotides [316].

The function of the polyol pathway in tissues other than the seminal vesicles, where it provides a mechanism for the synthesis of seminal fluid fructose, is unknown. The sequence can function as a transhydrogenation mechanism, and in some bacteria polyol formation and secretion serves as a means of disposing of metabolic hydrogen [708]. We have recently demonstrated that, in contrast to previous belief, polyol:NADP oxidoreductase is widely distributed in mammalial tissues [315], and it is possible that sorbitol formation from glucose is a normal process in many mammalian cells and is regulated by factors other than ambient substrate level. However, it is apparent from studies in the lens that tissues in which the intracellular transport of substrates for polyol:NADP oxidoreductase is not rate limiting are at risk when the plasma level of glucose is persistently elevated. This situation probably is prevalent in the aortic wall, although the specific cells that contain polyol:NADP oxidoreductase and in which sorbitol levels rise with increasing ambient glucose concentration have not been identified. The pathophysiologic consequences of polyol accumulation in the aortic wall remain to be documented, but the observations reported do indicate a potential biochemical mechanism by which hyperglycemia could lead to a significant derangement in the metabolism of the arterial wall.

ON THE ETIOLOGY AND PROPHYLAXIS OF ATHEROSCLEROSIS AND ISCHEMIC HEART DISEASE

V. V. Tyavokin

Comprehensive and specific prophylactic measures against atherosclerosis and ischemic heart disease are impossible without proper understanding of the etiology of these diseases. In considering the etiology of atherosclerosis and ischemic heart disease it would be rational to proceed on the basis of the following data:

1. Classical experiments of N. N. Anitschkov, S. S. Khalatov [52] and numerous investigations by their collaborators have clearly shown the contribution of cholesterol to the progression of atherosclerosis. The alimentary factor in human atherosclerosis is emphasized in numerous epidemiological investigations in this country and abroad [533, 1200].

2. Overstraining of the function of the central nervous system contributes to the progression of atherosclerosis [1075].

3. Oxygen shortage in the inspired air enhances the development of experimental cholesterol atherosclerosis [44, 802]; and conversely, systematic oxygen inhalations reduce or prevent the development of experimental atherosclerosis in rabbits [882, 883]. The important contribution of hypoxia to the development of human atherosclerosis is stated in a number of clinical investigations [995–997, 1489]. I. V. Maximova [944] demonstrated the favorable effect of oxygen therapy on the lipids, lipoproteins, and protein blood fraction of atherosclerotic patients.

4. Mental workers are more often affected by atherosclerosis and ischemic heart disease than manual workers [1074, 1179, 1211, 1423]. Stewart [1423] states that atherosclerosis of mental workers occurs five to eleven times more often than that of manual workers. I. A. Ryvkin [1273] states that myocardial infarction occurs two to three times more often among employees than among employers; the same proportion holds true for an urban population as compared to a rural population.

5. Experimental atherosclerosis with coronary insufficiency is reproduced by restricting the mobility of rabbits without administering exogenous cholesterol [1482–1485]. In a short period (10 to 30 days) of restricted mobility substantial cardiac and aortic changes were produced: atherosclerotic protuberances, ulcerations, aortic aneurysm (Fig. 1), and stenosis or full closing of the coronary arteries (Fig. 2). The main etiological factor in these experiments responsible for development of coronary atherosclerosis and insufficiency is the restriction of muscular activity, hypodynamia [1485]. The pathogenesis of atherosclerosis and coronary insufficiency in experiments on rabbits with restricted mobility is very complex and demonstrates disturbances not only in lipid metabolism but also in protein, carbohydrate, and mineral metabolism which accompany the reduced function of the sympathetic-adrenal system and adrenal cortex.

Clinical, epidemiological, and experimental data indicate the multiple etiology of atherosclerosis and ischemic heart disease, revealing the following important factors: (1) restriction of muscular mobility (hypodynamia); (2) overstrain of central nervous function; (3) abundant food with excessive cholesterol content; (4) insufficient oxygen content of the inspired air.

Which of the factors is decisive in the development of human atherosclerosis and ischemic heart disease? Information gathered in recent years shows that the alimentary factor in the etiology of atherosclerosis cannot be considered decisive. The inhabitants of Mongolia are very seldom affected by atherosclerosis

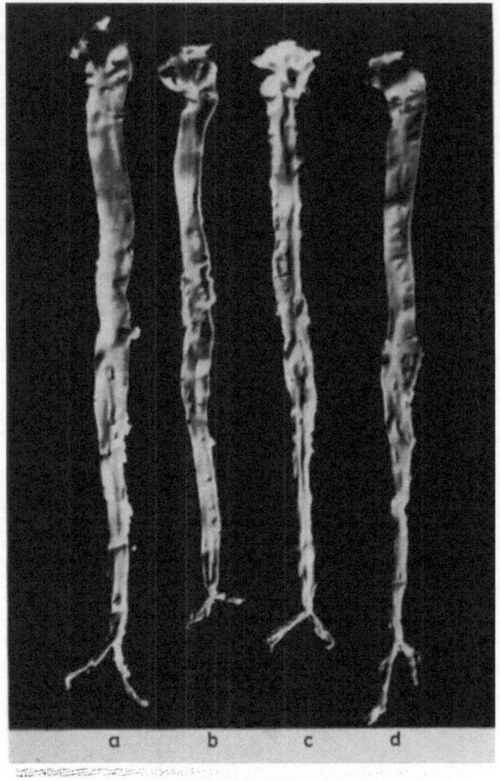

Fig. 1 a—d. Various extent of atherosclerotic changes in aortae of rabbits, occurring during the period of movement restriction. a Intima roughness in the pectoral and abdominal parts; b numerous protuberances in the aortic arch and ulceration in the abdominal part; c ulcerated protuberances in the pectoral and abdominal parts of aorta; d aorta aneurysm in the abdominal part; ulcer and ulcerated protuberances in the centre of the aneurysm

and myocardial infarction though their food is rich in animal fats; while Sahara shepherds never suffer from atherosclerosis, though their food ration comprises large amounts of camel milk with a high percentage of fat.

The nervous theory of atherosclerosis etiology [1075] also gives no explanation for the increase of atherosclerosis and ischemic heart disease in the postwar years. The attempt to explain this fact, from the point of view of the nervous theory, leads to the conclusion that people of all the countries suffered in the postwar years from greater nervous strain than they did in the years during World War II.

It is an established fact that during the war when nervous strain was very often excessive atherosclerosis and ischemic heart disease were seen less widely than in postwar years [276, 473, 498, 734, 1154, 1322]. The cause for expansion of these diseases in postwar years should be sought in the way people live. What are the changes in the way of life that characterize the postwar years? In recent years people are more often, and for a longer time, placed in conditions of restricted muscular activity.

Thus, based on clinical observations [1480]; on experimental data, in which the main factor causing atherosclerosis and coronary insufficiency is hypodynamia;

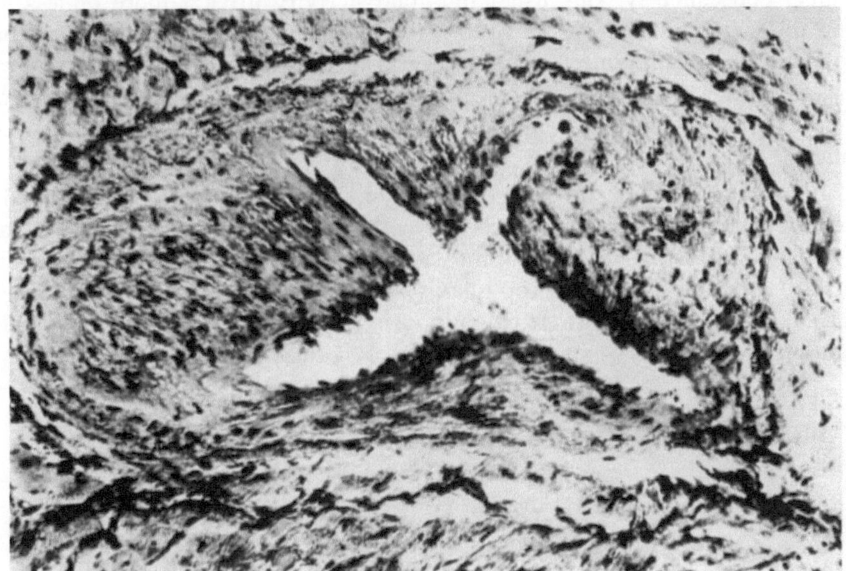

Fig. 2. Heart of the rabbit that perished in 12 days from the onset of movement restriction. Considerable stenosis of the coronary artery branch. Stained after Van Gieson, enlargement ×240

on comparatively frequent occurrences of atherosclerosis and ischemic heart disease in manual and mental workers; and on the expansion of these diseases in the postwar years, one can assume that the main etiological factor in the development of human atherosclerosis and ischemic heart disease is the restriction of muscular mobility (hypodynamia).

Our experimental data indicate that atherosclerosis and coronary heart disease should be considered as a unit; coronary heart disease must not be considered as simply a complication of coronary atherosclerosis. In our experiments with restricted mobility in rabbits, by varying the extent and duration of mobility, it becomes possible to deliberately reproduce in some cases coronary insufficiency without atherosclerosis and in others coronary insufficiency with atherosclerosis.

The present state of development of the problems of atherosclerosis and ischemic heart disease etiology allows us to undertake wider and more specific prophylactic measures against these diseases. Prophylaxis of atherosclerotic and ischemic heart disease comprises possible elimination or reduction of the deteriorating effect of the etiological factors, primarily the main one, i.e. restriction of muscular activity. The simultaneous action of all the preceding factors on the human organism is exceedingly dangerous.

In recent years both popular and scientific medical literature recommend physical exercise and sports as prophylactic measures against atherosclerosis and disturbances in coronary circulation. However, these exercises if carried out improperly can lead not only to the elimination but even to an enhancement of cardiovascular disturbances. In our experiment seven rabbits perished in conditions of their usual muscular activity after the end of a period of restricted mobility. Consequently, this usual muscular activity after a more or less long period of restricted mobility proved to be excessive. These experimental data have clinical confirmation; there are several instances of patients affected with myocardial infarction who pass more or less successfully through the acute and subacute periods of the disease but then perish after passing on to a less restricted regime.

Thus, the elimination or reduction of hypodynamia should be considered as a primary measure in the prophylaxis of atherosclerosis and ischemic heart disease. The development of corresponding measures is an urgent problem for hygienists, clinicians and physiologists. Prophylaxis of atherosclerotic and ischemic heart disease cannot be complete with only the preceding measures. While these measures are of primary importance, there are others that should be taken.

SYNTHESIS OF LIPIDS FROM GLUCOSE AND INCORPORATION OF PALMITATE IN ATHEROSCLEROTIC AND NORMAL RABBIT AORTA

S. BJØRKERUD

The definitive origin of lipids in atherosclerotic lesions is still uncertain. Thrombotic material, lipoproteins, and local synthesis have been suggested. Although, it now seems likely that the main part of the cholesterol in the atherosclerotic lesions is derived from plasma, it can be concluded from a multitude of evidence that the tissue of the artery wall is actively engaged in the atherosclerotic process (for review see Adams [13]).

Very little is known about the capacity of the arterial wall for the formation of lipids from glucose, an important question as a relationship between hyperglycemia and arterial disease has been found in population studies (for references see Stout [1425]). The scope of the present work was to study the incorporation of palmitate and glucose into different lipid classes in defined samples of atherosclerotic intima, underlying media, and normal aortic wall from normo-lipidemic rabbits.

MATERIAL AND METHODS

Atherosclerosis was induced in the aorta of male albino rabbits of the same strain, who were fed standard rabbit pellets and hay, by transverse, superficial, mechanical trauma as described by Bjørkerud [169, 170]. The abdominal aorta was injured at 2 cm intervals. In the injured segments nonregressive lesions developed which were morphologically very similar to early human atherosclerotic lesions [169].

From the atherosclerotic segments, samples of intima (denoted atherosclerotic intima) and of underlying media (denoted atherosclerotic media) were separated by means of microdissection in ice-cooled Krebs-Henseleit-original Ringer bicarbonate buffer (KRB) under a stereomicroscope. Samples of apparently normal wall between lesions served as one series of controls (denoted control media operated) and samples of unoperated animals as a second (denoted control media unoperated).

The samples were incubated at 37° C for four hours in KRB with addition of, for the glucose experiments, ^{14}C-U-glucose, and, for the palmitate experiments, ^{14}C-U-palmitate coupled to defatted, bovine serum albumin. After incubation, the samples were washed, extracted for lipids, freeze-dried, weighed [171] and their DNA content measured according to Kissane and Robins [805].

The lipid extracts were washed and fractionated on silicic acid thin-layer plates for different neutral and phospholipid classes [171]. The radioactivity of each lipid fraction and of aliquots of the total lipid extracts were measured in a Packard Tri-Carb liquid scintillation spectrometer. The lipid fractions were: lysolecithin, sphingomyelin, lecithin, phosphatidyl inositol, a fraction probably representing phosphatidyl ethanolamine, cholesterol and/or diglyceride, free fatty acids, triglycerides, cholesteryl ester, and two unidentified fractions.

RESULTS

The rates of incorporation for the different tissues of fatty acid and of glucose based on DNA are given in Table 1 (A). The incorporation of fatty acid was rapid in unoperated controls and in atherosclerotic intima, and was significantly slower in atherosclerotic media. Similarly, glucose was incorporated into total lipids at a lower rate in atherosclerotic media.

The incorporation rates of fatty acid into the different lipid classes did not differ for atherosclerotic intima and controls. In atherosclerotic media fatty acid incorporation occurred at a lower rate than in unoperated controls into the following lipid classes: cholesterol and/or diglycerides, triglycerides, lecithin, phosphatidyl inositol, sphingomyelin [as seen in Table 1(C)], and a fraction probably representing phosphatidyl ethanolamine. Glucose, on the other hand, was more rapidly incorporated into cholesteryl ester [Table 1(B)], sphingomyelin [Table 1(C)], and free fatty acids (Table 2) in both atherosclerotic intima and media than in unoperated controls. In addition, incorporation into lysolecithin and into triglyceride was more rapid and lecithin slower in atherosclerotic

Table 1. *Incorporation of palmitate and glucose into lipids in atherosclerotic and control tissues (mean ± S.D.)* [a]

Precursor	Control media unoperated	Control media operated	Atherosclerotic intima	Atherosclerotic media
(A) μμ Eq fatty acid or μμ moles glucose into total lipids/μg DNA/hour				
Fatty acid[1]	3.53 ± 1.06^{nx}	1.95 ± 0.82^{nm}	2.98 ± 1.57^{o}	0.68 ± 0.54^{xmo}
Glucose[2]	7.97 ± 1.88^{x}	6.25 ± 3.29^{a}	7.31 ± 1.94^{y}	3.75 ± 1.67^{xay}
(B) mμμ Eq fatty acid or mμμ moles glucose into cholesteryl ester/μg DNA/hour				
Fatty acid[1]	15 ± 18^{a}	99 ± 122^{a}	38 ± 40	48 ± 78
Glucose[3]	0 ± 0^{nm}	2 ± 3^{ao}	98 ± 107^{an}	197 ± 149mo
(C) mμμ Eq fatty acid or mμμ moles glucose into sphingomyelin/μg DNA/hour				
Fatty acid[4]	197 ± 62^{ax}	128 ± 84^{abc}	244 ± 145^{bn}	44 ± 46^{xcn}
Glucose[5]	0 ± 0^{anm}	77 ± 90^{abc}	374 ± 340^{bn}	442 ± 413^{cm}

[a] Values in the same row having the same superscript were different at the significance level indicated by the following: a, b, c, d = $p < 0.05$; n, m, o = $p < 0.01$; x, y, z = $p < 0.001$.

[1] Three unoperated animals with each four samples; four operated animals with duplicate samples of each tissue.

[2] Three unoperated animals with each four samples; six operated animals with duplicate samples of each tissue except for single sample and triplicate samples of control media operated from two animals.

[3] Three unoperated animals with each four samples; three operated animals with duplicate samples of each tissue and one animal with duplicate samples of atherosclerotic tissues.

[4] Three unoperated animals with each four samples; three operated animals with duplicate samples of each tissue and one animal with duplicate samples of atherosclerotic tissues.

[5] Three unoperated samples with each four samples; four operated with duplicate samples of each tissue except for atherosclerotic media with single samples in two animals.

Table 2. *Incorporation of glucose into free fatty acids, triglycerides, lecithin, and lysolecithin in atherosclerotic and control tissues*

	mμμ moles glucose/μg DNA/hour (mean ± S.D.)			
	Control media unoperated[2]	Control media operated[3]	Atherosclerotic intima[4]	Atherosclerotic media[5]
FFA[1]	33 ± 52^{nm}	226 ± 167	303 ± 209^{n}	288 ± 226^{m}
TG[1]	$2{,}336 \pm 1{,}274^{n}$	$1{,}739 \pm 1{,}397$	$1{,}726 \pm 1{,}300$	$1{,}144 \pm 533^{n}$
L[1]	$3{,}176 \pm 943^{abx}$	$2{,}076 \pm 1{,}219^{an}$	$2{,}236 \pm 1{,}049^{bm}$	569 ± 372^{xnm}
LL[1]	3 ± 10^{abn}	42 ± 43^{acd}	209 ± 235^{bc}	241 ± 223^{dn}

[1] FFA = free fatty acids; TG = triglycerides; L = lecithin; LL = lysolecithin.

[2] Three unoperated animals with four samples each.

[3] FFA: two animals with duplicate and single samples; TG: two animals with duplicate and one with single sample; L, LL: two animals with duplicate, one with triplicate and one with single sample.

[4] FFA: three animals with duplicate samples; TG, L, LL: four animals with duplicate samples.

[5] FFA: three animals with duplicate samples; TG, L, LL: three animals with duplicate and one with single sample. Superscripts of values: see Table 1.

Table 3. *DNA content in atherosclerotic and control tissues. µg DNA/mg dry defatted tissue (mean ± S.D.)*

Control media unoperated[1]	Control media operated[2]	Atherosclerotic intima[2]	Atherosclerotic media[2]
7.9 ± 0.9^{abn}	7.0 ± 2.3^{am}	9.7 ± 3.1^{nmo}	6.8 ± 2.7^{bo}

[1] Six animals with each four samples.

[2] Nine animals with duplicate and one animal with four samples of each tissue. Superscripts of values: see Table 1.

media than in unoperated controls (Table 2). Although, not significant, there was a trend for similar differences between unoperated controls and the two other tissues from operated animals (Table 2).

The relation between DNA content and dry defatted weight in the different tissues is given in Table 3. The DNA content was highest in atherosclerotic intima, intermediate in operated controls, and low in operated controls and atherosclerotic media.

DISCUSSION

The reciprocal findings with regard to lysolecithin and free fatty acids, on one hand, and triglycerides and lecithin, on the other, suggest the presence of lipases in the atherosclerotic tissues, although a decreased formation of triglycerides and lecithin cannot be ruled out. With regard to cholesteryl ester and sphingomyelin, however, the differences observed are likely to reflect different synthetic rates rather than differences with regard to decomposition since different positioning of label from the two precursors seems improbable within these molecules.

The relation between DNA content and dry defatted weight in the different tissues makes possible an evaluation as to the effect of differences observed for an atherosclerotic segment as a whole. For an atherosclerotic segment the high cellularity of the atherosclerotic intima tends to increase the differences found on a per cell basis. The lower cell content of the atherosclerotic media suggests, together with the lower rate of synthesis of total lipids from both precursors, tissue damage.

The rate of synthesis of cholesteryl ester and sphingomyelin from glucose was higher in the cells of both atherosclerotic tissues although total lipogenesis was lower in the media cells. As total lipogenesis was not higher in the atherosclerotic tissues than in controls, the composition of the lipid mixture formed from glucose was abnormal in the atherosclerotic tissues with a higher proportion of cholesteryl ester and sphingomyelin.

The results suggest that local synthesis may be responsible for accumulation in atherosclerotic lesions of cholesteryl ester and sphingomyelin, which together with cholesterol constitute the major atheroma lipids. Formation of lipids from carbohydrates seems to be a probable source.

THE INFLUENCE OF PROSTAGLANDIN E_1 ON EXPERIMENTAL PLATELET AGGREGATION IN RATS

J. JOHN GOTTENBOS and GERARD HORNSTRA

In our laboratory Kloeze [810] found that prostaglandin E_1 (PGE_1) inhibits the adenosine disphosphate (ADP)-induced platelet aggregation in citrated platelet rich plasma. We investigated the influence of PGE_1 on the hemostatic process in rats *in vivo*. To this end a curved polythene canula, the aorta loop, was inserted into the aorta between the spermatic and the iliolumbar arteries. This siliconized aortic loop remained patent for about five days. By continuous intravenous administration of 7.5 μg PGE_1/hr. this period was prolonged by 50% (e.g. from 5.3 to 7.9 days, $n=5$). From histological investigation it appeared that beginning proximally from the loop, the aortic lumen gradually became obstructed by a growing plug. This obstruction was initiated by the aggregation of platelets which then degenerated to form the plug.

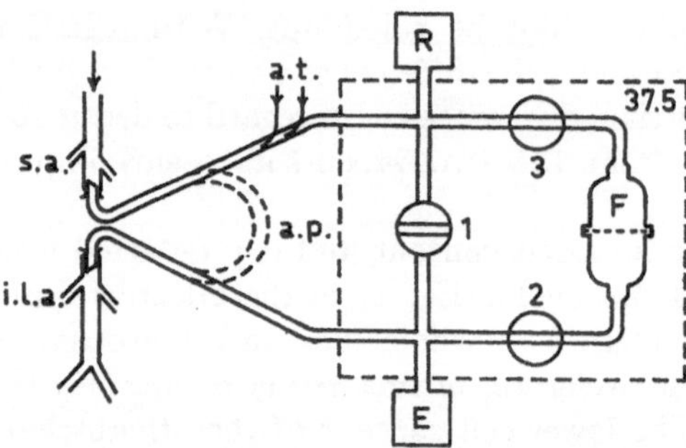

Fig. 1. Scheme of set-up for measuring thrombocyte aggregation: *a.p.* aorta prosthesis (cut through); *s.a.* spermatic artery; *i.l.a.* iliolumbar artery; *R* recording of reference pressure; *E* recording of experimental pressure; *F* filter; *a.t.* administration of test solutions; *1, 2, 3* clamps

In order to study the influence of PGE_1 on the initial phase of this intra-arterial thrombosis we developed a method for continuously measuring the degree of platelet aggregation and disaggregation in circulating blood of rats. By means of the aorta loop a filter (pore size 20 μm), as introduced by Swank [1446] for *in vitro* experiments, is connected to the arterial circulation of rats (see Fig. 1). The blood pressure is measured proximal and distal to the filter, and solutions are infused proximally. Filter and connecting tubes are siliconized and kept at 37.5° C. The blood stream can be directed via a by-pass or through the filter by means of clamps. Aggregates which occur in the blood stream obstruct the filter, as a result of which the pressure distal to the filter (the experimental pressure, EP) drops. The pressure proximal to the filter (the reference pressure, RP) increases slightly (see Fig. 2). The degree of aggregation, designated by the aggregation index A, is obtained by expressing the ratio of the minimal experimental and corresponding reference pressures after ADP administration (EP_2:RP_2) as a percentage of the ratio between experimental and reference pressure at the beginning of the ADP infusion (EP_1:RP_1) and subtracting it from 100. Therefore,

$$A = 100\left(1 - \frac{EP_2}{RP_2}\frac{RP_1}{EP_1}\right)$$

Microscopic examination of the material on the filter, as well as blood smears and thrombocyte-counts from blood taken proximal and distal to the filter

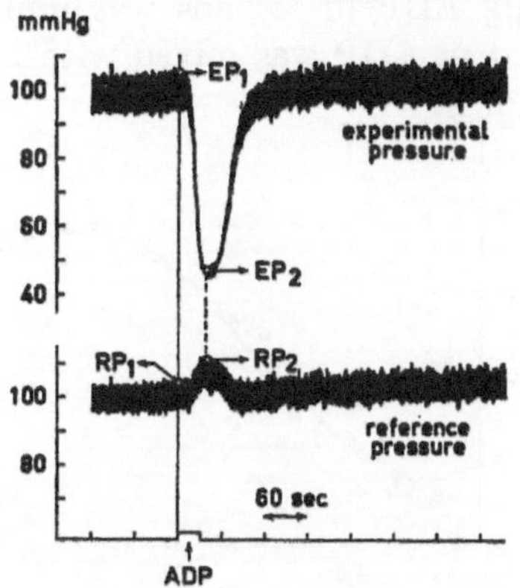

Fig. 2. Recording of an aggregation measurement

Table. *Aggregation inhibiting effect of increasing amounts of PGE_1 in circulating arterial rat blood ($n = 8$)* [a]

PGE_1 dose ($\times 10^{-2}$ µg/30 sec)	A_1	A_2	ΔA
0.00	78.9	77.4	1.5
0.16	76.1	69.6	6.5
0.31	68.5	57.8	10.6
0.62	63.0	42.9	20.1
1.25	66.0	43.0	23.0
2.50	69.0	26.9	42.1
5.00	61.7	18.1	43.6

[a] A_1: aggregation caused by ADP (0.06 µg/30 sec); A_2: aggregation caused by ADP + PGE_1; ΔA: inhibiting effect of PGE_1.

during ADP infusion, showed that occlusion of the filter is almost exclusively caused by thrombocytes. To induce thrombocyte aggregation an isotonic ADP solution is infused proximal to the filter at a rate of 0.1 ml/min for 30 seconds. After ADP administration, the pressure distal to the filter rapidly returns to its initial level, usually within a few minutes. This indicates a cleaning of the filter as a result of disaggregation. The time between two consecutive measurements is standardized at 10 minutes.

The degree of thrombocyte aggregation depends upon the dose of ADP. To obtain the dose-response curve each dose of ADP was administered twice to separate animals. Fig. 3 shows the relationship between the ADP dose and the aggregation index after the first and second measurement in the same animal. Statistical evaluation showed that there were no significant differences between the two dose-response curves, indicating that complete recovery of platelet response to ADP had occurred within the 10 minutes time lapse between the two measurements. After mixing PGE_1 with ADP, the aggregation-inhibiting action of PGE_1 can, therefore, be calculated simply by subtracting the aggregation index caused by the PGE_1/ADP mixture from that caused by the ADP alone. In all experiments 0.06 μg ADP/30 seconds was infused, while in the second determination this amount of ADP was mixed with increasing doses of PGE_1.

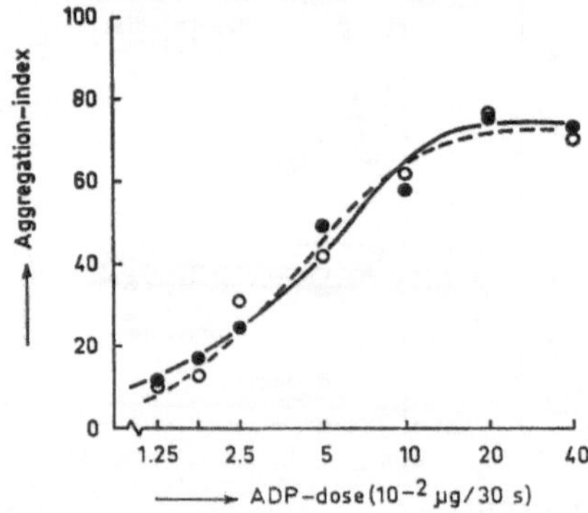

Fig. 3. Relation between ADP dose and aggregation index at the first (●——●) and second (○——○) measurement (mean of 10 experiments per dose)

The results are given in the Table and show a significant positive rectilinear relationship between the log dose PGE_1 and its aggregation inhibiting effect ($y = 71.4 + 26.8x$).

In clinical application of PGE_1 for the prevention of intravascular thrombosis, it is necessary to introduce the substance into the blood stream. Two important problems arise:

1. Because of the great hypotensive activity of PGE_1, the dose must be as low as possible.

2. Because of the rapid break down of PGE_1 in the body, a continuous supply to the blood stream is essential.

The method of aggregation measurement developed here makes it possible to determine how long the amount of PGE_1 which has been brought into a depot exerts its aggregation-inhibiting effect and what other effects the substance has, e.g. its influence on the blood pressure.

This has been investigated by a single subcutaneous, intramuscular or intraperitoneal administration of 50 μg PGE_1. In groups of six animals aggregation measurements were carried out every ten minutes with the standard dose of ADP (0.06 μg during 30 seconds). One minute before the second measurement PGE_1 dissolved in physiological saline was administered via one of the three routes mentioned. As a reference, the same number of animals were injected with an equal amount of physiological saline without PGE_1. An insight into the aggregation inhibiting effect of PGE_1 was then obtained by correcting the course of the aggregation index in the prostaglandin group for the course of the aggregation index in the reference group.

Fig. 4 shows the course of this inhibition with the time. The solid symbols indicate a significant aggregation inhibition, the open symbols a nonsignificant inhibition. It appears from the figure that after subcutaneous prostaglandin administration the effect is no longer significant within 21 minutes and that after intramuscular administration the significant inhibition period is < 31 minutes.

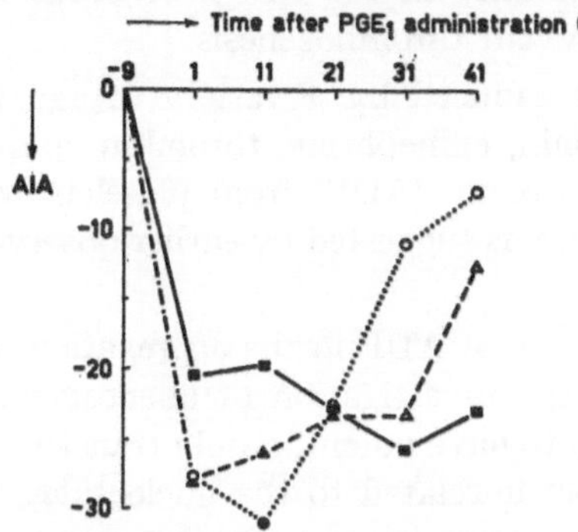

Fig. 4. Aggregation inhibiting action (AIA) of 50 μg PGE_1 administered subcutaneously (○····○), intramuscularly (■----■) and intraperitoneally (▲——▲)

The aggregation inhibition after intraperitoneal administration lasted longer than the experiment proper but remained significant for 70 minutes in later experiments.

The administration of PGE_1 invariably caused a mean drop in blood pressure of 20% with normal pressure completely restored within 11 minutes.

Further experiments showed that intraperitoneal administration of a dose of 12.5 μg PGE_1 did not influence the blood pressure whereas its aggregation-inhibiting effect was about the same as that induced by 50 μg PGE_1.

These results suggest that the application of PGE_1 for the prevention of intravascular thrombosis might be a useful extension of the existing therapeutic possibilities. An important application might also be found in the maintenance of thrombocytes otherwise lost to adhesion and aggregation in hemodialysis, heart-lung machines, etc.

BIOCHEMICAL ROLE OF PROSTAGLANDIN E_1 IN THE INHIBITION OF PLATELET AGGREGATION

NORMAN R. MARQUIS, ROGER L. VIGDAHL and PETER A. TAVORMINA

The vital role of blood platelets in the initiation of thrombogenesis suggests that the prevention of platelet cohesion or aggregation should lead to the prevention of thrombosis. Therefore, an understanding of the mechanism of aggregation seems of paramount importance in the design of drugs which will specifically inhibit aggregation and prevent thrombogenesis.

Platelet aggregation is induced by a variety of agents; some of the more physiological ones—serotonin, epinephrine, thrombin, and collagen—initiate the release of adenosine diphosphate (ADP) from platelets which in turn initiates the aggregation phenomenon as suggested by earlier observations of Hellem [657] and Gaarder [508].

Because of the implication of ADP in the aggregation mechanism, the search for inhibitors has led to the investigation of adenosine derivatives [205, 982] some of which have proven to have potent, if only transient, inhibitory properties. Several agents, structurally unrelated to the nucleotides (prostaglandin E_1 and 8-iso-prostaglandin E_1) have been found to inhibit aggregation at very low concentrations [1338], indicating that perhaps a regulatory mechanism may be involved. Consequently, we have investigated the mechanism by which one of the more potent prostaglandins (PGE_1) inhibits platelet aggregation.

MATERIALS AND METHODS

The processing of human blood, the preparation of isolated platelets and platelet membrane fractions, the assay of platelet phosphodiesterase and adenyl cyclase [824] have been described in a preliminary communication by Marquis [931]. Platelet aggregation was assayed by a modification of the method of Born [215] to be described in another communication (Marquis, unpublished data).

RESULTS AND DISCUSSION

Inhibition of Aggregation by Cyclic AMP. We have observed that cyclic AMP (C-AMP) or its dibutyryl derivative inhibits the aggregation of human platelets induced by ADP (Fig. 1), collagen and epinephrine (unpublished observation). The high concentrations necessary for inhibition are probably a result of the relative impermeability of the cell membrane. Dibutyryl C-AMP exhibits a greater activity than C-AMP per se, probably because it is more lipophilic or less susceptible to degradation.

Effects of PGE_1 on Isolated Platelet Membrane Adenyl Cyclase. Since it has recently been shown by Butcher [273] that PGE_1 affects the adenyl cyclase system in certain tissues, we examined the possibility that the prostaglandin effected the inhibition of platelet aggregation by altering adenyl cyclase activity.

Platelet adenyl cyclase is associated with the membrane fraction and is not detectable in the cytoplasmic fraction. C-AMP synthesis by membrane fractions is stimulated by NaF and PGE_1 and increases linearly with time, with the concentration of enzyme protein, and with the level of PGE_1 added [931]. Levels

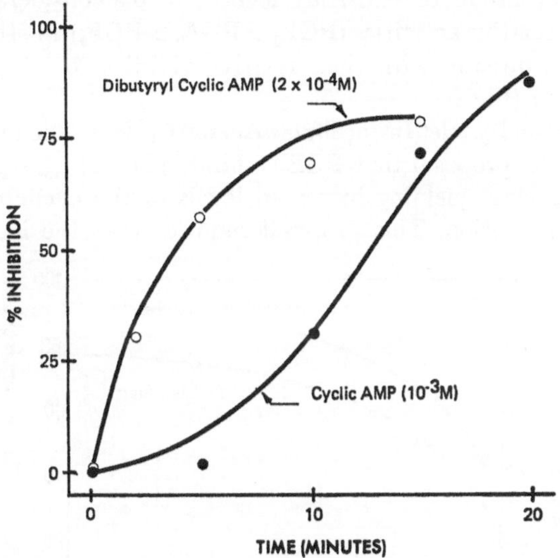

Fig. 1. The inhibition of ADP-induced platelet aggregation by cyclic AMP or its dibutyryl derivative

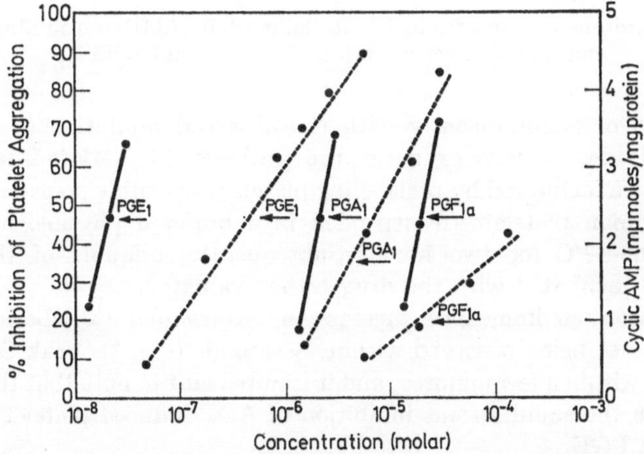

Fig. 2. The relative activities of several prostaglandins in inhibiting aggregation and stimulating cyclic AMP synthesis. Solid lines, platelet aggregation; broken lines, C-AMP synthesis

of PGE_1 as low as 10^{-8} M, significantly stimulated C-AMP synthesis; increases of up to twentyfold were observed with higher concentrations.

The increased synthesis of C-AMP observed with PGE_1 may result from the direct or indirect stimulation of adenyl cyclase or from the blockade of phosphodiesterase. However, the latter possibility may be excluded since PGE_1 does not affect platelet phosphodiesterase; whereas caffeine inhibits and imidazole stimulates this enzyme. We have observed that PGE_1 and caffeine behave synergistically in increasing C-AMP synthesis [931].

PGA_1 and PGF_1 also increase C-AMP levels but to a considerably lesser degree than PGE_1. Their relative activities ($PGE_1 > PGA_1 > PGF_1$) in stimulating C-AMP synthesis correlate directly with their relative abilities to inhibit ADP-induced platelet aggregation (Fig. 2).

Effects of PGE_1 on Platelet Intracellular Adenyl Cyclase. The preceding observations have led to the proposal that PGE_1 inhibits platelet aggregation via stimulation of adenyl cyclase yielding increased levels of the cyclic nucleotide which in turn blocks aggregation. This proposal requires that the increase in C-AMP

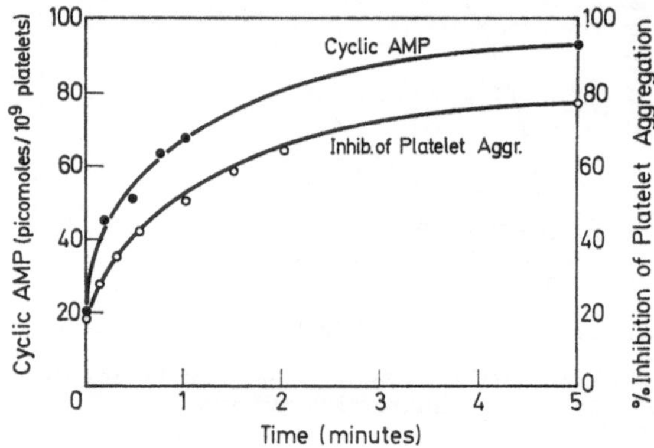

Fig. 3. The simultaneous increase in intracellular cyclic AMP and inhibition of ADP-induced aggregation effected by prostaglandin E_1

occur prior to or simultaneously with the observed inhibition of aggregation. To explore this idea, we have examined the synthesis of C-AMP in intact platelets. Our studies were facilitated by prelabeling platelet nucleotide pools via incubation of isolated human platelets (resuspended in a buffered physiological medium) with adenosine-8-^{14}C for two hours. Subsequently, aliquots of these labeled platelets were incubated with the drug to be evaluated.

PGE_1 induces an immediate increase in intracellular ^{14}C-labeled C-AMP, a threefold increase being observed within 15 seconds (Fig. 3). Peak C-AMP levels were attained within a few minutes; and it is important to note that this correlates very well with the simultaneous inhibition of ADP-induced platelet aggregation observed with PGE_1.

These observations, therefore, fulfill all of the criteria of Sutherland [1443] for implicating C-AMP mediation of an hormonal effect.

Alpha Adrenergic Mediated Platelet Aggregation. The inhibition of platelet aggregation by PGE_1 regardless of the stimulating agent suggests that a common mechanism of inhibition exists, particularly since many of the inducing agents are structurally unrelated. In addition, since C-AMP per se inhibits aggregation induced by ADP, epinephrine, and collagen, it is likely that the adenyl cyclase system is centrally involved in this inhibitory mechanism.

Robison [1246] has proposed that adenyl cyclase may be considered synonymously with the beta-adrenergic receptor, yet O'Brien [1113] and MacMillan [899] have proposed that epinephrine-induced platelet aggregation is mediated by an alpha-adrenergic mechanism. Furthermore, Ardlie [59] and Mills [1005] demonstrated that epinephrine and norepinephrine, but not isoproterenol, induce, as well as potentiate, ADP-mediated aggregation and that phentolamine, an alpha-adrenergic antagonist, prevents epinephrine-induced aggregation whereas propranolol, a beta-adrenergic antagonist does not. Can the adenyl cyclase system be involved, therefore, in mediating alpha-adrenergic mechanisms as well? To

Table. *Effects of alpha- and beta-adrenergic agonists and antagonists on PGE_1-stimulated cyclic AMP synthesis in intact platelets*

Conditions[a]	Cyclic AMP (picomoles/10^9 platelets)
Control	12.4
Epinephrine	9.9
PGE_1	57.6
Phentolamine	15.5
Propranolol	13.1
PGE_1 + Epinephrine	26.9
PGE_1 + Epinephrine + Phentolamine	60.9
PGE_1 + Epinephrine + Propranolol	25.5

[a] Concentrations: PGE_1, 1×10^{-6}M; epinephrine, 2×10^{-6}M; phentolamine, 1×10^{-5}M; propranolol, 1×10^{-5}M.

explore this possibility, we have investigated the effects of epinephrine and adrenergic antagonists on the synthesis of C-AMP in intact platelets.

Indeed, we have found that epinephrine marginally decreases basal C-AMP synthesis but markedly inhibits PGE_1-stimulated C-AMP synthesis (Table). Phentolamine slightly, but consistently, stimulates basal C-AMP synthesis as well as prevents the inhibition of PGE_1-stimulated C-AMP synthesis by epinephrine. Propranolol is without activity.

While our results do not prove that the adenyl cyclase system is involved in mediating an alpha-adrenergic response, nevertheless, it is tempting to speculate that a decrease in C-AMP may lead to a potentiation and perhaps even to an induction of platelet aggregation. The converse, an increase in C-AMP level may lead to the inhibition of aggregation or induction of disaggregation. In fact, Abdulla [2] recently showed that dibutyryl C-AMP, as well as isoproterenol (a beta-agonist) induces the disaggregation of clumped platelets, an observation that we have confirmed.

Fig. 4 depicts the interrelations of adenyl cyclase and phosphodiesterase in regulating intracellular C-AMP levels. It can be seen that a number of agents can alter the level of C-AMP, all of them having been implicated in altering platelet responses. Agents which increase C-AMP by either stimulation of adenyl cyclase (PGE_1) or inhibition of phosphodiesterase (methyl xanthines) have been shown to inhibit platelet aggregation or to induce disaggregation. In contrast, agents which decrease C-AMP by affecting adenyl cyclase (epinephrine) or stimulating phosphodiesterase (imidazole [1260]) induce or potentiate aggregation.

In the platelet, therefore, an increase in C-AMP may mediate a beta-adrenergic response whereas a decrease in C-AMP may mediate an alpha-adrenergic response.

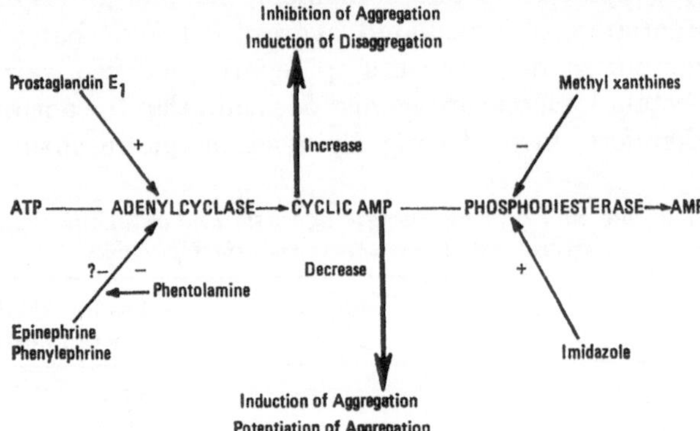

Fig. 4. The interrelations of adenyl cyclase and phosphodiesterase in the regulation of platelet cyclic AMP

Platelet C-AMP levels may thus be of importance in regulating the aggregatability of blood platelets in hemostasis and the pathological condition of thrombosis. We should emphasize, however, that agents which affect the adhesiveness of platelets need not necessarily affect adenyl cyclase nor phosphodiesterase.

Discussion Following Dr. Wanstrup's Paper

Dr. Adams: Has Dr. Wanstrup done any specific studies on the effect of hypoxia on lipid metabolism in the arterial wall? Is he able to tell us which specific part of the metabolic activity of the arterial wall is most altered?

Dr. Kjeldsen (for Dr. Wanstrup): No.

Dr. Wissler: I am certainly impressed with the differences in blood lipid values, although I am not convinced that they are large enough to account for the differences in lesions. I have also been impressed with some of Dr. Mustard's data on platelet stickiness and smoking. Have you tested the effects of carbon monoxide on platelet stickiness?

Dr. Kjeldsen: So far we have only investigated six students, who were exposed to 15% carboxyhemoglobin for six hours. An increase in platelet stickiness was observed in four of them, while no change was seen in the other two.

Discussion Following Dr. Day's Paper

Dr. O. Stein: With the help of high resolution radioautography following labeling with choline-^{3}H, we have demonstrated the localization of newly labeled lecithin to cells of the aortic media, in both the rat and the rabbit, with very little radioautographic reaction over the elastic laminae. These cells show an increase in phospholipid synthesis and their variations suggest the transformation of the smooth muscle cells of the media into foam cells.

Dr. ADAMS: I would like to add that we have seen a similar pattern by scintillation counting on multiple layers of the arterial wall, and I thoroughly agree with Dr. Stein's observation.

Dr. CHOBANIAN: I think Dr. Day's results are in agreement with our findings (see this volume, p. 000) demonstrating increased lipid synthesis in the human fatty streaks which show foam cell infiltration. What do you find in a perfectly normal human artery from a young individual where appreciable lipid synthesis can be demonstrated?

Dr. DAY: In the normal intima of both the rabbit and the human, there is uptake of fatty acid and incorporation mainly into phospholipid and triglyceride.

Where these intimas become atherosclerotic there is considerably more incorporation into cholesteryl ester. There are no foam cells, of course, in the normal intima, and my presentation is concerned primarily with the localization of lipid in the atherosclerotic intima to the foam cells that are present. In this regard the normal intima, of course, is not relevant.

Dr. CHANDLER: Cellular elements of thrombi, such as fragments of leukocytes, red cells or blood platelets, and lipid material derived from them, can be phagocytized by macrophages. Does Dr. Day think cholesterol thus ingested can be esterified by the macrophage?

Dr. DAY: We have not done experiments with phagocytized platelets. Isolated foam cells will take up lipid particles. They will take up a number of lipid precursors including fatty acids which they can incorporate into cholesteryl esters.

Discussion Following Dr. Kramsch's Paper

Dr. L. ROBERT: I am glad to see these results which confirm our predictions. I can report that *in vitro* experiments also show this association of lipid with elastin. Depolymerized elastin (K-elastin) has also high affinity for cholesterol.

These experiments may lead to a physical chemical basis for the understanding of lipid accumulation in elastic tissue.

Dr. AHRENS: Dr. Kramsch has alluded to *in vivo* experiments in man following administration of a pulse of radiocholesterol. Has he looked for this label in tissues other than artery tissue, such as connective tissue, which is present along with elastin in the artery wall?

Dr. KRAMSCH: No. We studied only arteries, and other tissues such as liver and kidney but not tissues that contain larger amounts of collagen or mucopolysaccharides.

Discussion Following Dr. Morrison's Paper

Dr. KEEN: I noticed that the Kinoshita data showed a sorbitol concentration of about 5 micromoles per lens, at the end of incubation, whereas the aorta showed a concentration of something like 50 millimicromoles per gram of tissue, which I imagine to be about the weight of a lens. Thus the aortic concentration is, perhaps, a hundredth that of the lens. Is one likely to get osmotic effects at such a low concentration?

Dr. MORRISON: The aorta is a relatively acellular organ. It has an extracellular fluid compartment of approximately 75% as shown by Dr. Winegrad in our laboratory. As for the effects of the polyol pathway in the aorta, we do not have the full answer to your question. It may serve several functions. It could serve purely as a transhydrogenase and yet if it were localized to a specific cell type or even a localized compartment within the cytoplasm, it is conceivable that it could alter the state of hydration in that cell. As mentioned, we do find small but consistent changes in the water content of the aorta.

Dr. ZEMPLENYI: Have you also studied the effect of insulin on the polyol pathway? Also, why did you use epinephrine? It leads to medial disease rather than lipid accumulation!

Dr. MORRISON: The aorta, provided that it has been stripped completely of adipose tissue and adventitia, is very permeable to glucose and is not an insulin sensitive organ; therefore, insulin would have no effect on the intracellular glucose concentration.

We chose epinephrine, because we were initially attempting to demonstrate acute changes in normal and diabetic animals. There were slight changes in the baseline without incubation which we felt could possibly be a hormonal effect.

Discussion Following Dr. Bjørkerud's Paper

Dr. ADAMS: I would like to ask for a little more detail about Dr. Bjørkerud's methods of causing experimental atherosclerosis.

Dr. BJØRKERUD: The instrument described was designed to enable induction of superficial mechanical trauma in rabbit aorta in an attempt to initate possible effects of hemodynamic strain due to, e.g., shear or turbulence. It was found that a nonatherosclerotic, proliferative repair reaction followed after the induction of a longitudinal, superficial defect in the aortic wall. The architecture of the wall was restored after eight weeks. After trauma performed in transverse direction to the length axis of the vessel, nonregressive lesions followed which were characterized by intimal thickening and accumulation of both intracellular and extracellular lipids. The different outcome of the two types of trauma seems to constitute another system for experimental atherosclerosis. This system may in some respects be advantageous to experimental atherosclerosis induced by dietary means. Nonatherosclerotic and atherosclerotic lesions can be induced in the same animal. The former may then serve as a control tissue in a very strict sense. In addition, no general metabolic change has been induced in the animals. The transverse type of trauma seems to be a very potent means for the production of atherosclerotic lesions. Recently, a member of our group, Dr. Bondjers, studied the effect of these types of trauma in the rat. The results were similar to those for rabbits. This is of interest as the rat is considered to be very resistant to atherosclerosis induced by dietary means.

Dr. BOWYER: I would like to report the results of an experiment on the incorporation of ^{32}P orthophosphate, in a perfusion experiment, into sphingomyelin, lecithin, and phosphatidylethanolamine in normal arterial wall and in adjacent diseased intima. There was a low rate of incorporation into sphingomyelin which was not significantly raised in the diseased tissue. There is, however, a slightly enhanced incorporation into lecithin of the diseased tissue.

A second comment: we know that the behavior of the fatty acid moiety in sphingomyelin is somewhat different from that of the ^{32}P. Thus, if we do an experiment in which we incubate together ^{32}P and ^{14}C fatty acid, then on increasing the concentration of fatty acid in the medium, there is increased ^{14}C fatty acid incorporation into lecithin but the ^{32}P incorporation is not enhanced.

Discussion Following Dr. Marquis' Paper

Dr. Schweppe: Dr. Jungman and I recently submitted a paper to *Nature* in which we described the influence of PGE_1 and PGF_2 on cholesterol to cholesteryl ester conversion. We found that between 250 to 500 ng of PGE_1 or PGF_2 there is about a 95% inhibition of the conversion of cholesterol to cholesteryl ester. This inhibition appeared to be a log-log function of dose. The influence of PGE_1 on lipolysis has been well established, but we feel that PGE may also possibly have a rather profound influence on cholesterol metabolism.

Dr. Paoletti: Are the effects of cyclic AMP shared by other nucleotides, notably by GMP and IMP?

Dr. Marquis: We have not examined GMP or IMP.

Dr. Mustard: One other point that I think should added to the discussion is that not only does PGE_1 inhibit ADP-induced platelets but it also inhibits platelet reaction, and this is interesting as well in terms of the cyclic AMP data that you have.

Dr. Butterfield: I would like to report a finding, based on work with my colleagues D. A. Smink and H. E. J. Kruisheer of the Gaubius Institute in Leiden, Holland and D. E. Fitzgerald of Guy's Hospital, London, of increased platelet adhesiveness after slowing blood flow in normal subjects; this is not found in patients with coronary artery disease.

Retrograde polythene catheters were placed in the brachial artery and an antecubital vein. Blood samples of 5 ml were taken first with the circulation free, and then when the arterial inflow was slowed by the following: elevation of the arm, occlusion of the circulation to the hand with a suitable pneumatic cuff, clenching the fist to contract the forearm muscles, and intermittant inflation of a sphygmomanometer cuff on the arm. Further blood samples were taken after eight minutes of slowed flow [*Angiology* *20*, 359 (1969)]. The samples were immediately studied for platelet adhesiveness using the Payling-Wright method. Twenty-seven patients with coronary artery disease ten days to one year previously and 15 controls of approximately the same ages have been investigated to date.

In subjects who displayed no clinical evidence of vascular disease with the circulation free, the mean platelet adhesiveness was 24.5% (S.E. $\pm$ 3.5) in arterial blood and 28% (S.E. $\pm$ 3.9) in the venous samples. After slowed flow, these levels rose to 75% (S.E. $\pm$ 4.3) in the arterial blood and 45% (S.E. $\pm$ 3.2) in the venous samples.

In marked contrast, in the coronary cases no such conspicuous rise of platelet adhesiveness was detected; the arterial blood platelet adhesiveness was 30.9% (S.E. ± 4.7) with the circulation free rising to only 33.8% (S.E. ± 4.0) after slowed flow. For venous samples the results were, with the circulation free, 29.9% (S.E. ± 4.5), after slowed flow, 30.6% (S.E. ± 5.9).

Comparing normals with coronary cases, with the circulation free, there was a slight but statistically insignificant increase of platelet adhesiveness in the coronary cases in both arterial and venous blood. But after slowed flow, to our surprise, the platelets in the coronary cases were less sticky. This result cannot be explained simply on the basis that the adhesive platelets in the coronary cases had stuck to the arterial wall and were not sampled, because there was less fall in total platelet count after slowed flow in these patients than in the controls. The mean platelet count in the normal subjects' arterial blood was 203,400 with the circulation free, falling to 119,100 after slowed flow, a statistically significant fall. But in the coronary cases, the mean count only fell from 175,000 to 156,300.

Some other explanation must, therefore, be sought for the highly significant differences between adhesiveness in the normals and coronary cases after slowed flow. Many can be advanced: perhaps prostaglandins are important. Alternatively, the peripheral arterial wall in coronary cases was also diseased, so that its demand for oxygen was reduced and less ADP accumulated in the blood *in vivo*. Another is that, in coronary cases, the platelets were less sensitive to ADP, which is known to accumulate under the circumstances of our study; we are investigating all these possibilities.

Looking at the total results, we were somewhat disappointed by the findings. We had hoped to discover more adhesive platelets in the patients with coronary heart disease than in the controls, then treat them with, perhaps, anticoagulants, or clofibrate or aspirin, or control their diabetes, and judge the effects of therapy by the improvement in platelet adhesiveness. Alas, if our results are confirmed, one wonders whether there is any value in reducing platelet stickiness in coronary cases. They seem to be naturally well protected for the important sequence of events, obstruction, atherosclerosis, slowing of flow and thrombosis! Of course it may be argued, and no doubt it will be, that our technique is not physiological. Our reply is that, at least, our work is *in vivo* and that slowed flow, possibly over longer periods, must occur in many parts of the body, e.g. in the fingers in cold weather or in diseased arteries particularly during the hypotension associated with sleep.

Dr. Mustard, how these results will be reconciled with your views about the role of platelet adhesiveness in the genesis of atherosclerosis, I do not know. If it will help you, one might argue that our adult controls were really subclinical cases of atherosclerosis! However, in conclusion, we believe these findings will be confirmed. They emphasize that we may get more insight into platelet behavior in arterial disease by studying arterial rather than venous blood.

Section V

SERUM LIPOPROTEINS

APOPROTEINS AND SUBSTRUCTURE OF HUMAN SERUM LIPOPROTEINS*

B. Shore and V. Shore

Isolation and characterization of the polypeptide components of the human serum lipoproteins are important for characterization of the lipoproteins themselves and for elucidation of their functions in health and disease. The lipoproteins, which vary greatly in size and density, normally show characteristic density distributions among four major classes: the very low density lipoproteins (VLDL, 0.94–1.006 g/ml), the low density lipoproteins (LDL, 1.006–1.063 g/ml), the high density lipoproteins (HDL, 1.063–1.20 g/ml), and the chylomicrons [1097, 1320]. Paper electrophoresis of plasma gives four lipoprotein bands called prebeta, beta, alpha and chylomicrons, which are correlated with the four density classes [853, 865]. The mobilities are related to the protein moieties, and the prebeta or VLDL lipoproteins can be dissociated into alpha and beta components by extraction of lipids [865]. Immunochemical studies indicate that VLDL contains a third protein component, apolipoprotein C [30], and the entire density spectrum of serum lipoproteins contains three [29, 30] or more distinct protein moieties.

Recent studies involving column chromatographic separation of the polypeptide components of lipoproteins [251, 1302, 1354, 1355, 1359] indicate more heterogeneity in the protein moieties than previous biophysical, chemical and immunochemical studies had indicated. In addition to diverse polypeptide moieties, polymorphisms are observed [40].

High Density Lipoprotein Proteins. The high density lipoproteins (HDL) of human serum range in density from 1.063 to 1.20 g/ml and in molecular weight from about 150,000 to 380,000 [1097]. The HDL spectrum is often partitioned into two subclasses: HDL_3, which are about one-half protein and 150,000–180,000 in molecular weight, and HDL_2, which are about one-third protein and 340,000 to 380,000 in molecular weight.

The protein moiety of HDL is readily obtained in a water-soluble, lipid-free form amenable to physical and chemical studies. Sedimentation equilibrium experiments on several different preparations of the unfractionated lipid-free protein in the presence of sodium dodecyl sulfate indicated homogeneity with respect to molecular weight and a molecular weight of about 30,000 [1358]. Inhomogeneity was observed in some preparations, but the presence of aggregates rather than more than one kind of protein was not ruled out. Earlier investigations of the terminal amino acids of HDL protein were consistent with one predominant polypeptide with amino-terminal aspartic acid and carboxyl-terminal

* The work herein was performed under the auspices of the U.S. Atomic Energy Commission.

threonine. More recently, carboxyl-terminal glutamine and threonine were found in comparable amounts equivalent to two moles of glutamine plus threonine per 30,000 g protein, and carboxyl-terminal alanine was present in minor amounts [1354, 1355].

The heterogeneity of HDL protein was also demonstrated by polyacrylamide gel disc electrophoresis of the protein in 8 M urea and by column chromatography on DEAE-cellulose [1354, 1355, 1359] and by fractionation on Sephadex G-200 [1302]. The major polypeptides R-gln and R-thr were isolated from both HDL_2 and HDL_3; other polypeptides were isolated in minor amounts, especially from HDL_2, which was more heterogeneous with respect to polypeptide content than HDL_3. In addition to heterogeneity with respect to polypeptide content, we found polymorphic variants of the polypeptides R-thr and R-ala and a polypeptide characterized by a high content of serine, glutamic acid and glycine [1355].

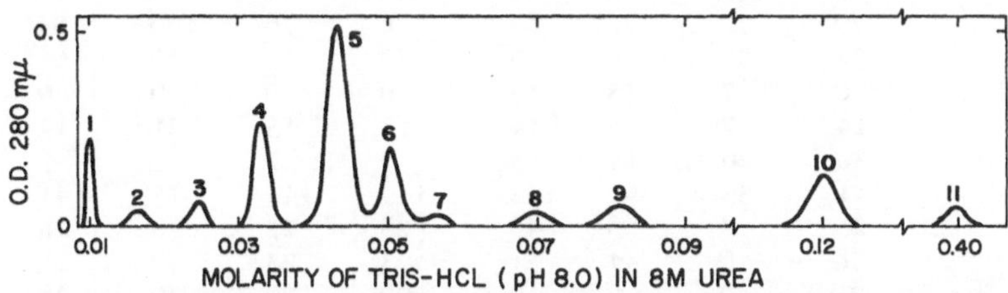

Fig. 1. Chromatographic separation of HDL protein on a DEAE-cellulose column (0.9 × 40 cm) equilibrated with starting buffer (0.01 M Tris-HCl at pH 8.0 in 8 M urea). The peptides were eluted with linear concentration gradients of Tris-HCl at constant pH at flow rate of 16 ml per hr and at 8° C

The polypeptide fractions from chromatography of HDL_2 protein in 8 M urea on DEAE-cellulose are shown in Fig. 1. Rechromatography of fractions 5, 6, 7, 8 and 9 was necessary to obtain one component per fraction as indicated by polyacrylamide gel electrophoresis. The major component of each of these fractions from rechromatography was eluted at the position of the corresponding fraction in Fig. 1. Fractions 5, 6 and 7, all characterized by 1 mole carboxyl-terminal threonine per 14,000 g protein, are polymorphic peptides that are not resolved by polyacrylamide gel electrophoresis. The major form of R-thr contains no isoleucine and the other two contain one isoleucine residue per molecule. Fractions 8 and 9 also appear to be polymorphic variants of the same peptide as are fractions 2 and 11. The amino acid compositions of the polypeptide components of HDL are shown in Table 1.

The two major polypeptide components of HDL, fractions 4 (R-gln) and 5 (R-thr), are very different in amino acid composition, but both peptides are about 15,000 in molecular weight [1302, 1359].

An HDL_3 molecule of molecular weight 170,000 and 53% protein would contain six polypeptide molecules of molecular weight 15,000, and an HDL_2 molecule of molecular weight 360,000 and 33% protein would contain eight. It is not known whether or not more than one kind of peptide is present in one lipoprotein subunit. Two polypeptides of molecular weight 15,000 may be present in a lipoprotein subunit, since electron microscope studies [481] by negative

Table 1. *Amino acid composition (moles/10^3 moles of amino acid) of polypeptides from HDL of normal human serum* [a]

Amino acid	Fraction from Fig. 1								
	1	2	3	4	5	6, 7	8, 9	10	11
Lys	101	74	100	116	79	80	73	79	74
His	13	30	7	0	22	22	15	14	27
Arg	65	16	13	0	67	66	32	52	16
Asp	87	69	53	41	95	96	88	85	68
Thr	38	41	65	81	38	38	60	48	37
Ser	108	210	114	81	62	57	121	70	204
Glu	156	165	186	198	183	184	152	189	163
Pro	24	22	46	52	38	38	30	42	21
Gly	55	188	78	43	45	44	56	49	201
Ala	79	72	76	67	76	76	106	83	74
Val	32	29	65	76	52	53	66	61	30
Cys ($^1/_2$)	0	7	15	15	0	0	0	0	6
Met	14	7	8	14	15	15	21	14	7
Ile	30	20	14	15	0	7	7	7	20
Leu	111	33	91	102	149	148	75	141	31
Tyr	25	8	28	46	28	27	28	28	7
Phe	38	16	41	51	23	23	40	28	16
Trp	25	0	0	0	29	29	29	28	0

[a] Values are the averages of two to six determinations for which standard errors were less than 5%. The compositions of fractions 6 and 7 were not significantly different, nor were those of fractions 8 and 9. Cystine was determined as cysteic acid after performic acid oxidation, and tryptophan was determined spectrophotometrically. Experimental values for cysteic acid, serine, and threonine were corrected for losses of 8%, 10% and 5%, respectively.

staining techniques show that an HDL_3 molecule is made up of three to four subunits and that an HDL_2 molecule usually contains five to six subunits, although as few as three are occasionally seen in HDL_2. It remains to be established that the two peptides R-gln and R-thr are in fact derived from the same parent lipoprotein molecule. In disc electrophoresis at pH 8.8 in $7^1/_2$% polyacrylamide gels containing 8M urea or 1% Triton X-100, HDL_3 gives two bands (stained with Amido Schwarz) as does the lipid-free protein [1359]. However, urea and Triton X-100 may dissociate the lipoprotein molecule as they do the lipid-free protein.

In any case, the roles of the two polypeptides R-gln and R-thr in the structure of HDL are of major interest in regard to the physiological function of lipid transport by these lipoproteins. Several different protein-lipid complexes are possible, e.g. P_1-L-P_1, P_1-L-P_2, P_2-L-P_2 and P_1-P_2-L, where P = polypeptide and L = lipid. On the basis of their striking differences in composition, the two peptides would be expected to have different affinities for lipids. From amino acid composition, the helical content would be expected to be 40 to 50% for the polypeptide R-gln and more than 90% for the polypeptide R-thr [552]. The prediction was qualitatively supported by the optical rotatory dispersion and circular dichroic spectra of the two peptides after chromatographic separation on DEAE-cellulose in 8M urea. The peptide R-gln may be more intimately involved than the peptide R-thr in interactions with the lipid moiety of HDL, since helical segments of most proteins are located at the surface and away from the hydrophobic interior.

The significance of the minor polypeptide components of HDL for its structure and function is largely unknown. It is possible that they are derived from lipoprotein species quite distinct from the major HDL lipoproteins containing the peptides R-gln and R-thr. It is also possible that lipid complexes of these peptides may associate with the more dense HDL molecules containing R-gln and/or R-thr to give larger, less dense HDL molecules.

Very Low Density Lipoproteins. The very low density lipoproteins (VLDL, S_f 20–400 and density 0.94–1.006 g/ml) contain a very high percentage of lipid of which the major component, triglyceride, increases with increasing S_f rate

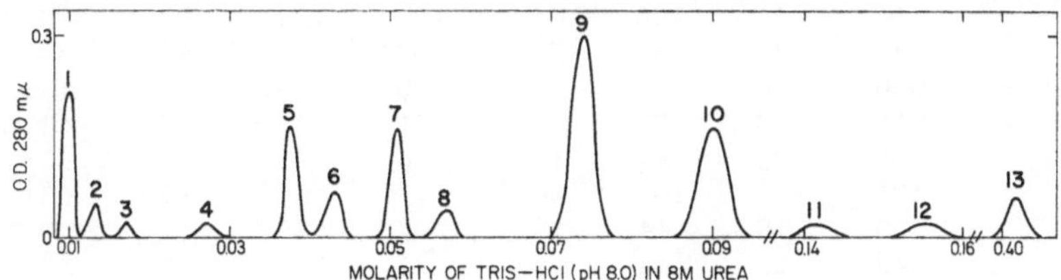

Fig. 2. Chromatographic separation on DEAE-cellulose of VLDL protein from hyperlipemic serum. The conditions were the same as in Fig. 1

[1097]. Electron microscope studies [480] indicate that VLDL are spherical structures with a wide range in size (>230 Å in diameter). No fine structure, either within or at the periphery of these lipoproteins, was revealed by the negative staining procedure used by Forte and coworkers. Immunochemical studies on the protein moiety of VLDL indicate that it is in part composed of LDL protein and HDL protein [590, 865], and that at least three different proteins are present in VLDL [30, 590].

More recently, some polypeptide components of VLDL have been isolated by column chromatography. In one study, two different polypeptides isolated from the protein moiety of VLDL from hyperlipemic serum were shown to differ immunochemically from the alpha and beta apoprotein moieties, which were also present in the VLDL protein [251]. These two peptides accounted for more than 50% of VLDL protein. One contained NH_2-terminal threonine but no histidine, tyrosine, cysteine or cystine. The other contained NH_2-terminal serine, COOH-terminal alanine but no isoleucine, cysteine or cystine. Both peptides were estimated from gel filtration to be smaller than a globular protein of molecular weight 25,000.

In another investigation of VLDL from hyperlipemic serum (Shore, unpublished data), these peptides and several other peptide components were isolated by column chromatography of the protein on DEAE-cellulose in the presence of 8 M urea (Fig. 2). Each of these fractions, except 2 and 13 which were not fixed, gave one protein band in polyacrylamide gel electrophoresis in 12% gels containing 8 M urea. These fractions account for approximately 60% of the protein applied to the column; the remainder of the protein was not eluted

Table 2. *Amino acid composition (moles/10^3 moles amino acids) of polypeptides of VLDL from hyperlipemic serum* [a]

Amino acid	Fraction from Fig. 2								
	1	3, 4	5, 6	7	8	9, 10	11	12	13
Lys	154	61	49	68	73	76	75	59	77
His	0	15	11	4	15	15	23	19	28
Arg	54	30	106	18	29	29	23	29	14
Asp	90	74	48	68	86	88	84	90	70
Thr	45	52	39	102	60	65	49	41	41
Ser	126	141	60	118	123	135	167	146	215
Glu	159	183	228	177	151	135	149	163	161
Pro	12	30	29	44	29	27	24	20	21
Gly	32	161	59	36	57	40	135	183	186
Ala	54	71	106	85	109	123	92	68	70
Val	35	46	67	54	67	73	46	38	29
Cys ($^1/_2$)	0	0	0	0	0	0	14	13	7
Met	15	8	23	23	21	24	8	13	7
Ile	48	25	11	12	8	0	15	30	19
Leu	104	63	108	94	73	65	52	63	35
Tyr	0	16	14	48	27	25	7	0	7
Phe	48	25	14	25	41	47	36	25	14
Trp	24		28	23	31	34			0

[a] Values are averages of three different samples of hyperlipemic serum analyzed separately. The compositions of corresponding fractions were within 5% of the average values. Fractions 3 and 4, 5 and 6, and 9 and 10 were not significantly different. Fraction 2 was essentially identical with fraction 13 except that it contained twice as much tyrosine. Cystine was determined as cysteic acid after performic acid oxidation, and tryptophan was determined spectrophotometrically. Experimental values for cysteic acid, serine, and threonine were corrected for losses of 8%, 10% and 5%, respectively.

from the column. The composition of the polypeptide components isolated from S_f 20–400 lipoproteins from hyperlipemic serum is shown in Table 2. Fractions 3 and 4 (Fig. 2) yielded the same amino acid composition as did fractions 5 and 6 and fractions 9 and 10.

The VLDL proteins from normal sera, in smaller amounts, were also fractionated by DEAE-cellulose chromatography [1355]. The major peptide components isolated from normal VLDL comprised two peptide fractions containing the carboxyl-terminal sequence R-ala-val-ala-ala (1 mole/11,000 g protein) and a fraction corresponding to fraction 13 of Fig. 2 and Table 2. The normal VLDL peptides with carboxyl-terminal alanine contained one or two isoleucine residues per molecule and were very similar if not identical in composition to fraction 8 of Table 2. Fractions 9 and 10 of Table 2, present in much greater amount than fraction 8 in VLDL of hyperlipemic serum, contained the carboxyl-sequence R-val-ala-ala (1 mole/11,000 g protein), but unlike the R-ala of normal VLDL, they contained no isoleucine.

None of the VLDL proteins yielded peptide fractions corresponding to the major HDL polypeptides R-gln and R-thr. The HDL and VLDL lipoproteins contained in common two polypeptides of very similar if not identical amino acid composition. One contained the carboxyl-terminal sequence R-ala-val-ala-ala (fractions 8 and 9 of Fig. 1 and Table 1 and fraction 8 of Fig. 2 and Table 2). The other contained a very high percentage (almost 60%) of serine, glutamic acid and glycine (fractions 2 and 11 of Fig. 1 and Table 1, and fractions 2 and 13 of Fig. 2 and Table 2). The high content of polar amino acids in the latter polypeptide suggests that it may confer aqueous solubility upon lipoprotein complexes that contain it.

The two peptides were minor components of HDL protein but major components of the S_f 20–400 lipoproteins of normal serum. However, normal serum contains more HDL protein (~100 mg/100ml) than S_f 20–400 lipoprotein protein (~10 mg/100 ml), so that the total amounts of these two peptides in HDL and in VLDL are similar. The roles of these two peptides in the structure of lipoproteins and in lipid transport are especially interesting, because they are found in lipoprotein classes of very different density. There is considerable evidence that HDL and VLDL are related structurally and metabolically [1097, 1320]. Immunochemical and paper electrophoresis studies [590, 865] indicate that both LDL and HDL proteins are present in VLDL.

Chylomicrons also appear to be related structurally to VLDL. Immunochemical studies show that chylomicrons contain all of the proteins of VLDL [30]. However, little information is available on chylomicron proteins, and their polypeptides have not been isolated.

The analyses of VLDL protein shown in Fig. 2 and Table 2 indicate that these lipoproteins may be heterogeneous with respect to protein moiety as well as to size and density. Although no subunit structures were seen in electron micrographs of VLDL [480], repeating structures of protein and lipid in these large molecules are possible. Each lipoprotein molecule contains a number of peptide molecules, since each of the peptides isolated from VLDL is much smaller ($10–15 \times 10^3$ g/mole) than the amount of protein in the lipoprotein (Shore, unpublished data). Further studies on the lipoproteins are necessary to determine whether two or more different peptides are derived from the same lipoprotein molecule and to elucidate the roles of the various peptides in VLDL structure. It would be interesting to know if heterogeneity in VLDL with respect to protein implies a multiplicity of VLDL functions in lipid-transport.

Low Density Lipoprotein Proteins. The low density lipoproteins (LDL) of density 1.006–1.063 g/ml are spherical molecules of mean diameter of 215–220 Å [480, 551]; they contain about 22% protein. For LDL, molecular weights of $2.1–2.3 \times 10^6$ have been obtained from sedimentation equilibrium [1301], 2.8 to 3.0×10^6 from light scattering [179], 3.3×10^6 from electron microscopy [480], and 3.5×10^6 from elution volumes using agarose gel columns [927]. Physical measurements on the apoprotein indicate a number of protein subunits in the lipoprotein molecule [130, 1353] although lipoprotein subunits were not seen in electron micrographs of negatively stained LDL [480].

Column chromatography of the lipid-free protein of an LDL fraction (1.029 to 1.039 g/ml or S_f 4–8) by the procedure used for HDL and VLDL proteins (Figs. 1 and 2) gave two different peptides, but none of the peptides obtained from HDL or VLDL [1355]. More recently, six peptide fractions, none similar in composition to those shown in Tables 1 and 2, were obtained from LDL (Shore, unpublished data). However, LDL of S_f 4–8 may be related to VLDL by common polypeptides, as yet not isolated, since about 70% and 40% respectively, of LDL and VLDL proteins were not eluted from the DEAE-cellulose columns. The S_f 4–8 lipoproteins do not appear to be related to HDL_2 and HDL_3 by common polypeptides. None of the peptides from HDL protein, which was recovered almost completely from the DEAE-cellulose column, was found on chromatography of the protein of LDL, nor were carboxyl-terminal glutamine, threonine and alanine found in S_f 4–8 LDL. A peptide with carboxyl-terminal alanine has been found, however, in LDL of density 1.050–1.063 g/ml and of density 1.007–1.019 g/ml (Shore, unpublished data).

Studies of LDL by optical rotatory dispersion and circular dichroism [385, 550, 1300] and by infrared spectroscopy [550, 1300] indicate that alpha-helix, beta and disordered conformations may be present in the protein moiety. Their presence was found to depend on temperature and on the lipid content of the lipoprotein fraction [385]. With increasing lipid content, the conformation appeared to become predominantly beta. The presence of lipid is important for the conformational state of the protein moiety, since removal of lipids causes conformational changes [550, 1300]. However, variations in conformational state of the protein moiety as a function of density of the LDL fraction may reflect differences in polypeptide composition of the protein moieties.

The presence of several polypeptides in multiple forms which are very similar but not identical in composition may be important in the physiological and biochemical functions of the lipoproteins. Small differences in amino acid sequences may affect the binding of lipids and the effectiveness of the polypeptide-lipid complex or lipoprotein in a lipid-transport system. The predominance in the VLDL of hyperlipemic serum of the form of the peptide R-ala containing no isoleucine and of the forms containing isoleucine in normal VLDL and HDL is very suggestive. However it may be a consequence of the fact that the average S_f rates of the VLDL fractions from hyperlipemic sera were higher than those of normal VLDL or it may be due to genetic differences among the limited number of individuals studied that have no bearing on the concentrations of VLDL in the plasma. Polymorphism could also be due to different sites of synthesis of the peptides, e.g. liver versus intestine.

At this point in the study of the apoproteins of the serum lipoproteins, increasing knowledge makes us increasingly aware of the complexity of the problem of apoproteins and substructure of the lipoproteins. Further studies on the lipoproteins themselves, with attempts to fractionate on the basis of peptide content and to obtain lipoprotein subunits, are very important for understanding the roles of the various peptides in lipoprotein structure and function. Such information, in conjunction with information on the amino acid sequences of the peptides and data (from optical rotatory dispersion, circular dichroism, and infrared spectroscopy studies) on the conformation of the purified polypeptides and lipoproteins, should give some insight into how the water-insoluble lipids are converted to soluble form. It is possible that some of the lipoprotein peptides serve primarily as lipid binders whereas others may serve primarily to confer the property of water-solubility on the lipid-peptide complex. Peptides may also play a role in the transfer of lipid from the transport molecule to the receptor site.

BIOSYNTHESIS AND SECRETION OF VERY LOW DENSITY LIPOPROTEINS

Y. STEIN and O. STEIN

Lipoproteins may be considered as the main building blocks of all living matter and thus form a very heterogenous group. In the animal kingdom, lipoproteins can be divided into two main classes: (1) those used for the formation of membranes which are the basic structures participating in the construction of subcellular components; and (2) those destined for secretion into the circulation.

While the lipoproteins of the first class are formed ubiquitously within all cells, the source of origin of the second class is mostly confined to the liver and, to a limited extent, to the intestine [1115, 1249]. The circulating lipoproteins can again be subdivided into groups on the basis of specific antigenicity, lipid composition, and density. The following groups are recognized and can be separated according to their density by ultracentrifugation: VLDL (very low-density lipoprotein) $d < 1.006$; LDL (low-density lipoprotein) $1.006 < d < 1.063$, and HDL (high-density lipoprotein) $d > 1.21$.

This review will be limited to the VLDL class only, the main components of which consist of protein, lipid and some carbohydrate. According to Granda and Scanu [560], the percentage of chemical composition of human serum VLDL $d < 1.006$ is the following: protein—10.0 ± 1.0, phospholipid—17.0 ± 1.0, total cholesterol—22.0 ± 1.0, and triglycerides—51.0 ± 2.0. This class of lipoproteins is considered to be the main carrier of triglyceride secreted from the liver into the circulation.

Some of the evidence which has accumulated with regard to the site of synthesis of the various components of VLDL, their transport in the liver cell, and the mode of their secretion into the circulation will be presented herein. The literature concerning the site of synthesis of the protein moiety of serum lipoproteins in the liver has recently been summarized [266]. The latter authors have studied incorporation of labeled amino acids into the protein moiety of both HDL and LDL by rat liver ribosomes *in vitro*, and have shown that it was necessary to add plasma or carrier lipid for the reisolation of immunologically reactive newly synthesized lipoprotein. Since formation of all serum proteins has been localized mainly to the membrane-bound ribosomes of liver (Fig. 1) [1217], it seems plausible that the protein moiety of VLDL is synthesized in the same manner on ribosomes attached to the membranes of the endoplasmic reticulum.

Another approach used to study the synthesis of the protein moiety of lipoproteins has been the use of different metabolic inhibitors. Thus, puromycin has been shown to interfere with the formation of VLDL, even though the synthesis of the lipid moiety has not been impaired (Table 1) [262, 754]. Actinomycin D decreased incorporation of lysine into VLDL, while synthesis of HDL was affected to a lesser extent [448] (Fig. 2). Feeding of orotic acid interfered primarily with the formation of beta lipoprotein, which is apparently obligatory for the release of triglycerides from the liver (Table 2, [1555]).

The synthesis of the lipid components, i.e., triglyceride, phospholipids and cholesterol, which participate in the formation of the VLDL has been studied extensively, and the earlier literature has been summarized by Stein and Stein [1417, 1418] and by Chesterton [303]. In these more recent studies, labeled

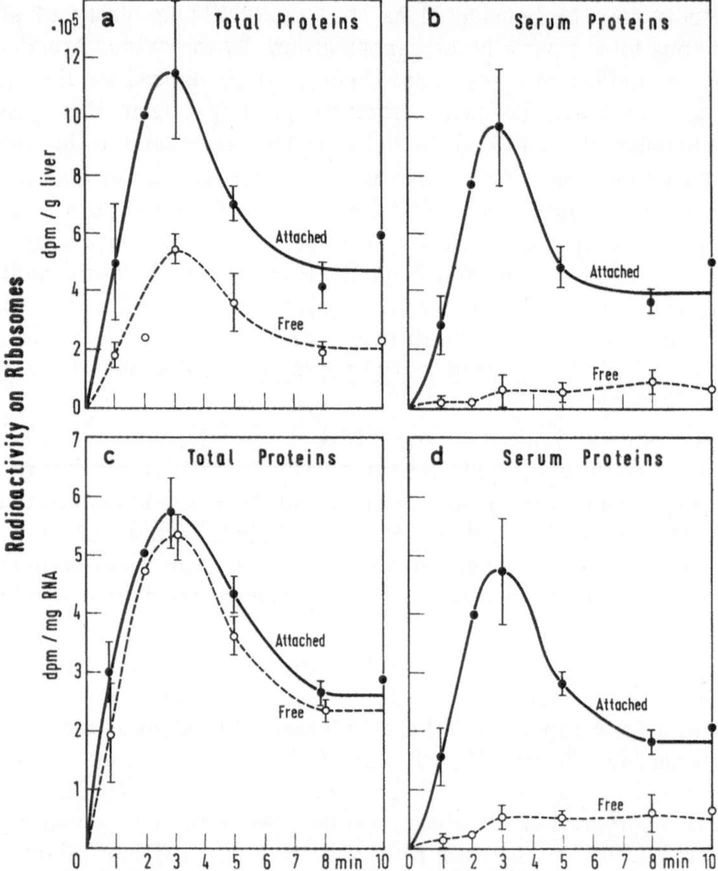

Fig. 1. The values given, except for the points at 2 and 10 minutes, are the mean of 3 experiments with the standard deviation. The points at 2 and 10 minutes are single observations. Total protein is TCA-insoluble materali. (Reprinted from Redman [121])

precursors were injected into intact animals and emphasis was placed on the more exact localization of the synthesis of specific lipid molecules to various cellular organelles. Use was made of radioautography at the electron microscope level [1417, 1418] and newer methods of subcellular fractionation [532]. The results obtained with different labeled precursors indicate that in the intact liver cell both the rough and the smooth endpolasmic reticulum participate to a similar extent in the synthesis of triglycerides [1417], phospholipids [1418] (Table 3), and cholesterol [303].

Table 1. *Effect of puromycin on incorporation of oleic acid-^{14}C and leucine-^{3}H into tissue and lipoprotein triglyceride and protein* [a]

	Radioactivity incorporated $10^{-3} \times$ dpm/g liver dry wt $\pm$ sem [b]		
	control	puromycin	P
Liver protein	$32{,}370 \pm 4{,}194$ ($n=6$)	451 ± 100 ($n=5$)	<0.001
Liver triglyceride	937 ± 250 ($n=6$)	956 ± 480 ($n=5$)	NS
Lipoprotein protein	410 ± 58 ($n=6$)	74.9 ± 50.0 ($n=4$) 24.5 ± 5.9 ($n=3$)	<0.005 <0.001
Lipoprotein triglyceride	18.0 ± 3.3 ($n=6$)	2.84 ± 1.9 ($n=5$) 1.0 ± 0.5 ($n=4$)	<0.005 <0.005

[a] Reprinted from Jones et al. [754].
[b] Corrected for differences in total radioactivity of initial medium.

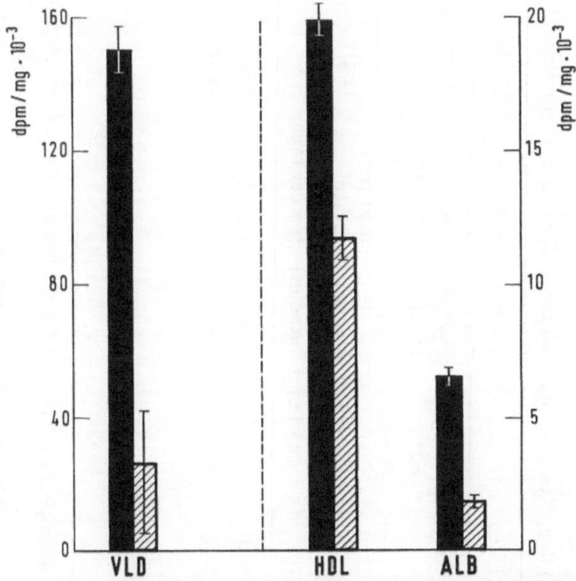

Fig. 2. L-[^{3}H]Lysine incorporation into VLDL, HDL, and albumin by isolated perfused rat livers. Liver donors were pretreated with actinomycin D, 0.2 mg/100 g at zero time and 0.1 mg/100 g at 6 and 9 hr. Controls received sham injections. At 10 hr livers were isolated and perfused. Data presented are from three actinomycin D treated livers (shaded bars) and three controls (solid bars) with the range of values indicated. (Reprinted from Faloona et al. [448])

It should be emphasized that so far, in the studies concerned with the synthesis of lipids, no separation has been made between structural and secretory lipids. Such a differentiation may become quite difficult owing to the growing realization that some phospholipid molecules of different cellular membranes do exchange quite rapidly [1418, 1560], and such an exchange could also take place between membrane and secretory phospholipid.

Table 2. *Synthesis and release of lipids and lipoproteins by perfused livers*[a]

Group	Addition to basal diet (for 8 to 11 days)	Appearance of livers	Liver		Fatty acid synthesized[b]	Fraction of synthesized fatty acid released into perfusate[c]	Net release into perfusate					
							lipids (μmoles)			total fatty acid	lipoproteins[d]	
			weight	total fatty acids			triglycerides	cholesterol	phospholipid		alpha	beta
			(g)	(μmoles/g)	(μmoles)	(percentage)						
I (8)[e]	none	normal	14.0	118	302	15.9	30.7	9.7	18.0	132.3	++	++++
II (4)	1 or 2% orotic acid[f]	uniformly fatty	15.5	456	36	0.3	0.0	2.5	5.7	−3.3	+	−
III (4)	1% orotic acid	variably fatty	17.2	403	122	4.5	6.6	5.1	11.7	27.4	+	+

[a] Livers of rats (270 to 300 g) were perfused *in situ* for six hours. Values are means of four to eight experiments. Reprinted from Windmueller and Levy [1555].

[b] Calculated from the incorporation of ^3H, from ^3H_2O, into liver and perfusate fatty acids.

[c] Fraction of the liver plus perfusate fatty acid radioactivity recovered in perfusate after sixt hours.

[d] Detected by immunoelectrophoresis; number of plus signs indicates relative quantities.

[e] Figures in parentheses represent number of experiments.

[f] Orotic acid, 1% in two experiments and 2% in two experiments.

Table 3. *Distribution of radioautographic reaction over subcellular elements in liver cells after labeling with choline-³H* [a]

In vivo labeling	Incubated in chase	Grains counted	Distribution of grains							
			RER [b]	SER [c]	mito-chondria	nucleus	Golgi	Cell boundary		
								bile capillary	sinusoid	lateral
(minutes)	(minutes)		(percentage)	(percentage)	(percentage)	(percentage)	(percentage)	(percentage)	(percentage)	(percentage)
5	0	500	33.8	28.6	13.0	1.4	3.2	7.2	7.8	5.0
5	10	488	37.1	25.3	13.5	1.4	2.8	5.3	11.3	3.3
5	25	430	30.0	30.0	13.0	1.0	3.8	6.6	11.0	4.6
5	115	860	30.2	27.0	17.4	0.6	3.4	6.7	11.7	3.0
60	0	430	31.0	24.1	17.0	1.1	6.0	7.0	11.0	2.8

[a] More than 95% of the radioactivity was in lecithin, reprinted from Stein and Stein [1418].
[b] RER = rough endoplasmic reticulum.
[c] SER = smooth endoplasmic reticulum.

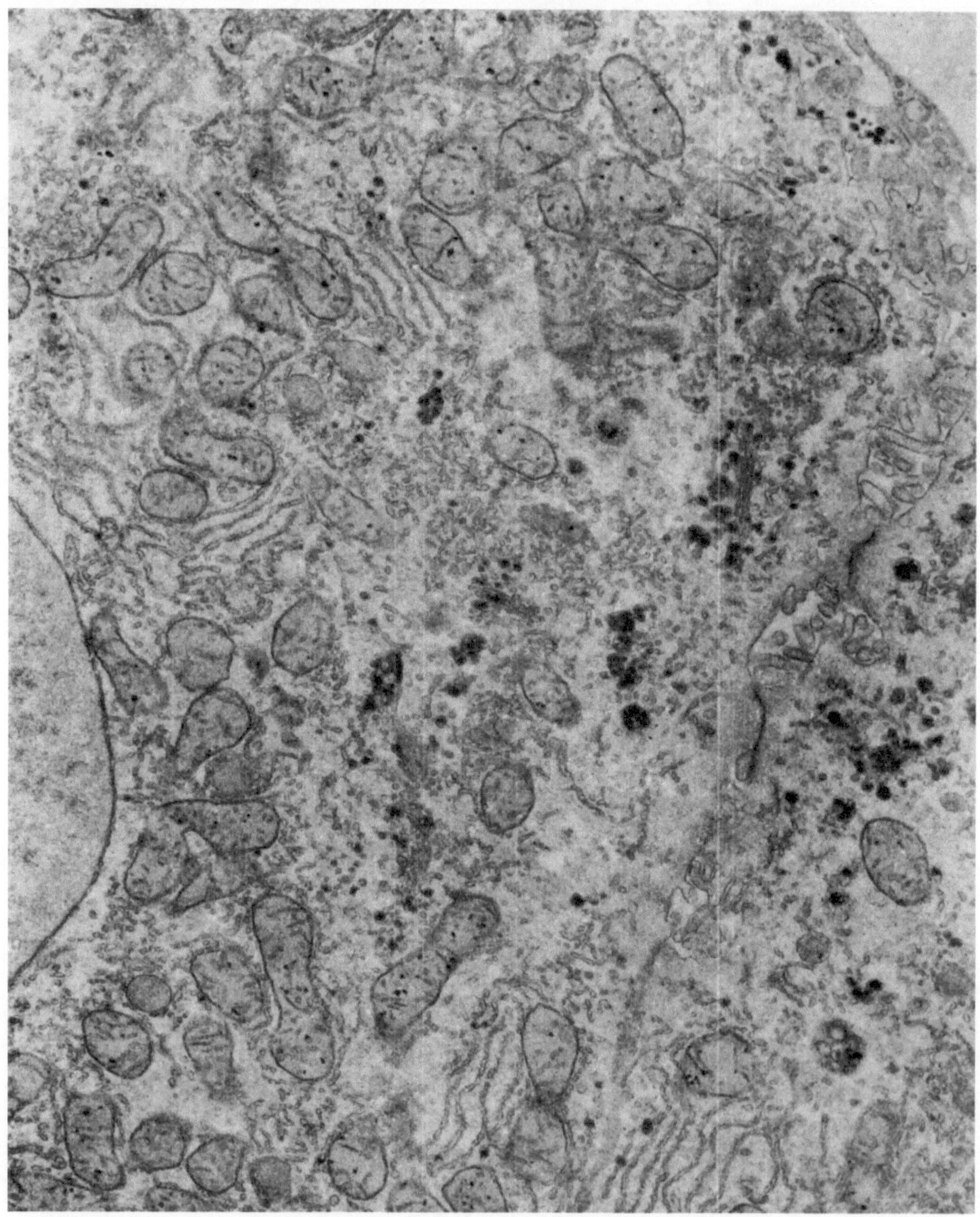

Fig. 3. Electron micrograph of liver of rat 4 hr after ethanol administration (0.6 g/100 g body weight). There are numerous lipoprotein granules in the cisternae of the endoplasmic reticulum, in the Golgi apparatus and in the space of Disse. ×16,000

Table 4. *Distribution of grains over liver subcellular structures after injection of 9,10-palmitic acid-^3H into rats fasted for 16 hours*

Time after injection (minutes)	Distribution of grains					Total grains counted
	endoplasmic reticulum [a] (percentage)	mitochondria (percentage)	Golgi region (percentage)	Disse space (percentage)	nucleus (percentage)	
2 [b]	87	6	1	4	2	243
5 [b]	86	7	2	3	2	242
10 [b]	67	15	11	5	2	434
20	65	16	11	6	2	297

[a] Includes cytoplasmic matrix.
[b] Samples obtained from the same rat.
Between 5 and 20 minutes more than 85% of the radioactivity was in triglyceride. Reprinted from Stein and Stein [1417].

Table 5. *Chemical composition of Golgi particles compared to very low density lipoproteins*

	Lipid analysis mg/100 mg lipid					Protein analysis, mg protein/100 mg dry weight	
	triglyceride	phospholipid	cholesteryl ester	free cholesterol	free fatty acids	Golgi particles	plasma VLDL
Golgi particles [a] ($d = 1.006$) Mean ± SE	59.8 ± 2.0	24.9 ± 0.9	8.3 ± 0.7	3.7 ± 0.6	3.4 ± 0.5	10.8	10.8
Plasma VLDL [b] (3½ hour fasted; $d = 1.006$) Mean ± SE	56.2 ± 2.3	24.9 ± 2.4	12.7 ± 2.9	6.2 ± 0.5	0.7 ± 0.1	8.9	9.4
Serum VLDL [c] (16 hours fasted; $d = 1.019$)	44.6	23.1	24.7	6.4	1.1	9.3	11.2

[a] Results obtained from 6 experiments.
[b] Results obtained from 4 of the 6 experiments reported for the Golgi particle lipid analysis.
[c] Calculated from Lombardi and Ugazio: J. Lipid Res. **6**, 498 (1965). Reprinted from Mahley et al. [903].

Another aspect of the problem of VLDL biosynthesis and secretion has been the visualization of the VLDL particle in the liver. The presence of electron opaque particles ranging in size between 300 and 1,000 Å in diameter in the cisternae of the endoplasmic reticulum, in the Golgi apparatus and in the space of Disse (Fig. 3) has been known for a number of years. Their nature as precursors of plasma VLDL was first postulated by the authors [1416], and a more firm identification was made by three groups of investigators, with the help of different techniques [600, 754, 1417]. In the liver of ethanol-fed rats, 10–20 minutes after injection with labeled glycerol or fatty acid, concentration of radioautographic grains was seen over clusters of particles, especially over the Golgi apparatus and near the sinusoidal cell surface (Fig. 4, Table 4). Enhanced production of these particles could be demonstrated in the rat liver during perfusion with a high load of free fatty acids [600, 754]. The particles isolated from the perfusate

Table 6. *Distribution of lipids and lipoproteins in hepatic perfusate after ultracentrifugation ($d = 1.016$)*

Feeding schedule	Perfusate fraction	Net release per liver during five-hour perfusion				
		lipids (μmoles)			lipoproteins[a]	
		tri-glycerides	phospho-lipid	choles-terol	α	β
Ad libitum (8)	$d < 1.016$	22.5	8.3	4.6	Tr	+
	$d > 1.016$	0.4	6.7	2.9	+	—
Fasted,	$d < 1.016$	56.2	10.3	9.0	Tr	+
re-fed (4)	$d > 1.016$	0.6	5.7	2.0	+	—

[a] Detected by immunoelectrophoresis; Tr = trace. Perfusate ($d = 1.016$ gm/ml) was centrifuged 16 hours at 143,000 g in a 40.3 rotor of a Beckman model-L ultracentrifuge. Floated ($d < 1.016$) and sedimented ($d > 1.016$) fractions were recovered after slicing the centrifuge tubes 18 mm from the top. Reprinted from Windmueller and Spaeth [1551].

morphologically resembled the VLDL of rat plasma. In a recent study these particles derived from isolated Golgi apparatus were analyzed, and their triglyceride and phospholipid composition and protein content were similar to that of the plasma VLDL particle (Table 5 [903]). The fine structure of the VLDL particles was investigated using negative staining and in contradistinction to the HDL particles, which were found to be composed of subunits, no substructure has been detected [480]. The electron opacity of the VLDL particle has been shown to be a function of the degree of unsaturation of dietary lipids. Thus, in mice fed a high carbohydrate, fat-free diet, the VLDL particles appear as electron translucent [1153] and similar observations were also made on VLDL particles of cortisone treated rabbits [903].

The VLDL particle does not have a fixed lipid composition and it may contain increasing amounts of triglycerides and cholesterol, depending on the nutritional state. Thus, under conditions of enhanced fatty acid synthesis as in fasted-refed animals the composition of the lipids released into the perfusate changes in favor of triglyceride (Table 6 [1557]). VLDL particles isolated from perfusates of rat liver after a considerable fatty acid load had a higher triglyceride to protein ratio and a larger average diameter than the VLDL particles derived from livers perfused with a lower load of fatty acid (Table 7 [1268]). An increase in the size of the VLDL particle has been described also in livers of rabbits treated with cortisone at a time when the animals developed a hypertriglyceridemia and their $d < 1.006$ serum fraction contained unusually large particles [902]. More recently an increase in the VLDL particle size has been shown to occur in some patients with carbohydrate-induced hypertriglyceridemia [1268].

Various metabolic inhibitors were used to study the transport and secretion of the VLDL particles. Backing up of the particles in the cisternae of the endoplasmic reticulum and formation of membrane-bound "liposomes" was caused by ethionine [86], which interferes with protein synthesis; engorgement of the

Table 7. *Size distribution of particles in lipoprotein pellets* [a]

Particle diameter	Total linoleate administered	
(Å)	40 μmoles (No. of particles)	480 μmoles [b] (No. of particles)
450	7	5
600	35	24
750	50	49
900	6	14
1,050	1	4
1,200	1	1
1,350	0	3
Mean particle diameter (A) ± SEM	693 ± 10	754 ± 16 [c]
Mean volume of 100 particles (A^3)	18.6×10^9	24.5×10^9

[a] For both groups of livers the diameters of 100 particles were estimated in two randomly chosen areas from the center of the pellet. Two pellets in each group were studied. Particle diameter was estimated to the nearest 150 Å.

[b] 120 μmoles added to initial medium plus 120 μmoles per hour by infusion.

[c] The significance of the difference in mean particle diameter was $P < 0.005$. Reprinted from Ruderman et al. [1268].

cisternae of the rough endoplasmic reticulum with lipid droplets was caused by orotic acid, which inhibits preferentially the synthesis of the protein moiety of beta lipoprotein [1555]. More puzzling is the impairment of VLDL secretion in choline deficiency [890] in which a reduction in the incorporation of glucosamine into $d < 1.21$ lipoproteins, which may affect the secretion of VLDL, was described [1019].

The route the VLDL particle traverses from its site of formation in the ER to the blood stream has been traced with the help of radioautography [1417] and it was proposed that the particles reach the Golgi vacuoles in which they are transported towards the cell surface and, after fusion of the vacuole membrane with the plasma membrane, the particles are released into the extracellular space of Disse (Fig. 4). Similar conclusions have also been drawn by Hamilton et al. [600] from experiments with liver perfusion.

The role of the Golgi apparatus in the secretory process of VLDL particles was studied in the liver of cortisone-treated rabbits [902]. The morphological findings in the liver were correlated with the changes in serum lipid levels (Table 8). The initial decrease in serum lipids was accompanied by engorgement of vacuoles with enlarged particles in the Golgi region. Some of the vacuoles seemed to

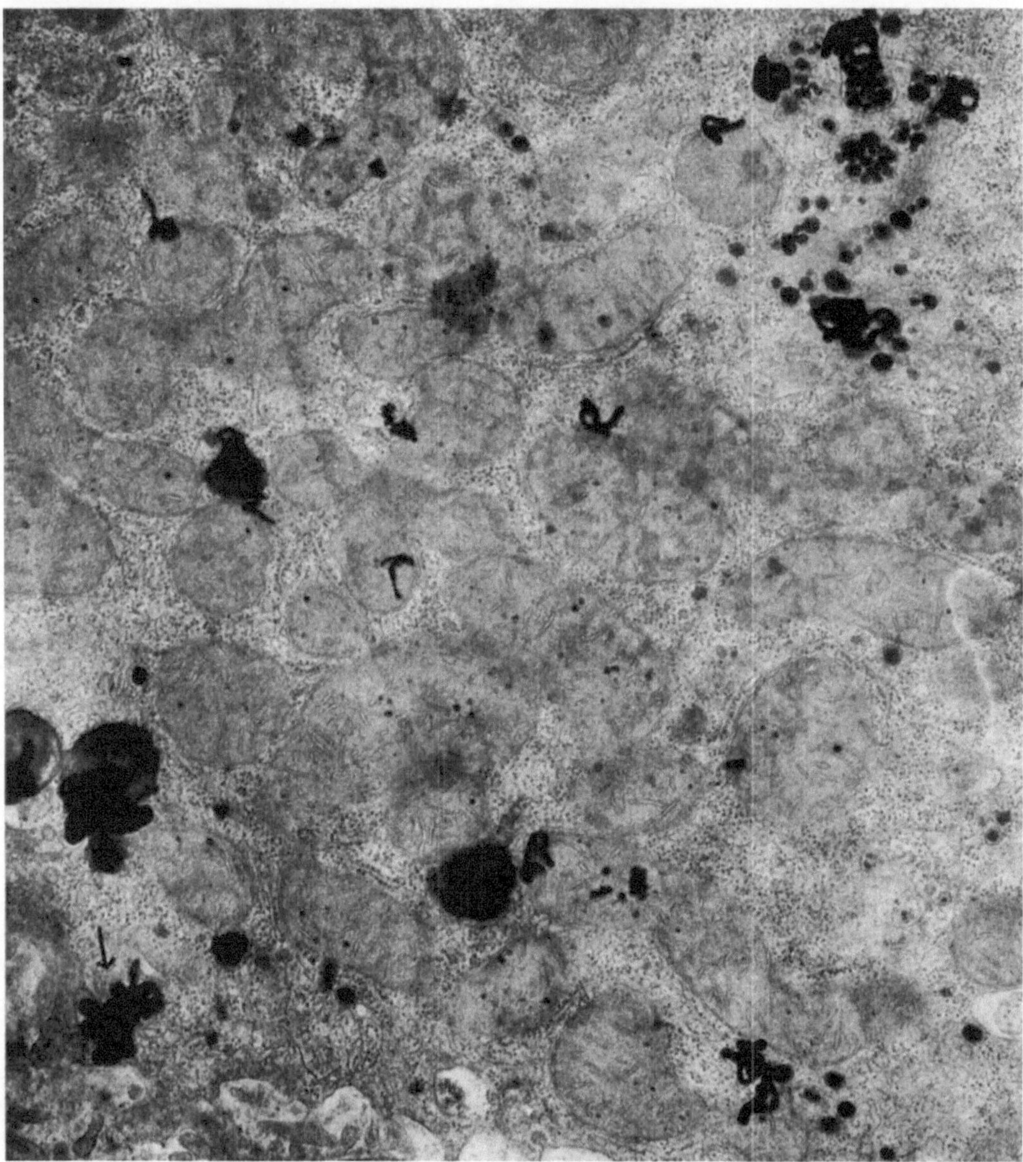

Fig. 4. Radioautograph of liver of rat 4 hr after ethanol administration, and 10 min after injection of oleic acid-^{3}H. The silver grains are concentrated over the Golgi vacuoles, lipoprotein granules in the space of Disse (arrow) and over lipid droplets. ×22,000

form lysosomes, suggestive of intracellular lipid catabolism. Two days after cortisone treatment there was an extreme paucity of Golgi elements, and four to six days after cortisone treatment the rapid rise in serum lipids was accompanied by a prominent increase in the Golgi apparatus and in the number of VLDL particles within secretory vacuoles.

Table 8. *Serum lipid levels in rabbits treated daily with cortisone*[a]

Treatment	Free fatty acid (μmoles/ml)	Total fatty acid (mg/100 ml)	Total cholesterol (mg/100 ml)	Phospholipid (mg/100 ml)
Controls				
8 hr., fasted	0.68 ± 0.19 (18)[b]	174 ± 63 (17)	36 ± 11 (13)	75 ± 36 (11)
Cortisone				
4 hr.	0.78 ± 0.05 (4)	53 ± 9 (4)	11 ± 2 (4)	50 ± 4 (4)
8 hr.	0.83 ± 0.20 (9)	85 ± 28 (10)	21 ± 8 (10)	69 ± 30 (10)
2 da.	0.50 ± 0.20 (11)	92 ± 25 (11)	18 ± 8 (11)	84 ± 37 (9)
4 da.	0.95 ± 0.34 (8)	519 ± 486 (8)	49 ± 36 (8)	123 ± 69 (8)
6 da.	1.07 ± 0.36 (9)	1,083 ± 1,000 (13)	102 ± 80 (13)	231 ± 151 (10)

[a] Rabbits were administered 50 mg of cortisone daily.

[b] Values are expressed as mean ± standard deviation. Numbers in parentheses respresent number of rabbits in each group. Reprinted from Mahley et al. [902].

An alternative to vesicular transport of VLDL particles has been proposed in which the Golgi apparatus is considered to be a multibranched tubular body with the dilated ends of the tubules making contact with the plasma membrane (D. J. Morré, personal communication).

This brief review covers only a small part of the information which has been added recently to knowledge of lipoprotein synthesis and secretion. The following constitute only a few of the numerous questions still unanswered: (1) the precise site and the sequence of the assembly of the complete VLDL particle; (2) the regulation of the direction of intracellular transport; and (3) the mechanisms operative in the final release of the VLDL particle from the cell into the circulation.

STUDIES ON A LOW DENSITY LIPOPROTEIN CHARACTERIZING OBSTRUCTIVE JAUNDICE*

D. Seidel, P. Alaupovic and R. H. Furman

It has been recognized for a long time that liver disorders are frequently accompanied by marked changes in plasma lipid concentrations. Flint [465] observed more than a century ago an increased blood cholesterol concentration in patients with obstructive jaundice. Subsequent studies correlating plasma

* The studies herein were supported in part by Grants HE-6221, HE-7005, and HE-2528 from the U. S. Public Health Service, and by the Oklahoma Heart Association and the American Heart Association. D. Seidel was supported by U. S. Public Health Service General Research Support Grant FRO 5538.

lipids with various liver diseases demonstrated dramatic changes in plasma lipids and lipoproteins in patients with intra- or extrahepatic biliary obstruction. Plasma lipid changes in subjects with biliary obstruction are characterized by increased concentrations of unesterified cholesterol and phospholipids resulting in an increased free/total cholesterol ratio and a diminished cholesterol/phospholipid ratio.

Kunkel and coworkers [833, 834] correlated increased plasma lipid and beta globulin concentrations and were first to suggest that the hyperlipoproteinemia and increased serum phospholipid concentrations in biliary obstruction were related. Several authors have proposed that phospholipids increase the stability of lipoproteins and, therefore, their capacity for cholesterol binding. Gofman and coworkers [542, 954, 1175] first described the marked increase of the serum

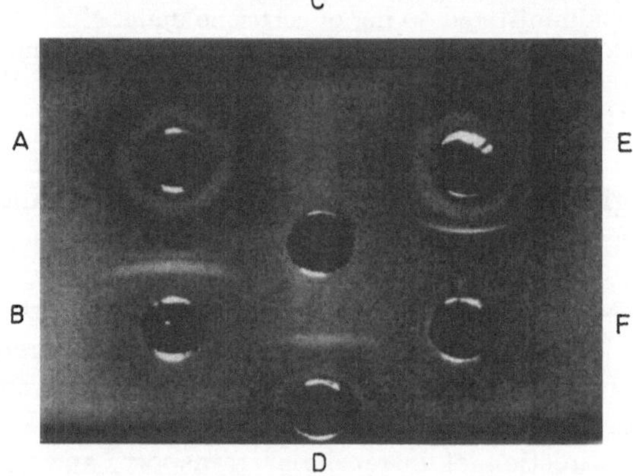

Fig. 1. Immunodiffusion patterns of LP-A (A), LP-B (E) and LP-X (C). Lower wells contain antibodies to LP-A (B), LP-X (D) and LP-B (F)

LDL fraction as a change characteristic of the ultracentrifugal lipoprotein pattern in patients with obstructive jaundice. Several investigators demonstrated that the increased concentration of LDL is accompanied by a decreased concentration of HDL. Eder and coworkers [420] found an increased concentration of serum lipoprotein in the Cohn fraction IV—VI. Russ and coworkers [1270] established the presence of an "abnormal" lipoprotein in Cohn fraction VI. Recently Switzer [1448] described the presence of an abnormal low-density lipoprotein (obstructive lipoprotein) which failed to react with antibodies to LDL. Burstein and Caroli [271] reported similar findings and discussed an abnormal alpha lipoprotein in these patients.

Although several investigators demonstrated immunochemically the presence of LP-A (LP-A is the predominant lipoprotein of the HDL ("alpha") lipoprotein fraction characterized by the presence of apolipoprotein A) in the LDL fraction, no quantitation of LP-A in the LDL fraction has been reported. Fredrickson and coworkers [489] suggested that the increased concentration of LDL in patients with biliary obstruction is caused by a shift of LP-A from the HDL into the LDL fraction. This presentation is the report of our studies on the isolation and characterization of plasma lipoproteins in patients with jaundice.

To achieve the separation of various plasma lipoproteins, including an abnormal lipoprotein (designated LP-X) in the LDL fraction and to determine the qualitative and quantitative distribution of lipoprotein families within the density ranged 1.006 to 1.063 g/ml, a procedure combining ultracentrifugation, heparin precipitation, and ethanol fractionation was developed in our laboratory (Seidel et al. [1337]). This procedure permits the separation and quantitative determination of three immunochemically distinct lipoproteins, LP-A, LP-B [LP-B is the predominant lipoprotein of the LDL ("beta") lipoprotein fraction characterized by apolipoprotein B] and LP-X (Fig. 1).

The LP-B and LP-X accounted for 98% and the LP-A for 2% of the total protein content of the LDL fraction. The LP-X/LP-B ratio varied in different patients from 0.2 to 0.6, probably with the degree and/or duration of biliary

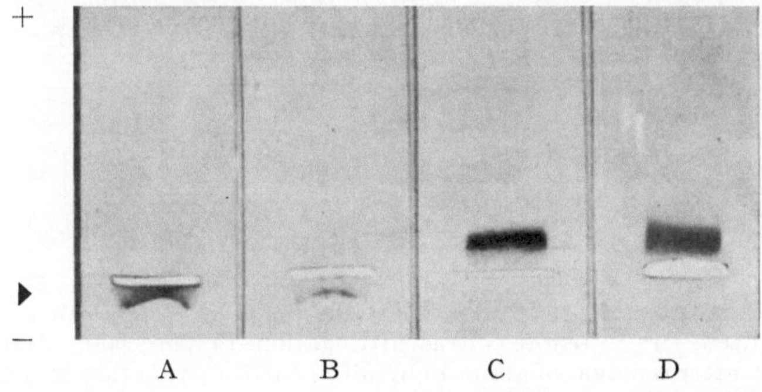

Fig. 2. Electrophoresis patterns of LP-X in 1% agar (A and B) and 1% agarose gel (C and D). A and D were stained with Oil Red O; B and C with Amido Black

obstruction. The protein-lipid composition of LP-X is unique and consists of 6% protein, 65% phospholipids, 25% cholesterol and 3% triglycerides. It is distinguished by the presence of cholesterol almost entirely in unesterified form (93% of total cholesterol) and by a high phospholipid/protein ratio of 11. The analysis of the two major low-density lipoproteins, LP-B and LP-X, revealed that the unique composition of the whole LDL fraction, and thus of whole serum, is attributable primarily to the presence of LP-X. The composition of LP-B is nearly normal with the possible exception of a slightly decreased amount of cholesteryl ester and increased content of unesterified cholesterol. LP-X is characterized, as are LDL and HDL, by lecithin (76%) and sphingomyelin (23%) as principal phosphatides. The high lecithin/sphingomyelin ratio of LP-X resembles that of HDL rather than LDL.

The ultracentrifugal analysis of the LDL fraction from patients with obstructive jaundice showed schlieren patterns with two peaks with flotation ratios of approximately S_f 8 and S_f 16–17. Subsequent studies on the separation and immunological characterization of these two components showed that the peak with an approximate S_f 8 correspond to LP-B and that with S_f 16–17 to LP-X.

The LP-X moves, under identical experimental conditions, toward the cathode in agar gel electrophoresis and toward the anode in agarose gel electrophoresis (Fig. 2). This is true for the isolated LP-X fraction as well as for LP-X in whole plasma. On paper and on starch gel electrophoresis LP-X migrates toward the anode, with a mobility slightly less than that of LP-B. The affinity of all electrophoretic bands of LP-X for lipid and protein stains indicates clearly its lipoprotein nature.

The extraction of LP-X by n-heptane resulted not only in a complete removal of neutral lipids, but also in a substantial removal of phospholipids; in contrast to a high phospholipid ratio of 11.5 for LP-X, the ratios for various preparations of partially delipidized LP-X varied between 1–2. The preferential extraction of lecithin, lysolecithin and cephalin was reflected in a decreased lecithin/sphingomyelin ratio of partially delipidized LP-X. Whereas LP-X showed single, slowly migrating bands in agar, agarose, paper and starch gel electrophoresis, and a single immunoprecipitin arc with anti-LP-X serum; the partially delipidized

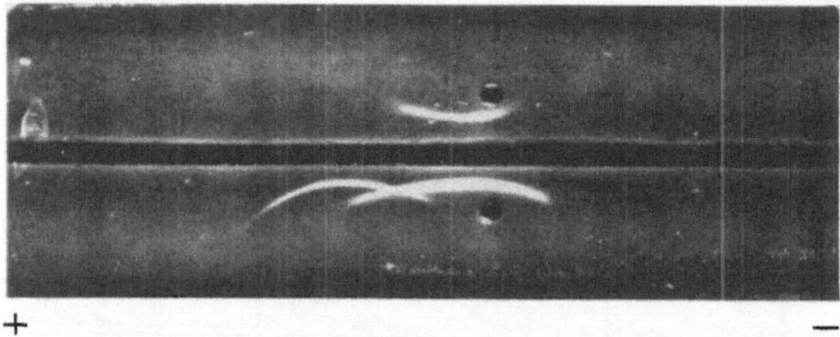

Fig. 3. Immunoelectrophoresis patterns of partially delipidized LP-X in 1% agar gel: partially delipidized LP-X before ultracentrifugation (upper well), and partially delipidized LP-X after removal of albumin by ultracentrifugation (lower well). Central trough contains antibodies to LP-X and albumin (Alaupovic et al. [33]; by courtesy of the FEBS Letters)

Fig. 4. Immunoelectrophoresis patterns of LP-X in 1% agar gel

LP-X fraction gave a positive immunoprecipitin reaction not only with antibodies to LP-X, but also with antibodies to albumin (Fig. 3). To separate albumin from the immunochemically characteristic protein of LP-X, the density of the partially delipidized lipoprotein solution was adjusted to 1.21 g/ml and the mixture was centrifuged at 105,000 × g for 44 hours. The top fraction contained immunoelectrophoretically-homogeneous partially delipidized LP-X, and the bottom fraction contained immunochemically identified albumin. Chloroform extraction of the albumin fraction revealed the presence of fatty acids (15 to 20 moles/mole albumin) and unidentified phospholipids (0.1–0.2 mg/ml albumin). The dissociation of LP-X by partial delipidization was reflected also in a changed electrophoretic mobility of the partially delipidized LP-X; intact LP-X migrated toward the cathode and partially delipidized LP-X toward the anode. The results of several separate quantitative analyses showed that albumin accounted for 40% and the nonalbumin protein moiety of LP-X for 60% of the total protein content of LP-X.

Total delipidization of the nonalbumin protein by extraction with ethanol-ether resulted in the isolation of a water soluble protein moiety, ApoX, which gave positive immunoprecipitin reaction with antibodies to LP-X. In agar gel electrophoresis ApoX displayed a higher mobility than the corresponding non-albumin protein after partial delipidization. The nonalbumin protein of LP-X contained no detectable anthrone positive carbohydrates or chloroform extractable fatty acids; it contained less than 0.1% of phospholipids. The nonalbumin protein, ApoX, contained serine and threonine as N-terminal and alanine as C-terminal amino acids; albumin was characterized by aspartic acid as the N-terminal and by leucine as the C-terminal amino acids.

The finding of a positive immunoprecipitin reaction of non-albumin protein with antibodies to VLDL, but not with antibodies to LP-A or LP-B, indicated

Table 1. *Immunochemical detection of LP-X in patients with jaundice*

Clinical diagnosis	Number of patients	Number of patients showing cross-reactions with anti LP-X serum
No cholestasis		
Hemolytic jaundice	26	0
Acute hepatitis	37	3
Chronic hepatitis	21	0
Laennec's cirrhosis	21	3
Cholestasis		
Biliary cirrhosis	15	14
Cholangiolitis	6	6
Tumor of the liver	8	8
Extrahepatic biliary obstruction	51	51
Biliary atresia	3	3
	Σ 188	

similarity with ApoC, the third typical apolipoprotein isolated first by Gustafson and coworkers [590] from plasma VLDL of hypertriglyceridemic patients and by Alaupovic and coworkers [31] from chyle VLDL of normal subjects. A direct comparison of nonalbumin protein ApoX and ApoC showed that these two proteins gave complete fusion of precipitin lines with antibodies to VLDL and LP-X. The results of chemical and immunological studies suggest strongly that non-albumin protein of LP-X and ApoC are similar if not identical.

Screening tests in 188 patients (Table 1) with various forms of jaundice indicated that a characteristic immunoelectrophoretic precipitin arc in agar gel (the immunoprecipitin arc extends from the antigen well toward the cathode) between plasma samples and purified antibodies to LP-X (Fig. 4) was observed only in patients in whom obstructive jaundice could be demonstrated by other tests (roentgenology, biopsy, surgery or autopsy).

In two of the three cases showing the presence of LP-X in a group of 58 patients with hepatitis, it was possible to demonstrate bile accumulation within the small bile ducts by biopsy; it was not possible to obtain a biopsy from the third patient.

In none of the biopsies from the hepatitis group with LP-X negative but increased alkaline phosphatase activity could evidence of an obstructive component be demonstrated (Table 2). It is noteworthy that in patients with jaundice not due to cholestasis, increased plasma alkaline phosphatase activity and the presence of LP-X in plasma show no necessary correlation. It appears that the immunological test for LP-X is highly specific for the detection of biliary obstruction.

Table 2. *Differential diagnosis of jaundice. (Percentage of total number of patients in the group)*

	Positive LP-X	Alkaline phosphatase		Transaminase		Number of patients
		> 50 mU	> 100 mU	> 15 mU	> 50 mU	
Jaundice due to cholestasis	99	95	68	88	53	84
Jaundice not due to cholestasis	3	82	42	96	76	102

We are proposing as a working hypothesis that the formation and accumulation in serum of LP-X may be the result of an impaired catabolism of ApoC-containing lipoproteins caused by inhibitory action of increased concentrations of bile salts in the liver.

AUTOIMMUNE HYPERLIPIDEMIA*

J. L. BEAUMONT

In autoimmune hyperlipidemia (AIH), *an atherogenic metabolic disease of immune origin*, soluble complexes made of antibodies bound to serum lipoproteins, accumulate in the circulating blood [121]. At first, autoantibodies of the IgA type reacting with serum alpha and beta lipoproteins were found [107, 109]. Now several types of antibodies which react with different lipoprotein sites are known [111, 112]. Obviously, like in autoimmune anemias, there are different types of AIH and most of them remain unknown.

The demonstration in 1964–1965 of the antilipoprotein activity of the myeloma protein, in one case of myelomatosis associated with hyperlipidemia and xanthomatosis, was the first step on the way to the AIH concept [121]. It was followed by the detection of similar antibodies, first in common hyperlipidemias of various

* The author wishes to thank M. Anthonucci, M. F. Baudet, V. Beaumont, C. Dachet, B. Delplanque, M. D. Ferry, T. Ghembaza, B. Jacotot, N. Lemort, L. Lorenzelli and D. Peron for their valuable help.

types, without myelomatosis in man [106] and more recently in hyperlipidemias induced in rabbits by immunization [127]. Data available today show that AIH may be frequent and is highly atherogenic.

In spite of its importance, AIH is not widely known by those who work in the atherosclerosis field. Therefore, the knowledge collected during the last five years on AIH in monoclonal gammapathies, in ordinary hyperlipidemias and in immunized animals will be summarized herein. Thereafter, the mechanisms and consequences in connection with this new metabolic disease of immune origin will also be presented.

AUTOIMMUNE HYPERLIPIDEMIA IN MONOCLONAL GAMMAPATHIES

Hyperlipidemia may occur in myeloma and in macroglobulinemia, but evidence for an antilipoprotein activity of the M protein was given only for myelomas.

Myelomas. Lipidemia is normal and often reduced in myeloma [577, 774, 868, 871, 1182, 1516], sometimes it is highly increased [237, 344, 345, 452, 681, 1182, 1274, 1309] and quite unusually this increase is associated with cutaneous xanthomatosis [74, 120, 265, 317, 318, 482, 671, 783, 856, 860, 869, 1297]. Since the case studied by Hill, Mulligan and Dunlop in 1948 [681], about 30 cases of myeloma with hyperlipidemia were reported, half of them with xanthomatosis. Chance can hardly explain the simultaneous occurrence of two rare disorders and the idea that in these patients myeloma and xanthomatosis were linked was expressed by Lennard-Jones in 1960 [856]. With regard to this idea, the molecular interaction seen in some cases between the myeloma protein (M protein) and lipoproteins gave the first physicochemical support. Accordingly Heremans [671] felt that the association of IgA myeloma, hyperlipidemia, and xanthomatosis was the result of a special attribute of the IgA M protein. Later on, Cohen [318] demonstrated that the serum of an IgG myeloma with hyperlipidemia contained a factor which prevented the alpha and beta lipoproteins of a normal serum from moving into a starch gel under electrophoresis. The name of "serum lipoprotein altering factor" as proposed for it by Spikes [1397].

Since 1964 the specific antilipoprotein activity of the serum of an IgA myeloma has been studied [12]. After purification, it was related to the IgA M protein which behaved like an auto-antibody reacting with a site common to serum alpha and beta lipoproteins, site P.G. [107, 109]. This myeloma was called anti-Lp.P.G. and a second case of this type was found [112]. Recently in an IgG myeloma, the purified M protein was found to react with a lipoprotein site different than site Lp.P.G., which was called site Lp.A.S. This myeloma was called anti-Lp.A.S. [111].

Before describing these two well defined types of antilipoprotein myeloma we will summarize the main characteristics of the reported cases of myeloma with hyperlipidemia.

Myelomas with Hyperlipidemia. A review of the studied cases shows that they belong to several types. Among 16 cases in which the type of the M component was clearly established (Table 1) seven are IgA (with surely 2 kappa and 1 lambda chains); nine are IgG (with surely kappa and lambda varieties). Among the IgG some move on electrophoresis as $gamma_1$ and others as $gamma_2$ globulins.

Table 1. *Myelomas with major hyperlipidemia*

References[a]	M Protein		Hyperlipidemia			Xanthomatosis			Atherosclerosis	Miscellaneous
	immunologic type	electrophoretic type	serum aspect	cholesterol	triglycerides	cutaneous		tendinous		
						tuberous	plane			
Lennard-Jones [856]	IgA	$gamma_1$	Milky	↑	↑	+	+	−	+	
Heremans [671]	IgA	$gamma_1$	Milky	↑	↑	+	+[b]	−	+	
Kayden [783]	IgG	?	Milky	↑	↑	−	+	−	−	
Levin [860]	IgG kappa	$gamma_2$	?	↑	↑	−	+	−	?	
Cohen [317]	IgG lambda	$gamma_1$	Milky	↑	↑	+	+	−	+	
Spikes [1397]	IgA lambda	$gamma_1$	Milky	↑	↑	−	−	−	−	Diabetes
Savin [1297]	IgA	$gamma_1$	Milky	↑	↑	+	−	−	−	Purpura
Lewis [869]	IgA	$gamma_1$	Milky	↑	↑	+	+	−	+	
Yaguinuma [c]	VIgG lambda	$gamma_1$	Milky	↑	↑	−	−	−		
Beaumont [120]	IgA kappa	$gamma_1$	Milky	↑	↑	+	+[b]	+	+	
Beaumont [74, 112]	IgA kappa	$gamma_1$	Milky	↑	↑	+	+[b]	−	+	
Beaumont [111][d]	IgG kappa	$gamma_1$	Milky	↑	↑	−	−	−	−	
Beaumont [111][d]	IgG	$gamma_1$	Clear	↑	Normal	−	+	−	+	
Beaumont [111][d]	IgG	$gamma_2$	Clear	↑	Normal	−	+	−	+	Cryoglobulin
Beaumont [111][d]	IgG	$gamma_1$	Milky	↑	↑	−	−	−	+	
Beaumont [111][d]	IgG	$gamma_2$	Clear	↑	Normal	−	+	−	−	

[a] Only references with complete data have been quoted.
[b] Palmo-plantar.
[c] Personal communication.
[d] Previously unpublished data.

The xanthomata are usually cutaneous, either tuberous on the knees, elbows, and buttocks with sometimes plane palmo-plantar spreading; or plane on the breast, abdomen, and the upper part of the limbs. Tendons are rarely involved. Atherosclerosis, which is rather unusual in myeloma [1392], is frequent in these cases.

The hyperlipidemia is chiefly of the mixed type; total cholesterol and triglycerides are increased, and the serum is milky. Sometimes hypercholesterolemia or hypertriglyceridemia may be predominant or even isolated. Especially in the mixed type, very high levels may be seen with total cholesterol above 1,000 mg and triglycerides above 2,000 mg/100 ml serum.

The lipoproteinemia which is greatly increased differs from one case to another. Usually in the ultracentrifuge, very low density lipoproteins prevail with or without a concomitant increase in chylomicra. On the other hand, high density lipoproteins may also be increased [120]. After electrophoresis we have seen different patterns which would be classified at present as Fredrickson type I, III, IV or V, according to the increase of either chylomicra, broad beta, prebeta, and chylomicra with prebeta lipoproteins.

Signs of a molecular interaction between the M protein and the circulating lipoproteins are often, but not always, detected. The most common are abnormal electrophoretic migration of lipoproteins which may precipitate or trail especially in agar or paper [125, 318] and sometimes do not enter into starch gel [318]. On immunoelectrophoresis, lengthened and distorted precipitin lines may be seen [120, 125]. In the ultracentrifuge, part of the M protein may float with the lipoproteins; and in contrast, in some cases, lipoproteins may coprecipitate with the M protein, either by dilution, cooling (cryoprecipitation) or salting out. In many cases the links between the M protein and the lipoproteins are strong, but in other cases they seem to be rather weak or they were not detected at all.

In short, the analysis of the reported cases suggests two important views:

(1) There are several types of myeloma with hyperlipidemia. Three of them, at least, may be individualized: IgA myeloma with mixed hyperlipidemia and cutaneous, tuberous and plane palmo-plantar xanthomas; the IgG myeloma with predominant hypercholesterolemia and plane cutaneous xanthomas; and the IgG myeloma with predominant hypertriglyceridemia and no xanthomas. It must be recalled that several cases cannot be included in those three types and that cases of myeloma with xanthomatosis and no hyperlipidemia have been described [801, 933, 1450].

(2) There are obviously from one case to another different kinds of links. These views are easily explained in the light of the characteristics of the antilipoproteins myeloma, which will now be reviewed.

Antilipoprotein Myelomas. Today, two types of myeloma with hyperlipidemia are known in which the M protein behaves like an antilipoprotein autoantibody. One is the IgA anti-Lp.P.G myeloma, of which two cases were studied [112, 121], and the other is IgG anti-Lp.A.S. myeloma, of which one case was recently studied [111]. In these two types, the serum is milky, and the lipidemia is highly increased and of the mixed type (Table 2). This hyperlipidemia is made essentially of very low density lipoproteins and chylomicra. High density lipoproteins may also be increased. All the circulating lipoproteins are complexed with the M protein. The vitamin A tolerance test [115] shows that the clearing of freshly absorbed lipids, coming from the intestine and carried by the lipoproteins, is very slow.

In vivo, the M protein of these patients is linked to the circulating lipoproteins. *In vitro*, this link remains strong and the whole serum has no visible activity against added lipoproteins. In the first case studied, some activity was found after the lipoproteins had been withdrawn by flotation. However, the antilipoprotein activity of the M protein is usually unmasked only after it is purified and separated from the lipoproteins to which it is linked. For this purpose, a potent method is necessary and many procedures have been tried in the last four years. Three were reported [118, 123, 124], the last one, in which the M protein is separated from the lipoproteins by ultracentrifugation in a medium containing sodium oleate, is preferred [124].

Table 2. *Anti-Lp Myelomas*

	Anti-LpP.G. IgA (2a, 35)		Anti-LpA.S. IgG (4)
	case Ger...	case Sor...	case Sa...
Sex	male	male	female
Age	57	62	52
Serum			
Aspect	milky	milky	milky
Cholesterol (mg/percent 100 ml)	400 to 900	770 to 1,120	360
Triglycerides (mg/percent 100 ml)	180 to 1,440	430 to 1,350	400
Phospholipids (mg/percent 100 ml)	400 to 900	290 to 670	—
M Protein			
Immunologic type	IgA kappa	IgA kappa	IgG kappa
Electrophoretic type	$gamma_1$	$gamma_1$	$gamma_1$
Active papaine fragment	Fab	Fab	Fab
Polymerization	+++	+	—
Lipoprotein reacting site	Lp P.G.	Lp P.G.	Lp A.S.
Presence of reacting site in			
human serum	+	+	+
beta-Lp	+	+	+
alpha-Lp	+	+	+
animal sera	+	+	—
Number of sites for 1 mole.			
of reacting beta-Lp	64	64	57
of reacting alpha-Lp	21	21	22

To detect the reaction between the purified M proteins and the lipoproteins, it was also necessary to develop methods for the purification of serum alpha [122] and beta lipoproteins [1194] as well as sensitive procedures; because, except for the first case studied, there is no precipitation. The following tests were routinely tried with each new pure M protein studied and purified: precipitation in saline [765], precipitation by double diffusion in agarose gels [1134], passive hemagglutination with red cells sensitized with diazotized benzidine [125] or chromium chloride [114], and filtration on dextran gels (Sephadex) [111]. This last method is highly sensitive, because it is able to demonstrate the primary reaction between the M protein and the lipoprotein (Lp). From it, the number of reacting sites on the lipoprotein molecule can be calculated. In the preceding tests fragments of the M proteins obtained after papain digestion were also used.

a) Anti-Lp.P.G. IgA Myeloma. In this type, the purified M.IgA is a gamma$_1$-globulin with a kappa light chain. It reacts with the alpha and beta lipoproteins [107] of all the human beings and all the animals studied (rabbit, rat, guinea pig, chicken and even carp). There are about 64 reacting sites on the human beta-Lp and 21 on the alpha-Lp molecules. Part of the reacting site can be extracted by ether and contains a phospholipid [113]. This site was called Lp.P.G.: Lp for lipoprotein, P for phylotypic, because it is present in many animal species, and G to remind us of the name of the first patient in whom a reacting M protein was found. After papain digestion, the Fab fragment of the anti-Lp.P.G. IgA reacts and not the Fc fragment. Although primary reaction with site Lp.P.G. seems exactly the same in a gel filtration test, there is some difference between the M protein of the two cases of anti-Lp.P.G. IgA myeloma studied. In the first case (Ger...), the IgA M is highly polymerized and gives with the lipoproteins heavy secondary reactions, precipitation occurs in agarose gels and, even in saline, the lipoproteins cannot enter into starch gels. Passive hemagglutination is still positive (+++) with 0.0001 μg of pure protein. In the second case (Sor...) the IgA M is only partially polymerized and gives only little secondary reaction. No precipitation occurs in gels or saline; the lipoprotein can enter into starch gel and 0.06 μg of pure protein is necessary to give positive passive hemagglutinations. A small difference in the structure of a part of the molecules distinct for the antibody site may explain the difference in their degree of polymerization. This is supported by the fact that the monomers have different electric charges.

b) Anti-Lp A.S. IgG Myeloma. In this type the purified M IgG is a gamma$_1$ globulin with a kappa light chain. It reacts with the alpha and beta lipoproteins of the patient's serum in two out of 35 human serums studied. It does not react with the rabbit lipoproteins studied. In one of the two reactive serums, all the alpha and beta lipoprotein molecules react; in the other, only part of them (about 30%). On each beta-Lp molecule, about 57 reacting sites were found and 22 on the alpha lipoprotein. This site is obviously different from the Lp P.G. site and was called Lp A.S. The Lp indicates lipoprotein, A because it corresponds to an allotypic character common to alpha and beta lipoproteins, and S to remind us of the name of the first patient in whom a reacting M protein was found. After papain digestion of the IgG M, only the Fab fragment was found to react with the Lp A.S. site.

c) Implications of Existence of Antilipoprotein Myelomas with Hyperlipidemias. There is no doubt that in the two types of myeloma with hyperlipidemia which have been described, the myeloma protein is an antilipoprotein antibody. The characteristics of the reaction are quite convincing; and the antigenic-reacting sites are well defined. As expected, they are different for the IgA and the IgG M proteins, and they are the same for the two IgA M proteins studied. The antibody-reacting site is part of the Fab fragment of the M proteins. In their monomer form, the antibodies are bivalent and their Fab fragments are monovalent.

As antibodies, these antilipoprotein M proteins take a place in the still short list of myeloma antibodies [427, 829, 975, 1339]. They support a hypothesis of Burnet's theory [270] which predicts that every M protein should have antibody activity. Their study will be useful for the understanding of the production and properties of antibodies [764].

As myelomas, the anti-Lp P.G. and anti-Lp A.S. types are probably the first examples of a longer series of anti-Lp myelomas [111]. Indeed it can be foreseen, without great risk of error, that the patient analysis of other cases of myelomas with hyperlipidemias will find M proteins which will react with lipoprotein sites unknown today. The grouping of the clinical and biological signs shows that there are surely more than three types in these series. In the same way one could explain hyperlipidemia being altogether rare and diverse in myeloma. It is rare because each M protein can only have one antibody activity [270, 764] so that the chances of seeing M proteins with antilipoprotein activity are not great. It is diverse because several M proteins can react with different lipoprotein sites.

The anti-Lp P.G. and anti-Lp A.S. myelomas also show that the specific activity of the M protein may explain part of the diversity of signs and disorders encountered in myeloma [109] such as hyperlipidemia, xanthomas, and atherosclerosis in the present cases and, for instance, bleeding [539] or anemias in others.

The occurrence of hyperlipidemia in anti-Lp P.G. and anti-Lp A.S. myelomas suggests that hyperlipidemia is partly independent of the lipoprotein site involved in the antibody reaction. To explain this it must be assumed that the enzymatic mechanisms which govern the clearing of the lipids carried by the lipoproteins can be blocked by different (more or less) specific reactions. In the same way, antibodies reacting with other proteins and with enzymes may, perhaps, induce hyperlipidemia in myelomas. Inhibition of heparin, and consequently lipoprotein lipase activity, by an M protein was recently described [538]. Accordingly the field of autoimmune hyperlipidemia is not restricted to cases with antilipoprotein antibodies and must be extended to all hyperlipidemias induced by antibodies which impair the clearing of blood lipids.

Macroglobulinemias. Hyperlipidemia is very unusual in Waldenström's macroglobulinemia. Among 25 cases, Hartmann [624] found only one in which the cholesterol level was higher than 300 mg/100 ml. On the other hand, hypolipidemia is usual [624, 837, 983, 1125, 1182]. At present there is no proof for an antilipoprotein antibody activity of the Waldenström's IgM. But this hypothesis must be kept in mind, because (1) several M proteins of this type were found to have auto-antibody activity reacting with an IgG-like rheumatoid factor [829]; (2) in another case, the IgM reacted with cardiolipin, a phospholipid [531]. (3) In one case, the IgM was linked to the circulating lipoproteins and cryoprecipitated with them [870].

However, it is well known that many of the Waldenström's IgM are stained by lipophilic dyes [621, 622, 910]. The frequency of this staining together with the fact that normal IgM contains lipids [623] suggests that in many cases physicochemical links (which are different than antigen-antibody links) interfere. Such links have already been studied *in vitro* [929].

Dyslipidemias in Monoclonal Gammapathies. If the antilipoprotein antibody activity of many M proteins can be proven, it will probably appear that in some cases hypolipidemia rather than hyperlipidemia is induced. Then a larger concept including autoimmune hyperlipidemias and hypolipidemias will be needed, in other words *autoimmune dyslipidemias*. However, this is pure hypothesis.

AUTOIMMUNE HYPERLIPIDEMIA IN ORDINARY HYPERLIPIDEMIAS WITHOUT MYELOMAS

"Ordinary" AIH. After the discovery of the antilipoprotein activity in one case of IgA myeloma with hyperlipidemia, research on antilipoprotein immunoglobulins in ordinary hyperlipidemia was immediately begun. They were found rather easily in a first case [106], and since then in several other cases [110, 119]. Today there is evidence for their presence in nine cases of which four were thoroughly studied. These figures give no information on the frequency of the disease, because the antibodies are still much more difficult to isolate and study in ordinary hyperlipidemia than in myeloma. We have spent years on only a few cases.

The hyperlipidemia is usually of the mixed type, made up of cholesterol and triglycerides, which can reach very high values. It is sometimes variable and may temporarily return to normal without any treatment. In some cases it seems to depend on the diet and in others not at all. During electrophoresis, the alpha and beta lipoproteins often enter uneasily into starch gel and may precipitate or trail in agar gels. In agarose with an albumin buffer [1106] several different aspects may be seen from one case to another: a broad beta band (type III), a predominant prebeta band (type IV), a prebeta and a chylomicra band (type V). On immunoelectrophoresis, the alpha and beta precipitin lines may be lengthened and distorted. In the ultracentrifuge, the VLDL and chylomicra are increased, the LDL may be decreased or normal, and the HDL may be slightly increased. The vitamin A tolerance test shows a great prolongation of the hypervitaminemia. The clearing rate of alimentary particles is very slow.

The antilipoprotein autoantibodies are linked to the circulating lipoproteins in soluble complexes and their activity can be demonstrated only after separation and extraction. This can be done with the methods used for studying antilipoprotein M proteins. The extracted antibodies are usually not precipitating but give positive passive hemagglutininations with red blood cells sensitized by beta or alpha lipoproteins. In all the cases studied, the reacting sites are common to alpha and beta lipoproteins, but their identity with site Lp.P.G. or site Lp.A.S. has yet to be proven. An Ig which mixes *in vitro* with lipoproteins is always present in the active extracts. In most cases it is an IgG or an IgA. One IgM was also found mixed with an IgG. However the type of reacting antibody was not exactly determined, because in "ordinary" AIH there is much less circulating antibody than in AIH with myeloma. However it is obvious that, like in myeloma AIH, several antibody types reacting with different sites can induce the disease.

Xanthomatosis, especially cutaneous or tuberous, was present in some of the first cases studied, but it may also be absent. Atherosclerosis seems very frequent and severe, three of the first four patients studied had ischemic diseases, two of which began early, at ages 33 and 35.

Situation of AIH among Hyperlipidemias. Lacking a convenient test for its detection on a large scale, we can give no figure for the frequency of AIH in the population. However, many facts suggest that this metabolic disorder of immune origin may be one of the most important causes of primary and secondary hyperlipidemias. Indeed the presence of antibodies and immune disorders are well known in the nephrotic syndrome and in biliary cirrhosis [1519, 1520], and the possibility of AIH is here very credible. AIH would also fit well into "primary" hyperlipidemias of the mixed type and especially when broad beta and prebeta lipoproteins are present (types III, IV, and V). In these three frequent types, beta and prebeta particles containing alpha and beta lipoproteins [507, 864] were found which also contain other proteins. One of these proteins called Apolipoprotein C has some characteristics of a gamma globulin: MW = 180,000 and a 7 S sedimentation coefficient. The presence of antilipoprotein antibodies would easily explain the structure of these complexes, which is still open to question. It is felt that when enough is known about AIH, a new classification of hyperlipidemias based on the types of antibodies involved will be necessary.

AUTOIMMUNE HYPERLIPIDEMIA IN IMMUNIZED ANIMALS

It is known that immunization of animals, for the purpose of inducing heteroantibodies, often produces a hyperlipidemia with a milky serum [88, 1008, 1305, 1452]. This is particularly true in rabbits [127] and chickens [1493]. This hyperlipidemia appears in rabbits [127] on a normal diet. It may happen early, beginning during the fourth to the sixth weeks of the immunization course. It is then usually transient and lasts only a few weeks. It may be late, beginning twelve weeks or more after the end of the immunization course. It is then permanent and looks very much like AIH in man. Cholesterol and triglycerides are increased together and may reach very high levels. Figures of 320 mg/100 ml for the cholesterol and 800 mg/100 ml of triglycerides were found in rabbits having a normal diet without any lipid supplement. Broad beta, prebeta lipoproteins and chylomicra are present giving types that differ from one case to another. Arterial lesions are usually present in these animals [127]. However hyperlipidemia is not absolutely necessary to produce them [240, 862, 1008, 1295, 1304, 1305].

In a rabbit which became highly hyperlipidemic six weeks after several injections of Freund's adjuvant, an Ig which behaved like an antilipoprotein autoantibody was extracted [116]. This antibody was linked *in vivo* to the circulating lipoproteins. To prove its presence and activity, it was necessary to use the purification methods already applied in human AIH. It reacts with a lipoprotein site which is not present in all rabbits and is probably allotypic. Accordingly it can be stated that a truly experimental AIH was induced in this animal, and it is likely that immunization hyperlipidemias are usually AIH. A thorough study of this condition will perhaps cast same light on the origin of human AIH. At present we only state that many different antigens can induce experimental hyperlipidemia in rabbits [127].

Also AIH is probably the cause of hyperlipidemia which develops in chickens. It would easily explain the fact that after immunizing with albumin, the beta lipoproteins will coprecipitate with the heterologous albumin-antialbumin complexes in hyperlipidemic animals [1493].

CONCLUSIONS

It is obvious that many hyperlipidemias are not AIH, e.g., familial hypercholesterolemia without hypertriglyceridemia which is sometimes called pure type II. The existence and importance of AIH are now well documented.

Its existence relies on three basic facts which strenghten each other: (a) in several myelomas with hyperlipidemia, the M protein is an auto-antibody to lipoproteins; (b) in ordinary hyperlipidemias in man, auto-antibodies to lipoproteins were found; and (c) in hyperlipidemias induced in rabbits by immunization, the presence of an antilipoprotein auto-antibody was once proved.

The importance of the AIH concept is illustrated by the great number of questions it can answer and also by the questions it raises, not only in the field of immunology, but also in the very practical fields of hyperlipidemias and atherosclerosis. The different types of antibodies involved in AIH will probably explain the origin and mechanism of many "primary" and "secondary" hyperlipidemias as well as the occurrence in many cases of an associated hyperglycemia or hyperuricemia and many other more or less rare associations. The structure of several different types of abnormal lipoproteins and particles which can be found in the serum, and the variable frequency of xanthomas of different types and of atherosclerosis in hyperlipidemias may also be thus explained. In the future, when more is known about the antibodies, a classification of hyperlipidemias including AIH types will probably be useful. Among the numerous new questions raised by the existence of AIH, three are specially important: (1) what is the mechanism of hyperlipidemia in AIH; (2) what is the mechanism of atherosclerosis in AIH; and (3) what is the treatment of AIH?

To understand the probable mechanism of hyperlipidemia in AIH, two facts must be recalled: (1) the circulating lipoproteins are trapped in big complexes, and (2) the lipids which are transported in these complexes remain longer in the vascular bed than when they are transported by free lipoproteins. These two facts suggest that the mechanism which release the transported lipids in the tissues are impaired. In this hypothesis, AIH is a consequence of a blockade of the enzymes which attack the lipoprotein molecules, and indeed we have found recently in several cases a great inhibition of lipoprotein lipase activity. However, the exact mechanism is surely more complex, because the inhibition of the enzymes must depend on the connection between their reacting sites and the site recognized by the antibody. Many advances can be made in the understanding of normal lipolysis by studying the different antibodies involved in AIH.

The mechanism of atherosclerosis in AIH deserves a thorough study. First we do not wish to imply that atherosclerosis in AIH is a direct autoimmune disease. This was said about many experimental types of atherosclerosis in which "antiarterial" antibodies were found, but it was never proved that these antibodies could be harmful to the vessel wall. In AIH, which is a spontaneous disease in man, there are no "antiarterial" antibodies but only soluble circulating autoimmune complexes. These complexes very probably move slowly through the arterial wall as nearly all circulating macromolecules do. Then as they are rather unstable, they may precipitate in this poorly vascularized tissue and become the first step of atherosclerosis. In this hypothesis, atherosclerosis, secondary to AIH, is an indirect autoimmune disease and could be classified as an "immune complex disease" like the arteriopathies of serum sickness [523]. Atherosclerosis in AIH differs from the arteriopathy of serum sickness by the autoimmune origin of the circulating complexes and by their big lipid load [127]. It may be called an "autoimmune complex disease".

The existence of AIH opens a new way in which to search for new antilipidemic drugs. After having tried penicillamine with very incomplete results [117], we now use with some success immunodepressing drugs. However, it is too soon to make any definitive statement on the value of these treatments. It is still an experimental field and one must remain very cautions in the use of these rather dangerous drugs.

Discussion Following Dr. Stein's Paper

Dr. AHRENS: Dr. Stein has very clearly shown the way in which lipids are released from the Golgi apparatus into the space of Disse. Can he tell us anything about the process of discrimination which allows cholesterol and phospholipids of a different type to be secreted into the biliary canaliculi?

Dr. STEIN: Dr. Ahrens is alluding to the unusual segregation of lipids within the liver cell by which only lecithin and cholesterol reach the biliary canaliculi: the lecithin belongs to one family type, mainly the palmitoyl-linoleoyl.

We assume, and I think Dr. Zilversmit will agree, that there is some carrier protein which is specific for this type of lecithin and which brings this molecule to the biliary canaliculus. During our radioautographic studies, we were not able to show independent synthesis of lecithin in the region of the biliary canaliculi.

Dr. STEINBERG: Many of us are wondering about the importance of the lecithin-cholesterol acyl transferase (LCAT) in relation to the cholesteryl esters of plasma lipoproteins. Dr. Stein showed data suggesting that the VLDL gets out of the Golgi apparatus with a high fraction of cholesterol present in the ester form. Would Dr. Stein (or anybody else) comment on whether that means the newly secreted lipoprotein already has the ester and doesn't have to acquire it as a result of LCAT in the plasma?

Dr. STEIN: The studies I have referred to were undertaken by the group from Vanderbilt University, who have shown the presence of cholesteryl ester in the granules isolated from the Golgi apparatus. I understand that these studies have now been repeated by Drs. Hamilton and Havel.

Dr. HAVEL: The fatty acid composition of the cholesteryl esters in Golgi particules is very similar to those of cholesteryl esters in VLDL of plasma and differ greatly from those in LDL and HDL. As has been postulated before, it appears that cholesteryl esters of VLDL in the rat are synthesized in the liver whereas those in HDL are produced by the LCAT reaction.

Dr. SEIDEL: Dr. Stein, do you believe that all of the circulating plasma lipoproteins derive from either liver or intestinal cells by *de novo* synthesis. In other words, do you think these cells are required for the synthesis of plasma lipoproteins, or would you believe that at least a partial formation of lipoproteins could occur within the plasma?

Dr. Stein: I believe that the evidence we have at the moment indicates that only the liver and the intestine form very low density lipoproteins. How the other lipoproteins which appear in the plasma may be formed is still disputed.

Dr. Fredrickson: I think I omitted in my summary a statement to the effect that there are no apolipoproteins within the plasma. Dr. Lees has presented some evidence, based on immunochemical studies of derivatives of low density lipoproteins, that, in fact, such apoproteins may circulate.

In our laboratory Dr. Gotto has extensively examined plasma from normal subjects and is unable to find a circulating apolipoprotein similar to the one which is obtained by delipidation of beta lipoprotein *in vitro*. Thus, a partial answer is that there is uncertainty regarding the presence of circulating apolipoproteins which would allow for the formation of lipoprotein within the plasma by combination of lipids with protein.

Dr. Boyle: In 1954 we published a paper with Drs. Bradgon and Brown on the production *in vitro* of $alpha_1$ lipoproteins from a system consisting only of plasma, with no liver cells. I would like to hear some comment on this.

Dr. Fredrickson: I have always interpreted the experiments of Dr. Boyle, and still do, in the light of current developments, as the first indication that one could move peptides or partially hydrolyzed products from VLDL to HDL. I think that the presence in both of these families of the same peptides, as described, corroborates those original observations.

Dr. Scanu: Dr. Shore, how do you assess the purity of the peptides before their analysis?

Dr. Shore: First, when there seems to be reason to do so, we rechromatograph the peptide in our 8M Urea-Tris system. On rechromatography, the peptide invariably comes off the column as a single peak at the same place it did before rechromatography.

We do disc electrophoresis in polyacrylamide gels containing 8M urea, terminal amino acid analyses by the dansylation and hydrazinolysis techniques, quantitative carboxyl-terminal amino acid analysis with carboxypeptidases A and B before and after fractionation, and sedimentation equilibrium studies in the analytical ultracentrifuge. We compare the molecular weight obtained in the centrifuge experiments with that obtained from carboxyl-terminal amino acid analysis. The use of centrifuge data alone (linearity of LNC versus R^2 plot) is not a sure way to demonstrate homogeneity since the molecular weights of most of the peptides, and there seem to be several, is of the order of 10 to 15,000.

Also, we are encouraged when we isolate a peptide deficient in an amino acid, and there are several peptides that are deficient, since this argues for purity rather than the presence of a contaminating protein. If all these methods and approaches indicate purity, we are reasonably happy.

Dr. Scanu: In your studies using the technique of circular dichroism did you take into account the fact that polypeptides with C-terminal glutamine and threonine have a different content of cystine? In other words, did you rule out the possibility that one of the peptides contains cystine and the other does not?

Dr. SHORE: There is a difference of 1.5 M% in half cystine content. I don't think it is great enough to account for the difference in helicity between the two, 50% in one case and 33% in the other; but it may be possible. I think the important point is that the two polypeptides seem to be different in alpha-helical content, no matter what brings about that difference.

Dr. SCANU: We agree with your differences, but I think the cystine content has something to do with it.

Discussion Following Dr. Beaumont's Paper

Dr. STEIN: Dr. Seidel, did you study the fatty acid composition of the lecithin to see whether this is the protein that carries the lecithin from the liver cell to the bile?

Dr. SEIDEL: We did not do any fatty acid determination; only phospholipid determinations.

Dr. KRITCHEVSKY: Did you do any determinations of the LCAT enzyme in the serum of these patients? That, perhaps, could give you some clue as to the site where the cholesteryl ester might be added to the lipoprotein?

Dr. SEIDEL: No.

Dr. AHRENS: Dr. Seidel, in view of the fact that you have found this new lipoprotein in all forms of biliary stasis, it would appear that the liver may be adding something that is responsible for the elaboration of this lipoprotein.

Have you looked to see whether the protein that you have isolated may have an increased content of bile acids? Might this account for some of the unusual physicochemical characteristics of this material?

Dr. SEIDEL: We haven't looked into that, but I believe the characteristic behavior of this lipoprotein is due to two facts. First, this lipoprotein has a content of 65% phospholipids. If you remove the phospholipids, the apolipoprotein behaves more or less as other apolipoproteins behave. Second, the behavior of the LP-X is probably also determined by the presence of albumin. Of the protein content of LP-X 40% arises from albumin. My feeling is that the increased concentration of bile salts may impair the metabolism of lipoproteins, in particular the catabolism of the VLDL fraction, rather than act as a moiety of LP-X.

Dr. BOYLE: Dr. Seidel, when a patient with primary biliary cirrhosis is treated with methyl testosterone, usually to relieve the itching of that disease, a new component appears that floats at a density of 1.063. It is a separate band from the S_f 0–10 low-density lipoproteins and has a flotation rate of S_f 16–17. I wonder if that is an LP-X or another lipoprotein of a different nature?

Dr. SEIDEL: Yes, your findings are correct. As a matter of fact, together with Dr. Mills, we have described these centrifugal patterns in a paper which will be out soon in *Clinica Chimica Acta*.

Dr. ENGELBERG: Dr. Seidel: In one of the slides the electrophoretic pattern was reminiscent of that seen in broad beta disease, Type III. I wonder if any studies have been done to examine the possibility that LP-X or a lipoprotein similar to it, might be the one that is giving that broad beta pattern?

Dr. Seidel: I think this is just a coincidence, because broad beta disease is caused by a VLDL with a beta lipoprotein mobility, while this broad beta band is caused by two low-density lipoproteins, LP-B and LP-X.

Dr. Connor: I wonder if Dr. Beaumont has seen this lipoprotein immunoglobulin in patients with transient infectious diseases?

Dr. Beaumont: Indeed, I am looking for it.

Dr. Magnani: I have studied cellulose acetate electrophoresis, and I have found on this particular medium that common lipid stains do not necessarily stain just lipid but will equally well stain certain proteins, particularly the more hydrophobic proteins such as those which make up the globulin complex. I also studied one patient with myelomatosis who had hyperlipidemia, and whose electrophoretic pattern showed a gamma M peak which stained well with one lipid stain. However, using a more selective stain, a chemical stain which particularly binds fatty acid double bonds, I was able to show that this gamma M peak contained no lipid whatsoever.

I would like to ask Dr. Beaumont what evidence he has that all these complexes do in fact contain lipid, and what evidence has he that the stains he uses on starch gel stain only lipid?

Dr. Beaumont: The demonstration of the lipoprotein-immunoglobulin interactions reported here does not depend upon lipid staining.

Section VI

SELECTED PAPERS ON LIPOPROTEINS AND ATHEROSCLEROSIS

STUDY OF THE PROTEIN MOIETY OF LOW AND HIGH DENSITY LIPOPROTEINS*

H. PEETERS and V. BLATON

The protein components of low (LDL) and high density (HDL) lipoproteins are now under investigation in several laboratories. The complete removal of all lipids from LDL produces irreversibly aggregated gel-like products [928, 1301]. This hampers the further characterization of the physical, chemical properties of the lipid-free apoprotein B. In the presence of sodium dodecyl sulphate (SDS) Granda [560] obtained a water-soluble phospholipid containing apoprotein and showed two fractions in free-boundary electrophoresis. We demonstrated the existence of two subunits in this modified apoprotein B after electrofocusing [188, 189].

A water-soluble, essentially lipid-free protein from human HDL was reported by Scanu [1299] and showed three bands in starch gel electrophoresis, all three reacting to rabbit antihuman serum. In the presence of 0.05% SDS, however, the three bands sedimented as a single component. Thus they concluded that alpha protein is an aggregate of one subunit. An analogous conclusion was obtained by Sodhi [1382]. However, the amino acid composition of the protein moiety obtained from alpha lipoprotein (LP) subclasses seems to imply several polypeptides [32, 1358]. We described four subfractions after electrofocusing [188, 189]. Recently Scanu [1302] demonstrated polypeptide heterogeneity of apo-HDL after urea treatment.

In this work the LDL subunits from man and baboon apoprotein B and the human HDL_2 subunits are described and compared.

MATERIALS AND METHODS

Lipoproteins were separated from the plasma of normal male students (20 to 22 years of age) and normal male baboons (4–5 years of age). The plasma lipids were determined and differentiated as described earlier [186, 187]. The low density fractions LDL_1 and LDL_2 were prepared as described by Scanu [1301]. Some experiments on beta-LDL were done on a commercial Cohn III-0 fraction (NBC) made soluble in Tris Buffer of pH 8.1, $\mu = 0.1$ containing M NaCl and 1% glycine and purified by molecular sieving on Sephadex G-150. An HDL 2 fraction (d. 1.063–1.125) was obtained from Scanu.

The lipoproteins and their apoproteins were submitted to gel filtration on Sephadex G-150 and G-100, to ion exchange cellulose chromatography on DEAE 25 C wet, and to electrofocusing in ampholine gradients 3–10, 4–6 and 6–8 (LKB).

* The authors are indebted to Tech. Ing. D. Vandamme and to Miss M. Lemahieu and Miss N. Vandecasteele for their skillful technical assistance. This work was supported by Grant No. 1153 of the N.F.W.G.O.

The purity of each preparation was verified by paper electrophoresis [853], by immunoelectrophoresis and immunodiffusion in agarose (Seravac) against rabbit antihuman alpha lipoprotein, antihuman beta lipoprotein and antihuman serum (Behringwerke).

The low density lipoproteins separated by centrifugation were delipidated according to a slightly modified method used by Day at a temperature of −16° C. The purified beta lipoprotein, obtained from Cohn III-0, and the HDL 2 fraction were delipidated according to Scanu [1298, 1299].

RESULTS

Subunits of Low Density Lipoproteins:

Subunits of LDL from Cohn III-0 Fraction. On Sephadex G-100 the SDS-apoprotein B still containing 2% phosphatidylcholine separates in two components neither of which precipitates against rabbit antihuman serum nor against

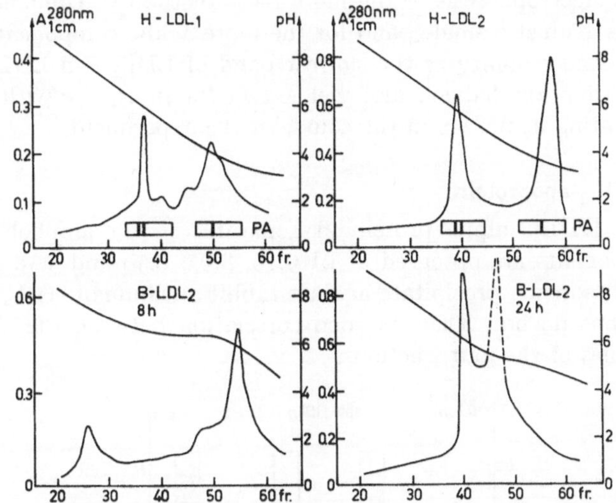

Fig. 1. Electrofocusing of human apo-LDL 1 and LDL 2 and of Baboon apo-LDL 2. The human (H-) fractions (LDL 1 and LDL 2) are shown with their polyacrylamide (PA) control. The baboon (B-) fraction (LDL 2) is shown after 8 and 24 hours. There is a precipitate around pH 5.5 after 24 hours

rabbit antihuman LDL. The separation improves with increasing pH, and there is a shift in the ratio between the fractions as a function of the apoprotein concentration. The same material gives two sharp main peaks with a pI value of 5.36 and of 6.12 after electrofocusing in a pH 3–10 gradient. These fractions do not precipitate against rabbit antihuman LDL.

In order to establish whether two different polypeptides or two polymers of the same polypeptide are present, the apoprotein is treated with 8M urea during the 24 hours before a separation on a Sephadex G-100 and on a DEAE cellulose column. On the two columns only two fractions are found. The absorption curves of these two fragments have the same maximal absorbance peak at 275 nm, a wavelength different from that of usual proteins, and a different slope with an intersect at 295 nm.

Molecular weights, determined on Sephadex G-100 against two calibration curves, established with and without SDS are 141,000 and 73,000. After correction for a 5% carbohydrate and a 2% residual lipid content plus an amount of 20% SDS by weight [381] molecular weights of 102,000 and of 53,000 are calculated.

We conclude that the apoprotein B from Cohn III-0 contains two polypeptides different in pI, U.V. absorption, and molecular weight. Due to the fact that the Cohn III-0 is derived from pooled plasma, a definite statement about the proportion of these two subunits in individual patients cannot be made.

Subunits of LDL from Ultracentrifuge (UCF) Fractions. In a second set of experiments apoprotein B from UCF fractions of individual human and baboon plasma was submitted to electrofocusing.

The apoprotein from the human LDL_1 shows two main fractions with pI 5.65 and 4.1. In LDL_2 there are also two fractions but at pI 6.4 and 3.65. The polyacrylamide gel electrophoresis of the more basic of the two compounds shows a double band as against a single band for the more acidic component. This single band has the same mobility as the slowest band of LDL_1 and LDL_2.

The LDL_2 from the baboon also yields two fractions, one with pI 6.15 and a zone precipitating at pH 5.5 in the course of the experiment.

Subunits of HDL_2-apoprotein:

Apoprotein HDL_2 (alpha protein 2) separates in an ampholyte gradient, and four components are observed at pI 9.16, 8.97, 6.36 and 5.38 (Fig. 2). The two central components precipitate against rabbit antihuman HDL, but the two extreme fractions do not. There is good correlation between the agar mobility and the pI values of the four fractions.

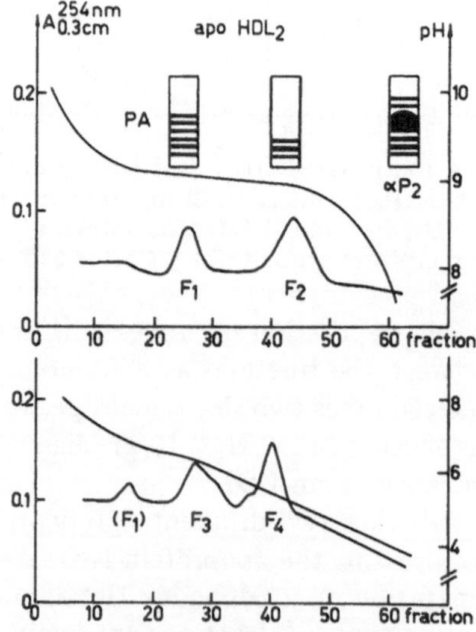

Fig. 2. Electrofocusing of human apo-HDL_2 between pH 8–10 and 4–8. The polyacrylamide (PA) fractionation is shown in regard to the fractions F_1 and F_2 and compared to the total apoprotein (alpha P_2). At lower pH an unidentified fraction (F_1) is seen next to F_3 and F_4

Further heterogeneity of the whole alpha $protein_2$ and of the fractions separated at pI 9.16 and 8.97 was demonstrated on polyacrylamide gel electrophoresis. Whole alpha $protein_2$ shows six bands with bands three and four as major components. The fraction obtained at pI 9.16 shows six bands of similar concentration. The fraction obtained at pI 8.97 has three bands, two of which coincide with those of the major component.

DISCUSSION

Apoprotein B from Cohn-precipitation and from ultracentrifugal origin contains two polypeptides with slightly different pI values. The difference may be ascribed to the method of separation of the protein and of delipidation of the apoprotein, as well as to differences in amino acid composition. There is an analogy between the two fractions found in baboon and in human LDL_2, and their primary structure must be compared. Antisera against these subunits could be of help in resolving their relationship to one another and to the total apoprotein. The fact that these subunits do not react to an antiserum against the total lipoprotein suggests that apoprotein LDL_1 and apoprotein LDL_2 are built up from subunits with a proper and characteristic structure.

The concept of four subunits for apoprotein HDL_2 after electrofocusing is insufficient in the face of the further heterogeneity on polyacrylamide.

Analogies in the pI values between the most acidic component of HDL_2 and the more basic component of LDL_1 suggests the existence of a common piece. This is, however, not confirmed by the polyacrylamide electrophoresis of these fractions which rather confirms a separate identity for alpha and beta lipoproteins and their individual behavior regarding lipid load as a function of age, disease or drug therapy [186–189, 1161, 1162].

Insofar as these subunits are important to the lipid composition and the stability of lipoproteins, they may provide a clue to the genesis of atheromatosis. The evidence for molecular variation within an individual, as shown for LDL_1 and LDL_2, and for the phylogeny, as shown in human and baboon LDL_2, must be confirmed by a complete identification (including the amino acid sequence) of apoprotein subunits obtained from individual patient and animal sera. The metabolic turnover of the apoproteins and their subunits, and the factors influencing their loading and unloading of lipid must also be compared in normals and in patients possessing atheromatous lesions.

LOW DENSITY LIPOPROTEIN STRUCTURE AND ITS RELATION TO ATHEROGENESIS*

ROBERT S. LEVY and CHARLES E. DAY

A wealth of information has accumulated which strongly indicates that the low density lipoprotein (LDL) is one of the primary components in the atherogenic process. However, no one has yet succeeded in demonstrating exactly how LDL is involved in this process or why it is this particular molecule instead of another of the many serum proteins. Information obtained in our laboratory about the charge distribution on the LDL molecule sheds some new light on these two important questions.

That LDL is selectively precipitated from human serum by sulfated polysaccharides has been known for many years. Although it has long been thought that the interaction of LDL with polyanions is essentially electrostatic in nature, this has not been sufficiently demonstrated. Indeed, LDL is not even a basic molecule since its isoelectric point is around pH 5.7. However, the molecules causing precipitation of LDL are macromolecular and for that reason have access only to the charged groups at the surface of the LDL molecule. It is quite possible that there exists an uneven charge distribution between the outside surface and the interior, that part inaccessible to macromolecules, of the LDL. If this were the case, then LDL would be regarded as a polycation by macromolecular polyanions. The purpose of the investigation described herein was to test this charge distribution hypothesis.

LDL contains a number of components which possess positively charged groups. These include the amino acids, arginine and lysine, and the phospholipids lecithin, lysolecithin, sphingomyelin and cephalin. By selectively modifying some of these charged moieties, it was possible to test the preceding hypothesis.

MATERIALS AND METHODS

Human serum LDL was isolated from outdated pooled serum by a combination of amylopectin sulfate (APS) precipitation and preparative ultracentrifugation between the densities 1.019 and 1.063 g/ml. The reaction of LDL with APS was carried out in 0.05 M sodium phosphate buffer, pH 7.4, and the extent of reaction was determined by measuring the absorbance at 680 mμ. Each tube contained 2–5 mg LDL protein (LDL_p) and a variable amount of APS in a total volume of 4.0 ml phosphate buffer. The APS/LDL_p ratios were in a range of 10^{-3} to 10^1. Precipitation at various pH values was studied at given APS/LDL_p ratios in phosphate buffers at a constant ionic strength of 0.1. Variation with temperature was studied by successively raising the temperature of the same samples from 0 to 50° C.

* The work herein was supported by Grant 68–702 of the American and Kentucky Heart Associations and Grant 583104 of the National Heart Institute. The authors wish to thank Dr. John Yankeelov, Department of Biochemistry, for the generous gift of the trimer of biacetyl (TB).

LDL was modified with succinic anhydride according to the method of Scanu et al., [1301] and with the trimer of biacetyl (2,3-butanedione) according to the method of Yankeelov et al., [1583]. Partial delipidation by ether extraction was carried out by extracting LDL (10 mg LDL_p/ml of phosphate buffer, pH 7.4) with 15 volumes of peroxide-free diethyl ether for 96 hours in the cold, the ether being changed every 24 hours.

RESULTS AND DISCUSSION

Succinic anhydride reacts with free amino groups on the LDL protein and replaces the positive charge of an amino group with the negative charge of a carboxyl group. If the interaction between LDL and APS is ionic in nature and

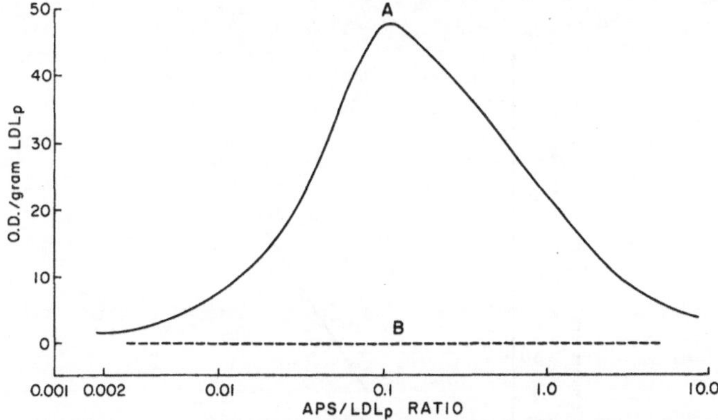

Fig. 1. The precipitation of native and modified LDL with APS. (A) native LDL, pH 7.4; (B) native LDL, pH 11; succinylated LDL, pH 7.4; TB modified LDL, pH 7.4

Table. *Interaction of amylopectin sulfate with low density lipoprotein under different conditions*[a]

Condition of LDL	pH	O.D./g LDL_p
Native	7.4	41
Native	8.3	20
Native	10.8	0
Ether extracted	7.4	68
Succinylated	7.4	0
TB modified	7.4	0

[a] APS/LDL_p ratio = 0.10.

amino groups contribute all or part of the positive charges, then the interaction of the succinylated LDL with APS should be reduced as is shown in Fig. 1 and the table. In fact, the precipitation of LDL with APS was completely eliminated by succinylation.

The trimer of biacetyl (TB) is a specific reagent for arginine modification in proteins under mild conditions [1583] although the structure of the reaction product has not yet been definitely established. Since arginine is a significant contributor to the positive charges in the LDL, treatment of this protein with TB should also reduce the precipitation reaction. It was found that TB modification had practically the same effect as succinylation as seen also in Fig. 1 and the table.

The effect of pH on precipitation was studied over a range of pH values from 6 to 11. The precipitation was maximal at pH 6 and eliminated at pH 11. Some of the pH data is shown in Fig. 1 and the table. These results are to be expected if the LDL-APS interaction is purely ionic. In the pH region of 9–11, LDL should lose the positive charge on lysine and gain a negative charge on tyrosine, thereby completely changing the charge profile and eliminating electrostatic attractions. Choline-containing phospholipids and arginine should maintain their charge at pH 11.

LDL modified by ether extraction showed an increased binding affinity for APS (table) probably indicating an uncovering of binding sites by the removal of neutral lipid. Ether extraction carried out in this manner also removes about

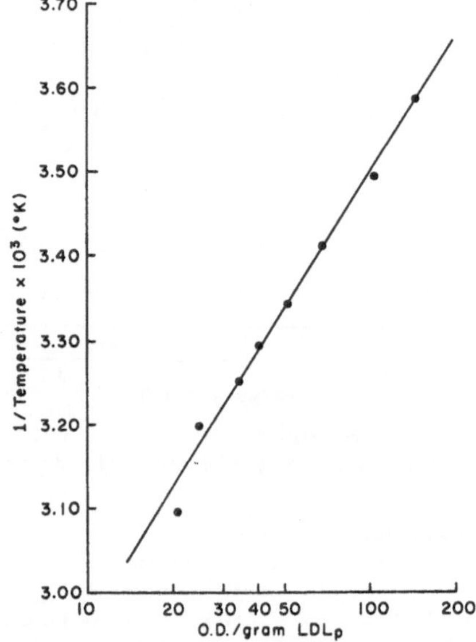

Fig. 2. Effect of temperature on the APS-LDL precipitation reaction

30% of the phospholipids indicating, along with the pH data, that phospholipids play only a minor role in the precipitation of LDL with APS.

This investigation demonstrates that the interaction of LDL with polyanions is an electrostatic phenomenon and that the positive charges on the LDL necessary for the reaction are contributed largely by lysine and arginine. The temperature data seen in Fig. 2 are consistent with an electrostatic interaction mechanism. Thus, the original hypothesis that the LDL possesses a net surface positive charge is substantiated.

The implications of this structural property of LDL toward the process of atherogenesis is quite obvious. The arterial intima is a tissue rich in charged macromolecular colloids, including acid mucopolysaccharides, collagen and elastin. Any LDL passing the lumenal-intimal barrier would be trapped in this briar patch of charged macromolecules, whereas other serum proteins would be unhindered because of their difference in surface charges. The deposition of LDL in the arterial wall may well be due to a nonspecific electrostatic enmeshment of this molecule with its cationic surface property. It seems certainly more than coincidental that fibrinogen is precipitated by polyanions in a manner completely analogous to LDL and that fibrinogen, too, is strongly involved in the genesis of atherosclerosis.

ANOMALOUS LOW DENSITY LIPOPROTEINS IN FAMILIAL HYPERBETALIPOPROTEINEMIA

JOAN SLACK and GERVASE L. MILLS

The high risk of ischemic heart disease associated with hypercholesterolemia has been well documented, and more recently it has become apparent that the risks are greater among patients with hypercholesterolemia associated with familial hyperbetalipoproteinemia than with hypercholesterolemia associated with hypertriglyceridemia [1007, 1374]. Familial hyperbetalipoproteinemia is inherited as an autosomal dominant characteristic resulting in a high concentration of beta lipoprotein, but there has been some doubt as to whether this beta lipoprotein is of normal composition [126, 488].

We have therefore examined the lipid composition of the S_f 0–20 substances in 32 carefully selected, untreated patients known to be heterozygous for familial hyperbetalipoproteinemia [1090] and compared the results with 35 controls of similar age and sex. In addition, the low density lipoprotein levels and the S_f 0–20 peak flotation rate have been determined for 15 of these patients and 20 controls. All the index patients had xanthoma tendinosum and total serum cholesterol levels over 325 mg/100 ml; none had total triglyceride levels greater than 200 mg/100 ml. First-degree relatives of the index patients were included if their cholesterol level was over 325 mg/100 ml. One girl of 11 years, the daughter of an index patient was included with a total serum cholesterol level of 315 mg/100 ml. The mean age of the patients was 31.3 years. In addition three patients known to be homozygotes were examined and their results reported separately. No patient was taking cholesterol-lowering drugs but some, on their own initiative, were using corn oil in their diet, some were deliberately cutting down the fat in their diet, but none was under any supervised dietary control. The controls were 16 men and 19 women volunteers some of whom were spouses of patients. All considered themselves to be in good health. Their mean age was 32.9 years.

Venous blood samples were obtained from patients and controls after an overnight fast. The distribution of the low density lipoproteins (density 1.007 to 1.063 gm/ml) was measured by the method of De Lalla et al. [386], and the S_f 0–20 lipoproteins were prepared for chemical analysis by the method of Havel et al. [649]. The lipid classes were separated by the chromatographic method of Hirsch and Ahrens [684]. Cholesterol and cholesteryl ester (without hydrolysis)

Table 1. *Lipoprotein distribution in patients and controls*

	S_f 0–12 mg/100 ml ± SD	S_f 12–20 mg/100 ml ± SD	S_f 20–100 mg/100 ml ± SD	S_f 100–400 mg/100 ml ± SD	Peak S_f rate ± SD
Controls					
Males (10)	355.90 ± 106.46	42.40 ± 17.40	92.50 ± 47.12	29.80 ± 32.68	6.33 ± 0.63
Females (10)	276.90 ± 55.28	44.20 ± 25.44	30.60 ± 20.87	2.00 ± 2.54	7.88 ± 0.81
Patients					
Males (5)	737.80 ± 177.68[a]	96.00 ± 21.37[a]	85.80 ± 36.97	16.00 ± 35.22	7.66 ± 0.73[a]
Females (10)	676.40 ± 155.72[a]	118.30 ± 100.11	47.70 ± 60.28	5.60 ± 15.02	8.33 ± 0.64

[a] Significance of difference from controls of same sex, $p < 0.001$.

Table 2. *Lipid composition of S_f 0–20 lipoprotein expressed as weight percentage of S_f 0–20 lipid*

	Cholesteryl ester ± SD	Free cholesterol ± SD	Triglyceride ± SD	Phospholipid ± SD
Controls				
Males (16)	50.35 ± 2.83	11.96 ± 2.92	8.46 ± 2.43	28.88 ± 2.88
Females (19)	51.46 ± 3.57	11.55 ± 1.40	7.17 ± 2.55	29.83 ± 4.56
Patients				
Males (12)	52.42 ± 4.63	12.90 ± 0.91	5.13 ± 1.46[a]	29.58 ± 5.55
Females (20)	53.88 ± 4.34	12.20 ± 1.36	4.27 ± 1.40[a]	29.61 ± 4.70

[a] $p < 0.001$ significance of difference from controls of same sex.

were measured by the Bloor [196] method, triglycerides according to Van Handel and Zilversmit [1492] and phospholipids by the method of Allen [39].

Table 1 shows that there is an increase in the concentration of lipoproteins in the S_f 0–20 range in both male and female patients but those of the S_f 20–400 range are similar to the controls. The method of selection of our index patients, which was adopted in order to exclude any patient with xanthoma tendinosum associated with Fredrickson Type III and IV hyperlipoproteinemia, ensured that the increase in their lipoprotein levels would be confined to the S_f 0–20 fraction.

There is a diminution of percentage triglyceride composition in the S_f 0–20 lipoprotein which is highly significant in both male and female patients, and there is a small increase in cholesteryl ester content which, however, fails to reach a significant level unless male and female patients are considered together. There is no difference in the proportion of free cholesterol or phospholipid. In the three homozygotes examined the mean triglyceride composition was 3.2%, and the content of cholesteryl ester was 53%.

Fig. 1 (a, b, and c) show representative photographs of the S_f 0–20 lipoprotein distributions from the model-E ultracentrifuge. There are characteristic differences in the contours of the peaks. Whereas the homozygote is characterized

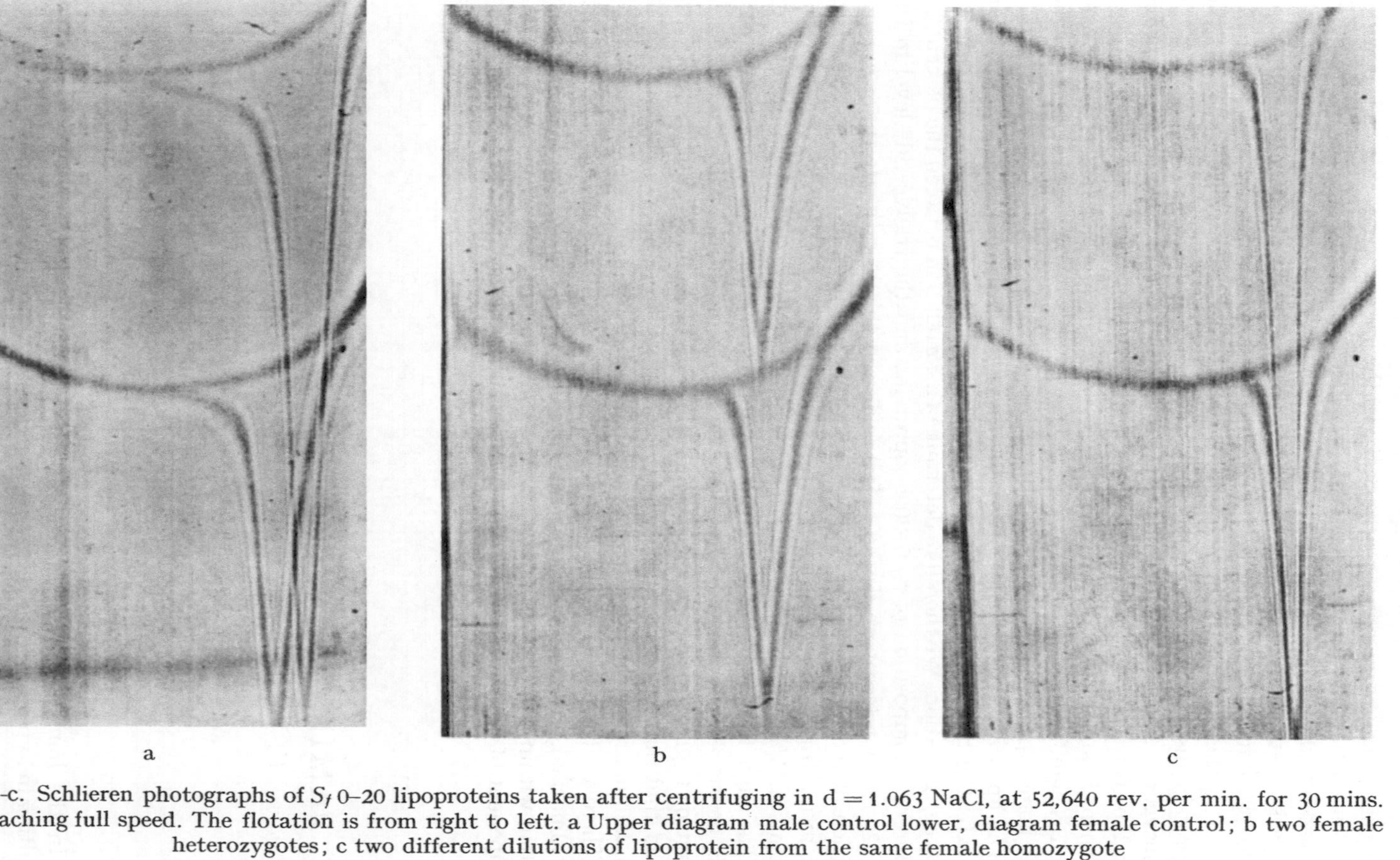

Fig. 1a–c. Schlieren photographs of S_f 0–20 lipoproteins taken after centrifuging in d = 1.063 NaCl, at 52,640 rev. per min. for 30 mins. after reaching full speed. The flotation is from right to left. a Upper diagram male control lower, diagram female control; b two female heterozygotes; c two different dilutions of lipoprotein from the same female homozygote

by a very narrow and symmetrical peak, in the heterozygote the peak is wider and skewed towards the trailing edge. In both homozygotes and heterozygotes the leading edge falls abruptly from the baseline. By contrast, in the controls the peak is still wider and the separation of the leading edge at the baseline is less precipitous, producing a triangular element at this point which is more marked in the male. The absence of this area seems to be characteristic of the lipoprotein distribution in our patients. The narrow symmetrical peak in the homozygotes suggests that their S_f 0–20 lipoproteins are more homogeneous than those of the controls or the heterozygotes.

There is an increase in the mean peak S_f rate in the patients of both sexes which is significant only in the males ($t=3.6570$, $p<0.001$; see Table 1). In the three homozygotes the mean peak S_f rate was 8.5 s.

The apparent triglyceride content of the S_f 0–20 lipoproteins depends upon the extent of their contamination with lipoproteins of $S_f>20$ during preparative ultracentrifugation. We therefore determined a correlation between the percentage triglyceride composition of S_f 0–20 lipoproteins and the triglyceride level in the $S_f>20$ fraction (compare Ewing [444]) and used this to estimate the true composition of the S_f 0–20 lipoproteins at zero concentration of $S_f>20$ substances. The mean triglyceride composition for controls was then 6.11% and for the patients 3.65%. This difference is highly significant ($t=5.5363$, $p<0.001$).

The high flotation rate of the lipoproteins from the patients suggests that their density is diminished. However, this is incompatible with the observed deficit of triglyceride but could result from an alteration of protein-lipid ratio of the kind that Beaumont [126] has reported in S_f 0–12 lipoproteins of patients with familial hypercholesterolemic xanthomatosis.

There is, therefore, evidence that the S_f 0–20 lipoproteins in the patients are abnormal. However, whether the genetic disorder produces a unique lipoprotein within the S_f 0–20 range or causes a disproportionate increase in a minor component of the natural spectrum still has to be investigated.

FAMILIAL HYPERBETALIPOPROTEINEMIA (TYPE II HYPERLIPOPROTEINEMIA) IN THE RHESUS MONKEY*

M. D. MORRIS and W. E. GREER

In the human, at least five heritable disorders of lipoprotein metabolism resulting in hyperlipoproteinemia have been described [489]. One of these, Type II,

* The authors wish to thank Mrs. Ann Kane and Mrs. Sara Smith for their excellent technical assistance. This work was supported by Grant MET 11811 from the U.S. Public Health Service, National Institutes of Health.

is found in association with an elevation of serum cholesterol and beta lipoproteins. Hyperbetalipoproteinemia, similar to that found in human Type II patients, has been previously reported in the Rhesus monkey [1040]. This paper reports the transmission of this defect to progeny of the affected male and affords the first evidence of an heritable defect of lipoprotein metabolism in the subhuman primate.

TREATMENT OF ANIMALS

Indian Rhesus monkeys were individually caged in an air-conditioned building and tuberculin tested every three months. The index male with hyperbetalipoproteinemia, Monkey No. 263, had been in the colony for four years. The female monkeys were shipped directly to our colony from the importer. All were post pubertal but precyclical when received. Prior to breeding each female had at least three menstrual cycles and had been in the colony from nine to eleven months. After breeding with the index male, the females were again individually caged.

Six of the eight females in the breeding study conceived, and dropped four live male term infants with birth weights between 303 and 342 g. One immature female infant (b.w. 210 g) died at birth, and one gravid female aborted spontaneously.

METHODS

Blood was drawn from the study infants at one to two days of age and at various intervals thereafter. No attempt was made to fast the infants prior to bleeding.

Plasma total cholesterol was determined as described previously [1038, 1041]. Agarose electrophoresis of the serum lipoproteins was done according to the method of Noble[1] et al.

RESULTS

A summary of the plasma lipid studies on Monkey No. 263 and control Rhesus monkeys is presented in Table 1. The persistent elevation of plasma cholesterol and beta lipoproteins observed in Monkey No. 263, and the absence of other common secondary causes of hyperbetalipoproteinemia fullfills the major criteria for Type II hyperlipoproteinemia.

Table 2 depicts the total serum cholesterol at various ages of the four male term offspring of the hyperbetalipoproteinemic male and age matched controls[2]. Infants of the index male had increased serum cholesterol content when compared to control infants during the first nine days of life. Infant No. 691 had an elevated serum cholesterol through the first month of life. Only infant No. 694 had increasing serum cholesterol through the first 60 days which reached a value of 367 mg/100 ml. Unfortunately this infant drowned at 90 days of age.

---

1 The authors wish to thank Dr. R. P. Noble for making this method available prior to its publication.

2 Some of the control sera were kindly supplied by Dr. David Valerio of Bionetics Research Labs.

Table 1. *Plasma lipids in monkey 263 (hyperbetalipoproteinemia) and control rhesus monkeys*

Plasma lipid	Mg/100 ml or percentage of total	
	No. 263	controls
Total cholesterol	266–723	144 ± 28
Phospholipids	360–560	225–265
Triglycerides	102–160	< 100
Total cholesterol/phospholipid	0.97–1.25	0.55–0.65
Alpha lipoprotein cholesterol	25–55	45–95
Cholesteryl esters (percentage of total cholesterol)	69–74	50–85
S_f 0–12 lipoprotein cholesterol (percentage of total cholesterol)	79–83	50–70

Table 2. *Total serum content of cholesterol in offspring of male rhesus monkey with hyperbetalipoproteinemia and age-matched controls*

Animal number	Age					
	< 33 hours	1–2 days	5–9 days	28–30 days	44–45 days	60–61 days
691			220	210		172
692		90		118	147	158
694	115			215	341	367
699	151					
Controls	51	57	88	127	133	115
ave range						
	42–62	36–89	71–110	98–151		111–120
N=	7	6	4	3	1	2

Fig. 1 shows that infant No. 691 at six days of age had an increased staining in both beta and prebeta lipoprotein bands when compared to an age-matched control. In Fig. 2, the remarkable qualitative similarity of the beta lipoprotein pattern of monkey No. 263 and his offspring, No. 694, at 44 days of age is evident[3].

DISCUSSION

The finding of progressively elevated cholesterol values and an increased beta lipoprotein by agarose electrophoresis from birth in one of the four progeny of the index hyperbetalipoproteinemic male provides strong evidence for the genetic transmission of Type II hyperbetalipoproteinemia in Rhesus monkeys. The serum cholesterol value of 367 mg/100 ml at 60 days of age of infant No. 694, is significantly higher than any value we have observed in a survey of more than 500 infant and adult Rhesus monkeys.

3 Infant 699, who expired suddenly at ten days of age after his mother rejected him, had a high serum cholesterol at 26 hours of age, and the lipoprotein pattern by electrophoresis was quite similar to that of infant No. 694.

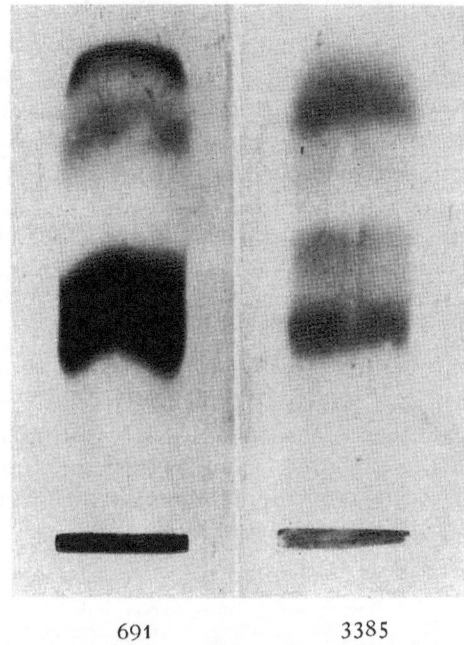

Fig. 1. Agarose electrophoresis of serum lipoproteins of offspring of Type II male rhesus monkey (No. 691) and age matched control (No. 3385). Total serum cholesterol: No. 691: 220 mg/100 ml; No. 3385: 78 mg/100 ml

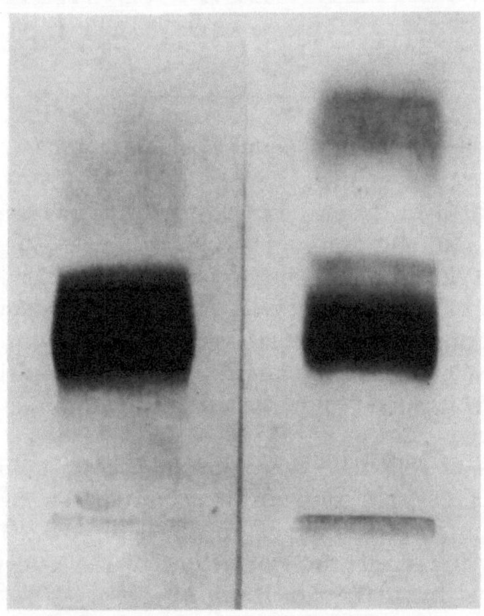

Fig. 2. Agarose electrophoresis of serum lipoproteins of offspring (No. 694) and Type II male rhesus monkey (No. 263). Total serum cholesterol: No. 694: 341 mg/100 ml; No. 263: 585 mg/100 ml

The other offspring of male No. 263, although found to have initial cholesterol values which were higher than age-matched controls, did not have a progressive increase in cholesterol as did infant No. 694. All of these infants, however, had beta lipoprotein which was elevated as judged by comparison of agarose electrophoretic patterns with age-matched controls. By two months the serum cholesterol values were considered to be in the normal range for all infants except No. 694.

Although the expression of the plasma lipid abnormality in the Rhesus monkey is very similar to that in the human, additional studies are essential to establish further likeness of the two conditions.

SUMMARY

Each of four infant Rhesus offspring from a male with hyperbetalipoproteinemia had elevated serum cholesterol soon after birth. One infant had an increased plasma cholesterol and beta lipoprotein during the first 60 days of life.

The transmittance of hyperbetalipoproteinemia (Type II) in the Rhesus monkey is clearly demonstrated by these studies.

SYNTHESIS OF LOW DENSITY LIPOPROTEINS BY ISOLATED CELL PREPARATIONS OF GUINEA PIG LIVER

G. L. MILLS and M. J. CHAPMAN

The ability of the liver to synthesize lipoproteins has been studied by several investigators, e.g., Radding et al. [1208], Haft et al. [592], Marsh [932], and Jones et al. [754]. Prior to an evaluation of the role of this activity of the liver in the maintenance of serum lipoprotein patterns, the following study has been undertaken to determine whether: (a) synthesis of lipoprotein will take place in preparations of isolated cells, as judged by the incorporation of labelled amino acid in the protein moiety, and (b) whether these lipoproteins can be characterized as serum lipoproteins.

The suspensions of cells have been prepared from guinea pig liver by the method of Ontko [1128], and respired at an initial rate of 20 µl O_2/10 mg dry weight in a medium of 0.02 M Tris, 0.1 M KCl, pH 7.4 at 37°. This had fallen by 50% after four hours, by which time there was evidence that the cells were becoming permeable to Trypan Blue.

In an effort to ensure that active lipoprotein synthesis was taking place before the liver was excised, the animal was first fed for six days on a high fat diet. This consisted of the normal diet pellets augmented by the addition of 15.0% corn oil and 1.7% cholesterol, and brought about a twenty fold rise in the serum

Table 1. *The gross chemical composition, percentage by weight, of guinea pig serum lipoproteins and of fractions isolated from liver cell preparations*

	Mean concen. mg/10 ml	^{3}H counts dpm/μg	Cholesterol[a]	Phospholipid	Triglyceride	Protein	CE/FC[a]
			Hepatic lipids				
Intracellular lipid	11.3	0.81	12.0	4.7	80.2	3.0	7.2
Lipomicrons	1.1	1.6	20.9	7.3	68.9	2.8	3.5
VLDL	0.07	8.3	56.5	13.8	26.0	3.7	5.0
LDL	0.06	5.6	37.6	22.5	27.6	12.2	2.0
			Serum lipoprotein lipids				
Serum VLDL (prediet)			10.6	13.8	64.5	10.6	1.5
Serum LDL (prediet)			40.6	16.3	14.3	28.9	8.4
Serum VLDL (postdiet)			19.1	8.0	65.8	7.1	2.3
Serum LDL (postdiet)			57.1	17.3	1.0	24.9	5.3

[a] The value termed "cholesterol" represents the sum of cholesteryl ester and the free sterol; CE/FC represents the ratio of these two.

levels of low density lipoproteins. Liver cells from one of these stimulated animals (45 ml of suspension containing 4 mg protein/ml) were incubated at 37° for four hours in the presence of ^{3}H-Leucine; a control was also made in the presence of 0.2 mM cycloheximide. After the incubation, three fractions were isolated from the medium and a fourth from the residual cells.

1. Lipomicrons: isolated by centrifuging for 20 minutes at 39,000 rev/min in solution of density 1.007 gm/ml.

2. VLDL: isolated by 16 hour centrifugation at 30,000 rev/min in solution of density 1.007 gm/ml.

3. LDL: isolated by 16 hour centrifugation at 30,000 rev/min at density 1.063 gm/ml.

4. Intracellular Lipid Material: isolated from homogenates of the cells by the method used for fraction 1.

Each fraction was then chemically analyzed, and the incorporation of label into the protein determined by scintillation counting.

The results summarized in Table 1 show that incorporation of ^{3}H-Leucine proceeded at a significant rate in the LDL and VLDL fractions but, perhaps because of the pool size, was barely detectable in the other two fractions. As expected, the intracellular lipid had a very high proportion of triglyceride, being slightly less in the lipomicrons. With decreasing molecular size and increasing density, however, the triglyceride level diminished while the content of cholesterol, phospholipid and protein tended to rise. However, the VLDL fraction contained more cholesterol and less phospholipid than the average guinea pig serum VLDL, while in the LDL fraction there was more triglyceride but less protein and cholesterol than in the corresponding serum lipoprotein. It may also be observed that more than 80% of the cholesterol in the intracellular lipid was esterified and that this proportion diminished to about 55% in the LDL fraction. The ratio of esterified to unesterified cholesterol in the latter was therefore significantly less than in the serum LDL.

Table 2. *Average distribution of fatty acids in lipoproteins from serum of guinea pigs before and after feeding a corn oil/cholesterol diet, and in lipoproteins isolated from liver preparations of fed animals*[a]

	Fatty acid distribution					
Carbons: double bonds	16:0	16:1	18:0	18:1	18:2	18:3
Corn oil	8.3	0.5	2.0	31.5	56.7	0.0
	Hepatic triglyceride					
Intracell. triglyceride	15.9	1.9	3.7	23.2	49.9	4.2
Lipomicron triglyceride	20.1	3.9	7.3	26.7	32.7	3.9
VLDL triglyceride	19.5	5.0	11.3	30.5	26.4	2.3
LDL triglyceride	27.3	8.3	17.4	28.3	8.0	2.4
	Serum lipoprotein triglyceride					
Serum VLDL (prediet)	17.4	2.0	4.3	20.9	36.2	15.3
Serum VLDL (postdiet)	12.0	1.0	3.7	22.1	58.7	2.4
Serum LDL (prediet)	21.6	3.0	8.1	25.7	23.9	8.6
Serum LDL (postdiet)	12.6	2.2	7.5	29.9	46.5	1.3
	Hepatic cholesteryl esters					
Intracell.	17.0	3.1	6.6	35.5	29.0	5.0
Lipomicron	21.0	5.3	12.6	29.4	18.4	5.2
VLDL	17.1	3.6	10.8	34.6	25.8	3.9
LDL	18.3	6.7	11.7	30.3	21.3	3.8
	Serum lipoprotein cholesteryl esters					
Serum VLDL (prediet)	19.1	4.5	12.7	25.8	14.5	1.7
Serum VLDL (postdiet)	10.6	1.7	3.0	32.3	50.6	1.8
Serum LDL (prediet)	11.7	2.7	13.2	62.9	6.2	0.0
Serum LDL (postdiet)	7.9	2.4	3.4	14.6	64.1	2.5

[a] The values are the weight percentage of each fatty acid, minor components being omitted.

Although the proportion of linoleic acid in the serum phospholipids was slightly higher in treated than in untreated guinea pigs, the diet was administered for too short a time to bring about any marked change in their fatty acid composition. It is, therefore, significant that the distribution of fatty acids in the phospholipids of the isolated liver fractions resembles that of the serum phospholipid from untreated animals. Furthermore, there is little systematic change in the fatty acid distribution of the phospholipids of one fraction compared with that of another, although there may be some increase in arachidonic acid towards the LDL fraction. The phospholipids have accordingly been omitted from Table 2, which presents the mean fatty acid composition of the other three isolated fractions.

The distribution of fatty acids in the intracellular triglycerides resembles that of the corn oil added to the diet in its high content of linoleic acid and low level of stearic acid. It differs, however, in having a higher level of palmitic and linolenic acids. Moreover, in the transition towards the LDL, the level of linoleic acid in the triglyceride falls, while that of palmitoleic and stearic acids rises. By comparison with serum lipoproteins, the triglycerides of the VLDL and LDL fractions are richer in stearic acid than those from either treated or untreated animals. By contrast, the level of linoleic acid in these fractions was markedly less than in serum lipoproteins from either source.

Like the phospholipids, the cholesteryl esters of all the fractions have similar fatty acid patterns. However, the proportion of oleic and linoleic acids in the VLDL and LDL fractions was intermediate between that in esters from serum lipoproteins from "normal" and diet-fed guinea pigs.

From this evidence, we conclude that the four fractions isolated from incubated cells differ in their lipid composition, not only from each other, but also from serum lipoproteins.

The possibility that the fractions might also differ from the serum lipoproteins in the identity of their protein moieties has been tested immunochemically on the LDL, the concentration of protein in the VLDL fraction being too small to produce clear cut reactions. An antiserum was prepared in rabbits to a purified specimen of LDL isolated from sera of untreated guinea pigs, and a second to whole guinea pig serum. The LDL fraction from an incubation experiment was concentrated to about 0.1 ml and allowed to react with the antisera by double diffusion in agarose gel. The heavy precipitin line characteristic of serum LDL was formed against the anti-LDL. No additional lines were produced by the antiguinea pig serum. It is not certain whether a second, very faint line produced by the anti-LDL serum was due to contamination with a trace of an antiglobulin, or to very small amounts of a lipoprotein with a secondary protein component. This analysis indicates however, that the principal serum protein component of this liver fraction was immunochemically indistinguishable from the serum apolipoprotein.

Finally therefore, we conclude that isolated guinea pig liver cells actively incorporate labelled amino acid into the protein moiety of lipoproteins which have the physical and immunochemical properties of serum low-density lipoproteins. Nonetheless, both in their gross lipid composition and in the distribution of their fatty acids, these substances differ from the circulating serum lipoproteins, and therefore cannot contribute directly to the serum lipoprotein pool. If these substances are also produced *in vivo* by the intact liver, this organ is either a minor source of serum lipoproteins by comparison with, e.g. the intestine, or the substances we have isolated are precursors of the circulating lipoproteins. In this case their synthesis might be completed in the liver prior to secretion via the Golgi apparatus [903], or their reconstruction could take place either within the vascular system or by passage through another organ.

Evidence that beta lipoproteins can be synthesized by the intestine of rat and man has been obtained by Windmueller and Levy [1556] and by Alaupovic et al. [31]. However, the latter showed that the composition of their chyle LDL differed from that of human serum LDL (and also from that of the guinea pig liver LDL). Consequently it appears that in this case also modification of the nascent lipoprotein may occur after secretion.

At least two mechanisms are known which could lead to modification within the blood stream. The plasma lecithin-cholesterol acyl transferase has been said [535] to be responsible for the esterification of most of the cholesteryl esters found in serum, and the low proportion of esterified sterol in the liver LDL fraction relative to the serum LDL is consistent with this view. Likewise, the action of the so-called "lipoprotein lipase" may reduce the high triglyceride content of the liver LDL to that of the serum lipoprotein. However, it may be observed that the secreted LDL and VLDL had a different pattern of fatty acids from that of the intracellular lipid fraction. This, with the evidence of the relative proportions of stearic and linoleic acids in the fractions and in the serum lipoproteins, suggests that the system examined was not in a steadystate condition. Further studies will, therefore, be needed before these results can properly be interpreted.

ON THE POSITIONAL SPECIFICITY OF "LIPOPROTEIN LIPASE"

Heiner Greten, Robert I. Levy, Henry Fales and Donald S. Fredrickson

It has been previously demonstrated that postheparin plasma contains separate triglyceride lipase (TGL) and monoglyceride hydrolase (MGH) activities [570, 1352]. TGL is more sensitive to heat and certain inhibitors; it is also reduced in the postheparin plasma of patients with Type I hyperlipoproteinemia, while MGH activity is normal.

We herein report further studies of lipolytic activity in plasma and tissues with reference to lipolysis of diglyceride and the positional specificity of the triglyceride lipase. For these purposes the following substrates were synthesized: ^{3}H-glycerol dioleate and two labeled diether monoesters of glycerol, glycerol-1,2-dioctadecylether-3-^{3}H-oleate and 1,3-dioctadecylether-2-^{14}C-oleate.

METHODS

Synthesis. Glycerol-^{3}H dioleate was synthesized by acylation of randomly labeled glycerol-^{3}H with oleyl chloride. The resulting diglyceride was separated from mono-and triglyceride by column chromatography [684]. It was found to be chemically and radiochemically pure by thin-layer chromatography. Its specific activity was 29.3 mC/mM.

D-alpha,beta-dioctadecyl glyceryl ether was synthesized as described by Kates et al. [780]. The diether was purified by crystallization from ethyl acetate and then acylated with ^{3}H-oleyl chloride to glyceryl-1,2-dioctadecylether-3-^{3}H-oleate. After purification by preparative thin-layer chromatography it was found to be chemically and radiochemically pure. Its specific activity was 1.0 mC/mmole.

D-alpha,alpha'-dioctadecyl glyceryl ether was a generous gift by Dr. W. Baumann (The Hormel Institute). It was acylated with ^{14}C- oleyl chloride to glyceryl-1,3-dioctadecyl-2-^{14}C oleate and purified correspondingly. Its specific activity was 0.1 mC/mmole.

Enzyme Preparations. Rat adipose and heart tissue lipoprotein lipase were prepared as described previously [569]. Postheparin plasma samples were obtained as described by Fredrickson et al. [490]. Four patients (P. P., J. P., L. W., D. T.) with familial Type I hyperlipoproteinemia [489] were used as sources for postheparin plasma in addition to 20 normal volunteers. All normal subjects and patients were hospitalized on a metabolic ward.

Enzyme Assays. Diglyceride Lipase Activity (DGL). In a total volume of 0.60 ml, each vial contained 0.64 μmoles of glycerol-^{3}H-dioleate (5.3×10^5 DPM); 333 μg of unlabeled diolein; 0.2 ml of a 10% sodium taurodeoxycholate solution; and 0.4 ml of 0.1 M Tris buffer (pH 8.6). Each incubation mixture was sonicated for exactly 30 seconds at 6.6 A and 4° using a Branson sonifier.

Diether Monoester Activity. Enzyme assays were carried out as previously described for TGL [569, 570]. In a total volume of 1.0 ml each vial contained: (1) 41.2 nmoles of either the alpha- or beta-acylated glycerol ether; (2) 0.9 ml of 1.35 M Tris buffer (pH 8.6); (3) 0.05 ml of 1% albumin solution; (4) 0.05 ml of a 1:100 diluted Triton X-100 solution. For assay of rat heart and adipose tissue lipoprotein lipase the following additions were made: (1) sodium heparin, 1 unit and, (2) 0.05 ml of preheparin plasma from a normal subject.

Incubation, extraction, and separation of the lipid extracts were performed as previously described for radioactive monoglyceride and triglyceride, respectively [570]. The radioactivity was measured using a Tricarb liquid scintillation spectrometer (Packard, Model 3375) provided with an external standard for quenching correction. When glycerol di-ether monoesters were used both compounds were incubated simultaneously under the same conditions, using the same source and amount of enzyme. All incubations were run in duplicate and agreement between paired samples was always greater than 94%. Hydrolysis was calculated in nmoles of ^{3}H-glycerol; nmoles of ^{3}H-oleic acid (alpha position) or nmoles of ^{14}C-oleic acid (beta position).

RESULTS

Postheparin TGL was distinctly inhibited by NaCl (1 M), sodium pyrophosphate (1×10^{-5} M) and protamine sulfate (150 μg/ml) whereas DGL and MGH activity were unaffected (table). DGL and MGH also differed from TGL in temperature stability (table). While TGL was partially inactivated at 37° for one hour, both DGL and MGH remained stable at this temperature. At 54° all lipolytic activities were decreased, but DGL and MGH remained more stable than TGL.

In the four patients with familial Type I hyperlipoproteinemia normal activities were found for both DGL and MGH activity while TGL activity was markedly decreased. Diglyceride lipase activity in 20 normal subjects was found to be 270 nmoles ^{3}H-glycerol/ml/h (range 150–570). In four patients with Type I hyperlipoproteinemia it was found to be 421 nmoles ^{3}H-glycerol/ml/h (range 212–596). As previously shown, normal TGL activity was found to be 9.3 nmoles ^{14}C-FFA/ml/h (range 6.3–13.0) while in four patients with Type I hyperlipoproteinemia only 2.8 nmoles ^{14}C-FFA/ml/h (range 1.9–3.7) were measured.

In order to investigate the positional sepcificity of TGL activity it was assumed that the ether linkages in alpha and beta, or alpha and alpha', respec-

Table. *For comparison of TGL, DGL, and MGH the same sample of postheparin plasma was used in each experiment. Postheparin plasma was heated prior to its addition to the incubation mixture. Figures represent mean of three experiments*

	TGL		DGL		MGH	
	mμmoles ^{14}C FFA per ml/hr	Percentage of inhibition	mμmoles ^{3}H glycerol per ml/hr	Percentage of inhibition	mμmoles ^{3}H glycerol per ml/hr	Percentage of inhibition
			Inhibitors			
No inhibitors	21.7	—	280	—	4,600	—
Sodium chloride (1 M)	7.0	68	300	—	4,310	—
Sodium pyrophosphate (10 μM)	10.8	50	270	—	4,700	—
Protamine sulfate (150 μg/ml)	9.1	58	290	—	4,300	—
		Percentage of expected activity		Percentage of expected activity		Percentage of expected activity
			Heat			
No preincubation	19.6	100	370	100	3,900	100
60′ preincubation at 37°	7.2	37	380	100	3,930	100
15′ preincubation at 54°	2.0	10	114	30	1,950	50
15′ preincubation at 60°	0	0	0	0	0	0

tively, were not hydrolyzed enzymatically. This assumption was confirmed by assaying for radioactivity in the position of chromatographic plate corresponding to glyceryl monoester monoether. Approximately 2% of the total radioactivity applied from samples before incubation was present in this region and no increase occurred during any of the incubations.

When glyceryl-1,2-dioctadecylether-3-^{3}H-oleate was incubated with postheparin plasma, the radioactive free fatty acid (FFA) released by 60 minutes was directly proportional to the amount of added postheparin plasma over a range of 0.05 to 0.3 ml. The FFA release was also linearly proportional with adipose tissue lipoprotein lipase between concentrations of 0.8 and 4.0 mg of proteins in the NH_4OH extract. Using either enzyme source the pH optimum for hydrolysis of glyceryl-1,2-dioctadecylether-3-^{3}H-oleate was 8.6. This is comparable to the pH optimum of TGL activity in plasma or adipose tissue [569].

Both the tissue and postheparin plasma enzymes were distinctly inhibited by added NaCl (1 M), sodium pyrophosphate (1×10^{-5} M) and protamine sulfate (150 μg/ml) when the substrates containing the fatty acid ester in either the alpha or beta position were used.

The relative rates of hydrolysis of the fatty acid ester linkage in the alpha or beta positions were compared using either postheparin plasma or tissue extracts. In experiments using five different sources of human postheparin plasma the

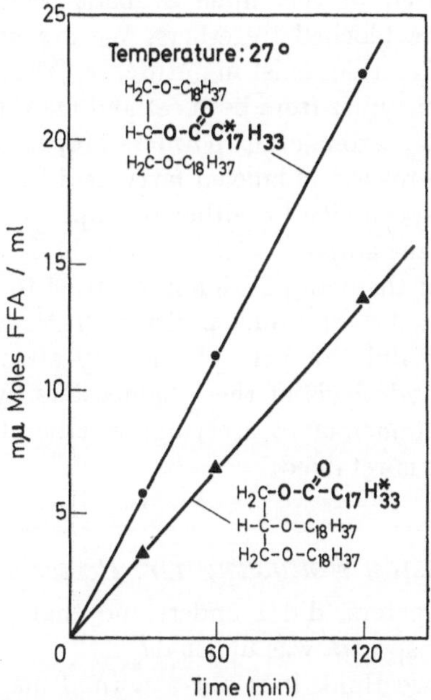

Fig. 1. Hydrolysis of glycerol-1,2-dioctadecylether-3-^{3}H-oleate and glycerol-1,3-dioctadecylether-2-^{14}C-oleate with postheparin plasma from the same normal subject

mean hydrolysis of glyceryl-1,3-dioctadecylether-2-^{14}C-oleate was 10.2 nmoles FFA/ml plasma/h. For glyceryl-1,2-dioctadecylether-3-^{3}H-oleate the mean activity was 6.2 nmoles FFA/ml plasma/h. This apparent preference for the beta position was also evident when the rate of hydrolysis was measured over a period of 120 minutes (Fig. 1). In three experiments with rat heart and adipose tissue lipoprotein lipase the mean total hydrolysis after 60 minutes of incubation was 9.5 nmoles FFA/ml extract (heart) and 11.5 nmoles FFA/ml extract (adipose tissue) from the substrates containing the beta-ester and 3.5 nmole FFA/ml extract (heart) and 5.1 nmoles FFA/ml extract (adipose tissue) from the substrate containing the alpha ester.

DISCUSSION

These experiments demonstrate that postheparin plasma contains diglyceride lipase (DGL) activity that is different from TGL in its relative stability at 37° and resistance to inhibition by NaCl, pyrophosphate, and protamine sulfate. Furthermore, DGL activity is not reduced in the postheparin plasma of patients with Type I. This, added to previous information, indicates that the enzyme or enzymes catalyzing the hydrolysis of diglyceride and monoglyceride are distinct from the enzyme or enzymes attacking the initial ester bond in triglycerides. It is not possible to ascertain from the available data whether the DGL and MGH activities represent separate enzymes.

The demonstration that the metabolic block in Type I hyperlipoproteinemia appears to involve hydrolysis of the initial ester linkage in triglyceride led to the examination of possible positional specificity of TGL activity. Synthetic glycerol monoesters were prepared in the alpha or beta position, the remaining two glycerol hydroxyls being blocked by ethers. We are unaware of evidence that glycerol di-ether monoglycerides exist in nature, but they proved to be hydrolyzed at the ester linkage by enzymes from both rat and man. Both postheparin plasma and NH_4OH extracts of acetone-ether powders prepared from rat adipose tissue and heart catalyzed the release of labeled fatty acid from either substrate. Thus, there was no absolute specificity for either the alpha or beta position in accord with previous studies of the adipose tissue enzymes by Korn [818]. There appeared to be some preference for the beta position in contrast to evidence that pancreatic lipase preferentially attacks the alpha position [942]. NaCl (1 M) inhibited the hydrolysis of either the alpha or beta position by about 30%. It will be interesting to examine the hydrolysis of these monoesters by postheparin enzyme(s) in Type I hyperlipoproteinemia to ascertain whether the ability to hydrolyze the alpha or beta bonds is retained.

Discussion Following Dr. Peeter's Paper

Dr. Benditt: Dr. Peeters, did I understand that you thought the 275 mμ absorption peak in your spectra was unusual?

Dr. Peeters: Yes, we think it is not a normal maximum usually obtained in proteins.

Dr. Benditt: Have you tried raising the pH to 12 and checking the resolution? I suspect that will turn out to be due to the combination of tryptophan and tyrosine in the protein. Is there much in it?

Dr. Peeters: We do not know.

Dr. Scanu: Did you have any dissociating agents in your gels during the fractionation of the various lipoproteins?

Dr. Peeters: No.

Dr. Wissler: I am glad that Dr. Day has finally come to the problem of why low density lipoproteins seem to be preferentially selected by the artery wall; this is a substantial contribution to a working hypothesis. Dr. Gerő and some workers from our laboratory, did show a number of years ago that there was binding of low density lipoprotein by the polysacharides of the aorta. I think that Dr. Day's work helps to explain why.

Dr. Walton: Some years ago we looked at the interaction of both fibrinogen and lipoprotein with dextran sulfate, and our results agree with everything that Dr. Day has said.

I want to add that one can also dissociate complexes of this kind at a high concentration of salt, and I would assume that here one is simply swamping any net charge on the molecule by the great electrolyte concentration.

Dr. KRAMSCH: We mentioned, Dr. Day, that the LDL would accumulate in the arterial wall, because it is rich in positively charged macromolecules. Among the macromolecules which you mentioned was elastin. I would like to point out that in *in vitro* experiments we were unable to show that the protein moiety of low density lipoprotein is being transferred to plaque elastin or normal elastin in proportion to the transferred lipid moiety.

If you run a time course incubation study, for one or four hours of incubation, large amounts of cholesteryl esters are being transferred from LDL to elastin of the plaque, but no protein. Only after 24 hours of incubation do you find a very small amount of lipoprotein protein bound to elastin. By this time 74% of the cholesteryl ester has been transferred to the elastin, whereas only about 24% of the protein is associated with elastin.

I do not really know whether the precipitation of protein after 24 hours of incubation is due to a denaturation phenomenon of the LDL protein or whether it represents a real binding to arterial elastin.

Dr. DAY: We were interested in your data because of the increased concentration of ionic amino acids in plaque elastin, which you demonsrtated. I think there was a twofold increase in the negatively charged amino acids over the positively charged ones. Thus, LDL could possibly dock with elastin, and then there would be a hydrophobic transfer of cholesteryl esters from LDL to elastin.

Dr. SCANU: In this particular area there are two contributions from Dr. Nishida indicating that, following hydrolysis by phospholipase-A, the precipitating effect of dextran sulfate on LDL is reduced or abolished. Then we have the findings by Drs. Benfeld and Kelly who felt that phospholipids did play a role in this particular reaction.

Dr. DAY: Yes, Dr. Nishida demonstrated that effect of phospholipase-A. We have been able to incubate the LDL with free fatty acids, and find that this also will inhibit the reaction. I think the free fatty acids released in his experiments may account for his data.

Discussion Following Dr. Slack's Paper

Dr. FREDRICKSON: Dr. Slack, was the S_f 10–20 in the three heterozygote patients as low as in the controls? In your total mean group it was as low, but was that true for the ones that you showed S_f rate calculations on? In other words, do you think your slight increase in the S_f rate for S_f 0–10 in heterozygotes could be due to an increase in concentration of the S_f 10–20 in those particular patients as opposed to the controls?

Dr. SLACK: No. This is diminished rather than increased in the patients.

Dr. BEAUMONT: Dr. Slack, do you think there may be, in these familial hypercholesterolemic patients, several different types of lipoproteins varying genetically from one family to another?

Dr. SLACK: Yes. I think there are several indications that these families have certain familial patterns. For instance, in their risks of ischemic heart disease and the ages at which they develop ischemic heart disease, certain familial tendencies have led me to suppose that families breed true and that they are not all alike. We do not know, of course, whether these may be genetic or environmental differences.

Dr. WALTON: We have also been looking at families of this kind, with the cooperation of Great Ormond Street Hospital in London where they have a number of families with juvenile arteriosclerosis. We have been going about it in a slightly different way, using antiallotypic antisera to see whether we could characterize a particular variety of the protein which might be predominantly involved. So far, we can confirm whether the patient was homozygote or heterozygote, but we have not found one particular allotype predominating in these cases.

Discussion Following Dr. Morris' Paper

Dr. SCOTT: With respect to Dr. Morris' monkey that drowned at 90 days, what did the autopsy show? Did he have any arterial lesions?

Dr. MORRIS: No arterial disease of any kind was found. He was comparable to a control of the same age.

UNIDENTIFIED: Dr. Morris mentioned he was using a purified diet. In many species purified diets tend to produce hypercholesterolemia. Did this hypercholesterolemia occur on a natural diet as well?

Dr. MORRIS: Yes. He has been back on monkey chow, Purina 25, for about $3^1/_2$ years, and his hyperbetalipoproteinemia has persisted. In fact, his hyperbetalipoproteinemia is not altered by dietary modification.

Dr. FREDRICKSON: Dr. Morris, I want to point out one other interesting fact. It is very remarkable that your heterozygote monkeys actually achieved human serum beta lipoprotein levels, meaning that they are increased over the controls by nearly sixfold, compared to the usual $2^1/_2$ increase in human heterozygotes. It is exciting to contemplate what will happen when you breed some homozygotes.

Dr. MORRIS: The baseline value for beta lipoprotein of the human control population is higher than the control Rhesus monkey's, because the latter ingested a low cholesterol diet: less than 0.5 mg/kg/day. Our values for lipid composition of the hypercholesterolemic beta lipoprotein are almost identical to those for humans that Dr. Smith showed yesterday.

Dr. HAUST: Dr. Morris, on your Fig. 1 I noticed that the cholesterol level of monkey 694 was lower several days after birth than the levels of the other two baby monkeys whose values then decreased later. Do you have any explanation for this difference, i.e. the one going up and the other two going down with time?

Dr. MORRIS: We really don't have any explanation. It may have something to do with fasting condition or to some unknown factors.

However, in spite of the fact that our number of controls is small, every one of the infants of the propositus male have initial cholesterol values which are higher than the controls.

Discussion Following Dr. Mills' Paper

Dr. HAVEL: Dr. Mills, would you tell us more about your method for preparing isolated liver cells, and also whether you have done any morphological studies to indicate the state of the endoplasmic reticulum and the Golgi apparatus in these cells?

Dr. MILLS: The method of preparation is a mechanical one. The liver is first minced lightly and centrifuged, then filtered through a silk screen, and the cells are washed and suspended in the medium. We have looked, microscopically, at the intact cells, but we haven't any electron microscopic studies.

Dr. GETZ: Could you comment on the degree of incorporation that you observed in the presence of cyclohexamide. Did you, for example, find inhibitions of incorporation into other proteins parallel to those observed with the LDL?

Dr. MILLS: Yes, we thought that inhibition was genuine. We were a little surprised by the degree of activity that we found, but it is rather difficult to wash the fractions very thoroughly because of the small number of cells, we believe there was a certain amount of adsorbed label.

Dr. AHRENS: Dr. Mills, your abstract suggests that the pretreatment of the animals had a good deal to do with the lipoproteins elaborated by their liver cells? Could you comment on that point?

Dr. MILLS: I think it probably does have a good deal to do with it, though it is difficult to elaborate on this, because we have to go into all sorts of questions about the composition of the fractions.

The diet unquestionably changes the composition of the serum LDL. This encouraged us to think that we might, in fact, be looking at something that came from the intestine. The distribution of fatty acids also made us think that the fractions we isolated weren't always drawn from the same pool, but we are not really in a position to make any very profound statements about the effect of the diet on the product.

Discussion Following Dr. Greten's Paper

Dr. BIERMAN: We have studied the question of positional specificity of postheparin plasma lipolytic activity using triglyceride substrates which are unaltered, since there is always the possibility that these diether linkages in some way influence substrate-enzyme interaction.

In experiments done with cocoa butter as substrate for postheparin lipolytic activity, in conjunction with Vogel and Porte, we found that hydrolysis of the alpha positions with pancreatic lipase produces a pattern of fatty acid release reflecting the saturated fatty acids which are the predominant acids present in that position. Cocoa butter is an unusual substrate since oleic acid is confined almost entirely to the beta position. Calculation of the pattern that would be produced by random hydrolysis and comparison of that pattern with the actual experimental data obtained from postheparin plasma lipolysis of cocoa butter indicates that there is neither specificity for the alpha or beta positions, nor is the hydrolysis completely random. If anything, the relative increase in the proportion of oleic acid in fatty acids released suggests a slight preference for the beta position, in confirmation of the results presented by Dr. Greten.

Dr. BOBERG: I think that the last point that Dr. Greten made (to test his system on the type I hyperlipoproteinemias) is a very good one. One cannot be sure, when incubating these ethers with postheparin plasma that only the triglyceride lipase and no other lipase acts on these substrates. Furthermore, we have good evidence that the triglyceride lipase should be inhibited more efficiently in the lipoprotein lipase enzyme system by 1 Molar sodium chloride.

Dr. GRETEN: We never found much inhibition with 1 M sodium chloride solution, and we have done this repeatedly. But there clearly exists a difference between postheparin plasma and tissue extracts. With regard to the first point, we are absolutely aware of the difficulties that are involved when one uses artificial compounds in measuring enzymatic activity. On the other hand, we have demonstrated that these monoesterdiethers can be used to determine so called "lipoprotein lipase" activity. I think it is a very good point and further experiments with these synthesized compounds will eventually cast some light on the important question of the exact metabolic block in hydrolyzing chylomicrons in patients with familial Type I hyperlipoproteinemia.

Section VII

REGULATION OF TRIGLYCERIDES, INCLUDING CARBOHYDRATE-LIPID INTERACTION

METABOLISM OF PLASMA TRIGLYCERIDES*

RICHARD J. HAVEL

Transport of TG[1] formed in intestinal mucosa and liver is one of the major functions[2] of plasma lipoproteins [645]. Their peptides and complex lipids provide for aqueous miscibility and for interaction with sites from which removal of TG occurs. This paper reviews the attempts that have been made to quantify the rate at which TG enter the blood in the absence of transport of dietary fat. The methods that have been used to measure this rate depend in large measure on the correctness with which the pathways of transport have been defined. Therefore, the sites at which TG enter and leave the blood will first be outlined, together with certain relevant molecular events, emphasizing some recently appreciated complexities and areas of controversy.

Formation of Plasma Triglycerides. The intestinal pathway serves to transport dietary fat as chylomicrons into the lymphatic system. This is a high capacity system which functions intermittently in most mammals. However, at least in rats, some TG whose fatty acids are derived mainly from biliary phospholipids is continuously delivered into intestinal lymphatics in the absence of recent fat ingestion [104]. The molecular size of lipoproteins secreted from intestinal mucosa during fasting is generally smaller than that of chylomicrons and largely overlaps that of TG-rich lipoproteins secreted from the liver [1116]. The chemical composition of these particles also closely resembles that of hepatogenous particles. Therefore, if one uses the convention that chylomicrons are TG-rich lipoproteins derived from intestinal lymph which are larger than 800 Å in diameter and that those which are smaller are VLDL, the intestine secretes primarily chylomicrons during absorption of dietary fat and mainly VLDL in the post-absorptive state[3].

---

* The work herein was supported by USPHS Grants HE-06285 and FR-00079. Important contributors to various aspects of the studies performed in this laboratory include E. O. Balasse, L. V. Basso, D. Bier, J. M. Felts, R. L. Hamilton, J. P. Kane, N. Segel, J. Seymour, and B. Wolfe.

1 Abbreviations used herein are: TG = triglyceride(s); TGFA = triglyceride fatty acid; FFA = free fatty acid; VLDL = very low density lipoprotein; LDL = low density lipoprotein; HDL = high density lipoprotein; LPL = lipoprotein lipase; and LCAT = lecithin-cholesterol acyl-transferase.

2 Other functions include transport of certain fat-soluble vitamins and cholesterol. The latter appears to involve transfer of free cholesterol from cell membranes to HDL followed by transesterification with fatty acid from the beta-position of lecithin, catalyzed by LCAT; the cholesterol esters formed can be exchanged with TG in VLDL and, presumably, are catabolized in liver with other lipid and peptide constituents of lipoproteins. [534].

3 This arbitrary convention is operationally necessary with present techniques, but it must be clear that not only can the intestine secrete particles in the size range of VLDL but that the liver, especially during states of rapid formation of TG-rich lipoproteins, secretes particles in the size range of chylomicrons.

Thus the intestine functions both in exogenous and endogenous transport of TG and contributes to the pool of VLDL-TG present in blood plasma in the post-absorptive state and during ingestion of fat-free diets. The fraction derived from intestinal lymph is uncertain but is probably on the order of 10–30% in the rat. Whether it is this large in animals with a gall bladder is unknown.

The liver continuously secretes VLDL directly into the blood. No evidence for direct secretion of TG in LDL or HDL from liver has been obtained [646]. In fact, TG in these lipoproteins may represent residual material remaining after extrahepatic metabolism of VLDL-TG or may be derived from transfer of TG from VLDL related to reciprocal movement of cholesteryl esters formed by the LCAT reaction [534]. In the postabsorptive state, VLDL-TGFA are derived primarily from FFA taken up by the liver [650]. During absorption of carbohydrate, fatty acids newly synthesized from glucose in the liver contribute to the formation of VLDL-TGFA [1557]. During absorption of fat, fatty acids from chylomicron-TG enter the liver and may subsequently appear in VLDL. Since some VLDL presumably enter the blood from the intestine during fat absorption, the origin of VLDL-TGFA under these circumstances is complex and probably quite variable, depending upon the rate at which fat is absorbed and other factors.

Utilization of Plasma Triglycerides. There is abundant evidence that LPL, synthesized in parenchymal cells of various tissues but operationally active at the surface of blood capillaries, is of major importance[4] in uptake of TG from the blood [645]. TG in VLDL and chylomicrons are good substrates for the action of this enzyme; the FFA and glycerol which are produced enter pathways similar to those available when these molecules enter the blood after hydrolysis of TG in adipose tissue. A critical difference, however, relates to the fact that FFA produced in a tissue by action of LPL more readily enter cells locally. This phenomenon, which has been demonstrated particularly in adipose tissue and the lactating mammary gland, presumably results from the high concentration gradient between capillary and tissue cell created at sites of high enzyme activity, but it also requires rapid utilization of the FFA entering the cells in order to maintain a flux from blood to tissue [645].

Present evidence is that the liver has a minor role in direct uptake of chylomicron-TG from the blood. After pulse injection of chylomicrons containing labeled TGFA into experimental animals, a substantial fraction of the radioactivity rapidly appears in hepatic lipids. During continuous infusion of such chylomicrons, however, most of the TG appear to leave the blood in extrahepatic tissues [645]. Part of the difficulty in interpreting experiments with pulse injection results from the fact that the liver can take up intact chylomicrons in a reversible manner, perhaps by trapping them in the space of Disse. In perfused livers, uptake of chylomicron-TG is limited unless heparin is present in the

---

4 The observation that LPL activity in separated cellular elements of adipose tissue is associated almost entirely with the fat cells and not with the stromal-vascular components has challenged this interpretation. However, recent studies by Cunningham and Robinson [349] indicate that LPL not present in the fat cells is unstable and is inactivated by the collagenase used to separate the fat cells from the stroma. Moreover, the activity of only that enzyme present outside the fat cells decreases with fasting.

perfusion system [455]. Analysis of livers of rats injected with labeled chylomicrons for unhydrolyzed TG and TGFA produced by extrahepatic lipolysis, suggests that the liver may account for direct uptake of up to 20% of chylomicron TG leaving the blood [1316]. The differences between results with perfused livers and intact animals would be reconciled if it could be shown that the liver takes up TG from chylomicrons which have been modified by action of LPL in extrahepatic tissues. It is known that the liver is the major site of removal of chylomicron-cholesteryl esters. In hepatectomized dogs, cholesteryl esters contained in injected chylomicrons leave the blood much more slowly than constituent TG [645]. This suggests that, after removal of the bulk of TG in extrahepatic tissues, the remaining chylomicron constituents (possibly including some residual TG) rapidly enter the liver. Such a requirement for preliminary extrahepatic modification is consistent with the strikingly deficient utilization of chylomicron-TG in subjects with genetically determined deficiency of LPL.

The rate at which chylomicron-TG leave the blood is related inversely to the size of the particle in which they are contained [1206]. In extension of this phenomenon, VLDL-TGFA are removed from the blood more slowly than chylomicron-TGFA. Studies with TGFA-labeled VLDL suggest that their constituent TG are metabolized by pathways similar to those for chylomicrons. After pulse injection of such labeled VLDL, as with chylomicrons, a substantial fraction of the labeled fatty acid is present in hepatic lipids [650]. It is questionable whether, as suggested earlier [650], there is an extensive direct exchange of TG between liver and plasma VLDL since the phenomenon may well resemble that observed after pulse injection of labeled chylomicrons. It would also be rather out of keeping with the putative role of VLDL as the vehicle for transport of excess hepatic TG from liver to extrahepatic tissues. As will be shown, studies of release of VLDL into hepatic venous blood suggest that total and net fluxes of TGFA produced by the liver are equivalent.

Role of Nontriglyceride Constituents of Lipoproteins in Triglyceride Transport. Certain peptides of LDL and HDL are present in VLDL and, probably, in chylomicrons, at least when they are isolated from blood plasma [489]. The "B" peptide of LDL is almost certainly essential for formation of VLDL since it is present in nascent VLDL isolated from a Golgi apparatus-rich fraction of rat liver (Hamilton et al., 1969, unpublished data). In abetalipoproteinemia, neither VLDL nor chylomicrons are formed, which suggests that LDL or its peptide is required to produce TG-rich lipoproteins both in liver and intestinal mucosa [489]. Inhibitors of protein synthesis uniformly depress formation of VLDL from liver, but their effect on secretion of chylomicrons is less certain [1216]. The concentration of LDL varies greatly among mammals and is particularly low in those species which ingest or absorb little carbohydrate and have low rates of hepatic synthesis of fatty acids [1204]. Since there is no evidence that LDL are secreted as such under normal conditions *in vivo* nor that they are reutilized in the biosynthesis of VLDL, their formation may be related directly to transport of TG-rich lipoproteins and the action of LPL [647].

Although the "A" peptides of HDL are present in both VLDL and chylomicrons, they have not been shown to be essential for their formation. VLDL are actually present in increased amounts in Tangier disease, in which a genetically determined abnormality of "A" peptides is present and levels of HDL are very low [489]. A similar phenomenon is observed in genetically determined deficiency of LCAT [1084]. In a recent reinvestigation of "activation" of fat emulsions by plasma lipoproteins to permit interaction with LPL in cow's milk, we have observed that HDL contain most of the activity found in human serum, while LDL are virtually inactive (Bier and Havel, unpublished data). The remainder of the activity in fasting serum can be attributed to VLDL per unit weight of protein, VLDL are much more active than HDL. We have also found that serum from guinea pigs, a species in which HDL are almost undetectable, has almost no capacity to activate fat emulsions. These observations are consistent with the hypothesis that one function of peptides in HDL and VLDL is to alter the surface of TG-rich lipoproteins so that they can form a suitable complex with LPL.

Other peptides have been identified as uniform constituents of human VLDL [489]. Elucidation of their function would undoubtedly resolve many uncertainties concerning formation and disposal of plasma triglycerides.

MEASUREMENT OF RATE OF TRANSPORT OF ENDOGENOUS TRIGLYCERIDES[5]

From the large quantities of dietary fat that can be absorbed daily and the relatively low blood levels of chylomicrons during fat absorption, it is obvious that removal mechanisms operate at high efficiencies. In accord with this, intravenously injected chylomicrons are removed rapidly from the blood. Below a saturating level, removal is first order, and the capacity of the system in man can be shown with Intralipid, an artificial fat emulsion whose constituent TG are handled similarly to those of chylomicrons, to be on the order of 10 g TG/hr [199]. As indicated earlier, the rate of uptake of chylomicron TG from the blood is an inverse function of particle size, and the rate of removal of VLDL-TG is appreciably slower. In various experimental animals, including primates, the turnover time of VLDL-TG at normal blood levels appears to be about two to three times that of chylomicron-TG, or in the range of 10–40 minutes [646]. In contrast, from the compartment size and various estimates of production rate of VLDL-TG turnover times in man are in the range of one to three hours. As discussed in the following, this slow turnover rate is supported by some, but not all, studies in which biologically labeled endogenous triglycerides have been injected intravenously.

In 1961, it was shown that, in the postabsorptive state, plasma FFA are the major precursors of plasma TGFA in man [499, 644]. This observation, together with the ready availability of biologically labeled lipoprotein-TG, has provided the basis for most of the subsequent application of isotopic tracer techniques to quantitative estimation of TG transport.

Measurements of transport of endogenous TG in man have used several techniques and have provided values on the order of 10 to 50 μmoles of TGFA

5 Definitions used herein are: (1) inflow or outflow transport: the mass of material entering or leaving a compartment per unit time; (2) turnover rate: the fraction of material leaving a compartment per unit time (reciprocal of turnover time).

per minute in healthy adults in the postabsorptive state. The methods have, however, not given consistent results when applied to a comparison of normotriglyceridemic and hypertriglyceridemic subjects. Comparison of the various methods provides some insight into the reasons for these discrepancies. Four general isotopic methods and two nonisotopic methods have been used.

The earliest method was proposed by Friedberg and associates [499]. They estimated the fraction of FFA converted to plasma TGFA from kinetic analysis of the appearance and initial exponential decay of radioactivity in TGFA after injection of ^{14}C-palmitate. This fraction was multiplied by the estimated transport of FFA to calculate inflow transport of TGFA from FFA. The values obtained were not correlated with plasma level of TG. When plasma containing such labeled TG was injected into recipients, the initial exponential decay of radioactivity was similar to that observed in plasma TG of subjects injected with labeled FFA. It was recognized at this time that the liver secretes TG primarily in VLDL and that the turnover rate of TG in this lipoprotein fraction is larger than in LDL or HDL [644]. Subsequently, this approach was explored by Farquhar, Reaven and their associates who added two refinements [450]. First, they measured the rate constant specifically in VLDL-TG, which they also found provided a value similar to that obtained when labeled VLDL-TG were reinjected into subjects from whom they had been obtained two days earlier. Second, they used labeled glycerol rather than palmitate as the tracer, since it gave considerably less "recycling" of radioactivity in VLDL-TG. From their studies [1214], they concluded that primary forms of endogenous hypertriglyceridemia in man result from increased rate of entry of TG into the blood plasma and that mechanisms for their removal from the blood are unimpaired.

A second and even simpler method, proposed by Ryan and Schwartz [1272] has been applied extensively by Sailer, Sandhofer and Braunsteiner [1280]. This method depends upon the fact that 30–40 minutes after starting a constant intravenous infusion of ^{14}C-palmitate, ^{14}C appears in plasma TG and increases linearly for the next two to three hours. From this, the rate at which ^{14}C appears in TG can be expressed as a fraction of the rate of infusion of ^{14}C-palmitate. Under the assumption that no TG-radioactivity is removed from the plasma during this time, this fraction, multiplied by the net transport of FFA (estimated from the ratio of the infusion rate of ^{14}C-palmitate to the steady-state specific radioactivity of plasma FFA) provides a measure of the "production rate" of plasma TG. Applying this method to the study of primary endogenous hyperlipemia, Sailer and associates concluded that a defect in disposal of TG causes the hyperlipemia.

More recently, the method of multicompartmental analysis developed by Berman and associates (Simulation, Analysis, and Modeling: SAAM) has been applied by Baker and Schotz [89] in the rat and by Eaton and associates in man [418]. With this method, pulse injection or continuous infusion of labeled FFA is followed by measurement of radioactivity in FFA and plasma TGFA and the simplest model, which is consistent with known pathways of FFA and TG transport and provides a close fit to the observed data, is determined by an iterative procedure with a digital computer. This method permits estimation of rate of conversion of FFA to plasma TG as well as the net outflow transport of TG. In two of four normotriglyceridemic subjects, Eaton and associates found close agreement between these two values, suggesting that no other major source of plasma TG existed. However, in the two other subjects, the outflow transport of TG considerably exceeded the estimated conversion of FFA to plasma TG, suggesting that other important sources were present. In a single subject with mixed hyperlipemia, values for net outflow transport were so low that they could not be estimated, but conversion of FFA to plasma TG was in their normal range.

Our own studies of quantitative aspects of TG transport have used a different approach which requires catheterization of an artery and an hepatic vein, together with constant intravenous infusion of ^{14}C-palmitate. We embarked upon this more complicated approach, because studies in animals and in man suggested that techniques depending for their validation upon reinjection of biologically labeled TG might be in error [646]. In addition our approach provided an opportunity to observe whether altered rates of conversion of FFA to plasma TGFA are accompanied by changes in oxidative metabolism of FFA in the liver or in other aspects of splanchnic metabolism. Initially, we conducted studies in anesthetized dogs, fitted with an indwelling catheter in the portal vein several days earlier and with catheters in an artery and hepatic vein on the day of study [100]. By infusing these dogs with ^{14}C-palmitate and indocyanine green (to measure hepatic plasma flow), we could estimate hepatic uptake of FFA separately from extrahepatic splanchnic uptake and conversion of the FFA taken up to major metabolic products: TG (in VLDL), ketones and CO_2. We found that the specific activity of FFA entering and leaving the liver was virtually identical. In addition, the composition of FFA in arterial, portal venous, and hepatic venous blood plasma was closely similar. From these observations, we deduced that the liver takes up FFA but does not release them into hepatic venous blood. Since portal venous FFA had a lower specific activity than arterial FFA, we concluded that, in contrast, the extrahepatic splanchnic region both takes up and releases FFA. In normal dogs and dogs infused with norepinephrine, the specific activity of VLDL-TGFA rose to closely approximate that of FFA in blood entering the liver (or FFA in hepatic venous blood plasma). Thus, in these dogs, FFA appeared to be the major precursors of VLDL-TGFA and the specific activity of precursor could be measured in hepatic venous blood plasma without sampling portal venous blood.

From these studies, it appeared feasible to measure net splanchnic production of TG without sampling portal venous blood. To date, we have performed studies in several groups of humans in the postabsorptive state. In our initial studies, we compared seven healthy subjects with eight individuals with endogenous hyperlipemia [646]. All subjects were on weight-maintaining diets containing 40% calories from fat for at least three days. The last meal on the evening before the study contained no fat and infusion of 1-^{14}C-palmitate was given from about 15 up to 19 hours later. Net transport of FFA was similar in the two groups, but slightly more than half of plasma FFA was taken up in the splanchnic region in the hyperlipemic subjects and about 40% in the normotriglyceridemic ones. In both groups an average of 18% was secreted into hepatic venous blood in VLDL-TGFA. The same fraction was secreted into TGFA of unfractionated plasma, so that secretion of TG in LDL or HDL was not detectable. Calculated production of VLDL-TGFA was about 30% higher in the hyperlipemic group, owing to increased splanchnic uptake of FFA. In both groups, production of TGFA was directly correlated with splanchnic uptake of FFA. Production rate was also estimated independently from the rate of equilibration of product VLDL-TGFA with its precursor pool, assumed from our studies in dogs to be that of FFA in hepatic venous blood plasma. This assumption was supported in subjects with low concentrations of VLDL-TGFA by virtually complete equilibration of these two specific activities near the end of the four-hour period of study. The results of the two estimates agreed closely, and no systematic difference was found. No correlation was observed between plasma concentration and production rate of VLDL-TGFA in these 15 subjects, leading to the conclusion that impaired extrahepatic removal was the chief factor responsible for increasing levels of VLDL-TGFA. Splanchnic production of ketones could account for about one-third of the uptake of FFA and measurements of specific activities in hepatic venous blood indicated that FFA were the sole precursor of these ketones. Oxidation to CO_2 could account for only 10% of the ^{14}C-palmitate taken up in the splanchnic region.

Studies in three adults with increased fat mobilization and hyperlipemia related to glycogenesis type I demonstrated increased fractional conversion of FFA to VLDL-TGFA (mean value 28%) and decreased conversion to ketones (13%) [648]. Similarly, infusion of sufficient ethanol to saturate hepatic removal capacity abruptly increased fractional conversion of FFA to VLDL-TGFA and decreased conversion to ketones (Wolfe et al., unpublished data). Discussion of the mechanisms underlying these alterations of splanchnic metabolism of FFA is beyond the scope of this paper. However, it is clear that such alterations can produce hypertriglyceridemia by increasing production of VLDL-TG from liver. Since we observed that prolonged deficiency of insulin in the dog [100] produced an abnormality opposite to that observed in glucose-6-phosphatase deficiency in man, it may be concluded also that the pathogenesis of hyperlipemia in states of increased fat mobilization is complex and influenced by changes in hepatic handling of FFA and extrahepatic utilization of VLDL-TGFA.

Two nonisotopic methods have been used to measure production of plasma TG. Direct chemical measurement of splanchnic production rate (arteriovenous difference times blood flow) is feasible only in subjects with low plasma levels. From such measurements Carlson was able to conclude that less than 100 μmoles per minute of TGFA is produced in the splanchnic region [284]. In our healthy subjects with VLDL-TGFA levels below 3 μmoles/ml, duplicate analysis of nine samples taken over the four-hour period of study provided estimates that did not differ systematically from those provided by the two isotopic methods of analysis. Because of the large analytical error, this is not a practical method, but these results support further those obtained by the more precise isotopic techniques. Another nonisotopic method has been proposed by Porte and Bierman [1188]. In individuals infused intravenously with sufficient heparin to reduce plasma TG concentration to a lower, constant value, they observed a fairly steady rate of hydrolysis of these TG when the blood plasma was incubated *in vitro* at pH 7.4 and 37° C. Under the assumptions that all effective LPL was displaced into the blood by the heparin and that no other mechanisms for disposal of plasma TG exist, this lipolytic rate was considered to equal numerically removal of TG. Application of this method to healthy subjects with carbohydrate-augmented endogenous hyperlipemia led them to conclude that the plasma concentration of TG is a direct function of transport. In subjects with exogenous or mixed hyperlipemia, TG levels exceeded those expected from values for transport, suggesting that impaired removal mechanisms contributed to the hyperlipemia.

The various methods that have been used to measure irreversible turnover of plasma TG provide differing absolute rates for a given plasma level and lead

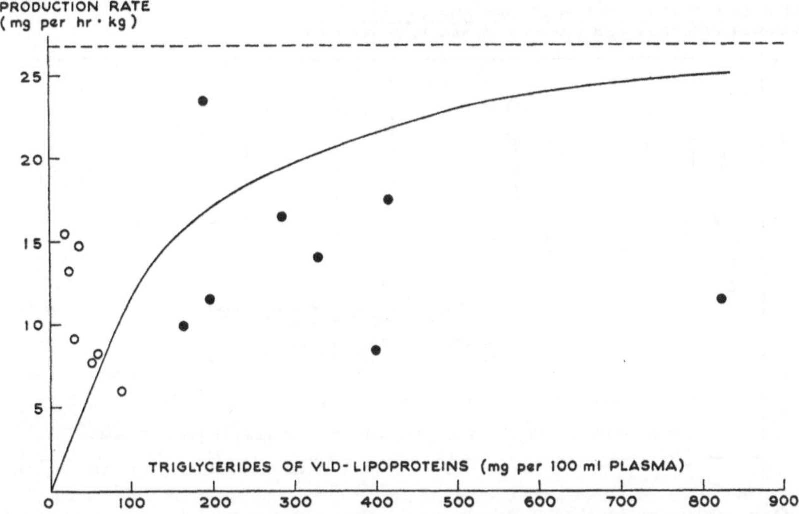

Fig. 1. Data obtained by hepatic venous catherization technique are plotted on graph with coordinates used by Reaven et al. [1214]. Open circles are values in normotriglyceridemic subjects and closed circles are those in hypertriglyceridemic subjects. Curving line is that fitted by Reaven et al. to their data

to different conclusions concerning mechanisms of primary endogenous hyperlipemia. Definitive elucidation of the reasons for these differences is not presently possible, but some can be attributed to faulty assumptions.

The most critical assumption underlying measurement of turnover rate from the decay of radioactivity in endogenously labeled TG is that this rate is determined by extrahepatic metabolism of VLDL-TG rather than by entry of tracer from liver. Although we have been unable to substantiate this assumption by injection of TGFA-labeled VLDL [646], the initial rate constant may not reflect net outflow transport; alternatively, the labeled TGFA may have been altered during preparation. Our values with the hepatic vein technique in healthy subjects are two to three times higher and those in our hyperlipemic subjects are slightly lower than those of Reaven and associates (Fig. 1). As discussed in the following, it is most unlikely that our results err on the high side. Therefore, it is reasonable to propose that the plasma compartment is not rate-determining for decay of radioactivity in VLDL-TGFA at low (normal) concentrations in man.

It follows that the method of pulse-labeling with a precursor may provide a valid measure of net outflow transport only in hyperlipemic subjects.

Two important assumptions are basic to the method proposed by Ryan and Schwartz. The first is that removal of ^{14}C-TGFA is negligible during the period of measurement. This is manifestly not the case and the extent of this error is inversely proportional to the turnover rate. Since our method also uses constant infusion of ^{14}C-palmitate, we have made such calculations in our subjects and compared them directly with those obtained by the hepatic vein technique [646]. This comparison shows that on this basis, the Ryan-Schwartz method provides

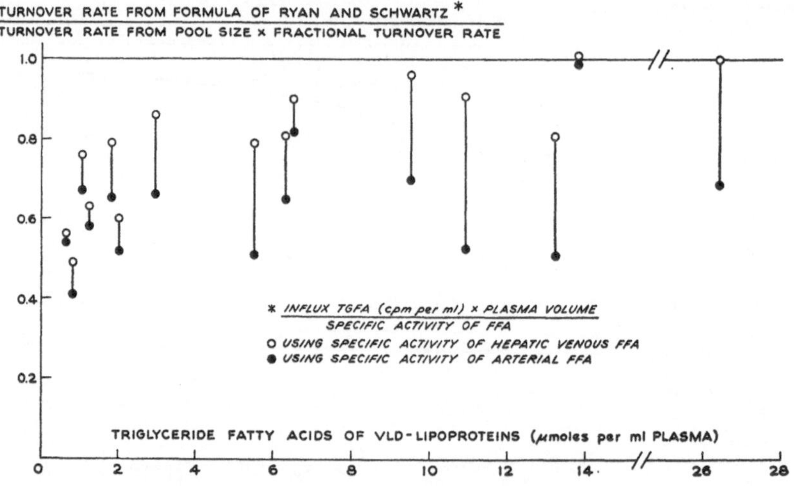

Fig. 2. Data obtained in the study shown in Fig. 1 were used to calculate net inflow transport of TGFA with the equation proposed by Ryan and Schwartz [1272], using either arterial or hepatic venous specific activities of FFA as the denominator. Values are plotted for each subject as a fraction of the value obtained from rate of equilibration of VLDL-TGFA with FFA in hepatic venous blood (see text)

a value approximately 25% low in normotriglyceridemic subjects (Fig. 2). The nature of this error is such that falsely positive correlations between concentration and disposal rate of TG may be obtained; such correlations have been observed by Sailer and associates [1280] and Nestel [1084]. The second assumption of this method is that arterial or peripheral venous FFA rather than hepatic venous FFA are in equilibrium with the precursor pool of VLDL-TGFA. This produces an additional error of about −10% in normotriglyceridemic and −25% in hypertriglyceridemic subjects (Fig. 2).

The method of multicompartmental analysis used by Eaton and associates involves the erroneous assumption that plasma TG constitute a homogenous pool. Measurement of ^{14}C in VLDL-TGFA should provide more precise information, although preliminary studies indicate that no large error is involved [418]. It is also assumed in this method (as well as other methods in which incorporation of ^{14}C-FFA into TGFA is measured) that delayed incorporation of radioactive precursors into VLDL-TGFA is insignificant. Comparison of their four with our seven healthy subjects shows a disturbing feature which is difficult to reconcile with similarity of dietary preparation and duration of experimental period. In their subjects, an average of 12% of FFA was converted to TGFA while in ours the corresponding value was only 7%. This would indicate that about 30% of FFA entering the splanchnic region of their subjects was secreted as TGFA (the values are even higher in their subject with mixed hyperlipemia). Hopefully, further studies will resolve these rather large discrepancies.

The method proposed by Porte and Bierman is attractive particularly because it allows repeated determinations to be made in a single subject. Since the values obtained with this method are higher than with any of the others, assumptions which might tend to minimize them will not be considered here. Values for transport of TGFA in their subjects with endogenous hyperlipemia are on the average about one-third of the net outflow transport of FFA that should obtain for the stated plasma levels. Since their subjects had been maintained on high-carbohydrate, fat-free diets for at least 10 days, direct comparison with our results is not possible, but the values are considerably higher than those reported by Reaven and associates in similar subjects on these diets. It is also noteworthy that Reaven and associates found that maximal outflow transport of VLDL-TG approached a limit of about 24 mg/kg an hour, while Porte and Bierman report no evidence for saturation of removal mechanisms at values up to three times greater (their highest subject's rate was 10 g TG/hour). The values obtained with this method might be excessively great because of perturbations produced by infusion of large quantities of heparin with displacement of LPL into the plasma compartment. It is assumed that triglycerides are hydrolyzed *in vivo* as completely and at the same rate as observed *in vitro* and are irreversibly removed from the blood. Possibly, some sort of accelerated turnover with a large component of recycling is involved.

Our method very likely provides reliable data for net outflow transport of VLDL-TG rapidly produced from hepatic uptake of FFA. It could err on the low side for at least two reasons. First, delayed incorporation of radioactivity could be missed, since it will provide low values to the extent that nonlabeled precursors contribute to VLDL-TGFA. One unlabeled or poorly labeled contributor of VLDL-TGFA that must be considered is VLDL of intestinal origin. Neither of these possibilities is likely when complete equilibration of precursor and product pools occurs, but this situation obtains only in some normotriglyceridemic subjects. It is unlikely that newly synthesized fatty acids contribute to production of VLDL-TG in either our normal or hyperlipemic subjects on ordinary diets, particularly since FFA appeared to be the sole precursors of blood ketones. Further studies are needed to determine whether the method is applicable to subjects on high carbohydrate diets or in the postprandial state.

CONCLUSIONS

The pathways for transport of TG in the blood are now sufficiently well defined to encourage attempts to measure their turnover under various conditions. The methods devised thus far have not given concordant results. Comparisons between some of these methods have defined certain limitations and clarified some discrepancies, but considerably more work is needed to determine their accuracy and range of applicability. Some of the isotopic methods have the virtue of providing information about the contributions of various precursors, the site of formation and associated alterations. The central role of transport of TG in the metabolism of all plasma lipoproteins underscores the importance of further studies of turnover and of mechanisms of physiologic and pathologic variations.

HYPERTRIGLYCERIDEMIA AND INSULIN SECRETION, A COMPLEX CAUSAL RELATIONSHIP*

ESKO A. NIKKILÄ and MARJA-RIITTA TASKINEN

Insulin has been originally implicated in the pathogenetic events of hyperglyceridemia on the basis of the frequent occurrence of glucose intolerance in this disorder [34, 769, 1213, 1511]. That a relative inefficiency of circulating insulin in promoting glucose uptake in hyperglyceridemia has been documented by several authors [366, 814, 1083], but whether this applies also to the antilipolytic action of insulin is uncertain. This insulin resistance is apparently the main factor in producing an impaired glucose tolerance, but the causal sequence of this abnormality and hyperglyceridemia has not been solved.

If not caused by a true insulin-deficient diabetic state, the glucose intolerance would be expected to be accompanied by elevated plasma insulin levels, which result from a normal insulin secretory response to an exaggerated hyperglycemic stimulus. In fact, hyperinsulinemia during glucose loading has been found to be common in patients with hyperglyceridemia [7, 367, 449, 478, 1099, 1278], although an abnormally low insulin response has also been reported [769]. A positive correlation between plasma triglyceride and immunoreactive insulin levels has been found in some studies [7, 449, 478, 1278], but not in others [537, 1100]. Detection of true correlations may be confused by obesity, which is often associated both with hyperglyceridemia and decreased glucose tolerance.

Another problem, still under dispute, is whether the insulin secretion per se is abnormal in hyperglyceridemia, i.e. is insulin output disproportionally high or low in relation to the blood glucose level? Evidence for this possibility has been provided by Reaven et al. [1215], who found the rise of plasma triglyceride level during high carbohydrate feeding to be highly (positively) correlated with the plasma insulin response but not with blood glucose. Furthermore, Sailer et al. [1278] have shown that the regression of plasma insulin versus blood glucose

* The study herein has been aided by grants from Sigrid Jusélius Foundation, Emil Aaltonen Foundation, Finnish Culture Fond and The Finnish State Medical Research Committee.

values during an oral glucose tolerance test is steeper in patients with carbohydrate-induced hyperglyceridemia than in matched controls.

Finally, the important question on causal relationships between hyperinsulinemia and hyperglyceridemia remains to be answered. If present, does the hypersecretion of insulin result directly or indirectly (via peripheral insulin resistance) from the hyperglyceridemia, or does it arise from some unrelated factor and secondarily lead to the increase of plasma triglyceride level? It is known that hyperglyceridemia is associated with elevated plasma free fatty acids (FFA) and that both FFA [567, 1340] and triglyceride [1163] are able to stimulate insulin output. On the other hand, evidence for a hypothesis that insulin increases the secretion of triglycerides into circulation is so far inconclusive and indirect.

It was thought that the series of studies reported here would solve some of the problems outlined. In order to distinguish a primary hyperinsulinemia (an exaggerated secretory response in relation to stimulus) from the secondary one (a normal response to exaggerated stimulus) a method was devised for the measurement of insulin secretion rate at different blood glucose levels. This method was used to study hyperglyceridemic patients and normoglyceridemic obese subjects under various conditions and to assess the possible influence of artificially elevated plasma FFA and triglyceride levels on insulin secretion. The results obtained do not prove that insulin is or is not involved in the genesis of hyperglyceridemia, but they allow a delineation of a tentative hypothesis on the complex relationships of insulin, glucose and triglyceride homeostasis.

METHODS

The determination of insulin secretion rate (ISR) was carried out by a method described in an earlier paper from this laboratory [1105]. The procedure includes a constant-rate infusion of ^{131}I-labeled bovine insulin and a subsequent assay of the specific activity of plasma immunoreactive insulin (IRI) and calculation of the ISR as the ratio of insulin infusion rate and the IRI specific activity. The limitations and sources of error of this method have been recently summarized [1104].

In all subjects the ISR was determined in the fasting state and at two additional blood glucose levels in the range of 120 to 200 mg/100 ml. These levels were reached and maintained constant by an intravenous primer dose of glucose followed by a constant-rate infusion (300 mg/min and 450 mg/min) of glucose delivered from a Braun Unita infusion pump. Each of the three periods lasted for 50 to 60 minutes and blood samples for the assay of glucose, IRI and IRI specific activity were withdrawn at ten minutes' intervals. The ISR was calculated separately for each sample and the mean of these values was used as the ISR of the corresponding period. Thus, three pairs of ISR and blood glucose values were obtained and when these were plotted against each other in a linear scale a regression of ISR versus blood glucose (ΔISR/Δglucose) described the increment of insulin secretion (units/min) produced by every increase of blood glucose (mg/100 ml). As will be shown, the regression was exactly linear in the large majority of cases.

The effect of artificially elevated plasma FFA level on the ISR was studied by injecting 50 mg of heparin intravenously during a constant-rate glucose infusion. Similarly, an acute increase of plasma triglyceride concentration was induced by intravenous infusion of a fat emulsion (Intralipid) during a constant hyperglycemia maintained by glucose infusion.

The radioimmunoassay of plasma IRI was carried out by the double antibody technique [1033] using ^{125}I-insulin and blood glucose by the o-toluidine method [732].

RESULTS

Plasma Insulin Response to Intravenous Glucose. The plasma IRI and glucose disappearance rate (K_G) were determined during a routine intravenous glucose

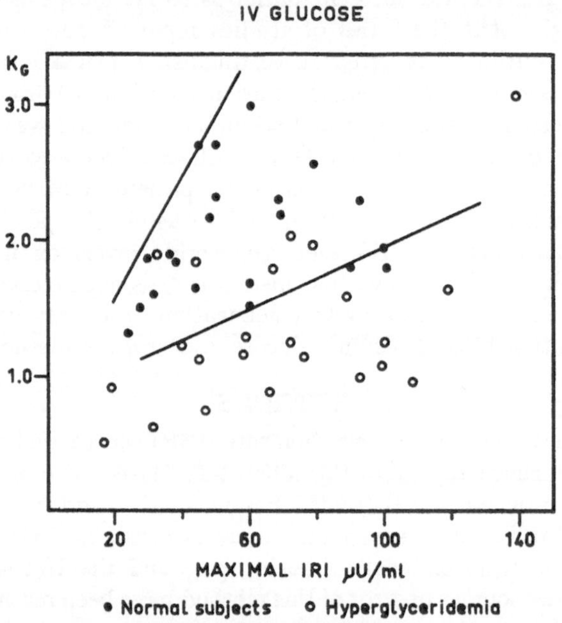

Fig. 1. Relationship of glucose disappearance rate (K_G) and maximal plasma insulin level in intravenous glucose tolerance test in healthy normal subjects and in patients with serum triglyceride exceeding 250 mg/100 ml. The samples for insulin assay were taken at 2, 5 and 10 minutes after the end of glucose infusion. Note the similar insulin responses of both groups and the low K_G of the majority of hyperglyceridemic subjects

tolerance test in 21 controls and in 23 patients with plasma triglyceride levels varying between 250 and 1,800 mg/100 ml. The results are illustrated as a plot (Fig. 1) of K_G versus the maximal plasma IRI observed during the test (a value recorded either two minutes or five minutes after the glucose bolus). As is evident from the figure, the plasma IRI responses were generally within normal range. An abnormally high response was found only in three and an abnormally low response in two instances. A most remarkable difference between the groups is noted, however, in the glucose removal rate elicited by a given plasma IRI level. A similar plasma IRI response was accompanied by a much smaller K_G-value in the hyperglyceridemic subjects than in the controls. Only six of the 23 patients with hyperglyceridemia had a completely normal glucose disappearance when related to the corresponding plasma IRI concentration. As the blood glucose values recorded at two minutes after the end of glucose infusion were not different in the two groups, the results may be taken to show that the insulin secretion remains normal in most cases of hyperglyceridemia while the efficiency of insulin to remove glucose from the circulation is decreased. In accordance with previous experience [1100], no correlation was found between the plasma triglyceride level on the one hand and plasma IRI response or glucose disappearance rate on the other.

Insulin Secretion Rate and Its Response to Increase of Blood Glucose. When the ISR was determined at three different constant blood glucose levels, a linear

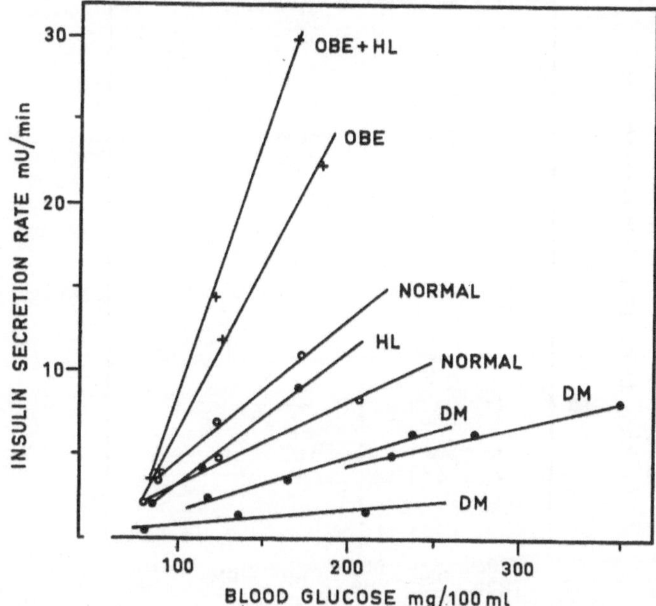

Fig. 2. Insulin secretion rate (actually the output of insulin from splanchnic to systemic circulation) at different sustained blood glucose levels. Note the linear correlation between ISR and glucose in all cases and the low response in three diabetics (DM), a normal curve in one normal weight hyperlipemic subject (HL) and the high responses in two overweight patients (OBE) one of which had hyperglyceridemia (OBE+HL)

correlation was found between these two variables in most cases. Representative curves of normal, obese, hyperglyceridemic, diabetic and obese hyperglyceridemic subjects are shown in Fig. 2. It will be seen that diabetics have a low insulin secretory response while obese subjects show a steep rise of the secretion rate on increasing blood glucose. The result agrees well with earlier knowledge derived from plasma insulin measurements.

There was no correlation between the basal (fasting) ISR and the serum triglyceride level. Many subjects with much elevated triglyceride values had an ISR within the normal range (1 to 3 mU/min) while others with only moderate hyperglyceridemia showed high ISR. The fasting IRI level showed no correlation to serum triglyceride either. The individual Δ ISR/Δ glucose values in different groups are presented in Fig. 3. With a few exceptions, obese normoglyceridemic subjects showed clearly elevated values and association of hyperglyceridemia with obesity did not essentially change the distribution pattern. Two cases of the latter group fell within a diabetic range. Of the eleven cases with hyperglyceridemia without obesity, four showed an elevated Δ ISR/Δ glucose values while the others were normal in this respect. In patients with a combination of diabetes, obesity and hyperglyceridemia the Δ ISR/Δ glucose was highly variable. It is evident that no uniform insulin secretion pattern emerged from patients with hyperglyceridemia. This fact is also apparent when the individual serum triglyceride and Δ ISR/Δ glucose recordings are correlated. Hyperglyceridemia may be combined

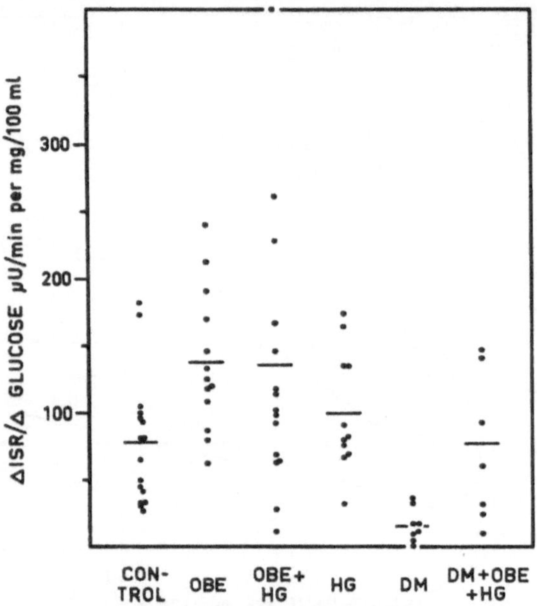

Fig. 3. Insulin secretory response to increments of blood glucose level (ΔISR/Δ glucose, i.e. the slope of the regression curves presented in Fig. 2). Note the exaggerated response in most, but not all, cases with overweight (OBE), and the similarity of distribution in obese normoglyceridemic and hyperglyceridemic subjects. Some cases with obesity and hyperglyceridemia had responses in diabetic range (DM) whereas others with obesity-hyperglyceridemia-diabetes combination had an increased insulin response

with a low, normal or high insulin secretory response while, on the other hand, a hypersecretion may occur without any increase of serum triglyceride concentration. The plasma IRI levels measured during the maintained hyperglycemia also did not correlate with the serum triglyceride values.

Effect of Caloric Restriction on Insulin Secretion. Serum triglyceride levels can be lowered in hyperglyceridemic subjects by reducing the caloric intake [1218]. In our experience, however, a normal range is seldom reached in true hyperglyceridemia on even total starvation. This may occur in obese patients with moderately elevated triglyceride values (pure secondary hyperglyceridemia?), but the majority of subjects with a visible hyperlipemia on a normal diet maintain a triglyceride level of 200 to 400 mg/100 ml during a total starvation or a 700 calorie diet. This finding clearly indicates that the basic metabolic error, at least in these cases, cannot be in the abnormal triglyceride response to dietary carbohydrate.

To find out whether the insulin secretion and plasma IRI behave differently in hyperglyceridemic as compared to normoglyceridemic subjects during caloric restriction, the plasma IRI, ISR and Δ ISR/Δ glucose were determined before and after a subtotal starvation (75 cal/day) period of one week. The summarized results appear in Table 1, which indicates that in all hyperglyceridemic cases the serum triglyceride remained at a higher level than in the normoglyceridemic subjects, in most instances attaining even higher levels than the latter group

Table 1. *Change of serum triglyceride, plasma insulin (IRI) and insulin secretion (ISR) during one week of subtotal fasting in obese subjects with and without hyperglyceridemia (mean values)*

	Normo-glyceridemic (6)		Hyper-glyceridemic (11)	
	before	after	before	after
Serum triglyceride, mg/100 ml	89	78	365	160
Fasting IRI μU/ml	22.3	14.0	21.8	17.6
Basal ISR mU/min	5.8	2.9	4.8	3.6
ΔISR/Δglucose, μU/min/mg/100 ml	165	95	163	65

reached during the isocaloric period. Also, the plasma insulin level and the insulin secretion rate diminished, on the average, less in the hyperglyceridemic group than in their controls but the difference is too small to account for the sustained hyperglyceridemia during the calorie restriction. In addition, no correlation was present between the individual IRI or ISR values and serum triglyceride level reached during the steady state starvation period. The insulin secretory response to glucose stimulus was reduced by fasting in all subjects, but it remained, in general, at a higher level in normoglyceridemic obese subjects than in the hyperglyceridemic ones. Also, in the nonobese hyperglyceridemic patients the plasma IRI content was reduced by a low calorie diet to a level not essentially different from that observed in subjects with normal serum triglyceride.

In conclusion, these results indicate that the response of insulin secretion and of plasma insulin concentration to prolonged fasting are similar in normoglyceridemic and hyperglyceridemic subjects and do not account for the differences in serum triglyceride level seen even under these conditions. This general conclusion does not exclude the possibility, however, that there are individual cases, in which the insulin response is abnormal.

Stimulation of Insulin Secretion by Elevated Plasma FFA. When heparin was given during a hyperglycemia maintained by a constant-rate glucose infusion, plasma FFA rose twofold to fourfold and the plasma IRI and ISR increased in all but one of eleven subjects studied. The mean values for blood glucose, plasma IRI and ISR before and after heparin are given in Table 2. Although

Table 2. *Effect of elevated plasma FFA (heparin) and triglyceride (Intralipid) levels on insulin secretion and plasma insulin during constant hyperglycemia*[a]

	Heparin		Intralipid	
	before[b]	after[c]	before[b]	after[c]
Glucose, mg/100 ml	200 ± 20	184 ± 16	197 ± 8	188 ± 11
IRI μU/ml	38.7 ± 4.0	72.7 ± 8.2	36.6 ± 4.1	49.2 ± 5.8
ISR mU/min	15.3 ± 3.0	28.5 ± 7.1	14.8 ± 3.8	21.6 ± 5.7

[a] The values are mean ± s.e.
[b] A period of 50 minutes.
[c] A period of 30 minutes.

the possible effect of heparin itself cannot be excluded it seems probable that a high FFA level promotes the stimulating action of hyperglycemia on insulin secretion.

Stimulation of Insulin Secretion by Acute Hyperglyceridemia. The effect of intravenous fat emulsion (Intralipid) administered during a sustained hyper-

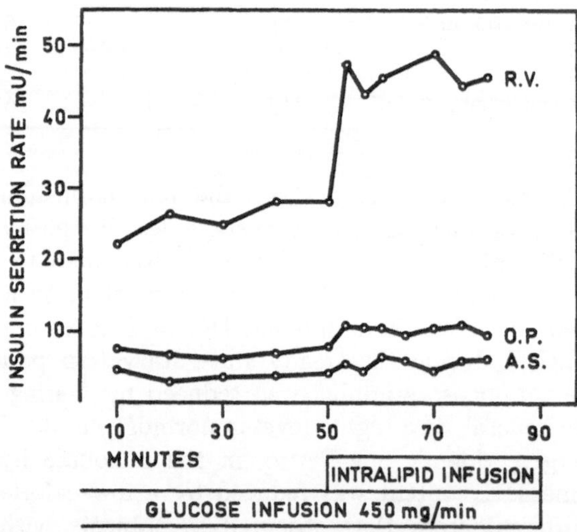

Fig. 4. Stimulation of insulin output rate by intravenous fat emulsion in three cases with different levels of insulin secretion before the fat infusion.

glycemia was very similar to that of heparin. In all of the eight subjects studied the ISR and plasma IRI increased more or less promptly after the beginning of the fat infusion while blood glucose concentration decreased slightly (Fig. 2). Again, the magnitude of the ISR response was positively correlated with the ISR level observed before the administration of fat, as shown by the three examples presented. The plasma FFA content increased during the fat infusion but this occurred more slowly than the stimulation of insulin output. It is thus evident, although not proven, that a high triglyceride level can also promote the secretion of insulin.

COMMENTS

When one attempts to test the hypothesis that hyperinsulinemia is the basic abnormality in many or most cases of so-called endogenous hyperglyceridemia, it is necessary to determine that (1) the occurrence of hyperinsulinemia is linked to the hyperglyceridemia and not to associated factors such as obesity and glucose intolerance; (2) hyperinsulinemia is not a mere consequence of hyperglyceridemia; and (3) increase of plasma insulin level is able to induce an elevation of plasma triglyceride concentration. It would then be necessary to determine whether the hyperinsulinemia is caused by a primary defect in peripheral glucose utilization or by factor(s) influencing directly the insulin secretory response.

Obesity is associated with both hyperinsulinemia and hyperglyceridemia and may form one of the links combining these chemical abnormalities. Moderately elevated serum triglyceride values are common among overweight subjects, particularly in those with an acquired type of obesity and with recent weight gain [36, 608]. In several studies a significant correlation has been found between the serum triglyceride level and the degree of obesity or magnitude of recent weight increase [36, 478, 608, 697, 1279]. However, in a population survey Abrams et al. [7] could not demonstrate a relationship between three measures of obesity (except ponderal index for men) and serum glyceride level. Also in a selected heterogeneous sample studied by Reaven et al. [1215], there was no correlation between the ponderal index and serum triglyceride. It is probable that some correlation between these two variables exists in an unselected population but within groups selected on the basis of either obesity or hyperglyceridemia this relationship disappears. Obesity is thus a contributing factor in the development of hyperglyceridemia but it does not account for more than mild or modest increases of serum triglyceride.

Hyperinsulinemia is a characteristic feature of obesity and both fasting plasma insulin and the insulin response to glucose are highly related to the degree of overweight [7, 82, 478]. It is remarkable that the insulin secretion (both basal and stimulated) is augmented in obesity without any impairment of glucose tolerance [823], and, as shown by the present data, remains abnormally high even on prolonged fasting. These observations suggest that factors other than hyperglycemia might be responsible for the chronic stimulation of beta-cells of the pancreatic islets in obesity. Even if plasma insulin and triglyceride levels are both separately correlated to the degree of obesity they need not be mutually interrelated. Actually, the lack of this correlation is clearly shown by the present study, in which obese patients were divided into two groups according to their triglyceride levels and no difference could be established between the groups in the insulin secretory response. Thus, a high insulin output rate (and a concomitant hyperinsulinemia) may be associated with a normal serum triglyceride and, conversely, hyperglyceridemia occurs in obese subjects without an exaggerated insulin secretory response. These studies were carried out with subjects on a standard diet containing 50% of calories as carbohydrate, and no prediction can be made on the possible correlation of triglyceride and insulin responses to a high carbohydrate diet. Thus, the results are not necessarily conflicting with those obtained by Farquhar et al. [449], who also could not observe any correlation between insulin and triglyceride levels when the patients were maintained on a low carbohydrate diet but demonstrated a parallel rise of both variables during high carbohydrate feeding.

Besides obesity, glucose intolerance is another factor which could explain the association of hyperinsulinemia with hyperglyceridemia. The reason for the common occurrence of an abnormal glucose tolerance in hyperglyceridemia is not known but the present finding of low *K*-values for glucose, in relation to the corresponding plasma insulin levels, and the resistance of blood glucose to exogenous insulin [366] and tolbutamide [814] in hyperglyceridemia strongly suggest that the error lies in the peripheral glucose uptake rather than in a deficient insulin secretion. Thus, the hyperinsulinemia might well be purely secondary to an increased hyperglycemic stimulus without any change in the secretory mechanism itself. Is then the impedance of glucose utilization a primary event leading to the development of hyperglyceridemia or is it secondary to the latter?

The first possibility is worth serious consideration since the metabolic situation in a carbohydrate intolerant, nondiabetic subject is very similar to that induced by a high carbohydrate diet in a normal individual. A correlation has been observed between serum triglyceride level and glucose tolerance in many studies [7, 34, 478, 608, 1102] but not in all [289, 1213]. However, the lack of this relationship does not necessarily form strong evidence against the hypothesis, since glucose tolerance is modified by insulin secretory response; also, inclusion of diabetic, insulin-deficient subjects in the material would readily disturb the correlation as indicated by earlier experiments of Reaven et al. [1215] on a heterogeneous group of diabetic and nondiabetic patients. The most significant evidence for a primary role of glucose intolerance in hyperglyceridemia is the observation of Farquhar et al. [449] that triglyceride response to a high carbohydrate diet is highly related to the glucose tolerance before the diet. This finding has not been confirmed by Belknap et al. [134], though one explanation for the discrepancy might be that their glucose intolerant patients may have been as heterogeneous as those of Reaven et al.

A second possibility, namely, that glucose intolerance is a consequence of elevated plasma triglyceride level, is also plausible. However, an acute exogenous hyperlipemia does not impair the glucose tolerance [1163, 1306] and in chronic fat-induced hyperglyceridemia glucose metabolism seems to be normal [489]. Since the plasma FFA level is also increased in hyperglyceridemia, the possibility cannot be excluded that this might lead to the reduced glucose tolerance. Whatever the exact relationship between glucose intolerance and hyperglyceridemia may be, it is apparent that either abnormality can occur without the other. High insulin secretory responses in proportion to a glycemic stimulus were found in some hyperglyceridemic nonobese subjects. An adequate explanation for this hyperinsulinemia might be derived from the observed direct stimulatory action of both triglyceride and FFA on insulin output. The stimulation of insulin release by FFA has been previously demonstrated *in vivo* in dogs [567, 1340] and in pancreatic slices of rat [906], and the observation is extended here to man. As plasma FFA content tends to be increased in obesity [397, 548], these findings could also offer an explanation for the hyperinsulinemia of obese people.

Finally, there remains the question whether hyperinsulinemia, with or without hyperglycemia, is able to increase the serum triglyceride level. The evidence related to this problem has been recently discussed and reviewed in detail [1098]. A number of data show that, on perfusion of the liver with increased concentrations of either insulin or glucose, fatty acid synthesis is stimulated, and this is accompanied by an enhanced hepatic secretion of triglycerides. On the other hand, it is well known that glucose and insulin at the same time tend to decrease the serum triglyceride by reducing the flux of FFA into the liver and by activating the removal mechanism (lipoprotein lipase) for circulating triglycerides. In view of these opposite effects it is easily understandable that the relationships between hyperinsulinemia and hyperglyceridemia are extremely complex and difficult to unravel.

CONCLUSIONS

Hyperglyceridemia is often, but not always, associated with hyperinsulinemia. In individual cases it is difficult to establish whether they are causally related or only coexistent disorders induced by a common underlying factor such as obesity or glucose intolerance. In patients who are hyperglyceridemic on consuming 200 to 250 g of carbohydrate daily, the plasma immunoreactive insulin level, insulin secretion rate and its response to graded hyperglycemia all may be normal, high or low. Thus, an exaggerated insulin secretion is not an absolute requirement for the development of hyperglyceridemia even though it may be a contributing factor.

When overweight subjects are divided into two groups, one with a normal serum triglyceride, another with hyperglyceridemia, there is no significant difference between the groups in plasma insulin, basal insulin secretion rate or, the insulin secretory response to graded hyperglycemic stimulus (Δ ISR/Δglucose). However, these three parameters of insulin output are significantly elevated in both groups as compared to nonobese controls. Thus, the hyperglyceridemia often accompanying obesity is not primarily caused by the hyperinsulinemia present in most overweight subjects. It is possible, nevertheless, that the secondary hyperinsulinemia and hyperglycemia caused by glucose intolerance may be partly responsible for the increased serum triglyceride in obese subjects. One additional and perhaps important factor in this respect is the increased flow of free fatty acids into the liver from adipose tissue of the mesenteric region, which could account for the observed correlation of serum triglyceride and truncal (acquired) obesity.

In subjects without overweight, a marked hyperglyceridemia may be combined with a normal basal plasma insulin, normal insulin secretion rate and a normal response of the latter to hyperglycemia. In some cases, however, the insulin secretion is increased and the possibility exists that this may be a significant factor in the genesis of hyperlipemia. Subjects with a manifest diabetes, defined here as fasting hyperglycemia, generally show an abnormally low insulin secretory response in proportion to glycemic stimulus (low Δ ISR/Δ glucose) but may still have a greatly elevated serum triglyceride level even in the absence of ketosis.

On intravenous glucose loading, hyperglyceridemic subjects, taken as a group, show a decreased rate of glucose disappearance in proportion to the corresponding plasma insulin levels. Thus, glucose intolerance is associated with hyperglyceridemia but whether this is a primary or secondary event cannot be stated.

An artificial elevation of plasma FFA by heparin and of plasma triglyceride by an intravenous fat emulsion during a sustained hyperglycemia is followed by a prompt increase of plasma insulin and insulin secretion rate without a concomitant increase of blood glucose. It is believed that this observation might partly explain the hyperresponsiveness of beta cells in obesity and hyperglyceridemia.

LIPOPROTEIN LIPASE AND PLASMA TRIGLYCERIDE*

EDWIN L. BIERMAN, DANIEL PORTE, JR., JOHN D. BAGDADE and WILLIAM R. HAZZARD

Evidence has accumulated supporting the role of lipoprotein lipase (LPL) in the regulation of the removal of triglycerides (TG) from plasma [1244]. Although the enzyme is present in a variety of tissues and is characteristically liberated from these tissue sites into the blood stream within a few seconds [1052] after the intravenous injection of highly charged molecules such as heparin, it is likely that its major physiologic site of action is adipose tissue. It has been suggested that the enzyme normally acts on its native substrates (chylomicrons and very-low density lipoproteins) at the endothelial cell lining the inner surface of capillaries [1244]. Consistent with this suggestion is the arrangement of chylomicrons at the endothelial cell surface observed by electron microscopy [1311] and the histochemical localization of lipase at adipose tissue capillaries [1044]. At this site the enzyme is available for combination with substrate. In accordance with formation of enzyme-substrate complex, low levels of lipolytic activity have been observed in the circulation during the absorption of a fatty meal and also have been related to the degree of hypertriglyceridemia in hyperlipemic subjects [1280].

Robinson [349] has presented evidence in the rat that lipoprotein lipase may exist at more than one site in adipose tissue and perhaps be present in more than one form. A stable form which can be isolated from fat cells of fed rats, represents a small proportion of the total activity of the whole tissue. Another form accounting for a larger proportion is unstable, may be located in the stromal-vascular cells, and varies with the nutritional state (increases with feeding, decreases with starvation). Thus a current concept suggests that in the fed

* The work herein has been supported by NIH Career Development Awards AM-28167, (Dr. Bierman) and AM-08865 (Dr. Porte), and NIH Research Project Grant AM-06670.

animal much of the lipoprotein lipase activity may reside in enzyme located outside the fat cells at an endothelial site [1245]. Therefore, although not all of the total enzyme activity assayable in tissue can be released by large doses of heparin, it is likely that only the releasable portion (presumably that associated with capillaries) is functional in the removal of triglyceride from plasma.

When heparin is administered intravenously as a single injection, lipolytic activity rapidly appears in the circulation and declines exponentially (Fig. 1). If heparin is continuously infused, either into the whole animal [1188] or the isolated perfused organ [200], enzyme activity is maintained in the circulation. Presumably this results from the saturation by heparin of hepatic inactivation

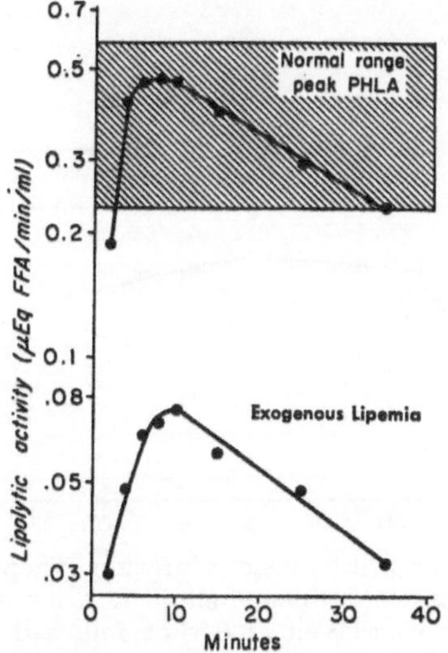

Fig. 1. Lipolytic activity in plasma (logarithmic scale) after an intravenous injection of heparin (380 units/M² at 0 time) in a normal subject (upper curve) and a subject with congenital exogenous lipemia (lower curve). The shaded zone indicates the normal range of peak postheparin lipolytic activity

systems [1540]. Several closely related enzymatic activities (phospholipases [1507] and monoglyceride hydrolase [570]) are also released by heparin. These may function in conjunction with triglyceride lipase activity in the dismantling and catabolism of lipoproteins.

Release of postheparin lipolytic activity (PHLA) into the circulation has been shown to be associated with a decline *in vivo* of plasma levels of very low-density lipoprotein triglyceride and lecithin and increases in free fatty acid, without any change in partial glycerides, cholesterol or other phospholipids (Fig. 2) [1188, 1508]. When large doses of heparin are given it is likely that most of the enzyme functional at tissue sites can be released into the circulation, since a reciprocal decrease in tissue activity has been shown [1160]. In addition, in cross circulation experiments in dogs, Hallberg [596] has shown that recipient dogs transfused with postheparin plasma have an increased maximal removal capacity for particulate triglyceride while donor dogs have a reduced maximal removal capacity.

Several lines of evidence solidify the relationship of lipoprotein lipase to the removal of triglyceride from plasma and assimilation of its constituent fatty acids. In a variety of species and experimental conditions, it has been shown that triglyceride uptake *in vitro* directly correlates with LPL activity in adipose tissue [76, 150, 513, 1180]. When LPL activity is stimulated by glucose, and even further by glucose and insulin, triglyceride uptake and incorporation increases. Although measurement of uptake includes several processes, both lipolysis and reesterification of fatty acids, it is likely that the relationship is, at least partly, due to changes in lipolysis, since actinomycin, which stimulates LPL activity presumably without effect on reesterification of fatty acids, has

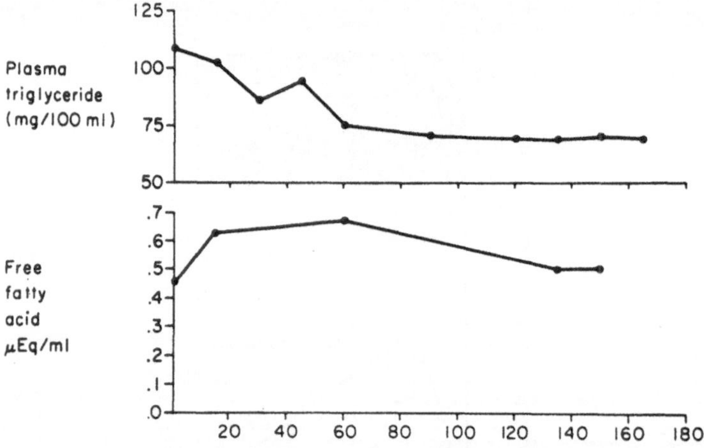

Fig. 2. The effect of a continuous intravenous infusion of heparin on plasma triglyceride and free fatty acid levels in a non-lipemic subject. A large loading intravenous dose of heparin (2,280 units/M^2) was given at 0 time followed by a constant infusion of 46.1 units/M^2/min from 10 to 165 minutes. In vitro lipolysis in blood samples was prevented by the inhibitor, paraoxan

been shown to be associated with increased triglyceride uptake [513]. In non-lipemic human subjects, despite the variety of determinants of both plasma TG concentration and lipolytic activity, a weak inverse correlation has been observed between plasma TG and either postheparin lipolytic activity [634] or lipoprotein lipase activity from human adipose tissue biopsy specimens [706]. However, much of the evidence linking LPL with plasma TG clearance in man has been derived from study of postheparin lipolytic activity in pathological states. A variety of disorders in humans have been described in which deficiency of PHLA has been coupled with exogenous lipemia and impaired removal of lipoprotein triglyceride [489]. In one such example, congenital lipoprotein lipase deficiency, severe exogenous lipemia has been associated with a marked deficiency of both PHLA [651], and adipose tissue LPL [609].

In general, individuals with impaired LPL activity, when maintained on fat-containing diets, have a preponderance in plasma of fat particles of dietary origin, which accounts for the bulk of plasma TG. They show responses to dietary changes typical of exogenous ("fat-induced") lipemia. However, even on fat-free diets, plasma TG levels are elevated. Thus when LPL deficiency in man has been observed, either primary (congenital) or secondary to other disorders, it is associated with both hyperchylomicronemia and increased endogenous triglycerides in very low-density lipoproteins. Lesser reduction of adipose tissue LPL activity may be associated with normal basal plasma TG levels, however impaired ability to assimilate an oral fat load can still be demonstrated [609]. The plasma lipoprotein pattern observed in an individual case thus appears to depend on the severity of the enzyme abnormality, the composition of the diet, and the inherent rate of endogenous TG production.

A reciprocal relationship between PHLA and plasma TG concentration also can be demonstrated in a variety of acquired hyperlipemic disorders. Two hormone

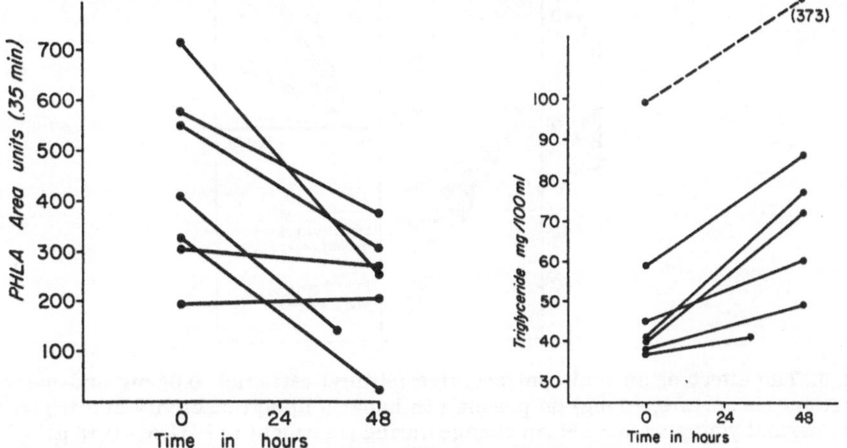

Fig. 3. Changes in plasma postheparin lipolytic activity (PHLA) (left panel) and triglyceride concentration (right panel) before and after insulin withdrawal in seven insulin-dependent diabetics

deficiency states have been associated with deficiencies of PHLA and hypertriglyceridemia. In hypothyroidism, both of these abnormalities revert to normal following the administration of thyroxin [1189]. In severe uncontrolled diabetes marked lipemia is associated with decreased PHLA and impaired ability to secrete insulin. Insulin administration reverses these abnormalities in parallel [83]. Insulin withdrawal reproduces both abnormalities. These results in man parallel the effect of insulin on adipose tissue LPL activity in experimental animals [634]. Thus, insulin withdrawal from insulin-dependent diabetic subjects produces a decline of PHLA associated with a reciprocal increase in plasma TG concentration (Fig. 3) [84]. Progestational agents given to certain individuals with evidence of a TG removal defect will lower plasma TG concentrations while raising PHLA [536]. These reciprocal relationships between PHLA and plasma TG concentration are not always quantitative, however, since in several situations circulating competitive inhibitors of PHLA and/or heparin have been described which result in marked depression of PHLA associated with variably increased plasma TG levels. Examples of this phenomenon include the decreased PHLA associated with oral contraceptives and estrogen (Fig. 4) [653], uremia [85] and the decreased PHLA associated with immunoglobulin disorders [538]. Furthermore, although the enzyme assay usually employed, using coconut oil emulsion as substrate, correlates well with activity measured using chylomicrons as substrate [1549], it is possible that functional abnormalities of TG clearing may exist without any decrease in assayable PHLA [570, 1188, 1421].

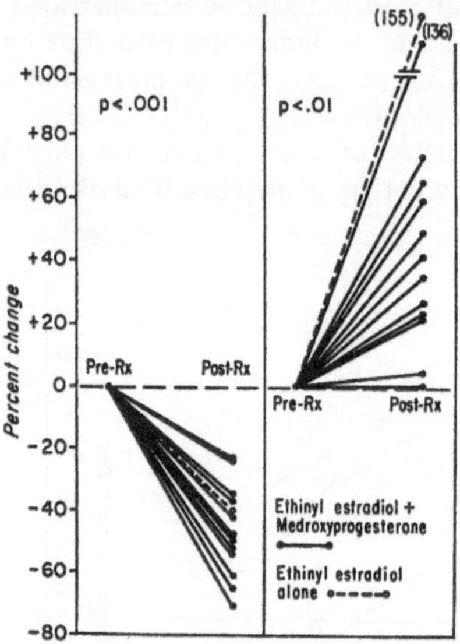

Fig. 4. The effect of an oral contraceptive (ethinyl estradiol, 0.05 mg and medroxyprogesterone acetate, 10 mg) on plasma postheparin lipolytic activity and triglyceride in 12 normal young women. Mean change during treatment in PHLA, −0.18 μEq/FFA/ml/min (baseline, 0.37) and in TG, +19 mg/100 ml (baseline, 45)

In summary, evidence accumulated thus far supports a critical physiological role for lipoprotein lipase in the dismantling of lipoproteins and the breakdown of constituent triglyceride for assimilation of component fatty acids. In addition to the role of reduced lipoprotein lipase in the gross lipemia of the congenital deficiency state, pathological changes related to this enzyme system have been implicated in a variety of acquired hyperlipemic disorders in man.

Discussion Following Dr. Bierman's Paper

Dr. STEINBERG: I would mention some studies that were done by Drs. Frank, Quarfordt, Shames and Bierman in Bethesda that are in agreement with Dr. Havel's results.

We used a multicompartmental kinetic analysis to determine triglyceride turnover in VLDL in two normal subjects and five Type IV hyperglycemics given a pulse of labelled palmitate. We found a net flux that was not clearly different between the two. That is, we did not find an overproduction of triglyceride. Even though the pool size was large, the fractional turnover was so very low that the net flux in the Type IV's was in the same range as that in the normals. Thus, our results based on kinetic analysis are in agreement with these much more direct and clearcut results of Dr. Havel's.

I might just add that we did four paired studies in which the VLDL-TGFA flux was determined on a balanced diet, and then again in the same subjects on a diet rich in carbohydrates. In those studies, the flux of triglyceride increased on the high carbohydrate diet, and there was no apparent difference between the controls and the Type IV patients with regard to the magnitude of that increment. In other words, a high carbohydrate diet does seem to increase triglyceride flux, but not in an exaggerated way, in the Type IV. Thus, their larger triglyceride response would seem to relate to a defect in rate of removal rather than to overproduction.

Dr. Bowyer: Dr. Bierman, showed that in a number of hypertriglyceridemias there is a decrease in the postheparin lipoprotein lipase. Is this a decrease in the triglyceride hydrolase activity alone, or is there also a decrease in a phospholipase activity?

Dr. Bierman: In most of the hypertriglyceridemics we studied, only triglyceride substrate was used. However, in a few cases we measured phospholipase activity as well, and in those, the two enzymes appear to be reduced in parallel. However, this question is currently under study, and we can not yet be certain about this parallelism in all types of hyperlipemia.

Dr. Sailer: I would like to add two points indicating that insulin is not absolutely a primary factor for hypertriglyceridemia. The first is that in patients with insulinoma we never see a true hypertriglyceridemia; secondly, there are many patients with very high levels of triglycerides and glucosuria who have very low insulin levels in the blood. Therefore, I think we are in agreement with Dr. Nikkilä.

Dr. Wellborn: I would like to differ with Dr. Nikkilä's use of the term "insulin secretion rate" because it is an "insulin escape rate", from the liver, and, as he pointed out, not a true pancreatic insulin secretion rate. Therefore, I would like to differ with his conclusion that triglyceride production is not related essentially to the insulin secretion rate; because, until we can actually measure pancreatic insulin secretion rate, we won't know the answer to that particular question.

Dr. Nikkilä: Of course, you are quite right, but I think that it is very difficult to measure the real rate of insulin release from the pancreas in man. On the other hand, we reasoned that, if the liver always takes up a constant fraction of insulin secreted into it, the output of insulin into the systemic circulation should measure indirectly the amount of insulin which perfuses the liver.

Dr. Wellborn: I don't think we know if the liver does remove a constant amount in different individuals.

I would just like to respond to Dr. Sailer's comment that insulin-deficient diabetics have triglyceridemia. I believe that the hyperglyceridemia of frank insulin deficiency may be related to the fact that insulin activates lipoprotein lipase, and in true insulin deficiency the hypertriglyceridemia is due to a decreased activity of lipoprotein lipase.

Dr. Boberg: Dr. Havel, how did you measure the uptake of fatty acids by the liver? It seems to me rather difficult to differentiate between the uptake over the omental region and the liver.

Dr. HAVEL: We cannot directly measure hepatic uptake of free fatty acids in man but rather uptake in the region drained by the hepatic vein. However, we have utilized our results in dogs to provide an estimate of the quantity of unlabeled fatty acid released from the splanchnic adipose tissue which does not reach the general circulation, because it is taken up by the liver. This estimate depends upon our measurements of the extraction fraction for FFA in extra hepatic splanchnic tissues and in the liver of dogs and upon measurements of fatty acid released from the splanchnic region into the general circulation in man. The calculations indicate that total splanchnic uptake of FFA (including those released from splanchnic adipose tissue) exceeds by 5 to 60% the estimate of splanchnic uptake of FFA from arterial blood plasma. The total transport of FFA in the blood is from 2 to 25% higher than the value calculated from specific activity of FFA in arterial blood plasma.

Our estimates of splanchnic release of FFA, derived from the dilution of specific activity of FFA between artery and hepatic vein, suggest that the release is primarily a function of obesity in man. Our hyperlipemic subjects were, on the whole, more obese than the control group. This accounts, in part, for the greater total splanchnic uptake of FFA, which amounted to an average of 57% of total outflow transport of FFA. In the control group this value was 42%. An additional factor was an increased extraction fraction of FFA in the splanchnic region of the hyperlipemic patients.

Dr. KEEN: Is it fair to extrapolate back from what one observes in the true insulin-dependent diabetic to the much larger number of older people who also have the same diagnostic connotation attached to them, but who are not insulin-requiring diabetics but who, in fact, are insulin-producers and in some cases hyperproducers?

Dr. BIERMAN: You have introduced a common complicating feature, since most of the subjects you refer to are diabetics who are also obese. Obesity affects insulin secretion independently of diabetes, producing hyperinsulinism. The severe diabetics with lipemia and low PHLA to which I referred had markedly impaired insulin responses. Thus individual differences and patient selection are extraordinarily important before general conclusions about groups of diabetics can be drawn. In any individual, triglyceride transport is influenced by a variety of factors which include effects of insulin on production as well as removal and, therefore, it is difficult to generalize.

Dr. OLIVER: Does heparin have the same effect on insulin secretion rate when given in the fasting state as in the nonfasting state?

Also, does intralipid and heparin, when given together, have an incremental effect on insulin secretion rate?

Dr. NIKKILÄ: The answer to the first question is no. The influence is much less if heparin is given in the fasting state. It increases with increasing blood glucose levels, which suggests that one must have first a basal stimulation of insulin secretion by glucose before obtaining a significant response.

We don't know the answer to the other question. We have not measured the effect of the combined administration.

Section VIII

STEROL BALANCE AND METABOLISM

INTRODUCTION TO THE RELATIONSHIPS OF STEROL BALANCE AND METABOLISM TO ATHEROSCLEROSIS*

IVAN D. FRANTZ, JR.

The purpose of this introductory paper is to examine the assumptions and premises on which current studies of sterol balance and metabolism are based. I will pose a number of questions which hang constantly over the head of the investigator who chooses to work in this field. These questions cannot be answered with certainty at the present time. Upon the answers to them depend the interpretation, significance, and relevance to atherosclerosis of research on sterol balance and metabolism.

Is Cholesterol Concentration in Plasma Causally Related to Atherogenesis? The Framingham Study [773] has left little doubt that the concentration of cholesterol in the plasma and the development of coronary heart disease are associated in a statistical sense. One of the principal conclusions of the Cooperative Study on Lipoproteins and Atherosclerosis [541] was: "The use of S_f 12–20 and S_f 20–100 lipoprotein measures, or the related Atherogenic Index (A.I.), had no advantage over the simpler measurement of cholesterol in the characterization of men prone to develop coronary heart disease". This conclusion, although disputed by some of the participants in the study, fostered the view that attention could be safely focused on cholesterol itself, as opposed to the form in which the cholesterol is combined. Nevertheless, the metabolism of the lipoproteins has not been neglected, as is apparent from other sections of this symposium.

Despite the inconclusive outcome of the Cooperative Study, it seems to me that the relationship of certain lipoprotein fractions to atherogenesis and the importance of the form in which the cholesterol is combined were established beyond reasonable doubt by earlier work in animals. Duff and McMillan [405] discovered that rabbits could be protected from the atherogenic effect of cholesterol feeding by pretreatment with alloxan, despite the usual great rise in plasma cholesterol concentration. In an attempt to explain this protection, Duff and Payne [407] showed that the rabbit in the alloxan-induced diabetic state had an unusually large rise in plasma phospholipids and triglycerides accompanying the rise in cholesterol produced by cholesterol feeding. Pierce [1174] studied the lipoprotein patterns of animals treated in this way, and found that most of the cholesterol was carried in fractions above S_f 100. The latter displayed no positive correlation with atherosclerosis, in contrast to the S_f 12–30 class, which was

* The original work from this laboratory mentioned herein was supported by a grant from the Life Insurance Medical Research Fund, and by Grants No. HE-07410, HE-05695, HE-01875, and HE-09686, National Heart Institute, U.S. Public Health Service.

strongly correlated. In this experimental situation, total plasma cholesterol and atherosclerosis actually showed a negative correlation.

I conclude from these observations that we must not become unduly preoccupied with cholesterol *per se*. Interpretation of experiments on sterol balance, and particularly on the regulation of the plasma cholesterol concentration, should be tempered by the realization that effects on total concentration may be less important than accompanying effects on the lipoprotein spectrum.

Is Total Exchangeable Cholesterol Pool of Body Related to Cholesterol Content of Arteries? Several investigators [546, 1546] (see also Moore herein) attempted to measure cholesterol pool sizes under various circumstances. In the following section we will consider some of the limitations of these measurements. Just now, let us assume that an accurate measurement can be made and inquire into the possible implications of a large total pool with respect to the amount of cholesterol in the walls of the arteries, the location that really matters. Data are lacking to permit a reliable answer to this question, but such information as does exist seems to point away from any very close association. Whyte, Nestel, and Goodman [1546] estimated cholesterol pool sizes in 22 persons and derived equations to relate these quantities to plasma cholesterol concentration and excess body weight. Their results pointed clearly to a strong dependence of total exchangeable body cholesterol on excess weight but no correlation at all with plasma cholesterol (except for the small increment in the rapidly exchangeable pool due to the increased amount of cholesterol in the plasma itself). We know from the Framingham Study [773] that the clinical manifestations of atherosclerosis correlate strongly with plasma cholesterol concentration but only weakly or not at all with moderate degrees of obesity. It is difficult to believe that in the subjects studied by Whyte et al., there would have been a significant degree of correlation between atherosclerosis and total exchangeable cholesterol.

This tentative conclusion does not render worthless the measurement of cholesterol pool sizes in the evaluation of hypercholesteremic patients and the effectiveness of treatment. Moore et al. [1027] calculated that the total exchangeable pool in three patients subjected to partial ileal bypass had fallen some 34% one year after surgery. To the extent that this estimate is correct, it provides knowledge of the amount of cholesterol that has been "pulled out" of the tissues. Excretion of cholesterol after ileal bypass has been estimated to increase nearly fourfold [1027]. The relatively smaller fall in plasma cholesterol concentration and total body pool is indicative of the effectiveness of homeostatic mechanisms at work to maintain the constancy of tissue and blood cholesterol. It will be of interest to learn whether there are circumstances in which the magnitude of changes in total pool are clearly dissociated from changes in plasma concentration. Unfortunately, information concerning concomitant changes in the cholesterol content of the arteries is not likely to be forthcoming, at least for man.

How Reliable are Measurements of Cholesterol Pool Size? Estimates of cholesterol pool size depend on an elaboration of the isotope dilution technique. After labeled cholesterol is administered intravenously, the fall in specific activity of the plasma cholesterol has been found by several groups of investigators [308, 578, 1026, 1087] to follow a curve which can be closely approximated as the sum of two exponential functions. Such a curve is suggestive of a model in which the exchangeable cholesterol is divided between two pools, one of which turns over more rapidly than the other. The details of this model are not determined uniquely, however, if no information is available other than the curve of plasma specific activity. Gurpide, Mann, and Sandberg [588] have presented a full explanation of the extent to which the parameters of the model can be calculated, and the effect of making simplifying assumptions. Goodman and Noble [546] have applied their analysis to the problem of cholesterol pools. In brief, the size of the rapidly miscible pool can be calculated but that of the slowly miscible pool cannot be calculated unless the rate of synthesis in one or the other pool is zero, and the loss of cholesterol from the body out of that pool is also zero. Most investigators who have carried out such calculations have assumed that no newly synthesized cholesterol is introduced directly into the slowly miscible pool, and no cholesterol is excreted directly out of the body from it. Although these assumptions are certainly incorrect, the weight of evidence points towards the conclusion that in many circumstances they are sufficiently closely approximated so that calculations based on them are not greatly in error. The rapidly miscible pool appears to include the cholesterol of the plasma, erythrocytes, liver, part of the intestine, and a small fraction of the cholesterol of some other organs [309]. Dietschy and Wilson [393], using acetate-2-^{14}C and the tissue slice technique, estimated that 97% of the cholesterol synthesized by the squirrel monkey originates in the liver and intestine, both of which belong to the rapidly miscible pool. Excretion from the body also takes place almost entirely through these organs, with only a small loss by way of the skin and the adrenal glands.

Whyte et al. [1546] calculated the size of the slowly miscible pool for their 22 human subjects assuming first, as mentioned, that no newly synthesized cholesterol entered it directly. They then made a second calculation on the assumption that all of the newly synthesized cholesterol entered the slowly miscible pool. This latter calculation gave values for the size of the slowly miscible pool that were some 40 to 60% higher than the values calculated in the more usual method.

The evidence favoring little synthesis and excretion by the slowly miscible pool lends a certain degree of confidence to calculations of cholesterol pool size, but some doubt remains. In the absence of proof to the contrary, one is free to speculate that a stimulus which apparently caused a change in cholesterol pool size actually produced instead a shift in the percentage of the newly synthesized cholesterol that was entering the slowly miscible pool directly.

Can We Measure Cholesterol Excretion? Early attempts to measure cholesterol excretion products in the stools, on which preliminary conclusions concerning the effect of polyunsaturated fats in the diet were based, made use of analytical methods that were not sufficiently specific to yield valid results. Probably the first reasonably reliable measurements were made by Hellman, Rosenfeld, Insull, and Ahrens [660]. These investigators administered labeled cholesterol and then followed the specific activity of the plasma cholesterol and the total radioactivity in the feces. The total cholesterol excreted, regardless of its chemical form, could then be calculated by making use of the fact that the specific activity of the cholesterol excretion products is about the same as that of the plasma cholesterol. This clever approach circumvented the problem of recovering quantitatively and in pure form the various components of the complex mixture of cholesterol derivatives in the stools. It has been used by other investigators [1024, 1568] but, as pointed out in Ahrens' paper in this Symposium it suffers from the defect that steroid may be lost through some as yet unidentified mechanism.

Ahrens and his coworkers [581, 993] have perfected methods which now permit valid, quantitative chemical analyses to be made on the mixture of cholesterol excretion products. They correct for destruction of the steroid nucleus by monitoring the loss of plant sterols, which seem to disappear in a parallel fashion [582]. Studies in which such corrections have not been made must be regarded with some suspicion at the present time. It may also be pointed out that even with the best available techniques, the intrusion of new phenomena can conceivably lead to false conclusions. It is manifestly impossible to check to see, each time that an experimental condition is changed, that the assumption concerning parallel loss of plant and animal sterols is still valid. Furthermore, dietary changes that alter the intestinal flora may possibly produce changes in the spectrum of excretion products, such that one is misled in the interpretation of the chromatographic separations.

The answer to our question "Can we measure cholesterol excretion?" is, then, a hesitant affirmative. Precise and even elegant methods are available, but the task is so complex that the investigator must be ever on the alert to avoid error.

Can We Measure Cholesterol Synthesis? The measurement of cholesterol synthesis presents problems that are, if anything, more serious than those surrounding the measurement of cholesterol excretion. The techniques that have been used with some success are the administration of acetate labeled with ^{13}C or ^{14}C, and the administration of water labeled with deuterium or tritium. It seems clear that mevalonate as a precursor for such measurements is of little value. The time required for it to enter the cells in which synthesis is taking place and for the cholesterol synthesized to become accessible in the plasma is too great compared with the time required for the biochemical conversion. At first glance it might appear that similar objections would apply to acetate. The situation with this precursor is different, however, in that only a small fraction of it is converted to cholesterol. Most of the administered dose is rapidly burned to carbon dioxide and water. If the rate of the latter reaction remains constant, any change in the rate of cholesterol synthesis should be reflected in a change in the fraction of the dose that ultimately finds its way into cholesterol. Calculation of absolute rates of synthesis, however, is impossible, because the extent to which the tracer is diluted by endogenous acetyl-CoA cannot be assessed. Tritiated water is theoretically more appealing as a precursor, because its specific activity in the body can be accurately measured. Here the only possibly serious flaw is that the constancy of the percentage of the hydrogen atoms in cholesterol that are derived from water has not been established under all circumstances. Some seemingly reasonable values have been obtained for the rate of cholesterol synthesis in human beings by the use of tritiated water.

One of the most encouraging features of the complicated picture is that it has been possible to demonstrate fairly good agreement among the three methods of measuring cholesterol metabolism: (1) excretion by the isotopic method; (2) synthesis by incorporation of tritium from body water; and (3) turnover based on the slope of the curve of plasma cholesterol specific activity (Moore, see this Symposium). This apparent agreement under a limited number of sets of circumstances does not constitute grounds for dismissing as unimportant the deficiencies in our methods previously outlined.

THE MEASUREMENT OF CHOLESTEROL POOLS AND TURNOVER IN MAN*

DEWITT S. GOODMAN

During the past three years a useful kinetic approach has been developed to obtain information about cholesterol pools and turnover in man. It has been known for several years that when isotopically labeled cholesterol is injected intravenously, the semilogarithmic plot of cholesterol specific activity versus time describes a curve during the first four to six weeks, whereas beyond this time the plot is linear. Two years ago we reported that the plasma cholesterol specific radioactivity-time curves obtained in such experiments could be resolved precisely into two exponential functions, as shown in Fig. 1 [546]. This indicated that the turnover of plasma cholesterol conformed to a simple two-pool model (see Fig. 2), and that the turnover curve could be characterized by

$$a = C_A e^{-\alpha t} + C_B e^{-\beta t}$$

in which a = specific activity in pool A; C_A, C_B, α, and β are constants, and t = time. The fact that this model, and this equation, satisfactorily characterize turnover curves of plasma cholesterol in man was subsequently confirmed by Samuel et al. [1288], Grundy and Ahrens [579], and Nestel, Whyte and Goodman [1088]. In the reported studies the two-pool model was found to be suitable and adequate for every one of 53 studies carried out in 41 subjects.

From the analysis of the specific radioactivity-time curve the values of several constants (including C_A, C_B, α, and β) are readily obtained. From these, a number of model parameters can be calculated, namely M_A, the size of pool A; $-k_{AA}$, the rate constant for total removal of cholesterol from pool A, which includes transfer into pool B (k_{AB}) and excretion from pool A (k_A); $-k_{BB}$, the rate constant for total removal from pool B; and PR_A, the production rate of cholesterol in pool A, defined as the rate of entry of "new" cholesterol into pool A, excluding recycled material originating in pool A. The formulas for M_A and PR_A are

$$M_A = \frac{R_A}{C_A + C_B}; \; PR_A = \frac{R_A \alpha\beta}{\alpha C_B + \beta C_A}.$$

* The work herein was supported by Grant AM-05968 from the National Institutes of Health. Fig. 1—4 originally appeared in the *Journal of Clinical Investigation*, and are reproduced here with permission of the editors of that journal.

As discussed previously [546] inferences can be drawn about the tissue locations of the cholesterol molecules which comprise the two pools (A and B). Pool A probably includes plasma, red cell and liver cholesterol, and most of the cholesterol in other viscera such as intestines, lung, spleen, and kidneys. Pool B is probably mainly in peripheral tissues, particularly muscle, and also adipose tissue, and probably includes some of the cholesterol in the viscera. In addition, there is a

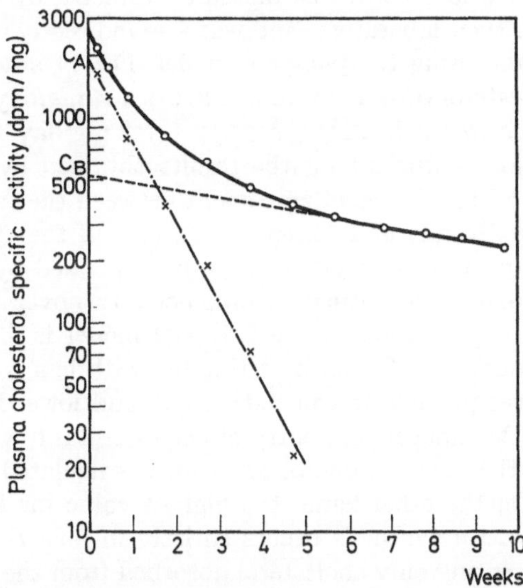

Fig. 1. The turnover of plasma cholesterol in a normal subject injected with 30 μc ^{14}C-cholesterol i.v. The experimental curve (circles and solid line) is resolved into two exponential functions with y-intercepts C_A and C_B [546]

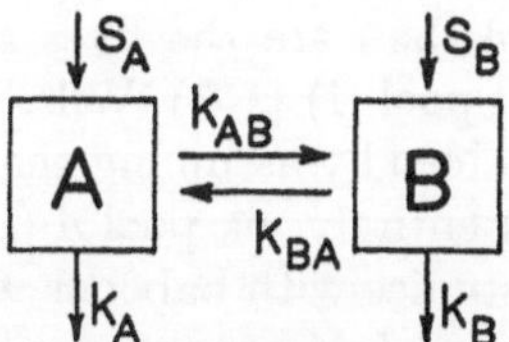

Fig. 2. General two-pool model. Rate constants are denoted by the k values; s_A and s_B are the rates of entry of material into the pools from outside the system. For the model of cholesterol turnover, k_B is assumed to be 0 (see text) [546]

considerable amount of cholesterol in the body which is not exchangeable with plasma, and would not be included in either pools A or B; this nonmiscible cholesterol is mainly in the central nervous system.

From our current knowledge of cholesterol metabolism, it is likely that almost all of cholesterol catabolism and excretion occurs via the tissues which comprise pool A. We have therefore assumed that $k_B = 0$ in the two pool model for cholesterol turnover (Fig. 2). With this assumption it is possible to calculate the individual rate constants k_{BA}, k_{AB}, and k_A. The assumption that $k_B = 0$ also make it possible to determine the metabolic turnover rate, that is the rate of cholesterol degradation in the whole body, since in this case the metabolic turnover rate (the rate of entry into and loss from the system) will be identical with PR_A. The two-pool model (with $k_B = 0$) thus permits one to estimate the total body turnover of cholesterol in the intact subject from the plasma turnover curve.

Evidence for the validity of this approach has been presented by Grundy and Ahrens [579]. These workers conducted several studies in which the cholesterol turnover rate in the whole body was measured directly by the sterol balance method developed in their laboratory, and was also indirectly calculated from the plasma turnover curve using the two-pool model. For 11 studies carried out in 10 patients, the cholesterol turnover rate was 876 ± 304 mg/day when determined by the sterol balance method, and was $1{,}017 \pm 348$ mg/day from the two-pool model. The correlation coefficient for the results obtained by the two methods was 0.90, indicating a high degree of agreement between the two methods. Moreover, as indicated by Grundy and Ahrens [579], part of the 15% discrepancy in the results obtained by the two methods may be explained by the fact that the two-pool model probably overestimates total body turnover by 3–11% [1288].

Another important parameter of the two-pool model is M_B, the size of the second pool. Unfortunately, M_B can be estimated with less confidence than M_A or PR_A. It is however possible to calculate upper and lower limiting values for M_B [1088]. Thus, if the independent entry of cholesterol into pool B is negligibly small (i.e. if $s_B = 0$) the lowest value of M_B can be calculated from the formula $M_B = M_A k_{AB}/k_{BA}$. On the other hand, the highest value for M_B is obtained by assuming that cholesterol synthesis occurs entirely in pool B, i.e. is represented by s_B, with s_A representing only cholesterol absorbed from the diet. The mean of the two limiting values for M_B was used in a recent study which examined the correlation between body weight and the parameters of cholesterol metabolism [1088]. The true value for M_B is probably much closer to the lower than to the upper limiting value, since the tissues which comprise pool B are much less active in the synthesis of cholesterol than are the liver and the gastrointestinal tract (which are presumably part of pool A) [393]. Wilson [1551] has in fact suggested that the estimate for M_B, obtained by assuming that the entry of new cholesterol into the system occurs almost entirely via pool A (i.e. that $s_B = 0$), may be fairly reliable, and has carried out studies with baboons which support this suggestion. This approach to the estimation of M_B may prove useful for lean (although not for obese) human subjects.

Nestel, Whyte, and Goodman [1088] recently examined the relationship between some parameters of cholesterol metabolism and body weight in 22 subjects. The amount of cholesterol in the more rapidly turning over pool A (M_A) varied from 14.9 to 32.7 g. The mean value for the extra-plasma part of pool A was 17.9 g. The mean upper and lower limiting values for the size of pool B (M_B) were 32.0 and 52.9 g respectively. The metabolic turnover of cholesterol (PR_A) varied between 0.73 and 1.68 g/day. Both the production rate (PR_A) and the size of pool B were found to be significantly related to total body, and particularly to excess body, weight. Fig. 3 illustrates the relationship between PR_A and total body weight. When the plasma content was excluded, the amount of cholesterol in pool A was not related to weight. For a body of ideal weight the production rate was 1.10 g/day and the size of pool B a mean of 42 g. For each kilogram of excess body weight the expected increments in PR_A and M_B were 0.022 g/day and 0.90 g, respectively.

The plasma cholesterol concentration was not related to the production rate, nor to the size of pool B or of the extraplasma part of pool A. It was, however, inversely related to the fractional turnover rate of cholesterol in pool A, and to the "metabolic clearance rate" of cholesterol (defined as the volume of plasma which contains the amount of cholesterol turned-over each day). It thus appears that elevated levels of plasma cholesterol are not associated with an increase in the cholesterol content of other pools, nor in the rate at which cholesterol is produced or acquired (or excreted) by the body. This suggests that abnormally

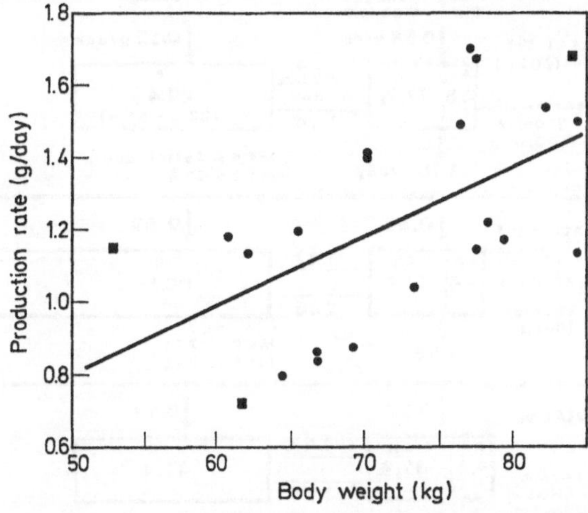

Fig. 3. Relationship between the production rate of cholesterol (PR_A) and total body weight. Circles refer to male and squares to female subjects [1088]

high plasma cholesterol levels are due to defects specifically involving the metabolism of plasma cholesterol, and not affecting the major parameters of cholesterol metabolism in the whole body. This conclusion is consistent with the recent report of Langer, Strober and Levy [840] which proposed that the elevated levels of beta lipoprotein seen in patients with type II hyperlipoproteinemia might be due to an abnormally slow rate of catabolism of the apoprotein of the beta lipoprotein.

Fig. 4 summarizes the values for cholesterol metabolism calculated by Nestel et al. [1088] for three sets of circumstances, in which the body weight and plasma cholesterol are being varied. The values for the parameters of the two-pool model for a subject at an ideal weight of 60 kg, with a plasma cholesterol level of 200 mg/100 ml are illustrated in the upper panel. The middle panel shows the effect of excess weight, and the lower panel the effect of hypercholesterolemia.

The two-pool model can readily be used to examine the effects of drug therapy or other perturbations on the various parameters of cholesterol metabolism. Thus, the effects of cholestyramine were assessed by comparing the results obtained without therapy with those obtained during therapy in five subjects studied under both conditions [546]. Cholestyramine produced a large increase in PR_A (from a mean of 0.98 to 1.98 g/day) and in the rate of removal of cholesterol from pool *A*. Cholestyramine did not, however, significantly alter the size of pool *A*. In contrast, neomycin therapy reduced the size of pool *A* from 33 to 44% (mean 38%) in four subjects studied with and without therapy [1288]. The effect of neomycin on M_A was larger than its effect on the serum cholesterol level, which was reduced 20 to 29% (mean 24%) in the four subjects under study.

In discussing the turnover of plasma cholesterol in terms of the two-pool model, it must of course be recognized that the two pools (*A* and *B*) represent mathematical constructs and do not have precise physical meaning. It is, for

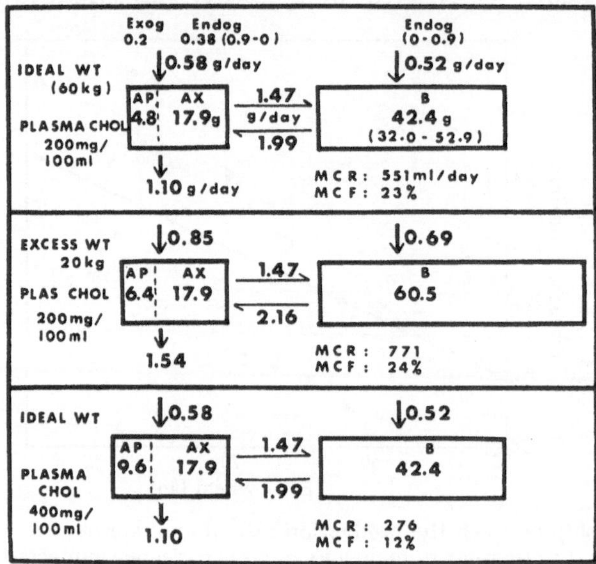

Fig. 4. Hypothetical models of cholesterol turnover, for a subject with a normal plasma cholesterol level and at ideal weight (top panel), and showing the effects of excess weight (middle panel) and of hypercholesterolemia (bottom panel). *AP* cholesterol in plasma (gm); *AX* cholesterol in pool *A* excluding plasma; *MCR* metabolic clearance rate (see text); *MCF* metabolic clearance fraction (% plasma volume per day) [1080]

example, clear that the *in vivo* turnover of cholesterol in man involves a large number of metabolically heterogeneous pools of cholesterol in different tissues, and within given tissues. The finding that the turnover of plasma total cholesterol conforms to a two-pool model hence means that the various tissue pools of cholesterol fall into two groups in terms of the rates at which they equilibrate with plasma cholesterol. One group of pools is apparently in fairly rapid equilibrium (in terms of hours to days) with plasma cholesterol, whereas the second group of pools is in fairly slow equilibrium (in terms of days to weeks) with plasma cholesterol. Within each group, the rates of equilibration of the different pools with plasma cholesterol are apparently sufficiently similar so that the group behaves as a single pool, when analyzed in terms of the turnover curve of plasma total cholesterol.

It is now well established that within plasma itself four metabolically heterogeneous pools of cholesterol can be distinguished. These pools consist of plasma free cholesterol, and esterified cholesterol in each of three plasma lipoprotein fractions. This conclusion derives from studies of the turnover rates of individual cholesteryl esters in whole plasma and in each of three plasma lipoprotein fractions in man [545]. These studies demonstrated that in whole plasma, and in each of three lipoprotein fractions (HDL $= D > 1.063$; LDL $= D$ 1.019–1.063; VLDL $= D < 1.019$) all of the different cholesteryl esters (i.e. palmitate vs. oleate vs. linoleate) turned over at the same fractional rate. The fractional turnover rate of the cholesteryl esters differed, however, from lipoprotein to lipoprotein, with the highest fractional turnover rate being present in the HDL cholesteryl esters, and the smallest fractional turnover rate in the LDL cholesteryl esters.

The finding that heterogeneity among plasma cholesteryl esters in man exists between the different plasma lipoproteins, rather than between the different esters in a given lipoprotein, has been confirmed by Nestel, Couzens and Hirsch [1086]. These workers, moreover, obtained similar findings in subjects with normal and with high plasma cholesterol levels. Nestel et al. [1086] also examined the effect of diet on the turnover of individual cholesteryl esters, using diets rich in carbohydrate, saturated fat, or safflower oil. Although the composition of the plasma cholesteryl esters was altered by changing the diet, under each condition the fractional turnover rates of the different individual cholesteryl esters were all the same.

We have recently studied the effects of cholestyramine and of clofibrate therapy on the turnover of individual cholesteryl esters in different plasma lipoproteins (Goodman and Noble[1]). These two drugs were selected because cholestyramine greatly increases the total body turnover of cholesterol but has very little effect on the plasma cholesteryl ester composition, whereas clofibrate. strikingly alters the composition of the plasma cholesteryl esters. Two subjects were studied during a period of cholestyramine therapy, and two while on clofibrate. In all four subjects, the fractional turnover rates of the different individual cholesteryl esters were the same in whole plasma, and in each of the three plasma lipoprotein fractions. These results were similar to those previously obtained with normal subjects. The relative turnover rates of the cholesteryl esters in the different plasma lipoproteins were also similar to those observed in normal subjects. These results demonstrate that neither drug has a markedly selective effect on the turnover of one particular cholesteryl ester or of the cholesteryl esters in one particular lipoprotein fraction.

Summary. The turnover of plasma cholesterol in man conforms to a simple two-pool model. When a known amount of labeled cholesterol is injected intravenously the model permits calculation of the size of the first pool (M_A) and of the Production Rate in this pool (PR_A). The average size of M_A was 26 g in a series of 22 subjects. Upper and lower limiting values can be calculated for the size of the second pool (M_B), and the pool size then estimated. Both PR_A and M_B are significantly related to total and to excess body weight. At ideal weight, M_B is ca. 32–53 g and PR_A ca 1.1 g/day. The value of PR_A provides a good quantitative estimate for the total body metabolic turnover (i.e. degradation

1 Goodman, DeW. S., Noble, R. P.: Cholesteryl ester turnover in human plasma lipoproteins during cholestyramine and clofibrate therapy. J. Lipid Res., in press, (May) 1970.

plus excretion) of cholesterol. This conclusion has been validated by simultaneous turnover and total balance studies carried out in 10 subjects by Grundy and Ahrens. The effects of various perturbations on the parameters of cholesterol metabolism can be examined readily with the two-pool model. Such studies have shown, for example, that cholestyramine mainly increases PR_A, whereas neomycin reduces M_A.

Plasma cholesteryl esters (CE) are metabolically heterogeneous and can be separated into three pools corresponding to the three classes of plasma lipoproteins. HDL CE show the greatest, and LDL CE the smallest, fractional turnover rate. Within each lipoprotein, all the different CE turn over at the same fractional rate. The relative turnover rates of the CE in the different plasma lipoproteins are not altered by therapy with either cholestyramine or clofibrate.

A REVIEW OF THE EVIDENCE THAT DEPENDABLE STEROL BALANCE STUDIES REQUIRE A CORRECTION FOR THE LOSSES OF NEUTRAL STEROLS THAT OCCUR DURING INTESTINAL TRANSIT

E. H. AHRENS, JR.

Grundy, Ahrens and Salen [582] reported that losses of neutral sterols (cholesterol and plant sterols) occur during their movement through the intestinal tract (but no losses of bile acids); that these losses frequently are large (up to 60% of the neutral sterols in transit); and that the losses of plant sterols and of cholesterol are equal. Therefore, since the absorption of plant sterols in man occurs to only a negligible degree [554–55], the cholesterol losses can be dependably corrected according to the percentage recovery of dietary plant sterols in the feces. All our findings were made in patients maintained solely on liquid formula feedings.

These losses are presumed to be due to degradation of the ring structure of these 3βOH,Δ^5-sterols by intestinal bacteria. However, proof has not yet been obtained that the process is bacterial, nor have we been able to identify the fragments into which the ring structure is split. Thus, while the evidence for neutral sterol degradation is inferential, our conclusion is supported by many interlocking findings; taking cognizance of all the data, we can offer no alternative explanation. The evidence at hand today (November, 1969) is presented in this report.

New lines of evidence have recently been obtained in this laboratory [1284] that show the absorption of beta sitosterol in man is less than 5% of its dietary intake (regardless of the magnitude of that intake). There was no measurable endogenous synthesis of beta sitosterol in the patients we studied. Thus, if there is no degradative loss of beta sitosterol in the course of the transit of this sterol through the intestinal tract, 95% or more of the beta sitosterol fed will be recoverable in the feces. In some patients this indeed is found to be true; but in others the losses of dietary beta sitosterol may range as high as 60%. Our recent studies on beta sitosterol absorption in man rule out the possibility that losses of this magnitude can be ascribed to absorption.

Patients fed radiocholesterol daily for many weeks to attain the isotopic steady state [1553] must, by definition, excrete as much isotope in cholesterol or its products as they ingest. Some patients readily attain this isotopic balance, and in these patients the recovery of both radioactivity and dietary beta sitosterol is quantitative. However, in other patients in whom the recovery of unlabeled beta sitosterol is not complete, there is also an incomplete recovery of radioactive cholesterol. Furthermore, the percentage losses of radioactivity precisely match the percentage losses of beta sitosterol. In other words, whatever causes a loss of cholesterol during its intestinal transit causes an equal loss of beta sitosterol. When the recovery of radioactive sterols in the feces is corrected according to the percentage recovery of dietary beta sitosterol, the excretion of radioactivity now matches the intake of radioactivity, thus satisfying the definition of the isotopic steady state and signifying its attainment in our patients.

Large losses of neutral sterols are demonstrable even when the recovery of bile acids in the feces is complete. In experiments examining this important methodologic point, radioactive bile acids are fed daily to achieve the isotopic steady state [1553] in which, by definition, each unit of radioactivity fed must be matched by a unit excreted. Radioactive bile acids are completely recovered even in patients in whom neutral sterol losses are large during the same study periods [582].

If mixtures of radiocholesterol and radio-beta sitosterol (labeled with different isotopes) are instilled into the proximal colon (distal to which there is no sterol absorption), the radiosterols should be completely recovered in the feces over the next week or 10 days if there is no degradation of the sterols in the colon. In two such experiments the recovery of the two isotopic compounds was incomplete; moreover, the percentage loss of each radiosterol was exactly the same [582]. In another study we found that the longer the colonic contents are retained in the colon, the greater the chance for degradative losses to occur [369].

These four findings indicate that sizable losses of neutral sterols can occur during intestinal transit; presumably, the enzymes causing neutral sterol losses in the intestinal lumen fail to discriminate between $3\beta OH,\Delta^5$-sterols differing in sidechain structure. Apparently the enzymatic attack occurs at the A ring end of the molecule containing a double bond at C_{5-6}, but not when the A and B rings are in cis configuration (as in the case of the bile acids).

The performance of dependable sterol balance studies depends on having methods which allow accurate measurements of all neutral and acidic steroids in feces (Δ^5, 5α- and 5β-compounds) with clean distinction between cholesterol and plant sterols. The (TLC-GLC)[1] methods developed in this laboratory [581, 993] meet these criteria. It is critical to the present argument to reiterate the

1 Thin layer chromatography, gas liquid chromatography.

published evidence [582] that, when radioactive cholesterol is given to patients by pulse labeling intravenously or by continuous daily oral administration, the total isotopic content (^3H or ^{14}C) of feces is recoverable entirely in the two steroid fractions of feces (neutral and acidic); in other words, the total isotopic content of feces obtained by combustion analysis of the fecal homogenate equals the sum of the radiosterols in the two fecal steroid fractions isolated from that homogenate by our TLC-GLC methods.

Large losses of neutral sterols are demonstrable even when the recovery of the inert indicator Cr_2O_3 is quantitative [582]. Thus, the losses cannot be ascribed to incomplete collections of feces.

In some patients there are no detectable losses of neutral sterols during their intestinal transit, while in others these losses are consistent, week after week, so long as any one diet is fed [582].

These three findings strongly support our concept that the losses of neutral sterols during intestinal transit are due to biological factors and cannot be ascribed to methodologic errors, either on the metabolic ward or in the laboratory.

Turnover data for cholesterol in man are obtainable through application of the sterol balance method [579], but also by mathematical analysis of isotope kinetics after pulse labeling with radiocholesterol by the intravenous route; equations for a two-pool model [546] have been used for this calculation. These two independent approaches yield turnover data which are very similar [579], but they approximate each other only if neutral sterol losses determined by the balance method are corrected by the percentage recovery of fed beta sitosterol. If this correction is not applied to the data obtained by the balance method, the turnover data obtained by the two approaches are grossly dissimilar. Uncorrected results obtained by the sterol balance method are, of course, consistently smaller (the larger the degradation of neutral sterols in transit through the intestine, the smaller the recovery of those sterols in feces). But also, if this degradation takes place proximal to sites of reabsorption of endogenous cholesterol, less endogenous cholesterol will be reabsorbed, and this in turn will lead to a more rapid decay curve and a falsely high calculation of cholesterol turnover by kinetic analysis of that curve. Thus, the greater the degradation and the higher in the intestinal lumen this occurs, the more disparate the estimates of cholesterol turnover by these two approaches will be. These considerations weigh heavily in the decision that neutral sterol losses must be corrected according to the recovery of the internal standard, beta sitosterol, fed daily in constant amounts.

Data for daily beta sitosterol turnover obtained mathematically according to the two-pool model after intravenous pulse labeling with radioactive beta sitosterol correspond closely to data obtained by the isotopic balance method [1284]. The latter technique is similar to that which has been described previously for cholesterol [579]; it depends on chemical isolation of fecal steroids. The excretion of radioisotopic materials in the neutral and acidic steroid fractions is translated into milligrams by dividing the radioactivity excreted daily in each fraction by the specific activity of plasma beta sitosterol. The correspondence of data obtained by kinetic analysis and by the isotopic balance method is very close, but only if the losses of neutral sterols during intestinal transit are corrected according to the percentage recovery of fed nonisotopic beta sitosterol.

These two findings indicate that the turnovers of cholesterol and of beta sitosterol in man can be calculated by two independent methods, but that the results correspond closely only when the sterol balance data are corrected for neutral sterol losses during intestinal transit.

In experiments on rats in this laboratory, Miettinen, and later Quintao consistently noted complete neutral sterol recoveries (unpublished data). However, in six dogs fed a refined diet of known composition and studied repeatedly over a two-year period, my colleagues Pertsemlidis and Kirchman have found neutral sterol losses ranging from 0 to 20% (unpublished data). These losses were characteristic of each animal; simultaneously the recovery of Cr_2O_3 was always greater than 90% of the daily dose.

Connor et al. [324] have confirmed that neutral sterols can be lost during intestinal transit in man; they used our TLC-GLC methods. They noted reasonably quantitative recoveries of fed beta sitosterol in four of six formula-fed normal men and losses up to 58% in one patient. In further studies carried out on this latter patient with formula feedings, Connor has repeatedly confirmed the finding of large neutral sterol losses and noted that these losses were greatly reduced by adding cellulose to the formula (personal communication). This new finding raises the question as to whether neutral sterol losses ever occur in patients fed solid foods, a question that we have not explored. However, Borgström [201] has recently reported significant losses of radio-beta sitosterol fed as a single test dose in six of 19 normal young men maintained on *ad libitum* diets, and Miettinen has encountered losses of beta sitosterol ranging from 30–60% in four patients fed diets comprised of solid foods (personal communication).

Counter-Evidence. The evidence that degradation of the ring structure of sterols does not occur in mammalian organisms has been obtained in two studies in rats [298, 1368] and one in man [659]. All of these reports were based on experiments in which ^{14}C-4-cholesterol was administered as a single dose and respired gases were then examined for the presence of $^{14}CO_2$; in no case was a significant amount of labeled carbon dioxide formed. As noted, we also have failed to find neutral sterol losses in rats through application of the same sterol balance techniques by means of which we have demonstrated large losses in our clinical studies; hence, we take no issue with the published findings in rats. Nor have we been able to detect $^{14}CO_2$ in respired gases in man even when the sterol balance data indicated large losses of ^{14}C-4-cholesterol; hence, we take no issue with Hellman's conclusion [659]. Since we have not been able to demonstrate respiratory $^{14}CO_2$ in our "degraders", we have proposed that fragments other than $^{14}CO_2$ are formed when the sterol ring structure is degraded (see below).

It is worth noting that reference is made frequently to the fact that Schönheimer failed to find any evidence of the degradation of cholesterol and plant sterols in his classic balance studies in rabbits and mice. On careful review of the literature it becomes clear that Schönheimer never addressed this question. A quotation from one of his last papers on sterols [1314] is in order: "It is a problem of future investigation to establish whether a rupture of a ring or only a less drastic change in the molecule takes place". This "study for the future" was never undertaken by him.

DISCUSSION

Taking note of all the evidence, we conclude that neutral sterols need not be, but can be degraded during their transit through the intestinal tract. This is not a radically new proposal, since in 1935 Nékam and Ottenstein [1081] noted that cholesterol incubated with human intestinal contents was altered to products not precipitated with digitonin, and in 1952 Curran and Brewster [351] isolated a strain of *E. coli* from the duodenum of a patient with chronic cholecystitis that could be shown on culture to utilize cholesterol as its sole source of carbon.

Since the degradation of the ring structure of a wide variety of closely related sterols by soil bacteria is understood in detail, we suggest that similar processes may occur in the mammalian intestine. In reviewing this topic, Sih and Whitlock [1363] describe the voluminous evidence showing that an attack on the ring structure takes place with oxidation of ring A and subsequent opening of ring B to form 9,10-seco compounds, followed by further fragmentation to produce branched-chain volatile compounds. If these volatile fragments were excreted with the feces or passed in the intestinal flatus, they would be lost to combustion analysis; if aminated [334] and absorbed, they might be incorporated into protein biosynthetic pathways. Since metabolism in the large intestine is largely anaerobic, we would not be surprised if these products were excreted in the respiratory gases as compounds other than CO_2, such as methane.

There are many experimental approaches to this important question that remain to be explored. An animal model must be sought in which large losses of neutral sterols occur; a search could then be made in various tissues for radioactive materials derived from ingested radiosterols. *In vitro* experiments with feces obtained from patients who are known "degraders" have not been illuminating in our hands, but negative experiments of this kind may mean only that the correct experimental conditions have not been used; a positive result could, of course, give an important foothold for learning whether the process is bacterial or host-initiated, as well as offering opportunities for study of the enzymatic reactions involved.

CONCLUSION

Investigators studying excretion either by sterol balance techniques or by isotopic balance methods should not overlook the possibility that neutral sterol losses of sizable magnitude can occur in the intestinal tract. Indeed, we think it mandatory that appropriate steps be taken to determine whether this phenomenon occurs in any animal or man studied by sterol balance techniques, so as to make corrections when they are needed. To dismiss the possibility of sterol degradation on the basis that final proof has not yet been obtained through isolation of the split fragments seems to us to give undue weight to experiments conducted years ago that do not bear directly on the question under study.

THE EFFECTS OF DIETARY LIPID AND STEROLS ON THE STEROL BALANCE*

WILLIAM E. CONNOR

The sterol balance concept has special usefulness because the steroid nucleus cannot be oxidized by the tissues of the body. Although oxidations, reductions and hydroxylations within the steroid nucleus or in the side chain may occur, the basic molecular structure of the nucleus is preserved indefinitely in the body. The stability of the four-membered ring means that its accumulation within the body and in certain individual tissues including arteries may occur if the input into the system exceeds its capacity for appropriate compensation in the output. In fact, the disease atherosclerosis represents in part a positive sterol balance of the arterial wall. With a greater flux of cholesterol into the arterial intima than that amount leaving, the gradual storage of cholesterol in the artery ultimately leads to progressively severe atherosclerosis.

Table 1. *The sterol balance*

Sources of sterol input	Output of sterols
1. From the diet Cholesterol Plant sterols, seafood sterols 2. Synthesis in liver and intestinal mucosa	1. Fecal cholesterol: From the bile and intestinal mucosa 2. Fecal bile acids 3. Skin losses: sebum and squamous cells 4. The fetus and the milk under the special circumstances of pregnancy and lactation

The input of sterol into the body pools is derived from two sources: (1) the diet, and (2) the synthesis of cholesterol in the body from acetate (Table 1). Since sterols are necessary constituents of all living cells, they are generally found in foodstuffs derived from both animals and plants. Cholesterol, a 27-carbon molecule, is the chief animal sterol and beta sitosterol, a 29-carbon sterol, is the most common plant sterol (see Fig. 1 for structural comparisons). Although plant sterols have a discrete metabolism of their own, from the quantitative point of view they provide almost no input into the body because they are poorly absorbed by the intestine (less than 5% of the intake). Cholesterol thus provides the only important dietary input of sterols in a range from 0–1,500 mg/day. The intake may be zero because cholesterol is not an obligatory nutrient.

Even the absorption of dietary cholesterol is incomplete, being only 20 to 40% of the intake in man [201] and may vary from time to time, perhaps dependent upon the quantity of cholesterol contained in the plasma-liver-intestinal pool (pool A). There is some evidence that absorption becomes less after an

* The work herein was supported by Public Health Service Research Grants HE-11, 485, by the American and Iowa Heart Associations, and by the Clinical Research Center Grant MOl-FR-59.

increased amount of dietary cholesterol has elevated the plasma cholesterol level [580].

In Western man at any rate, with regard to the sterol balance, the amount of cholesterol in the diet is additive to the amount synthesized in the liver and intestinal mucosa [1455]. The reason for this additive effect is that the total amount of synthesized cholesterol entering pool A is not affected by the "feed-back inhibitory" action which entering dietary cholesterol has in some animals. This failure is, in part, responsible for the rise of plasma cholesterol when choles-

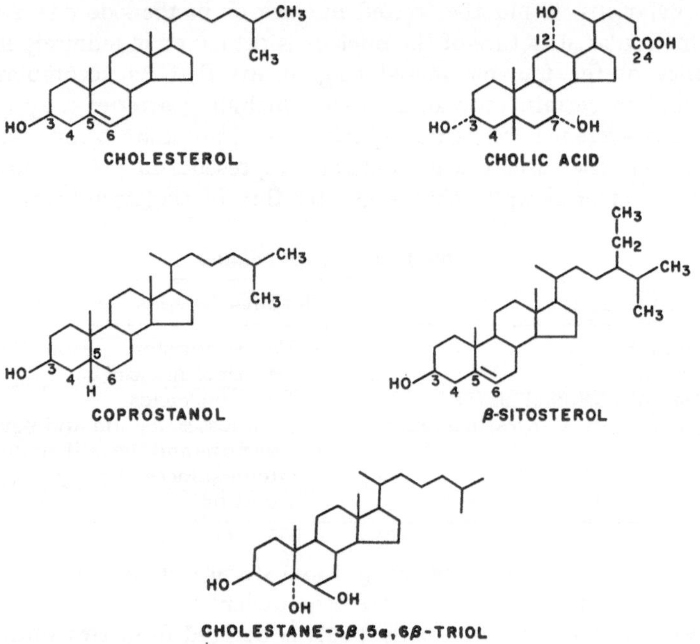

Fig. 1. The chemical structures of various sterols and steroids important in the "sterol balance"

terol-containing foods are added to the diet. Synthesized cholesterol usually ranges from 500 to 1,000 mg/day.

The output component of the sterol balance is almost entirely through the stool, either as cholesterol and its chief bacterially altered product, coprostanol, or as bile acids converted from cholesterol in the liver. The fecal cholesterol is derived from cholesterol secreted into the bile, cholesterol excreted by the mucosal cells (the latter component perhaps the result of continual cell sloughing), and unabsorbed dietary cholesterol. The excreted cholesterol mixes with the cholesterol consumed in the diet and probably has the same possibility for limited absorption which would return it to pool A. On the other hand, bile acids are reabsorbed into the enterohepatic circulation most efficiently with only a small quantity (5% or less) of the total amount excreted into the bile having a final fecal pathway [140].

The skin may participate to a limited extent in the sterol balance. The sebum secreted by the sebaceous glands of the dermis contains sterols as well as squalene. Likewise, the cholesterol of the stratified squamous epithelial cells which are constantly desquamating represents a constant loss from the body. Whether the excretion of cholesterol from the skin represents a net loss from the plasma cholesterol pool or whether that excretion is derived entirely from cholesterol synthesized in the dermis and not entering into more labile cholesterol pools is at the present time undetermined. The total twenty-four output of sterols from the skin in an adult man may range from 50–100 mg, a not inconsiderable quantity [328].

Dietary Sterols and Sterol Balance. Dietary sterols have a direct and measurable effect upon the sterol balance (Table 2). The consumption of dietary cholesterol in a digestible form such, as egg yolk or crystalline cholesterol dissolved in oil, and in amounts from 310 mg/day and above has the effects here listed.

Table 2. *Effects of dietary cholesterol on sterol balance in man*

1. Increases in the serum cholesterol levels (from 10 to 70%)
2. Expansion of body pool of cholesterol (plasma-tissue)
3. Total biosynthesis of cholesterol remains unchanged
4. Enhanced bile acid excretion (variable). 371 to 665 mg/day (a +79% change); 152 to 183 mg/day (+20%, a slight change)

We have found that amounts of dietary cholesterol from 475 to 3,600 mg/day have similar serum cholesterol raising effects. Invariably, the serum cholesterol rises; the range of increase is from 10 to 70%, with 20 to 30% changes being most common. Fig. 2 depicts these effects of dietary cholesterol upon the serum cholesterol levels [322].

Secondly, the body pool of cholesterol expands. Such an increase in cholesterol pool size is well known from cholesterol feeding in experimental animals [62]. In man the available evidence is meager. In the one appropriate study, dietary cholesterol led to an accumulation of some 20.5 g of cholesterol in the body [580]. Thirdly, we must appreciate again that biosynthesis of cholesterol is not altered in most men by dietary cholesterol. Finally, bile acid excretion may be typically increased but perhaps not always. Here are the results of three studies. In three men the mean increase in bile acid excretion from dietary cholesterol ingestion was from 371 to 665 mg/day (unpublished data). In another study the increase was not significant, from 152 to 183 mg/day [580]. In the third study subject A had an increase in bile acid output of 170 mg/day when dietary cholesterol was increased from 100 to 2,280 mg/day. A further increase to 2,780 mg/day augmented fecal bile acids only an additional 70 mg/day. Subject B had only a 50 mg/day increase in fecal bile acids when cholesterol was increased from 80 to 2,009 mg/day [1553].

Another effect of dietary cholesterol may be to change cholesterol absorption. Grundy, Ahrens and Davignon found, as is indicated in Fig. 3, that when challenged by a large increment of 1,600 mg of dietary cholesterol the intestine compensated by greatly reducing cholesterol absorption from an initially high level to successively lesser amounts [580].

The amounts of cholesterol in the diet which man will tolerate without increases in the plasma cholesterol concentration occurring is indicated in Table 3 (unpublished data). These 6 normal men had a baseline diet containing 10 mg

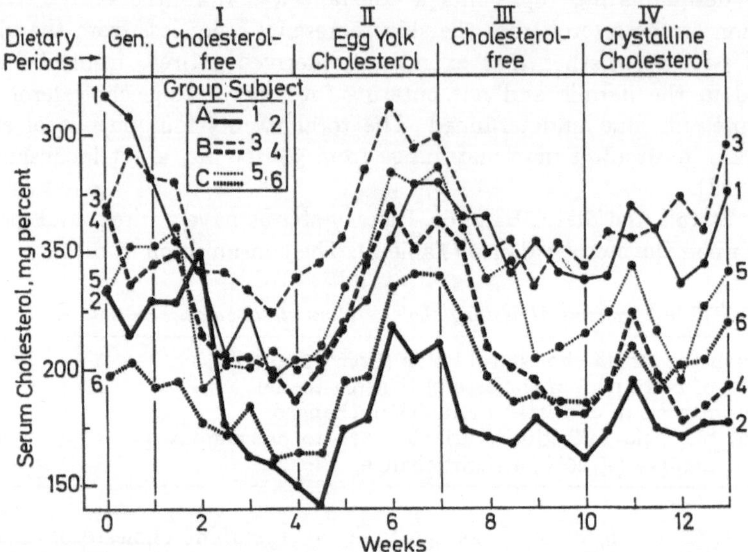

Fig. 2. The serum cholesterol values for each subject during the different dietary periods. In period II, group A subjects received 475 mg, group B, 950 mg and group C, 1,425 mg of egg yolk cholesterol. In period IV, group A subjects received 1,200 mg of crystalline cholesterol, group B, 2,400 mg, and group C, 3,600 mg

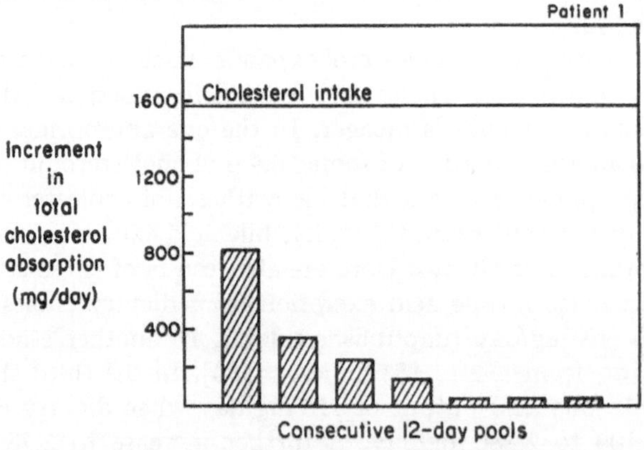

Fig. 3. Increment in absorption of total cholesterol (endogenous plus exogenous) in Patient 1 on a high cholesterol intake. Reproduced from reference [580]

of cholesterol. They then received challenges of dietary cholesterol in amounts from 110 to 610 mg/day. The 110 mg dietary level did not alter the baseline serum cholesterol. The amounts of 310 and 610 mg/day produced similar increases, plus 27 mg% and plus 32 mg%. This "cholesterol overload", as we would term these serum cholesterol increases, resulted from a certain intake of cholesterol in the diet, 310 and above. Data for intakes between 110 and 310 mg/day are not yet available but might establish the critical overload input in milligrams per day for human beings, information of considerable importance.

Dietary Fat and Sterol Balance. The fat of the human diet may affect cholesterol metabolism by virtue of its actual quantity and also through its fatty acid composition. Cholesterol absorption is especially reduced when dietary fat is absent or very low [1476]. However, within the usual range of fat intake in Americans it is unlikely that the amount of fat has a profound effect upon cholesterol absorption. How dietary fat might affect cholesterol synthesis in the intestinal mucosa remains an open question. Cholesterol, as an integral constituent of the chylomicron, must be supplied from some source (either the plasma or intestinal mucosa). It might well be that the greater the quantity of dietary fat

Table 3. *Dietary cholesterol and cholesterol overload*[a]

Amount of cholesterol in the diet (mg/day)	Serum cholesterol change % (mg)
110	− 1
310	+27
610	+32

[a] Six normal men.

being absorbed and stimulating chylomicron formation in the mucosal cell the greater quantity of cholesterol that would be required from synthesis. Dietary fat *per se* appears to have no direct effect upon the hepatic synthesis of cholesterol other than providing acetate substrate, as will also dietary carbohydrate and protein.

The quantity of dietary fat has importance in at least two other situations. In patients with Types I and V hyperlipoproteinemia the intense lipemia and the chylomicron band found at the origin on lipoprotein electrophoretic pattern are profoundly ameliorated by a sharp reduction of the dietary fat to a range of 5 to 10% of the total calories. The reduction of dietary fat improves the lipemia and concomitant hypertriglyceridemia so dramatically because the basic problem in these patients is impaired removal of chylomicrons from the blood. In some patients with Type IV hyperlipoproteinemia a reduction of fat calories with a concomitant increase of carbohydrate calories may intensify the prebeta lipoproteinemia (VLDL lipoproteins) and further elevate the serum lipids, particularly serum triglycerides and also the serum cholesterol level.

The fatty acid composition of the dietary fat invariably affects the serum lipids greatly. Since 1952 when this phenomenon was first demonstrated by Kinsell and coworkers, it has been shown repeatedly that the replacement of saturated fat in the diet by polyunsaturated fat greatly lowered plasma cholesterol levels [26]. The effects of polyunsaturated fat upon the sterol balance may be variable. The disposition of the considerable quantity of cholesterol leaving the plasma as the plasma cholesterol level declines might be twofold: (1) it might simply move into the tissues (an enrichment of one pool *vis à vis* another); or (2) this cholesterol might leave the body in the form of enhanced bile acid and neutral sterol excretion in the feces. Such excretion might occur because of enhanced bile acid or cholesterol secretion into the bile, or because of effects in the intestinal mucosa to prevent absorption or reabsorption of bile acids and cholesterol. If the sterol balance is actually altered by increased fecal excretion of bile acids and neutral sterols, is this only a consequence of the primary alteration of lipoprotein fatty acid composition which then enables less lipid to be carried in the plasma by the same quantity of protein [1401]? While there is a paucity of answers to some of these questions, many investigations have been made concerning the effects of polyunsaturated fat upon the excretion of fecal steroids and bile acids.

Problems of methodology have prevented precise and accurate measurement of the fecal steroids until recent years, but the development of the isotopic balance

Table 4. *Description of diets*[a] *used to determine effects of polyunsaturated fat on sterol balance*

Period	Source of fat	Iodine value of fat	Fatty acid composition (percentage of total)			Sterols (mg)	
			saturated	monounsaturated	polyunsaturated	cholesterol	plant sterol
I + III	Cocoa butter	32	61	34	3	0	398
II	Corn oil	127	12	31	56	0	345

[a] All subjects received the amount of calories to maintain body weight. The composition of all diets in percentage of total calories was 15 protein, 40 fat, 45 carbohydrate.

technique and the chemical determination of the mass of fecal steroids by Miettinen, Grundy and Ahrens [581, 993] have now made quantitative sterol balances possible. It is important in any such studies to know about the plant sterol dietary intake and fecal output in order to correct for intestinal tract losses of the neutral sterol nucleus [582].

A recent study is typical of those designed to provide information about the effects of polyunsaturated fat on the sterol balance [324]. Six normal men were given formula-type diets with the source of dietary fat being either cocoa butter (a predominately saturated fat) or the predominately polyunsaturated corn oil (see Table 4). The formula diets were cholesterol-free and had a constant amount of plant sterols. The three-week dietary periods in sequence were as follows: I cocoa butter, II corn oil, and III cocoa butter. The fecal neutral steroids and bile acids measured by the chemical techniques of the Rockefeller University investigators were correlated with the changes in the serum lipids. As expected with a baseline diet of predominately saturated fat, the substitution of polyunsaturated fat, corn oil in period II, reduced the serum cholesterol level from 222 to 177 mg% (Table 5). The following period of saturated fat feeding (period III) resulted in a serum cholesterol elevation, to 224 mg%, an almost exact return to the 222 mg% of the first period of saturated fat feeding.

The fecal steroid excretion in milligrams per day is summarized in Table 6. Mean values for the six subjects are listed. During the cocoa butter formula, in Period I, the neutral sterol excretion was 447 mg/day, the bile acid excretion 298 mg and the total excretion 745 mg. The neutral sterols consisted of cholesterol and its bacterially altered derivatives, coprostanol and coprostanone. For Period II during the corn oil formula, the neutral sterol excretion increased to 510 mg/day and bile acid output increased to 426, totaling 936 mg. In Period III, when cocoa butter replaced corn oil, the men returned to a fecal output similar to

Table 5. *Mean serum cholesterol concentrations during three dietary periods (mg/100 ml)* [a]

	General diet	277 ± 16 (S.E.)[b]	
Period I	Cocoa butter	222 ± 13	$p < 0.001$
Period II	Corn oil	177 ± 14	$p < 0.001$
Period III	Cocoa butter	225 ± 13	$p < 0.001$

[a] The average of two determinations of the serum lipids were made three days apart during the final week of Periods I, II and III.
[b] S.E. represents the standard error of the mean.

Table 6. *Fecal neutral sterol and bile acid excretion* [a]

	Dietary periods		
	I Cocoa butter	II Corn oil	III Cocoa butter
Neutral sterol			
Mean	447 ± 34 (S.E.)[b]	510 ± 20	429 ± 24
Probability		$p < 0.05$	$p < 0.01$
Bile acid			
Mean	298 ± 43	426 ± 49	243 ± 37
Probability		$p < 0.05$	$p < 0.05$
Total			
Mean	745 ± 42	936 ± 54	672 ± 41
Probability		$p < 0.02$	$p < 0.01$

[a] Mean values for the last two weeks (2 and 3) of each dietary period for all six subjects (mg/24 hrs).
[b] S.E. represents the standard error of the mean.

that of Period I. The steroid excretion uniformly decreased: neutral sterols declined to 429 mg, bile acids to 243, and the total to 672. Since the diets were cholesterol-free, the fecal neutral steroids and bile acids represented the excretion of cholesterol and its metabolites from the body. The fecal bile acid changes during these periods involved significant changes for both deoxycholic and lithocholic acids.

As Ahrens has described in the preceeding paper, we also failed to recover all ingested plant sterols from the stools of some subjects. When we corrected the neutral sterol excretion for plant sterol losses the neutral sterol excretions in all dietary periods were similar. This left the only significant change in the fecal bile acids which has constituted 60% of the increase in total fecal steroids brought about by the consumption of the diet high in polyunsaturated fat content.

If the total plasma cholesterol shifts occurring from one diet to another are calculated, then this figure can be compared with the changes in total fecal bile acid excretion (Table 7). From Period I and II (a change to the corn oil diet) the plasma compartment lost a total of 1,448 mg of cholesterol. At the same time the fecal bile acid excretion increased 1,778 mg. From Period II to III (a change back to cocoa butter) the total plasma cholesterol increased 1,629 mg while the fecal bile acids decreased 2,548 mg. Note the invariable reciprocal nature of these changes in plasma cholesterol and fecal bile acids, and that the fecal changes were always much greater than the plasma changes. We suggest that

Table 7. *Comparison of total plasma cholesterol shift with change in total fecal bile acid excretion (mean values)*

	From Period I to II (Cocoa butter to Corn oil)	From Period II to III (Corn oil to Cocoa butter)
Plasma cholesterol shift	−1,448 mg	+1,629 mg
Change in bile acids	+1,778	−2,548
Difference	330	919

Table 8. *Bile acid excretion: Polyunsaturated fat versus saturated fat*

Study	Type of patient	Bile acid mg/day	Percent change	Probability
A	Six normal men	+127	+ 42	$p<0.05$
		+182	+ 75	$p<0.02$
B	Five normal men	+ 91	+ 24	$p<0.05$
C	One normal woman	+209	+167	
D	Five hypercholesterolemic patients	−152	− 15	N.S.
E	Five Type II hypercholesterolemic patients	− 1	− 0.5	N.S.
F	One Type V hyperlipidemic patient	+392	+ 49	$p<0.01$

this difference might be accounted for by the movement of cholesterol from the liver and other tissues. Changes in synthesis rate of cholesterol or in the reabsorption of bile acids cannot be excluded as possible explanations of these findings.

The results of studies by others in normal men also show increased bile acid excretion from polyunsaturated fat feeding (Table 8). Study A which was just described involved two comparisons of polyunsaturated versus saturated fat, each leading to increased bile acid excretion. Study B reported by Moore, Anderson, Taylor, Keys and Franz yielded a similar result: a plus 91 mg/day excretion of bile acids or an increase of 24% from polyunsaturated fat feeding [1024]. In study C by Wood, Shioda and Kinsell a similar pattern of response resulted, an estimated 209 mg/day of additional bile acid excretion [1568].

The pattern of response in hypercholesterolemic patients, in contrast to the normal subjects, was quite different (Table 8). In study D, carried out by Avigan and Steinberg, five hypercholesterolemic patients fed polyunsaturated fat in the diet did not increase the bile acid excretion; the minus 15% change was not significant [77]. In study E bile acid excretion again did not increase when polyunsaturated fat was given to five patients with Type II hyperbetalipoproteinemia and hypercholesterolemia (unpublished data). The mean net change was minus 1 mg/day. A quite different response resulted in a Type V hyperlipoproteinemia patient in study F. This patient with hypertriglyceridemia was studied on two occasions, eight years apart by Hellman, Rosenfeld, Insull and Ahrens initially and later by Grundy and Ahrens [578]. The data from both studies indicated a great increase in fecal steroid excretion. For example, the fecal bile acids increased +392 mg/day in the second study from polyunsaturated fat feeding.

What these varying data may indicate is that metabolically different human beings may respond differently to polyunsaturated fat feeding: normal men and a Type V patient had increased fecal bile acid excretion; Type II patients did not. Perhaps these different responses represent a metabolic divergence of the Type II patient from the normal individual. From other studies it has been observed that the fecal bile acid excretion in the Type II patient appears to be low [820, 994]. The ultimate mechanisms responsible for the effects of dietary polyunsaturated fat feeding must be delineated by future studies.

SUMMARY

The sterol balance may be altered by both dietary cholesterol and polyunsaturated fat. Dietary cholesterol in amounts of 310 mg/day and above raised the serum cholesterol concentrations, increased the body pool of cholesterol, may change the amount of cholesterol absorbed and usually caused increased fecal bile acid excretion. Man, however, compensates inadequately to certain intake levels of dietary cholesterol. The resulting increased storage of cholesterol in the plasma and other body pools has been termed "cholesterol overload". In normal men, polyunsaturated fat in the diet increased fecal bile acid excretion as serum cholesterol levels were decreased. The amounts of bile acid found in the stool were sufficient to account for the total amount of cholesterol leaving the plasma. Polyunsaturated fat in the diet did not usually cause enhanced fecal bile acid excretion in Type II hypercholesterolemic patients. This divergence between the normal subject and the Type II patient may indicate one facet of the metabolic abnormality in the Type II patient.

CATABOLISM OF CHOLESTEROL BY WAY OF BILE ACIDS

Sven Lindstedt

Pathways in Formation of Bile Acids from Cholesterol[1]. Bloch, Berg and Rittenberg in 1943 [192] administered deuterium-labeled cholesterol to a dog with an anastomosis between the choledochus and the renal pelvis. Labeled cholic acid was isolated from the urine thus establishing for the first time the conversion of cholesterol into a bile acid. This conversion of cholesterol into cholic acid involves a number of modifications in the sterol skeleton: (1) hydroxylation at position 7, (2) inversion of the 3β-hydroxyl to the 3α-configuration, (3) saturation of the Δ^5 double bond, (4) hydroxylation at position 12, and (5) shortening of the side chain by three carbon atoms.

Work to elucidate the order in which these changes occur and the underlying enzymatic mechanisms started around 1950. A prerequisite for these studies was the availability of ^{14}C-labeled cholesterol, and the development of chromatographic methods for the separation of bile acids and of neutral steroids implicated in the reaction sequences. It was soon realized that administration of labeled cholesterol to rats did not result in an excretion of intermediates in the bile or an accumulation of intermediates in the liver to such an extent that conclusions could be drawn about the reaction sequences. Consequently, possible intermediates were synthesized in labeled form and administered to animals to establish if the naturally occurring bile acids were formed. By this technique one could determine how the remodelling of the steroid skeleton occurs. Subsequently, these studies have been supplemented with work on *in vitro* systems and in some cases the individual enzymes have been partially purified and studied in more detail. In the following an attempt will be made to summarize the present concept of the steps involved in the formation of the two main bile acids formed from cholesterol in the liver of humans, i.e. cholic acid and chenodeoxycholic acid (Fig. 1).

Reaction 1. It was realized at an early stage that rebuilding of the cholesterol skeleton started in the nucleus and not by degradation of the side chain, and it was established that cholest-5-ene-3β, 7α-diol (7α-hydroxycholesterol) gave rise to cholic and chenodeoxycholic acid in the bile fistula rat by a stereospecific hydroxylation reaction [141, 878]. Danielsson and Einarsson [356] identified cholest-5-ene-3β,7α-diol as a metabolite of cholesterol in an *in vitro* system. In a 20,000 × g supernatant of a homogenate from rat or human liver a conversion of about 2% of added cholesterol into 7α-hydroxycholesterol has been observed [176]. It should be stressed, however, that it may be very difficult to draw any quantitative conclusions about reaction rates (i.e. μmoles formed per g liver per min) from *in vitro* studies of this type in which the water-insoluble substrate is added to the reaction mixture in an acetone solution, making it impossible

1 Detailed discussions of the reactions and bibliography can be found in the literature [146, 173, 359, 426].

to know to what extent the added compound mixes with endogenously present cholesterol or the intermediates in the reaction sequence. The 7α-hydroxylation is catalyzed by a microsomal hydroxylase and soluble cofactor(s). With microsomes and reduced pyridine nucleotides, 7-ketocholesterol is the dominant product. The reason for this is not clear, and further work is needed to elucidate the

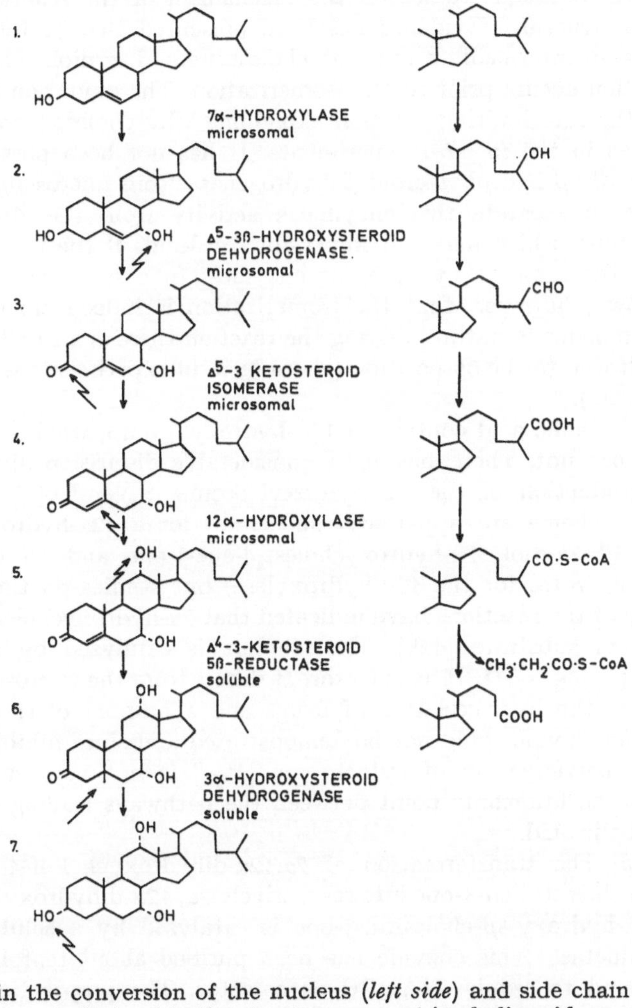

1. 7α-HYDROXYLASE microsomal

2. Δ5-3β-HYDROXYSTEROID DEHYDROGENASE. microsomal

3. Δ5-3 KETOSTEROID ISOMERASE microsomal

4. 12α-HYDROXYLASE microsomal

5. Δ4-3-KETOSTEROID 5β-REDUCTASE soluble

6. 3α-HYDROXYSTEROID DEHYDROGENASE soluble

7.

OH, CHO, COOH, CO·S-CoA, $CH_3 \cdot CH_2 \cdot CO \cdot S\text{-}CoA$, COOH

Fig. 1. Steps in the conversion of the nucleus (*left side*) and side chain (*right side*) of cholesterol to the structure present in cholic acid

mechanism of the reaction. Attempts to demonstrate a 7α-hydroperoxide as an initial product have not been successful [178]. As will be discussed in more detail later, the 7α-hydroxylation appears to be the rate limiting reaction in the conversion of cholesterol to bile acids and the reaction at which metabolic control occurs.

Reactions 2 and 3. Green and Samuelsson [566] have shown that a Δ^4-3-keto-compound is an intermediate in the conversion of cholesterol to cholic acid.

7α-Hydroxycholest-4-en-3-one is a major metabolite of cholesterol and of cholest-5-ene-3β,7α-diol *in vitro*, and it has been shown that the latter compound is converted to the Δ^4-3-keto configuration by liver microsomes in a NAD-requiring reaction. Also 7α-hydroxycholest-4-en-3-one is a precursor of cholic and chenodeoxycholic acids in the bile fistula rat [177, 356]. Recently, Björkhem [172, 174] has carried out detailed studies on the mechanism of the reaction leading to the Δ^4-3-keto structure. Evidence has been presented that 7α-hydroxycholest-5-ene-3-one is an intermediate but not cholest-4-en-3β,7α-diol. Thus, oxidation at the 3-position occurs prior to the isomerization. The oxidation has also been found to be the rate limiting reaction explaining why cholest-5-ene-3-one could not be isolated in the *in vitro* experiments. It has not been possible so far to solubilize the Δ^5-3β-hydroxysteroid dehydrogenase from microsomes, nor has it been possible to separate this enzymatic activity from the Δ^5-3-ketosteroid isomerase activity which makes it impossible to decide if the two reactions are catalyzed by the same or by different enzymes. In a series of experiments it has been shown, however, that the isomerization is indeed enzyme catalyzed and not spontaneous in nature. During the reaction there is a significant transfer of the 4β-hydrogen to the 6β-position (about 12% in experiments with deuterium labeled substrate).

Reaction 4. Cholic acid contains a 12α-hydroxyl group, whereas chenodeoxycholic acid does not. There has been considerable discussion about the stage at which introduction of the 12α-hydroxyl occurs. Several of the compounds shown in the scheme are apparently substrates for a 12α-hydroxylase. Thus, cholest-5-ene-3β 7α-diol, 7α-hydroxycholest-4-ene-3-one and 5β cholestane-3α, 7α-diol are substrates for the 12α-hydroxylase, but studies on the time course and efficiency of the reactions have indicated that 7α-hydroxycholest-4-ene-3-one is the preferred substrate [425]. The reaction is catalyzed by a microsomal oxygenase requiring NADPH as cofactor. It differs from the microsomal enzymes which catalyze the hydroxylation of drugs and a number of steroids, since a requirement for flavine could not be demonstrated and since inhibition with CO (showing the participation of cytochrome [P_{450}] is not very marked [178]). Reaction 4 is the branching point between the pathways leading to cholic and chenodeoxycholic acid.

Reaction 5. The transformation of 7α,12α-dihydroxycholest-4-en-3-one and of 7α-hydroxycholest-4-en-3-one into respectively 7α, 12α-dihydroxy-5β-cholestan-3-one and 7α-hydroxy-5β-cholestan-3-one is catalyzed by a soluble Δ^4-3-ketosteroid 5β-reductase. This enzyme has been purified about tenfold by Berséus [145] and found to require NADPH as cofactor. The preparation was active towards several substrates including 7α-hydroxycholest-4-en-3-one and, on the basis of inhibition studies, it was concluded that more than one reductase might have been present in the preparation. Further studies by Björkhem [174] have demonstrated that the reaction involves a transaxial addition of hydrogen in which hydrogen from the A position of NADP is incorporated into the 5β-position and a proton from water added at the 4β position.

Reaction 6. Reduction of the 3-keto group is catalyzed by a soluble enzyme which is fairly stable and which has been purified about 300 times (Berséus, personal communication) [145]. Its activity towards a number of substrates has been tested. Available data do not permit definite conclusions whether one or several 3α-hydroxysteroid dehydrogenases are present in liver. The enzyme involved in the degradation of cholesterol is more active with NADPH as cofactor than with NADH. The hydrogen from the A position of NADPH position is incorporated into the 3α-position. It has not been quite clear in which order reactions 5 and 6 occur. Thus Mendelsohn and coworkers [971] were of the opinion that reduction of the 3-keto groups was the first event whereas Hutton and Boyd [730] considered 7α-hydroxy-5β-cholestane-3-one as a likely intermediate. The problem has been studied in some detail by Danielsson and coworkers who studied the metabolism of Δ^4 cholestenols [175]. It was concluded from these studies that reduction of the Δ^4-double bond precedes the reduction of the 3-keto group.

Side Chain Degradation. The right-hand side of Fig. 1 illustrates the pathway for the degradation of the side chain. It is interesting to note that the bile acid with 27 carbon atoms 3α, 7α, 12α-trihydroxy-5β-cholestan-26-oic acid (trihydroxycoprostanic acid) which is the chief bile acid of alligators and crocodiles [631] has also been isolated from human bile [278]. It is formed from cholesterol in man and is metabolized to cholic acid [277].

Quantitative Aspects of Cholesterol Degradation to Bile Acids. Simultaneously with the elucidation of the mechanism of the conversion of cholesterol to bile acids there has been considerable interest in the quantitative aspects of this transformation. Cholesterol is synthesized mainly in the liver and the intestine, but appreciable synthesis occurs also in the skin and in most other tissues with the exception of the central nervous system. A detailed analysis of the contribution of different tissues to the total production of cholesterol in the squirrel monkey has been presented by Dietschy and Wilson [393]. Cholesterol absorbed from the intestine mixes with endogenously synthesized cholesterol in the tissues, but the rate of equilibration varies considerably for different tissues. Numerous attempts have been made to determine the turnover of cholesterol after injection or feeding of either labeled cholesterol precursors or of labeled cholesterol itself. It has, then, generally been observed that after a certain period of time the specific radioactivity of serum cholesterol declines in such a way that a straight line is obtained if the logarithm of the specific radioactivity is plotted versus time.

Attempts have been made to calculate turnover time and also total turnover from plots of this type. It is obvious, however, that cholesterol metabolism should be described by a multipool system and that the parameters of the specific radioactivity-time curve are, therefore, functions of the different rate constants for elimination and transfer between different pools of cholesterol in the body. Goodman and Noble [546] have recently shown that in humans the specific radioactivity-time curve for serum cholesterol which is obtained after administration of labeled cholesterol may be resolved into two linear components and that consequently a two-pool system may be used to describe cholesterol metabolism. This, in fact, means that the many different compartments may be lumped together into two pools, one with a slow turnover and one with a "fast" turnover. It was concluded that the "fast" pool (liver, intestine and blood) contained about 25 g of cholesterol and that the elimination of cholesterol from the body (i.e. not including unabsorbed dietary cholesterol) amounts to 1.35 g per day in normals and 0.98 g per day in hyperlipidemic subjects. In view of the theoretical objections which can be raised against procedures of this type many attempts have been made to measure directly the two main pathways for cholesterol elimination, i.e. the conversion to bile acids and the excretion of neutral steroids in feces. As mentioned, difficulties inherent in the *in vitro* technique with water insoluble substrates has made it difficult to measure reaction rates for the individual reactions in the transformation of cholesterol to bile acids. Thus, our present knowledge of the quantitative aspects of bile acid metabolism are based almost entirely on *in vivo* experiments in animals or humans. Three methods have been used to estimate the daily production of bile acids, i.e. measurement of the rate of excretion of bile acids in a bile fistula, measurement of the turnover of bile acids in the bile acid pool, and measurement of bile acid in feces.

Excretion of Bile Acids in Bile Fistulas. The most obvious way to measure the bile acid production would be to follow the rate of excretion from a bile fistula. It has been found, however, that when a bile fistula is established the rate of bile acid excretion first decreases during a period when the bile acid pool is eliminated and then increases as a consequence of the elimination of a feed-back control of cholesterol catabolism. In practice it has been difficult in experimental animals to distinguish an intermediate phase of minimum excretion which, in theory, should represent a normal rate of bile acid production. Recently, Scherstén and coworkers (personal communication) have studied bile acid production in patients operated upon for gallstone disease and provided a T-tube drainage which could be blocked in the efferent limb. Seven days after the operation the bile was drained and the rate of excretion determined. From the initial excretion phase and the phase of minimum rate of excretion which was well defined in these subjects, the following figures were obtained: total bile acid pool, 1.6 g (range: 0.6–2.5 g); cholic acid formation per day, 0.38 g (range: 0.31–0.48 g); and chenodeoxycholic acid formation per day, 0,32 g (range: 0.18–0.46 g).

Turnover of Bile Acids in Bile Acid Pool. This technique requires that the half-life time ($t_{1/2}$) [or the interconvertible parameters turnover time (t) or rate constant for the elimination (k)] and the pool size can be determined. In humans a direct approach to the measurement of the turnover of the bile acid pool has been possible [879]. Labeled bile acids have been administered and bile samples have been obtained at intervals of a few days by duodenal intubation after stimulation of bile secretion with cholecystokinine; the bile acids have been isolated and their specific radioactivities have been determined. In most instances the values for the specific radioactivity fall on a straight line when plotted on a semilogarithmic paper, which allows determination of the half-life. This technique has in several studies been used to follow the rate of conversion of cholesterol to cholic acid [663, 664, 880]. In eight medical students the average of half-lives was 2.8 days (range: 1.2–4.2 days).

Results from a study in which ^{14}C-labeled cholic acid and ^{3}H-labeled chenodeoxycholic acid was administered simultaneously to two subjects indicate that the half-life of chenodeoxycholic acid is close to that of cholic acid [358]. As a plot of the logarithms for specific radioactivity versus time yields a straight line, the bile acids which are located in the liver, gallbladder and duodenum, apparently form a one-pool system, which follows first-order kinetics. However, the first bile sample has been collected one to three days after the administration of the labeled compound, and it was considered important to obtain an estimate of the rate constant for the formation (=elimination in the steady state) by another technique. The ^{14}C-labeled cholesterol was, therefore, administered simultaneously with tritium-labeled cholic acid and the specific radioactivity determined in both cholesterol and in the doubly-labeled cholic acid isolated from bile samples. The rate constant for cholic acid formation was then determined from the ^{14}C-data

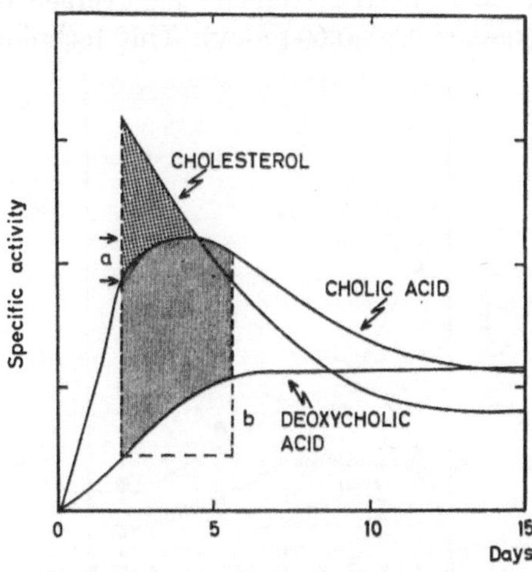

Fig. 2. Specific radioactivity of bile cholesterol, cholic acid, and deoxycholic acid after oral administration of ^{14}C-labeled cholesterol

Table 1. *Half-life of cholic acid calculated from specific activity-time curves obtained after simultaneous administration of cholesterol (^{14}C) and cholic acid (^{3}H)*

Case	Half-life of cholic acid	
	calculated from ^{14}C-cholesterol	calculated from ^{3}H-cholic acid
1	6.3	6.5
2	9.5	10.2
3	0.8	1.4
4	1.3	1.4

by the method of Zilversmit [1593] (Fig. 2) and the rate constant for cholic acid elimination from the tritium data as described previously. As almost identical values were obtained (Table 1) the results confirmed the hypothesis that the bile acid in the liver and duodenum form a one-pool system.

To determine the size of this one-pool system we have extrapolated the plot of specific radioactivity versus time to zero time and calculated the size from the dilution of the administered amount. This procedure should give a correct figure, if the labeled bile acid mixes "completely" with the pool. In eight medical students the average pool size for cholic acid was 1.38 g (range: 0.5–2.29 g). In many instances the ratio between cholic acid, chenodeoxycholic acid, and deoxycholic acid has been determined in the bile samples. Assuming that the relation between these acids is the same over the entire pool, it is possible to calculate the total size of this bile acid pool. In the students the average was 3.58 g (range: 1.88–4.97 g).

Combination of values for the rate constant for bile acid formation with values for pool size makes it possible to calculate the amount of cholesterol that is converted into bile cholic acid per day and to estimate also the conversion into chenodeoxycholic acid. In the students an average of 0.36 g cholic acid was formed per day (range: 0.26–0.69 g/day). This technique of measuring the

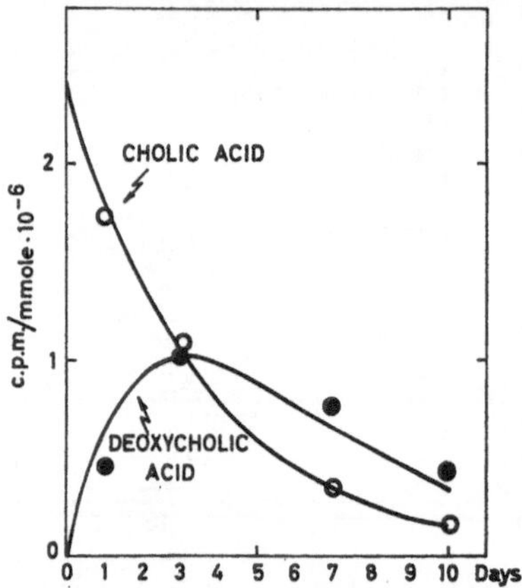

Fig. 3. Specific radioactivity of cholic- and deoxycholic acid after administration of ^{14}C-labeled cholic acid

Table 2. *Rate constants for the metabolism of cholic- and deoxycholic acid (see Fig. 4) calculated from four experiments in which ^{14}C-labeled cholic acid was administered*

Case	k_1	k_2	k_3	$\frac{k_1}{k_1+k_3}$
5	0.145	0.140	0.015	0.91
6	0.025	0.06	0.320	0.07
7	0.04	0.035	0.114	0.25
8	0.24	0.40	0.04	0.86

catabolism of cholesterol to bile acids has been used in studies on the effect of thyroid hormone and of various diets on cholesterol degradation to bile acids.

Deoxycholic acid accounts for about 20% of the bile acids in human bile, but it is formed from cholic acid in the enterohepatic circulation. From data on the relative specific radioactivities of cholic acid and deoxycholic acid in the enterohepatic circulation, obtained in experiments in which labeled cholesterol or labeled cholic acid was administered, it has been possible to calculate that from 10 to 90% of the cholic acid formed is converted to deoxycholic acid within the pool from which bile was sampled (Fig. 3, Table 2). As, however, cholic acid is present only in small amounts in the feces, these results indicate that in some subjects the deoxycholic acid formation occurs mainly at such a low level in the intestinal tract that reabsorption of deoxycholic acid does not occur, i.e. that bile acids in the distal part of the gut form a pool which is separate from the enterohepatic circulation. Evidence for this has also been obtained in rat experiments [881] (Fig. 4).

Excretion of Bile Acids in Feces. During the passage of bile through the gut, bacterial enzymes catalyze extensive modifications of the bile acids which result in the presence of a large number of bile acids in feces. To circumvent the analytical problems, Hellman and coworkers in 1957 [660] devised an isotope balance method, which is based on the following principles: after administration of

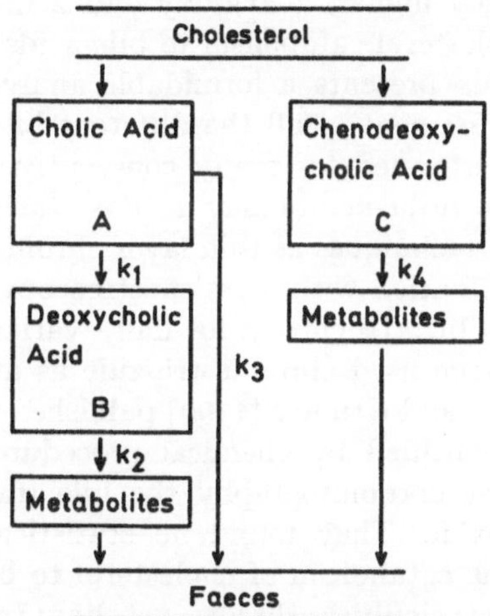

Fig. 4. Model for kinetic calculations of bile acid metabolism in man. k_1 is the rate constant for the conversion of cholic acid to deoxycholic acid in the enteropheatic circulation, k_2 the rate constant for the elimination of deoxycholic acid from the enterohepatic circulation and k_3 the rate constant for the elimination of that part of the cholic acid which is not converted to deoxycholic acid in the enterohepatic circulation. The expression k/k_1+k_3 gives the fraction of cholic acid converted to deoxycholic acid per day in the enterohepatic circulation

labeled cholesterol, the specific radioactivity of the serum cholesterol and the total radioactivity in acid and neutral steroids in the feces are determined over a period of time. By dividing the total fecal radioactivity with the specific radioactivity of serum cholesterol one obtains the amount of acidic and neutral fecal steroids. For the procedure to be valid the extraction of radioactive material from the feces must be complete, and the separation into acidic and neutral steroids must yield well defined fractions.

Furthermore, the specific radioactivity of the serum cholesterol must be the same as that of the fecal steroids. This assumption should preferably be tested in each experiment since the size of the bile acid pool in the distal part of the intestine may vary from one subject to another resulting in different relations between the specific radioactivity of serum cholesterol and fecal bile acids. The isotope balance method was first used by Hellman and coworkers in a study of the effect of unsaturated fat on the catabolism of cholesterol in a subject with hyperlipidemia. Ahrens and Grundy [578] used the same isotope balance method, but they also determined the bile acid excretion with a technique based on thin layer chromatography and gas liquid chromatography and obtained good agreement between the two methods. Avigan and Steinberg [77] have used the technique in six hypercholesterolemic patients on liquid formula diets containing either safflower oil or coconut oil. In five of the subjects, the bile acid excretion on the coconut oil diet was 0.80 g/day (range: 0.24–1.27) and on the safflower oil diet 0.54 g/day (range: 0.10–0.88). The bile acids accounted for 50.1% (range: 22.6–71.2) and 58.5% (range: 15.4–59.4%) of the total excretion of steroids derived from the body cholesterol. In the sixth patient the bile acid excretion was considerably higher, 2.20 g/day and 2.32 g/day on the two diets.

Determination of cholesterol catabolism to bile acids by determination of the individual fecal bile acids presents a formidable analytical problem. Not only does it require the measurement of all the different bile acids, but these determinations have to be performed for many consecutive days or on large pools of feces to eliminate the influence of day to day variation in fecal excretion. The introduction of such techniques as thin layer chromatography and gas liquid chromatography in combination with mass spectroscopy has, nevertheless, made such determinations possible. To correct for daily variations in defecation [369] Ahrens and coworkers have used chromic trioxide as an inert marker.

In 1965 Spritz, Ahrens and Grundy [1399] published their first study in which fecal bile acids were quantified by chemical procedures. After extraction and purification by thin-layer chromatography the bile fraction was titrated with ethanolic sodium hydroxide. They found no statistically significant effect of type of dietary fat on the catabolism of cholesterol to bile acids, but noted that the bile acid excretion was significantly lower on liquid formula diets completely devoid of steroids. When dietary steroids were present they determined the bile acid formation to be 247 ± 70 mg/day on a diet containing saturated fat and 271 ± 48 mg/day on a diet containing unsaturated fat. In a later version of the method the final quantification was carried out by gas-liquid chromatography [581].

Sjövall and coworkers [430, 431, 432] have carried out extensive work on the extraction, isolation, and identification of the acidic metabolites of cholesterol present in feces. The procedures were tested on feces from subjects which had received labeled bile acids. Purification of the bile acid fraction was achieved by chromatography on silicic acid columns, and the final quantification was then carried out by gas-liquid chromatography. Identification of bile acids was based on combined gas chromatography–mass spectroscopy. The amount of fecal bile acids was in the range 50–500 mg/day, but the actual number of samples examined was low, and no systematic study was carried out on the day to day variations in one and the same subject.

Bile acid excretions between 50 and 2,000 mg/day have been reported (for compilations, see literature [174, 426]). If one disregards data which have been obtained with obviously inadequate techniques, it appears that 400–700 mg/day is a plausible figure in a normal subject on a solid diet. Only in a few instances has more than one analytical technique been used in one and the same patient or have several consecutive studies been performed, and at the present time it is difficult to decide if the different methods yield results which differ in a systematic manner. Apparently, there are large individual variations in the excretion of bile acids, and it is not improbable that such factors as intestinal flora, type of food, defecation habits, etc. primarily affect the rate of bile acid elimination from the upper part of the intestinal tract. The rate of cholesterol catabolism to bile acids would then be adjusted accordingly, possibly by a feedback control at the first step in the degradation sequence, i.e. the 7α-hydroxylation.

It was suggested in 1958 [139] that bile acid formation is regulated by the concentration of bile acids in the portal blood, but Sjövall and Cronholm [347] determined portal bile acids in rats and obtained results which did not support this hypothesis. On the other hand, it has been conclusively shown that drainage of bile results both in an increase in the incorporation of acetate into liver cholesterol and in about an eightfold increase in the 7α-hydroxylation of cholesterol in a liver homogenate [357]. It appears likely that detailed studies in man of regulation mechanisms at the enzymatic level may yield more meaningful information than *in vivo* studies which, even if carried out with the most sophisticated analytical techniques, are influenced by several physiological factors.

OVERALL CONTROL OF STEROL SYNTHESIS IN ANIMALS AND MAN*

KANG-JEY HO, C. BRUCE TAYLOR and KURT BISS

The biosynthetic pathways of cholesterol and its mechanisms have been studied extensively since the elucidation of the molecular structure of cholesterol in the early 1930's [486]. Liver was believed to have been the main source of plasma cholesterol and its esters in mammals [1454]. Recently, however, it has been proven that the intestinal tract contributes cholesterol to the plasma [1550]. The skin is probably also important quantitatively in total body cholesterol synthesis [1550]. Thus, there are two sources of endogenous cholesterol: one is liver, and the other extrahepatic tissues. The physiological controls of cholesterol biosynthesis have been investigated rather thoroughly. The hepatic and extrahepatic cholesterologenesis seem to be under the control of different mechanisms. The purpose of this paper is to present a concise review of these control mechanisms.

Control of Hepatic Cholesterologenesis. Employing balance studies Schönheimer and Breusch [1314] first showed that cholesterol metabolism in animals

* This investigation was supported by grants from The Chicago, Illinois, and American Heart Associations; The Glenview Area and Arlington Heights United Funds; Public Health Service Grant HE-11029 from the National Heart Institute, and General Research Support Grant FR-05629 from the National Institutes of Health; the Thomas J. Dee and the George C. Moody Memorial Research Funds; and the Gladys Henry Dick Memorial Pathology Fund of Evanston Hospital, Evanston, Illinois.

is under homeostatic control. It remained, however, for the experiments of Taylor and Gould [1454] to prove conclusively that there is marked compensatory suppression of newly synthesized cholesterol in liver and plasma of dogs ingesting a high cholesterol diet. Hepatic cholesterologenesis was later shown to be inhibited by dietary cholesterol, bile salts, and starvation; their inhibitory mechanisms are different. The suppression of hepatic cholesterologenesis was roughly related to the amount of cholesterol in the diet [1371]. The inhibitor is cholesterol of exogenous origin which is in a low-density lipoprotein fraction of serum, appearing after cholesterol feeding. The major site of this inhibition is located at the reaction responsible for the conversion of beta-hydroxy-beta-methyl-glutarate to mevalonate, namely beta-hydroxy-beta-methyl-glutaryl CoA reductase which is located in microsomes bound to the membrane [1369]. This feedback regulation of hepatic cholesterologenesis has been suggested to involve direct endproduct inhibition rather than inhibition of enzyme synthesis or genetic repression [1369]. At least two minor sites of control for hepatic cholesterol synthesis exist between mevalonate and squalene [556]. Since these inhibitions are gradual and incomplete, it is likely that they are secondary to the primary inhibition of mevalonate synthesis. Actual measurement of the quantities of these enzymes will provide a definite conclusion.

Beher and Baker [132] demonstrated the inhibition of hepatic cholesterologenesis by bile salts. Fimognari and Rodwell [458] later showed that bile salts serve as endproduct inhibitors of the enzyme, beta-hydroxy-beta-methyl-glutaryl CoA reductase, by a competitive inhibitory mechanism.

Hepatic cholesterologenesis can be inhibited by fasting rats in as short a time as 24 hours. The activity of beta-hydroxy-beta-methyl-glutaryl CoA reductase is decreased in the liver of fasted rats and there is also a partial block between squalene and cholesterol [255]. The details of the mechanism still remain unclear.

Control of Extrahepatic Cholesterologenesis. Cholesterol synthesis in extrahepatic tissues is not affected by starvation or cholesterol intake. The intestine is the only extrahepatic tissue in which the control mechanism of cholesterol synthesis has been extensively studied [392]. The cholesterol synthesis of the gastrointestinal tract is under the control of bile salts which inhibit the conversion of beta-hydroxy-beta-methyl-glutarate to mevalonate through a possible mechanism of enzyme repression at the genetic level rather than competitive allosteric inhibition of the enzyme [392]. Very little is known about control mechanisms in tissues other than liver and the intestines. Bailey [87] studied *de novo* synthesis of cholesterol in several cell lines and found that the major block in cellular cholesterol synthesis produced by exogenous cholesterol was the conversion of acetate to acetyl CoA. Cristafalo et al. [346] suggested that the effectiveness of this negative feedback control varied among different cell lines.

Mammalian cholesterol biosynthesis is also under the control of hormones and a host of chemicals and drugs. The mechanisms of action of most of these factors are not clear and will not be discussed here.

Overall Control of Cholesterol Biosynthesis. Dietary cholesterol seems to be the most important factor in control of total body cholesterol synthesis; however, liver is the only organ under its control. The quantitative significance of this hepatic feedback control mechanism, *in vivo*, can be determined and has been shown to be different in various species of mammals and various ethnic groups of humans. During cholesterol feeding the percentages of body cholesterol of the exchangeable pool contributed by dietary cholesterol are 90–95% in dogs, [335, 1455], 80–90% in rats [1039], and 60–80% in monkeys [1552].

With regard to humans, Kaplan et al. [778] studied 24 healthy ambulatory Caucasians in an isotopic steady state, who were fed known constant dose levels of cholesterol and Cholesterol-4-^{14}C for eight-week periods. Their study showed that only 25% (20–33%) of plasma cholesterol was contributed by the diet when a person was on a diet containing 0.5 g or more of cholesterol per day. The other 75% of plasma cholesterol, or more precisely 75% of the total body exchangeable cholesterol, was not affected by the dietary cholesterol and presumably was derived from extrahepatic tissues.

Our recent study on cholesterol metabolism in the Masai in Kenya is quite interesting [691]. Despite their customary diet which is rich in animal fat and protein, Masai men and women, excluding pregnant women, have very low plasma cholesterol levels and no evidence of arteriosclerotic heart disease. The Masai do absorb more dietary cholesterol than Caucasians; however, their body cholesterol synthesis can be suppressed to 50% by cholesterol feeding [691]. This efficient feedback mechanism protects the Masai from developing hypercholesteremia.

Discussion Following Dr. Goodman's Paper

Dr. Connor: I would like to ask Dr. Goodman if, when dietary cholesterol is given to experimental animals and serum cholesterol concentration is increased, total body stores or pools of cholesterol are also increased, and if the same might apply to human beings given similar kinds of feeding. The reason I ask is that you didn't seem to indicate a correlation between serum cholesterol concentrations and total body pool.

Dr. Goodman: I don't know of any data from kinetic studies with which to answer that question. In our small group of human beings we found no such correlation. I suspect that in animals rendered hyperlipidemic by having been fed high cholesterol diets you would find such a correlation, but I am not sure that is the proper model for human hyperlipidemia.

Dr. Malinow: I would like to bring to your attention some experiments that seem to indicate that another factor is also very important in sterol balance, namely, physical activity.

It is very well known, since Chaikoff did it, that injection of cholesterol labeled in the 26-carbon atom produces labeled CO_2 in organisms. We have demonstrated that if we inject the labeled cholesterol into many species, including man, the amount of labeled CO_2 in the expired air is increased with exercise. Obviously, the rest of the molecule will contribute to synthesis of other substances, mainly bile acids.

Discussion Following Dr. Ho's Paper

Dr. Rodwell: I would like to comment on some points relating to regulation of HMG-CoA reductase. In part, I am afraid we have been responsible for some, perhaps, erroneous ideas in this area. We have recently shown that if you study HMG-CoA reductase activity in rat's liver, it is not inhibited by bile acids at any reasonable level. This was a surprise since we had suggested that was going to be the case. While I would not argue as to whether or not bile acids regulate cholesterol synthesis, I would say that they do not regulate it by inhibiting rat's liver HMG-CoA reductase.

A second point that was raised by Dr. Ho concerning the regulation of hepatic sterol synthesis may very well turn out to involve repression of enzyme synthesis. The activity of rat liver HMG-CoA reductase measured in isolated rat liver microsomes is a function of the time of day. We, and quite recently Lynen, have shown that the activity varies in a cyclical pattern with the time of day, the peak activity being at night. The activity of this enzyme goes up approximately nine fold to tenfold, in a 24-hour cycle. It is capable of very profound changes of activity in very short periods to time.

This rise in activity is dependent upon protein synthesis. If rats are treated with an inhibitor of protein synthesis, such as cyclohexamide, the normal rise in activity, which might have occurred between 4:00 and 8:00 p.m., is prevented. This suggests, then, that the rise which is seen is dependent upon protein synthesis and is due to synthesis of new HMG-CoA reductase.

Finally, the fall also must be dependent on the synthesis of new protein because, if cyclohexamide is injected into rats at the high point in the cycle, their HMG-CoA reductase levels remain high for the succeeding four hours while control animals show the diurnal fall in activity. This suggests, then, that there may also be either a specific degradative enzyme for HMG-CoA reductase or a specific inhibitory protein which is synthesized, perhaps cyclically, which has something to do with the regulation of its activity.

I point to these observations in order to get people thinking about regulations of protein synthesis as the basis for regulation and inhibition of this protein activity.

Section IX

SELECTED PAPERS ON LIPID METABOLISM

TRIGLYCERIDE TURNOVER MEASURED BY SPLANCHNIC PRODUCTION OF PLASMA TRIGLYCERIDE IN MAN*

Jonas Boberg, Ulla Freyschuss and Lars A. Carlson

In patients with various manifestations of atherosclerotic vascular disease, hypertriglyceridemia is very common. To determine whether the hypertriglyceridemia is caused by an increased influx or decreased removal of plasma TG requires a reliable method for estimating plasma TG turnover rate [197]. This study deals with the evaluation of such methods.

Table. *Methods for calculation of TG turnover*[a]

Methods	Calculations
1. Ryan-Schwartz [1272]	$\frac{(Ra_{TG_{120}} - Ra_{TG_{60}})\,PV}{60} : 3\,Sa_{FFA_A}$
2. Ryan-Schwartz [646] modified	$\frac{(Ra_{TG_{120}} - Ra_{TG_{60}})\,PV}{60} : 3\,Sa_{FFA_{HV}}$
3. Splanchnic production of labelled TG	$(Ra_{TG_{HV}} - Ra_{TG_A})\,F : 3\,Sa_{FFA_{HV}}$
4. Splanchnic production of unlabelled TG [197, 284]	$(C_{TG_{HV}} - C_{TG_A})\,F$
5. Efflux of labelled TG	$\frac{(Ra_{TG_{HV}} - Ra_{TG_A})\,F\,60 - (Ra_{TG_{300}} - Ra_{TG_{240}})\,PV}{60} : Sa_{VLD\,TG_{240-300}}$

[a] The symbols used herein are: Ra = radioactivity; A = arterial; Sa = specific radioactivity; PV = plasma volume; HV = hepatic venous; F = splanchnic blood plasma flow; TG = triglycerides; FFA = free fatty acids; C = concentration; and VLD TG = very low density triglycerides.

A constant infusion of Cardio-green, for estimation of splanchnic blood plasma flow, and of albumin bound ^{3}H-palmitate, precursor of plasma TG, was given to patients fasted overnight. By simultaneously taking arterial and hepatic venous blood for analysis of radioactivity, and chemical concentration of plasma triglycerides (TG), and free fatty acids (FFA), the splanchnic production of

* The work herein is preliminary and the completed study will be published elsewhere. Thus far it has been supported by grants from the Swedish Medical Research Council (19X-204-05 and- 06, B69-19P-2628-01, -02) and Reservationsanslagen, Karolinska Institutet.

plasma TG was estimated by five different methods of calculation shown in the Table. Methods 1 and 2, described by Ryan and Schwartz [1272], are based on several approximations and assumptions, methods 3, 4 and 5 require sampling of hepatic venous blood. In the chemical technique (method 4) the hepatic vein-arterial difference of plasma TG concentration was estimated and multiplied by

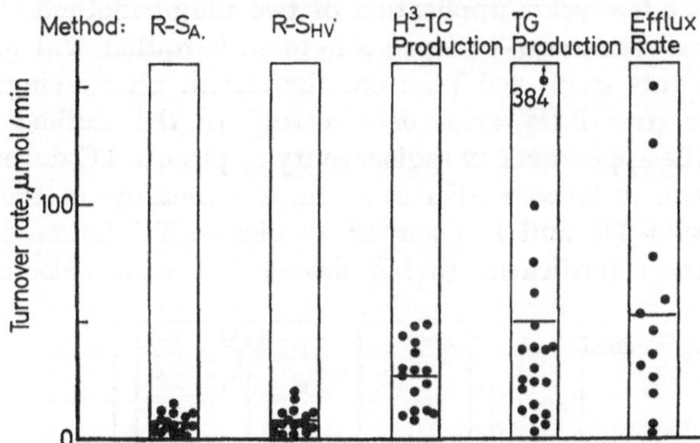

Fig. 1. Triglyceride turnover rate by different methods in 17 men. Five methods applied on each subject. Individual data (•) and mean value (—)

the splanchnic blood plasma flow. In the most reliable isotopic technique, method 3, the production of labelled plasma TG was estimated when a steady state condition of radioactivity in the TG production pool of the liver had been achieved (after three hours of constant infusion of labelled palmitate). To obtain values for the total TG production these figures were divided by three times the specific radioactivity of plasma FFA in the hepatic vein. As shown in Fig. 1, the values were higher in all cases with methods 3–5 than with the Ryan-Schwartz technique, even when the lower specific activity of FFA in the hepatic vein was used for the precursor of plasma TG synthesis.

INCORPORATION OF PLASMA GLUCOSE CARBON INTO PLASMA TRIGLYCERIDES IN NORMALS AND PATIENTS WITH HYPERTRIGLYCERIDEMIA (TYPE IV)

S. Sailer, F. Sandhofer, K. Bolzano and H. Braunsteiner

Increased concentration of plasma triglycerides (TG) and of very low density lipoproteins is found in nearly all cases of premature atherosclerosis. On the other hand, in patients with endogenous hypertriglyceridemia, signs of atherosclerosis are observed in a very high percentage. In order to study the mechanism which leads to the hypertriglyceridemia, a great deal work has been done. To approach this problem, different methods have been used. However, any method which estimates the TG flux into or out of the plasma is based on several assumptions. It is very often difficult or even impossible to verify them in man.

During the past few years application of two major methods has been used to measure the turnover rates of plasma TG in man. Farquhar et al. [450] measured the disappearance rate of labeled TG from the plasma after a single injection of labeled precursors (free fatty acids or glycerol). In the method of Ryan and Schwartz [1272] the appearance of radioactivity in plasma TG during a continous intravenous infusion of labeled FFA is taken as a measure of the plasma FFA converted to plasma TG and is regarded as plasma TG influx. During steady state conditions, the esterification rate of plasma FFA equals also the TG efflux.

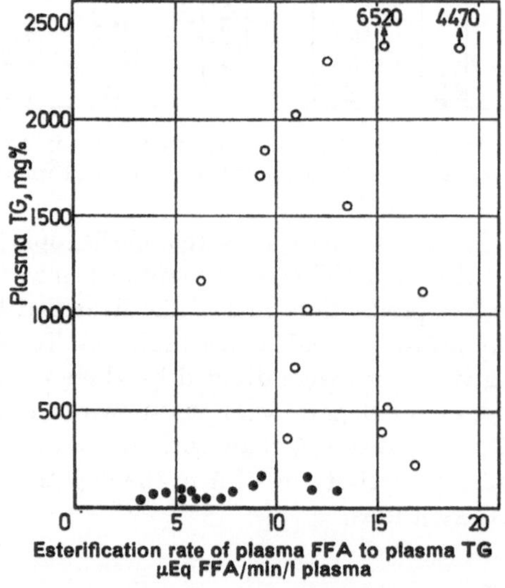

Fig. 1. Plasma triglyceride level is plotted against the esterification rate of plasma free fatty acids into triglyceride for normals (•) and hypertriglyceridemic patients (o)

Using a single injection of FFA or glycerol, it has been concluded that increased production of TG causes hypertriglyceridemia, and that the removal mechanism works normally [1214]. Using continous infusion of FFA and measuring the esterification rate of FFA to plasma TG, it has been concluded that the TG influx is not essentially increased in patients with hypertriglyceridemia so that an inefficient removal of plasma TG in these patients with endogenous hypertriglyceridemia must lead to the excessive plasma TG concentration [1280].

Using the method of Ryan and Schwartz [1272], three points may lead to an underestimation of total plasma TG influx:

1. Dilution of the specific activity of FFA taken up by the liver by nonlabeled FFA originated from splanchnic (adipose?) tissue. As shown by Havel [646], this error accounts for about 20% of the total plasma TG influx. But there is no

reason to assume a difference of this error between normals and hypertriglyceridemic patients.

2. The disappearance of labeled plasma TG from the blood is neglected. This fact underestimates the TG influx especially in persons with a small plasma TG pool, e.g. in normals, but to a much less extent in patients with hypertriglyceridemia.

3. Dilution of the specific activity of FFA in the liver by *de novo* synthesis of unlabeled FFA in the liver.

In order to eliminate the error caused by the efflux of labeled plasma during constant infusion of labeled FFA, we measured the radioactivity of plasma TG at short intervals and estimated the initial slope of the increase in radioactivity of arterial plasma TG which was used for the calculation of plasma FFA esterification to plasma TG. Further, the incorporation of plasma glucose carbon into plasma TG was measured in normals and in patients with endogenous hypertriglyceridemia (Type IV according to Fredrickson and Lees [487].

As shown in Fig. 1, the mean esterification rate of plasma FFA to plasma TG is only slightly increased over the control group in patients with endogenous hypertriglyceridemia. Their mean plasma TG level, however, was about 20 times higher. Therefore, we assumed that in endogenous hypertriglyceridemia not an increased synthesis but an insufficient removal of endogenous plasma TG was responsible for the hypertriglyceridemia. To avoid underestimation of TG influx by neglecting any *de novo* synthesis of fatty acids used for TG synthesis, the following questions were studied:

1. How much plasma glucose-C is incorporated into the plasma TG-FA respectively, TG-glycerol in the fasting state, and during a glucose load in normals and in patients with endogenous ("carbohydrate-induced") hypertriglyceridemia [28]?

2. What quantitative role does the incorporation rate of plasma-glucose-C into plasma TG play as compared with the esterification rate of plasma FFA to plasma TG?

The investigations were performed in normals and in patients with endogenous hypertriglyceridemia (no deficiency of lipoprotein lipase, plasma lipoprotein pattern according to Type IV). All persons investigated consumed an isocaloric carbohydrate-rich diet (85–90% carbohydrates, 3–5% fat and 7–10% protein) for five days prior the test. The esterification rate of plasma FFA to plasma TG was estimated by constant infusion of ^{3}H-labeled albumin-bound palmitic acid and the calculations were made from the specific activity of FFA in the arterial plasma and the initial slope of the increase of radioactivity in the plasma TG [1272, 1280, 1294]. Analogously, the incorporation of plasma glucose-C into plasma TG was calculated from the specific activity of plasma glucose-C in the arterial plasma [1293] and the initial slope of the increase of ^{14}C-radioactivity in plasma TG. After a priming dose, ^{14}C-U-glucose was infused concomitantly with the ^{3}H-labeled palmitic acid at a constant rate. To avoid dilution of the radioactive glucose taken up by the liver by "cold" glucose originating from absorption, the oral glucose load had the same specific activity as the plasma glucose.

As shown in Fig. 2, in the fasting state plasma glucose-C was incorporated only in plasma TG-glycerol, in normals as well as in patients with hypertriglyceridemia.

No incorporation into plasma TG-FA could be observed. If the incorporation rate of plasma glucose-C into plasma TG-glycerol is compared with the total glycerol used for the esterification of plasma FFA to plasma TG, it could be demonstrated that 30–40% of the glycerol used for the esterification of plasma FFA to plasma TG was derived from plasma glucose-C. There was no difference between normals and patients with endogenous hypertriglyceridemia.

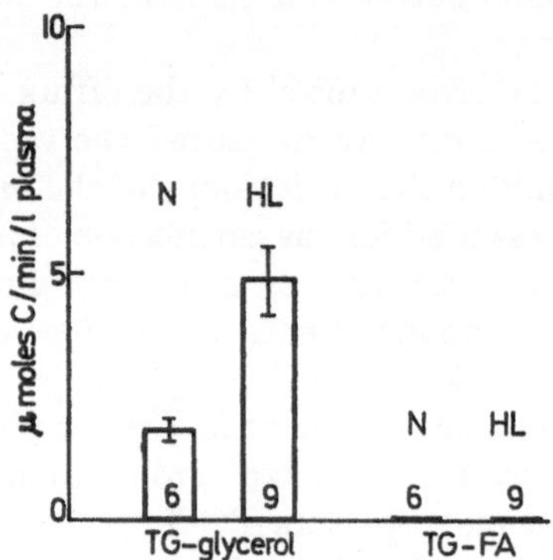

Fig. 2. The rate of incorporation of plasma glucose into plasma triglyceride glycerol and triglyceride fatty acids for normals (*N*) and hypertriglyceridemic (*HL*) patients in the fasting state

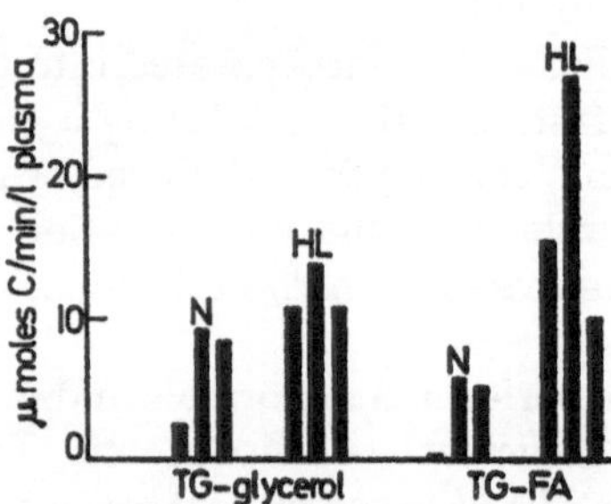

Fig. 3. Comparison between normals (*N*) and hypertriglyceridemic (*HL*) patients in the rate of incorporation of plasma glucose-C into triglyceride during a glucose load

In three normal persons and three patients with hypertriglyceridemia the incorporation rate of plasma glucose-C into plasma-TG was estimated during an oral glucose load of 40 g/hour, whereby the labeled glucose was also given orally. Under these conditions incorporation of plasma glucose-C into plasma TG-glycerol and TG-FA could be demonstrated (Fig. 3). Again, the incorporation of plasma glucose-C into plasma TG-glycerol was compared with the glycerol-C used for the esterification of plasma FFA to plasma TG. As shown in the left part of Fig. 4, during the oral glucose load in normals, as well as in patients with hypertriglyceridemia, a major part of the glycerol-C used for the esterification of plasma-FFA to plasma TG was derived from plasma glucose. In the same way, the incorporation of plasma glucose-C into plasma TG-FA was compared with the FFA-C used for the esterification of plasma FFA to plasma TG, assuming a mean chain length of 16 C-units of the plasma TG-FA. As shown in the right part of the figure, even under massive glucose loading, the synthesis of plasma TG-FA from plasma glucose is less than 10% of the esterification rate of plasma FFA to plasma TG (expressed in C-units). In other words, the *de novo* synthesis of plasma TG-FA from plasma glucose does not play any significant role in the plasma TG influx, even under a massive glucose load, either in normals or in patients with endogenous hypertriglyceridemia.

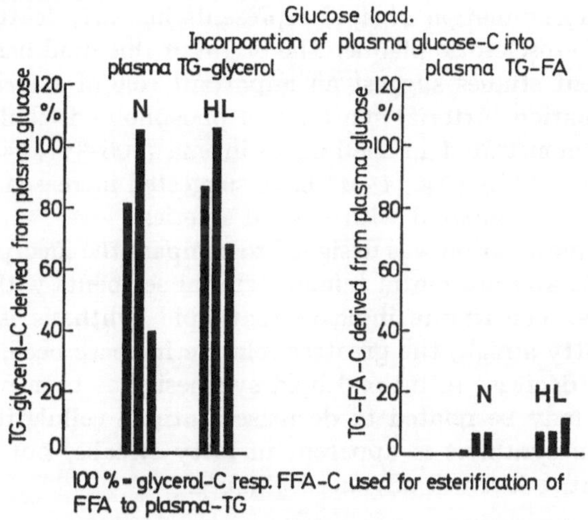

Fig. 4. The incorporation of plasma glucose-C into the glycerol and free fatty acid portions of plasma triglyceride during a glucose load. Normals (*N*) are compared on the left with hypertriglyceridemic (*HL*) patients on the right

From these investigations the following conclusions may be drawn:

1. In normals and in patients with endogenous hypertriglyceridemia there is no incorporation of plasma glucose-C into plasma TG-FA in the fasting state. Even during glucose loading only a very small, quantitatively insignificant amount of plasma glucose-C is incorporated into plasma TG-FA in both groups. However, a considerable amount of plasma TG-glycerol is derived from plasma glucose.

2. In the fasting state, as well as during glucose loading, plasma TG seem to be synthesized mainly by esterification of plasma FFA.

3. These findings support the hypothesis that an impaired fractional removal of endogenous plasma TG is mainly responsible for the excessive hypertriglyceridemia in these patients. The "carbohydrate-induction" is apparently not based on an increased synthesis of plasma TG from plasma glucose.

EFFECTS OF ATHEROSCLEROSIS ON LIPID AND PROTEIN SYNTHESIS IN HUMAN AORTA*

Aram V. Chobanian and Robert D. Lille

The intimal accumulation of lipid represents an early feature in the genesis of the human atherosclerotic plaque. The origin of this lipid has not been clearly defined, but recent studies suggest an important role of arterial metabolism in the lipid accumulation. Arterial synthesis of phospholipid, cholesterol, and fatty acid has been demonstrated in the human intima [306–311, 946] and studies in pigeons [888] and rabbits [946, 1541] have suggested increased synthesis of lipid in atherosclerotic as compared with normal arteries.

The present investigation was designed to compare the incorporation of labeled acetate into lipids and protein in human arterial segments with varying degrees of atherosclerosis. The results indicate that lipid synthesis is significantly increased in the fatty streak, the greatest relative increase occurring in the sterol ester fraction. A decrease in intimal lipid synthesis has been noted in advanced atheromata and may be related to decreased intimal cellularity. No significant change in protein synthesis is apparent in fatty streaks, but protein synthesis may be somewhat reduced in advanced plaques.

MATERIAL AND METHODS

Human aortas were obtained at post-mortem examination within six hours of death. The adventitia and most of the media were removed and discarded. Adjacent areas of normal-appearing intima, fatty streaks and advanced plaques were carefully dissected from one another and the individual lesions pooled together. The fatty streaks were identified as slightly raised, nonulcerated, yellowish segments present as scattered lesions or confluent aggregates. The tissues (0.08–0.30 g dry wt) were incubated for three hours in 3 ml Krebs bicarbonate buffer (pH 7.35) containing sodium acetate-2-^{14}C (1.0 μc/ml, specific activity 34.0 mC/mmole). Detailed descriptions of the procedures involved in the tissue incubations and in the lipid analyses have previously been published [307, 309, 311]. The arterial DNA contents and protein radioactivity were determined as recently described [306].

RESULTS

Lipid Synthesis in Normal Intima and Fatty Streaks. Incorporation of labeled acetate into total arterial lipids (Table 1) was significantly greater in the fatty streaks than in normal-appearing intima (Table 1, patients 1–6). The increase in incorporation in the fatty streak averaged 123% (range 13–262%, $P = 0.04$) when the results were compared on the basis of tissue weight. When related to arterial

* The authors wish to thank Hyo Young Chung and Kathleen Rudolph for their expert technical assistance. This study was supported in part by Grants HE-12869, HE-07299 and HE-1536 from the U.S. Public Health Service, and the U.A. Whitaker Fund.

Table 1. *Incorporation of acetate-2-^{14}C into lipid and protein by normal intima, fatty streaks, and severe atherosclerotic aorta*

Patient	Age and sex	Degree atherosclerosis	Cholesterol content (mg/g dry wt)	Incorporation of acetate-2-^{14}C			
				lipid		protein	
				(dpm/g dry wt)	(dpm/mg DNA)	(dpm/g dry wt)	(dpm/mg DNA)
1	26, M	0	14.1	7,400	7,480	24,000	13,900
		Fatty streak	24.5	8,360	8,670	27,600	13,900
2	54, F	0	10.0	8,100	6,800		
		Fatty streak	117.2	29,300	32,500		
3	57, F	0	8.9	19,100	19,100	53,200	53,200
		Fatty streak	57.0	29,300	35,100	51,200	62,000
4	58, M	0	30.5	17,700	21,600	4,260	5,180
		Fatty streak	156.1	57,300	88,900	26,400	41,000
5	27, M	0	11.6	12,300	16,500	11,500	15,300
		Fatty streak	45.5	15,500	23,100	5,200	7,780
6	51, F	0	16.0	13,100	10,200	85,500	66,300
		Fatty streak	53.4	33,700	20,900	38,000	21,100
7	49, F	0–2+	21.3	49,000	25,600	42,900	22,400
		3–4+	35.3	48,800	19,200	39,500	15,600
8	77, F	0–2+	53.6	116,000	111,000	50,800	48,200
		3–4+	59.2	30,500	72,400	18,900	44,800
9	75, F	0–1+	40.6	94,800	199,000	27,700	57,200
		4+	119.0	55,200	199,000	11,100	40,000
10	74, F	0–2+	27.5	29,000	19,200	14,900	9,870
		4+	61.2	14,400	13,800	6,470	6,230

DNA content, the mean increase in incorporation in the fatty streak was 156% (range 16–378%, $P=0.05$).

The cholesterol content of grossly normal intima (Table 1) averaged 15 mg/g dry wt (range 9–31) while that of adjacent fatty streaks averaged 76 mg/g dry wt (range 25–156). The largest percentage increase in incorporation of acetate to lipid occurred in the fatty streaks with the highest cholesterol content (patients 2, 3, 4 and 6). The DNA content of normal intima did not differ significantly from that in the fatty streak.

In both normal intima and fatty streak, the major incorporation of acetate to lipid occurred in the phospholipid fraction (Table 2). All lipid groups participated in the increased incorporation observed in the fatty streak lesions. The greatest numerical increase occurred in the phospholipid fraction and the largest proportionate increase in the sterol esters. Following saponification, greater than 93% of total lipid radioactivity was recovered in the fatty acid fraction.

Sterol ester radioactivity averaged 2.8% of total lipid radioactivity in the normal intima and 7.0% in the fatty streak. Greater than 95% of sterol ester radioactivity was recovered as fatty acid. The intimal free sterol fraction averaged 3.0% of intimal lipid radioactivity in normal intima and 3.5% in the fatty streak. Our previous studies have demonstrated that approximately 50% of the radioactivity of this sterol fraction is associated with cholesterol and cholestanol with the remainder as nonsterol material [307]. Because of the limited quantity of tissue, no attempt was made to purify the sterol moiety.

Table 2. *Incorporation of acetate-2-^{14}C into Individual lipids in normal intima and fatty streaks (percentage of total lipid radioactivity)*

Patient	Degree atherosclerosis	Phospholipid	Triglyceride	Free fatty acid	Sterol	Sterol ester
3	0	31.6	33.3	21.2	4.9	4.5
	Fatty streak	34.4	25.5	27.2	4.9	6.3
4	0	53.0	27.3	15.5	1.0	2.5
	Fatty streak	40.0	30.5	14.8	3.0	10.4
6	0	57.5	15.4	22.3	3.1	1.5
	Fatty streak	51.9	22.0	19.3	2.5	4.3

Lipid Synthesis in Normal and Severely Atherosclerotic Aorta. The mean incorporation of acetate into lipids of severely atherosclerotic segments was 48% less than that of relatively normal intima when related to tissue weight and 14% less when related to DNA content (Table 1, patients 7–10).

Aortic Protein Synthesis. The incorporation of acetate to protein was not significantly different in normal intima and fatty streaks when compared either on a weight basis ($P = 0.5$) or according to DNA content ($P = 0.5$). In the severely atherosclerotic intima, the mean incorporation of acetate to protein on a weight basis was 44% less than that in relatively normal intima. When related to arterial DNA content, the mean decrease was 22%.

DISCUSSION

These *in vitro* studies demonstrate for the first time an increased cellular synthesis of lipid in human fatty streaks and suggest an important role of arterial metabolism in lipid accumulation in the fatty streak lesion. The results are in agreement with recent animal studies indicating increased synthesis of fatty acid, phospholipid, and cholesteryl ester in atherosclerotic arteries of pigeons [888, 1281] and rabbits [378, 946, 1541]. The absence of increased lipid synthesis in advanced human atheromata differs from the reported findings in these experimental animals where lipid synthesis is apparently accelerated even in advanced lesions.

The significance of our observations with respect to the pathogenesis of atherosclerosis is uncertain. Examination by electron microscopy of human fatty streaks from young individuals has demonstrated an early intracellular accumulation of lipid in the smooth muscle cell [953]. Local intimal synthesis might represent an important source of this intracellular lipid. However, the fatty streaks utilized in the present studies were probably not representative of very early atherosclerotic lesions. Microscopic examination of comparable lesions from the same tissues in some instances demonstrated foam cell infiltration and extracellular lipid and fibrous tissue deposition. In view of recent studies in rabbit suggesting that the major synthesis of lipid in atheromata occurs in the foam cell [378], our observed increases in lipid synthesis might be related to an increased number of intimal foam cells in the fatty streak.

The greatest percentage increase in acetate incorporation in the fatty streak was apparent in the sterol ester fraction, although the sterol esters accounted for a relatively small percentage (less than 11%) of total intimal radioactivity. This increased incorporation may be secondary to an augmented activity of the lecithin-cholesterol acyl transferase enzyme in the human fatty streak [4]. Increased rates of cholesterol esterification in atherosclerotic arteries have previously been reported in pigeons [888] and rabbits [378]. The present results and the previous demonstration of differences in the fatty acid composition of cholesterol esters from human fatty streaks and plasma [516] suggest a role of arterial metabolism in cholesteryl ester accumulation. Reduction in cholesteryl ester hydrolyzing activity of atheromata [716] and increased binding capacity of diseased arterial elastin for cholesteryl esters [822] may also contribute to the markedly increased levels of these esters in atherosclerotic tissue.

The increased lipid synthesis of the fatty streak did not appear to reflect a generalized increase in metabolic activity since a similar acceleration in incorporation of acetate into proteins was not apparent. Both lipid and protein synthesis appeared somewhat reduced in some of the advanced plaques, the decrease appearing to relate in part to a diminished cellularity of the advanced lesions.

SUMMARY

The incorporation of acetate-2-^{14}C into individual lipids and protein has been examined in human arterial segments with varying degrees of atherosclerosis. The results indicate: (1) The synthesis of lipid is significantly greater in fatty streak lesions than in normal intima when compared either on the basis of arterial weight or DNA content. (2) Phospholipids are the major lipid synthesized in both normal intima and fatty streak, but all lipid groups appear to participate in the increased incorporation in the fatty streak. The greatest relative increase in incorporation in the fatty streak is apparent in the sterol ester fraction. (3) Incorporation of acetate to protein is not significantly different in normal intima and fatty streak. (4) Reductions in protein and lipid synthesis may occur in advanced lesions, the decreases relating in part to decreased tissue cellularity.

The findings have demonstrated an abnormality in lipid metabolism in the human fatty streak and suggest that intimal synthesis contributes to the marked accumulation of lipid in the fatty streak.

STUDIES ON THE CATABOLISM OF CHOLESTEROL TO BILE ACIDS IN LIVER: CHOLESTEROL-7α-HYDROXYLASE*

G. S. Boyd and Margaret E. Lawson

The breakdown of cholesterol to bile acids is quantitatively important, and the conversion of cholesterol to bile acids has been reviewed by Danielsson [355]. It has been shown that one possible sequence of events from cholesterol to cholic acid may involve the endoplasmic reticulum, the cell supernatant, and mitochondria acting sequentially as shown in Fig. 1. Lindstedt [878] showed that

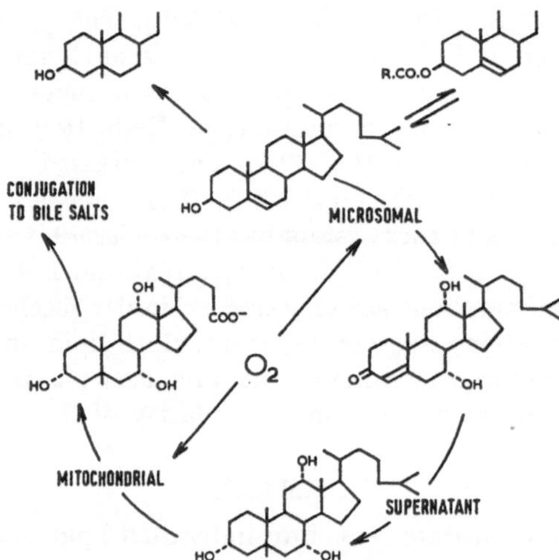

Fig. 1. Reactions involved in the conversion of cholesterol to cholic acid

one of the possible metabolites on this pathway was 7α-hydroxycholesterol. Bile acid synthesis occurs in the liver, and the hydroxylation of cholesterol to 7α-hydroxycholesterol has been shown to occur in the microsomal fraction of rat liver [355, 1015]. If 7α-hydroxylation is the initial step on the pathway of degradation of cholesterol to bile acids, then this reaction might be the rate-limiting reaction in the sequence.

Recent studies on the mechanism of biological hydroxylation reactions have shown that many of these enzymic reactions involving the introduction of hydroxyl-groups into sterols, fatty acids, amino acids or drugs belong to the class termed "mixed function oxidations" [938]. These enzymic reactions frequently involve an interaction of the substrate, molecular oxygen, NADPH and

* The studies herein were supported by a research grant from the Medical Research Council.

the enzyme system, in a complex reaction which results in the hydroxylation of the substrate and a simultaneous production of water:

$$RH + O_2 + NADPH \rightarrow ROH + H_2O + NADP^+$$

Summarized herein are some experiments on the liver cholesterol-7α-hydroxylase system enzyme and the effects of ablating certain endocrine organs on the activity of the liver microsomal cholesterol-7α-hydroxylase enzyme system.

MATERIALS AND METHODS

Cholesterol-4-^{14}C (50 mc/mM) was obtained from the Radiochemical Center, Amersham, England. D-glucose-6-phosphate, NADP and β-mercaptoethylamine hydrochloride were products of the Sigma Chemical Co., St. Louis, Missouri, and glucose-6-phosphate dehydrogenase (E.C.1.1.1.49) of Boehringer and Soehne, Mannheim, Germany. All other reagents and solvents were of analytic grade.

Male Wistar strain rats weighing about 200 g were used in all experiments. The animals were fed the stock diet as described by Boyd, Scholan and Mitton [234]. In the experiments involving removal of endocrine organs, such as the

Table. *Composition of reaction mixture*

Microsomal fraction	Equivalent to 1 g weight tissue	4.0 ml
Phosphate buffer (Na_2HPO_4:NaH_2PO_4) containing β-mercapto-ethylamine 10 mM	0.1 M pH 7.4	2.0 ml
NADP	5 μmoles	0.5 ml
Glucose-6-P	50 μmoles	0.5 ml
Glucose-6-P-dehydrogenase	1 I.U.	0.1 ml
Cholesterol-4-^{14}C	0.1 μc	0.05 ml

gonads, adrenals, or thyroid, these surgical procedures were conducted under clean but not aseptic conditions. Animals receiving the bile salt sequestering agent, cholestyramine (Cuemid), had this additive in the diet at a concentration of 4% w/w. The rat livers were perfused with 0.25 M sucrose or with 0.154 M KCl to remove contaminating haemoglobin, and 20% homogenates were prepared in either of these media using a low-speed glass-teflon homogenizer. The endoplasmic reticulum in the cell sap was isolated in the usual way. The microsomal fraction was incubated at 37° for 60 min, as shown in the table. The 7α-hydroxylase activity was assayed using cholesterol-4-^{14}C purified by thin-layer chromatography prior to use. The reaction was stopped with methanol, and lipid extracts were made with chloroform and ethylacetate; the products were separated by thin-layer chromatography on silica gel H in the solvent system benzene:ethylacetate: 7:13 [1312].

It is known that if cholesterol is incubated in air in certain solutions in the presence of traces of metallic ions or other catalysts then a variety of oxidation products is produced as discussed by Boyd, Scholan and Mitton [234]. In this microsomal preparation, only 7α-hydroxycholesterol can be considered as a physiological monohydroxylated derivative of cholesterol, and for this reason the other substances encountered in a typical incubation mixture were classified as "autoxidation products" to differentiate them from 7α-hydroxycholesterol. Following thin-layer chromatography of the products of the incubation mixture, the thin-layer chromatograms are either scanned in a windowless gas flow counter [1212] or the radioactivity on segments of the plate, established by elution of the radioactive sterols from the supporting material, and followed by liquid scintillation counting [234].

The most active cholesterol-7α-hydroxylase system was found to be the 18,000 g/15 min supernatant fortified with NADPH. Scholan and Boyd [1312] showed that it was possible to retain the cholesterol-7α-hydroxylase activity in the microsomal fraction provided it was resuspended in either a solution of the "boiled supernatant" or in a buffer solution containing β-mercaptoethylamine.

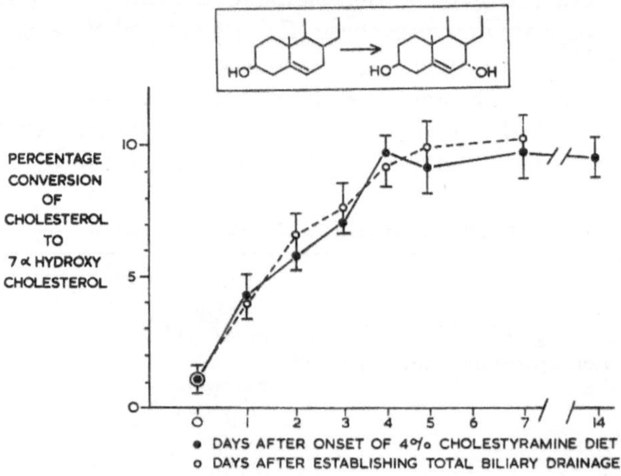

Fig. 2. Time course of the percentage conversion of hepatic cholesterol to 7α-hydroxy cholesterol in rats receiving cholestyramine (•) or carrying a bile fistula (o)

This thiol could replace the necessary cofactors in the cell supernatant [1313]. The results of the liver 7α-hydroxycholesterol enzyme assays conducted on various groups of animals subjected to endocrine ablation procedures have all been conducted on the liver microsomal fractions suspended in β-mercaptoethylamine with other additives as shown in the table. In normal rats, liver cholesterol-7α-hydroxylase activity was altered after breaking the enterohepatic circulation as shown in Fig. 2.

RESULTS

Male rats were thyroidectomized and maintained thereafter on the stock diet supplemented by calcium lactate in the drinking water. Twenty-one days later the animals were challenged with 4% cholestyramine in their diet. They were killed seven days later and the liver microsomal cholesterol-7α-hydroxylase activity determined as outlined previously. As shown in Fig. 3, although the average hydroxylase activity was lower in the thyroidectomized animals, the difference was not significant.

Male and female rats were gonadectomized and maintained thereafter on the stock diet. Twenty-eight days later the animals were challenged with cholestyramine in their diet as detailed above and then killed 7 days later for liver microsomal cholesterol-7α-hydroxylase activity determinations. The results of these experiments are shown in Fig. 3 where it can be seen that ablation of the gonads failed to influence this hepatic hydroxylase response to the bile salt sequestering agent.

Male rats were adrenalectomized and maintained thereafter on the stock diet supplemented with 1% sodium chloride and 10% glucose in the drinking water. Seven days later, cholestyramine was introduced into the diet as before and the animals were killed after a further seven days. The liver microsomal cholesterol-7α-hydroxylase activities are shown in Fig. 3 where it can be seen that the

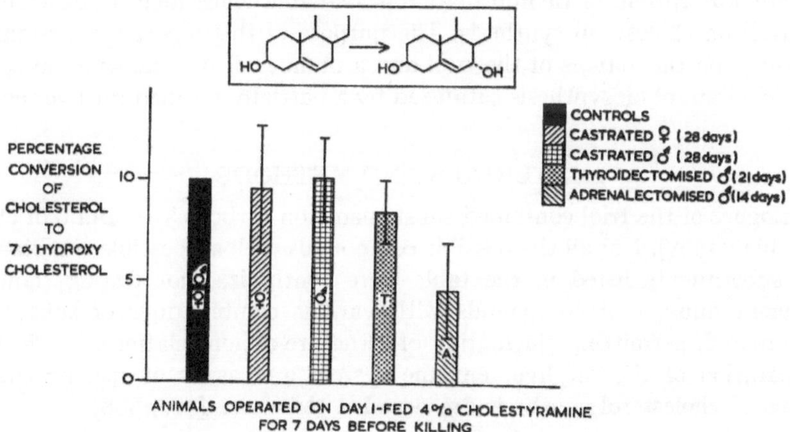

Fig. 3. Hepatic cholesterol conversion to 7α-hydroxy cholesterol after castration, thyroidectomy and adrenalectomy

response of the animals to this challenge is significantly lower in the animals which were deprived of their adrenals. The mechanism by which the cholesterol-7α-hydroxylase is controlled remains to be elucidated.

SUMMARY

In male and female rats when the entero-hepatic circulation of bile salts is broken by the introduction of the bile salt sequestering agent cholestyramine, there is a rapid increase in the hepatic cholesterol-7α-hydroxylase activity. Gonadectomy in the rat failed to influence the normal response of the animals to cholestyramine feeding. Similarly, under the conditions of this study thyroidectomy in the rat also failed to influence the normal response to cholestyramine feeding. Adrenalectomy in the rat produced a diminished response in the liver microsomal cholesterol-7α-hydroxylase activity as a result of cholestyramine feeding.

EFFECTS OF CHOLESTANE-3β,5α,6β-TRIOL AND ITS ANALOGUES ON CHOLESTEROL BIOSYNTHESIS IN VITRO*

MARY E. DEMPSEY, MARY C. RITTER, DONALD T. WITIAK and ROGER A. PARKER

Cholestane-3β,5α,6β-triol is a recognized hypocholesterolemic antiatherogenic agent [58, 322, 735]. One known mode of action of the triol is to block intestinal cholesterol absorption. Little information is available concerning the direct effects of the triol on cholesterol synthesis. The purpose of this report is to summarize our findings on the actions of the triol and a number of its analogues on specific steps of cholesterol biosynthesis catalyzed by a partially purified rat liver enzyme system.

MATERIALS AND METHODS

Analogues of the triol contained substituents on carbons 3, 5, and 6 of cholestane (table)[1565]. Not all the possible compounds with all possible combinations of the substituents listed in the table were synthesized for testing; however, a sufficient number of compounds with various combinations of substituents were prepared, permitting elucidation of structure-action relationships. Methods of preparation of the rat liver enzyme system and assay of specific enzymic reactions of cholesterol synthesis are detailed elsewhere [387, 388].

RESULTS AND DISCUSSION

Conversion of Acetate, Mevalonate, and Squalene to Sterols and Cholesterol. The data presented in Fig. 1 show that 50% inhibition of the conversion of acetate and mevalonate to cholesterol occurs in the presence of 5 μM cholestanetriol and inhibition is complete at 50 μM triol. A related finding is that there is no inhibition by the triol and usually a slight activation (15%) of the conversion of acetate and mevalonate to nonsaponifiable compounds. Inhibition of cholesterol synthesis by the triol resulted in the accumulation of a compound which migrated during silicic acid column chromatography as a 29–30 carbon atom sterol, slightly more polar than lanosterol. The compound is readily converted to cholesterol by an uninhibited enzyme preparation. It may contain a conjugated double bond system, i.e. it can be converted to an epiperoxide derivative [387, 388]. It did not migrate during chromatography with 4,4-dimethyl-$\Delta^{5,7}$-cholestadienol (gift of Drs. E. Paoletti and A. Fiecchi, University of Milan). One possible structure of the compound is 4,4-dimethyl-$\Delta^{8,14}$-cholestadienol, a product of lanosterol demethylation. The unknown compound also accumulated in the presence of a number of the analogues of the triol, in particular those in which the 5α, 6β, or 3α substituent is an amino group and the remaining substituents (R or R^1 and R^2, table) are hydroxyl groups. There was no accumula-

* The work herein has been supported by U.S.P.H.S. grants HE-8634 and HE-6314 from the National Heart Institute.

tion of $\Delta^{5,24}$-cholestadienol. Findings similar to those just described were obtained with squalene as substrate for the enzyme system.

With regard to structural requirements for inhibition of cholesterol synthesis from acetate and mevalonate, the data indicate that substituents on all three positions (3β, 5α, and 6β) of cholestane are necessary for maximum inhibition. Compounds such as the diols [$R=R^1=OH$, $R^2=H$ or $R=R^2=OH$, $R^1=H$ (table)] were considerably less active than the triol ($R=R^1=R^2=OH$). Cholestanol ($R=OH$, $R^1=R^2=H$) and cholestane ($R=R^1=R^2=H$) showed no inhibition; cholesterol slightly activated the conversions of acetate and mevalonate. Amino derivatives (e.g. $R=R^2=OH$, $R^1=NH_2$; $R=R^1=OH$, $R^2=NH_2$) showed the

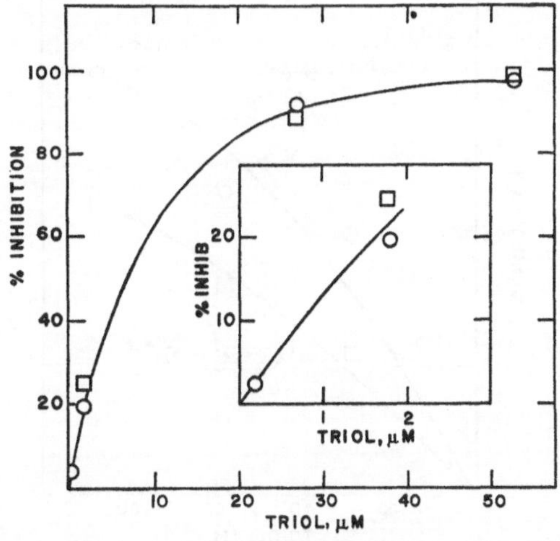

Fig. 1. Effects of varying concentrations of cholestane-3β, 5α, 6β-triol on the enzymic conversion of acetate and mevalonate to cholesterol. ○—○, conversion of mevalonate—2-^{14}C to cholesterol; □—□, conversion of acetate-2-^{14}C to cholesterol. Concentrations of the constituents of each incubation medium (total volume 1.35 ml) were 0.1 M phosphate buffer, pH 7.35, 2.3×10^5 dpm sodium acetate-2-^{14}C (2.0 mC per mole) or 3.9×10^5 dpm mevalonate-2-^{14}C (3.1 mC per mmole), 0.8 mM NADPH, NADP, and NAD, and 5 mM ATP, 5 mM $MgCl_2$, cholestane-triol, as indicated, and 22.5 mg protein from the 500×g supernatant fraction of a rat liver homogenate. Incubations were for 30 minutes at 37° under oxygen. Conversons to nonsaponifiable compounds, sterols, and cholesterol were determined as described elsewhere [387, 388]

same level of inhibition as the triol. The 3α-NH_2 analogue of the triol was also inhibitory; in contrast the 3β-NH_2 analogue ($R=NH_2$, $R^1=R^2=OH$) was considerably less inhibitory. Esterification of the triol (i.e. the triacetate analogue) eliminated the inhibitory action of the triol.

Conversion of Δ^7-Cholestenol and Δ^{5,7}-Cholestadienol to Cholesterol. The data presented in Fig. 2 show that cholestane-3β,5α,6β-triol is capable of inhibiting two partially purified enzymes catalyzing the final stages of cholesterol biosynthesis, i.e. Δ^7-sterol Δ^5-dehydrogenase and $\Delta^{5,7}$-sterol Δ^7-reductase. The triol and its analogues are more specific inhibitors of the Δ^7-reductase than of the Δ^5-dehydrogenase. Inhibition of the Δ^5-dehydrogenase could readily be overcome by increasing the substrate (Δ^7-cholestenol) levels. As indicated by the data presented in Fig. 3, inhibition of the Δ^7-reductase was not completely overcome by increasing the substrate ($\Delta^{5,7}$-cholestadienol) level. These findings (Fig. 3) also demonstrate that the 5αNH$_2$ [R=R^2=OH, R^1=NH$_2$ (table)] and the-3α-NH$_2$ (R=NH$_2^{(\alpha)}$, R^1=R^2=OH) analogues are more powerful inhibitors of the Δ^7-reductase than the triol.

With regard to structural requirements for inhibition of the Δ^7-reductase, our findings demonstrate that the 3 position of cholestane is more important than the 5 or 6 position. The order of effectiveness of substituents is NH$_2$(3α)> NH$_2$(3β)>OH(3β). The amino derivatives (i.e. 5α and 6β) are also more inhibitory than the corresponding hydroxyl substituted derivatives [e.g. R=R^2=OH,

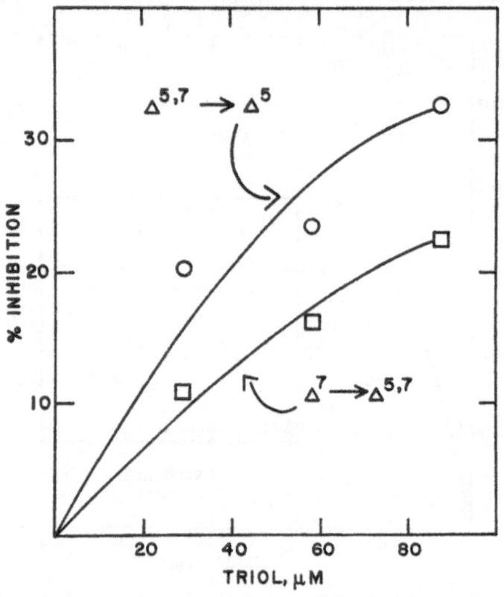

Fig. 2. Effects of varying concentrations of cholestane-3β, 5α, 6β-triol on purified Δ^7-sterol Δ^5-dehydrogenase and $\Delta^{5,7}$-sterol Δ^7-reductase of rat liver. O—O, conversion of $\Delta^{5,7}$-cholestadienol-4-^{14}C to cholesterol-4-^{14}C; □—□, conversion of Δ^7-cholestenol, 2,4-^{3}H to $\Delta^{5,7}$-cholestadienol-2,4-^{3}H. Concentrations of the constituents of each incubation medium (total volume, 2.45 ml) were 0.1 M phosphate buffer, pH 7.35, 1 mM NADPH and 31.8 μM $\Delta^{5,7}$-cholestadienol-4-^{14}C or 1 mM NAD, 31.7 μM Δ^7-cholestenol-2,4-^{3}H, and 0.1 mμM AY-9944, cholestane—triol as indicated, and 2.4 mg purified enzyme system protein and 30 mg activator protein. Incubations were for 45' at 37° under nitrogen ($\Delta^{5,7}\rightarrow\Delta^5$) or oxygen ($\Delta^7\rightarrow\Delta^{5,7}$). Preparation of the purified enzyme system and assays for enzymic activities were performed as described elswhere [387, 388]

R^1=NH$_2$>R=R^1=R^2=OH (the triol)]. Furthermore, cholestanol (R=OH, R^1=R^2=H) and cholesterol are more inhibitory than the diol derivative (R=R^1=OH, R^2=H) which is more inhibitory than the triol. However, the 5α-diol and the triol are more effective than the 6β-diol (R=R^2=OH, R^1=H), indicating that the 6 position is of least importance with regard to inhibition of the Δ^7-reductase. Stigmastane-triol is approximately as effective an inhibitor as the 5α-NH$_2$ derivative (R=R^2=OH, R^1=NH$_2$). Cholestane (R=R^1=R^2=H) has no effect on the Δ^7-reductase. An unexpected finding was that the triacetate) analogue of the triol and in particular the dioximino (R=R^2=NOH, R^1=OH and the azido (R=O—C(=O)—CH$_3$, R^1=N$_3$, R^2=OH) analogues are powerful activa-

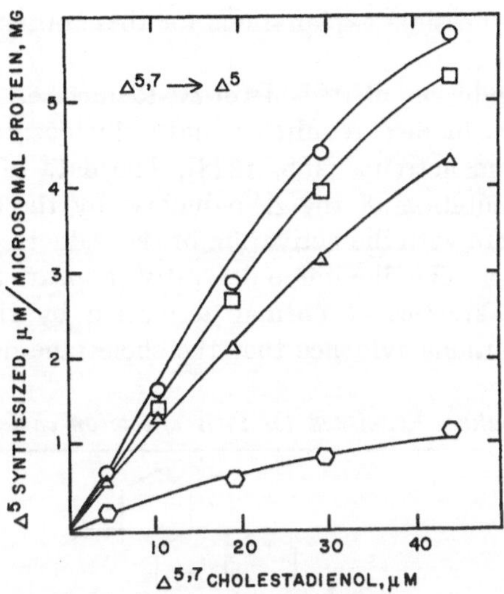

Fig. 3. Effect of varying concentrations of $\Delta^{5,7}$-cholestadienol-4-^{14}C on the inhibition of $\Delta^{5,7}$-sterol Δ^7-reductase by cholestane-3β, 5α, 6β-triol and some of its analogues. ○—○, Δ^7-reductase activity, no inhibitor; □—□, effect of cholestane-3β, 5α, 6β-triol; Δ—Δ, effect of 3β, 6β-hydroxy-5α-amino-cholestane; ⬡—⬡, effect of 3α-amino, 5α, 6β-hydroxy-cholestane. Concentrations of each incubation medium (total volume, 2.65 ml) were 0.1 M phosphate buffer, pH 7.35, 1 mM NADPH, with or without cholestane derivative (27 μM) as indicated, with $\Delta^{5,7}$-cholestadienol-4-^{14}C as indicated, and 5.2 mg microsomal enzyme protein and 30.6 mg activator protein. Incubations were for 45 minutes under nitrogen. Cholesterol-4-^{14}C synthesis was measured as described elsewhere [387, 388]

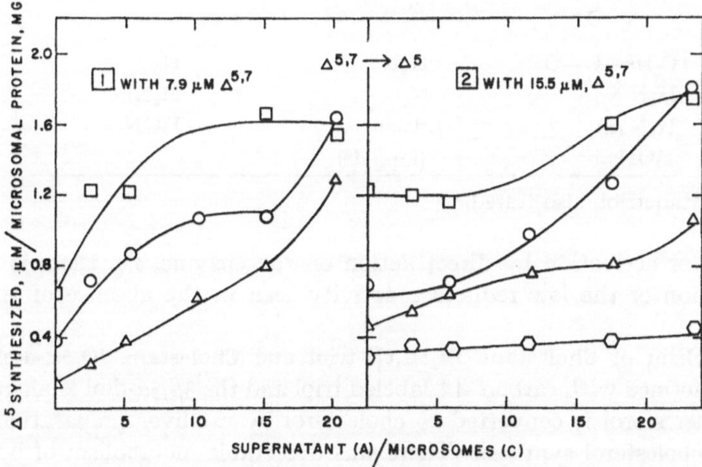

Fig. 4. Effects of varying the ratio of activator protein to microsomal enzyme protein on the inhibition or activation of $\Delta^{5,7}$-sterol Δ^7-reductase at two substrate levels by cholestane derivatives. Graph. 1 ○—○, Δ^7-reductase activity, no inhibitor or activator; □—□, effect of 3β, 6β-dioxoimino, 5α-hydroxy-cholestane; Δ—Δ, effect of 3β, 6β-hydroxy, 5α-amino-cholestane. Conditions were as given with Fig. 3, except that the ratio of activator protein to microsomal enzyme protein was varied as indicated. Graph 2. ⬡—⬡, effect of 3α-amino, 5α, 6β-hydroxy-cholestane; other symbols and conditions as indicated for Graph 1

tors of the reductase. Possible explanations for these observations are discussed in the following section.

Mechanisms of Inhibition of $\Delta^{5,7}$-Sterol Δ^7-Reductase. In recent studies, we showed that the Δ^7-reductase requires a naturally occurring liver protein as activator for maximum activity [388, 1228]. The data of Fig. 4 indicate that one mechanism of inhibition of the Δ^7-reductase by the amino derivatives of cholestane is to interfere with the activation of the reductase by increasing levels of the protein activator. The dioximino derivative appears to activate the reductase by altering the kinetics of normal activation by the protein activator. In addition, Fig. 4 contains evidence that the cholestane derivatives cause their

Table. *Cholestane derivatives examined for their effects on cholesterol biosynthesis*

R
R¹
R²

R	R_1	R_2
HO	HO	HO
CH_3—C(=O)—O	CH_3—C(=O)—O	CH_3—C(=O)—O
O=	H	O=
C_2H^5—C(=O)—O	H_2N	H
H_2N	N_3	H_2N
H_2N (α)	absent	HON=
HON=	(i.e., Δ^5)	

Stigmastanetriol, also tested.

inhibition or activation by direct action on the enzyme, i.e. there is inhibition or activation of the low reductase activity seen in the absence of the protein activator.

Metabolism of Cholestane-3β,5α,6β-triol and Cholestane-3β,5α-diol. Experiments performed with carbon -14 labeled triol and the 3β,5α-diol analogue showed that neither sterol is converted to cholesterol by rat liver preparations capable of active cholesterol synthesis. There was detectable metabolism of both sterols to compounds having the spectral characteristics of the Δ^4-3-ketone bond system, i.e. absorption maximum at 240 mμ. The metabolic product of the diol also migrated during silicic acid chromatography with unlabeled Δ^4-cholestene-3-one. Related experiments with the labeled diol and triol indicate that these compounds are irreversibly bound to the microsomal enzyme system, but not to its protein activator described in the previous section.

Effects of Cholestane-3β,5α,6β-triol on Cholesterol Synthesis by Intestinal Enzymes. In studies similar to those outlined in the conditions with Fig. 1, the triol was found to inhibit the conversion of acetate to cholesterol by rat intestinal slices and mucosal preparations. The other analogues (e.g. table) have not been tested for effects in the intestinal system.

SUMMARY

These studies *in vitro* with cholestane-3β,5α,6β-triol and its analogues offer new insights regarding mechanisms of specific enzymic reactions of cholesterol biosynthesis and the hypocholesterolemic, antiatherogenic actions of the triol and related compounds.

CHOLESTEROL DYNAMICS AFTER PARTIAL ILEAL BYPASS*

RICHARD B. MOORE, IVAN D. FRANTZ, JR., RICHARD L. VARCO and HENRY BUCHWALD

For over six years partial ileal bypass surgery has been employed as a powerful therapeutic weapon in the management of patients with various types of primary hypercholesterolemia. In our series of 70 patients there have been marked reductions in plasma cholesterol levels, averaging 53% from pretreatment levels or 40% from the preoperative values obtained after at least three months of treatment with a "cholesterol-lowering" dietary regimen. Body cholesterol is in a dynamic state and is continuously (a) lost from the body, primarily by fecal bile acid and neutral sterol excretion (with only minor losses from skin and minute losses in the urine), and (b) replenished by intestinal absorption of dietary cholesterol and by *de novo* cholesterol synthesis in various body tissues. The magnitude of the daily cholesterol turnover may be determined by examination of either of these two processes. The rationale of using distal ileal bypass in the treatment of hypercholesterolemia is the establishment of a twofold drain on the body cholesterol pool. First there is a direct drain resulting from increased fecal loss of normally absorbed (exogenous) and reabsorbed (endogenous) cholesterol, and secondly there is an indirect or metabolic drain resulting from reduced bile acid absorption, eliciting a compensatory increase in hepatic conversion of cholesterol to bile acids. Herein studies of several aspects of cholesterol dynamics before and at three and twelve months after partial ileal bypass are presented.

Cholesterol Biosynthesis. The incorporation of tritium from body water into serum cholesterol during the two days following a single oral tracer dose of

* The work herein has been in part by U.S. Public Health Grants No. HE 11901-01 and H-1875, American Heart Association Grant No. 64G168, and a grant from the Life Insurance Medicine Research Fund.

tritiated water was used as a measure of *in vivo* cholesterol synthesis in 15 patients before and three months after surgery (and again at one year in six patients). Specific activity (SA) measurements were made for serum cholesterol and body water (using distillates from timed one hour urine collections) at 0-, 12-, 24-, and 48-hours after isotope ingestion. An index of relative *in vivo* cholesterol synthesis at one day (R_1) was obtained by calculating the ratio of the 24-hour serum cholesterol SA to the 12-hour body water SA (representing the average body water SA during the 24-hour period). In a similar manner the two-day relative

Table 1. *24-Hour tritium incorporation ratio before and at three months and one year after partial ileal bypass* [a]

Patient	Before	Three months after	Increase (after/before)	One year after
1	134	725	5.4	—
2	302	790	2.6	—
3	155	851	5.5	—
4	218	1,224	5.6	914
5	151	648	4.3	777
6	97	731	7.5	636
7	119	1,184	9.9	—
8	257	866	3.4	1,353
9	121	435	3.6	—
10	90	1,160	12.8	857
11	54	639	11.8	629
12	140	1,228	8.8	—
13	143	223	1.6	—
14	126	1,032	8.2	—
15	124	1,090	8.8	—
Mean $\pm$ SD	149 ± 65	855 ± 301	—	—
Subgroup av. [b]	145	877	—	861

[a] Tritium incorporation ratio (R_1) $\times 10^4$.
[b] Subgroup of 6 patients studied at all three time periods.

synthesis index (R_2) was obtained by dividing the 48-hour serum cholesterol SA by the 24-hour body water SA. Before surgery the two-day index values (R_2), averaging 0.0282 (range 0.0087 to 0.0594), were found to be essentially double the corresponding one-day values (R_1) averaging 0.0149 (range 0.0054 to 0.0302). Similar relationships were found for the two ratios (R_1, R_2) in the postoperative studies.

The 24-hour ^{3}H-incorporation ratios are listed for each patient in Table 1. Although there was considerable inter-individual variability in each of the three studies, there was a highly significant difference ($p < 0.001$) between the pre-operative and the three-month postoperative studies, averaging 0.0149 ± 0.0065 and 0.0855 ± 0.0301, respectively. The magnitude of the postoperative increase in R_1 is listed in column 4, which shows that there was a definite increase in each patient; the overall group response was a 5.7-fold increase in this index of body cholesterol synthesis three months after ileal bypass. The six patients restudied one year after surgery (column 5, Table 1) show that this increased cholesterol synthesis persisted beyond the early postoperative period; the average values for R_1 were 0.0145 before, 0.0877 at three months, and 0.0861 at one year after surgery.

In order to quantitate the cholesterol synthesis rate the freely miscible cholesterol pool size was calculated as the combined cholesterol content of blood plasma, red cells, liver, and gastrointestinal tract, using the following assumptions: plasma volume = 45.2 ml/kg body weight [667]; red cell volume = 28.2 ml/kg [726] and cholesterol concentration = 1.38 mg/ml [914]: liver and GI tract cholesterol content = 72.9 and 54.3 mg/kg [328]. Blood and liver cholesterol are in rapid equilib-

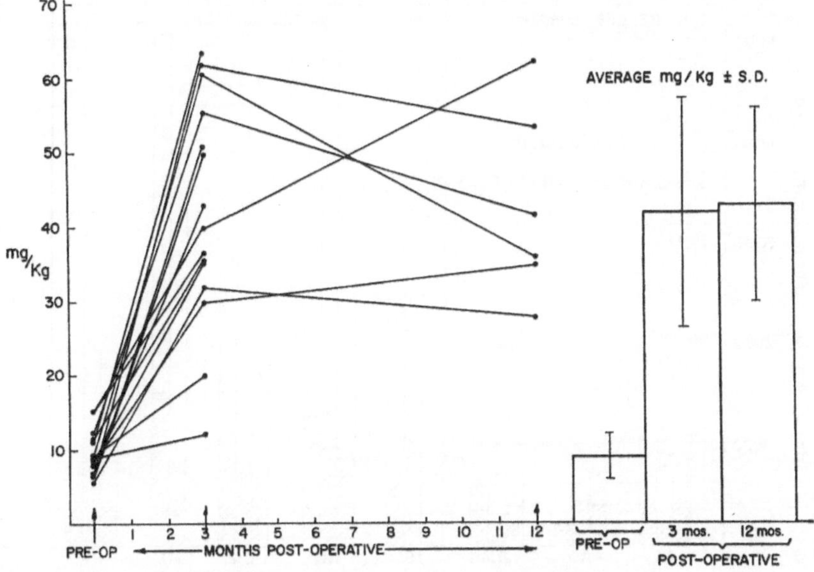

Fig. 1. Estimated cholesterol synthesis rate before and at 3 months and 1 year after surgery (mg/kg/day)

rium; the liver and gastrointestinal tract account for over 97% of the total cholesterol synthesized in the squirrel monkey [393], and the cholesterol synthesized in the intestinal wall rapidly enters the circulation via intestinal lymphatics [1550]. These findings give support to the concept that the freely miscible cholesterol pool includes the blood, liver, and intestine. The pool size averaged 23.836 g before and 18.068 g after surgery; these values are in the general neighborhood of values obtained by isotopic methods [546] but are lower than those mentioned later in this report. However, we believe their use as first approximations of the freely miscible pool can be tolerated. The pool size (in milligrams) was then multiplied by the tritium incorporation ratio (calculated using SA values in terms of cpm/per gram of cholesterol or water *hydrogen*) to give the estimated daily cholesterol synthesis rate. There was a highly significant difference ($p<0.001$) between the preoperative and postoperative periods (662 ± 328 versus 2753 ± 895 mg/day), and the average change was a 4.2-fold increase following surgery. Six patients had averages of 623, 2937, and 3,058 mg/day in studies before, at three months and one year after surgery. The synthesis rates for individual patients (in mg/kg/day) are shown graphically in Fig. 1. The preoperative study (9.07 ±

3.14) was significantly different ($p < 0.001$) from the postoperative study (41.45 ± 15.45), but in the subgroup of six patients there was no significant difference between the three month postoperative study (46.89 ± 14.84) and the one year postoperative study (48.03 ± 15.27).

Cholesterol Absorption. Cholesterol absorptive capacity, estimated from plasma radioactivity following an oral test dose of cholesterol-4-^{14}C [259] was reduced an average of 60% (range 37 to 95%) in 30 patients studied before and at three months after ileal bypass.

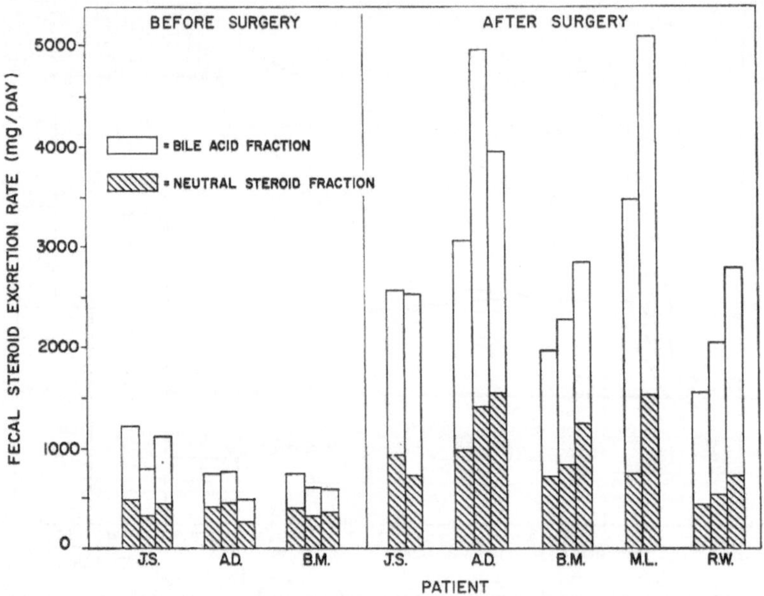

Fig. 2. Fecal steroid excretion rates before and after ileal bypass (mg/day)

Fecal Steroid Excretion. Fecal steroid excretion was measured in three patients before and again two months after ileal bypass using the isotope balance technique following a single intravenous injection of cholesterol-4-^{14}C; two additional patients were studied one year after surgery. Three four-day pooled feces collections were used in each patient for solvent extraction of bile acids and neutral steroids [1024] and ^{14}C measurement using wet carbon combustion and phenethylamine absorption of CO_2 [1025]. Serum cholesterol SA values 24 hours prior to the mid-point of each stool collection period were used in calculating fecal steroid excretion. The average daily fecal steroid excretion values for each patient are shown in Fig. 2. The total steroid excretion rate in the three patients before surgery (averaging 785 mg/day) was somewhat lower than observed in normal subjects using similar techniques (966 mg/day) [1024]; but the proportion of bile acids (average 49%) was the same as in normals, suggesting no significant loss of neutral steroids during intestinal transit. Following surgery in these three patients there was a 3.8-fold increase in total fecal steroid excretion (from 785 to 2,955 mg/day), with a much greater increase in bile acids (4.9-fold, from 399 to 1,934 mg/day) than in neutral steroids (2.7-fold, from 386 to 1,022 mg/day). Similar magnitudes of fecal steroid excretion were observed in the two patients studied at one year after operation (4,295 and 2,246 mg/day), showing persistence of augmented steroid losses beyond the early postoperative period.

Isotopic Cholesterol Turnover and Pool Size. Two months before surgery each of seven patients was given a single intravenous injection of labeled cholesterol and the serum cholesterol specific activity (SA) values during the succeeding four months were plotted on a semilogarithmic graph. The SA curves thus formed were seen to become linear after about 30 days; following surgery there was a more rapid rate of decline in SA values which again became linear after about three weeks but which had greater negative slopes (average half time of 36.1 days compared to 68.0 days before operation). In three patients the study was repeated one year after surgery when a second injection of labeled cholesterol was given. The second curves showed more rapid decline in SA values and the linear portions were steeper than in the preoperative studies (half-time averaged 23.4 days compared to 80.2 days in the same patients before surgery). These qualitative changes suggest that ileal bypass results in a marked and persistent increase in cholesterol turnover.

Table 2. *Cholesterol turnover rate before and after ileal bypass*

Patient	Cholesterol turnover rate			
	before		one year after	
	mg/day	mg/kg/day	mg/day	mg/kg/day
L	1,201	15.1	4,038	53.1
W	728	9.4	2,008	29.3
S	862	12.2	2,366	35.3
(Mean) [a]	(930)	(12.3)	(2,804)	(39.2)
P	997	13.4	—	—
D	856	13.8	—	—
M	598	10.5	—	—
PE	958	10.3	—	—
Mean	886	12.1	—	—

[a] Average values for three patients restudied one year after surgery.

Mathematical analysis of serum cholesterol SA curves [1027] was made using a two-compartment open mammillary system [941] as a model describing the behavior of labeled cholesterol and with the following assumptions: all new cholesterol enters the system and all cholesterol is lost from the system via compartment-1. This gives results similar to the method of Goodman and Nobel when S_b and k_b equal zero [546]. The turnover rates calculated in this manner are listed in Table 2. The preoperative values (average 886 mg/day) were similar to the fecal steroid excretion rates noted above (average 785 mg/day). After surgery there was a three-fold increase in cholesterol turnover (from 930 to 2,804 mg/day, or from 12.3 to 39.2 mg/kg/day). The calculated sizes of the exchangeable cholesterol pools before and one year after surgery are listed in Table 3. Both the freely miscible (34.5 g) and the total exchangable (83.0 g) pools were higher than

Table 3. *Exchangeable cholesterol pool sizes before and after partial ileal bypass*[a]

Patients	Freely miscible pool (P_1)		Slowly miscible pool (P_2)		Total exchangeable pool (P_T)	
	before	one-year after	before	one-year after	before	one-year after
L	37.97	29.45	56.73	33.26	94.71	62.72
W	33.19	26.86	47.03	22.56	80.22	49.42
S	32.24	28.33	41.75	22.97	73.96	51.30
Mean	34.47	28.21	48.73	26.27	82.96	54.48

[a] In grams.

values we have found in normal subjects using similar methods (21.9 and 69.2 g, respectively). Following surgery there were definite reductions in both the freely miscible (P_1) and the slowly miscible (P_2) pools, averaging 6.26 and 22.46 g, respectively. (When P_1 was estimated by calculating the combined plasma, red cell, liver, and GI tract cholesterol there was an average 5.77 g reduction in these same three patients after surgery). In each patient there was a relatively greater reduction in P_2 than P_1 suggesting loss of cholesterol from tissues other than the blood and liver. Diminution in xanthomata observed in such patients after surgery tend to confirm this concept.

SUMMARY

There were significant changes in all parameters of cholesterol dynamics studied; the average values for synthesis, fecal steroid excretion, and isotopic cholesterol turnover were respectively: 662, 785, and 930 mg/day before, and 2,753, 2,955, and 2,804 mg/day after surgery. These studies support the conclusion that distal ileal bypass produces a double drain on the body cholesterol pools (diminished intestinal absorption of cholesterol and bile acids, and increased conversion of cholesterol to bile acids). These changes appear to be permanent. A compensatory increase in *in vivo* cholesterol synthesis occurs following surgery but apparently not soon enough and/or large enough to prevent the significant reduction in plasma cholesterol concentration and to offset the augmented fecal steroid losses. In addition, there appears to be a significant reduction in the exchangeable cholesterol content in tissues other than the blood.

Discussion Following Dr. Sailer's Paper

Dr. Havel: I wish to comment that the term "carbohydrate-induced lipemia" has suggested to many that carbohydrate causes the hyperlipemia. I think that the present evidence, seems to dispel that notion.

It has been shown by many investigators that when high carbohydrate, low fat diets are fed to individuals with primary endogenous hyperlipemia, the absolute increase in triglyceride level is generally greater than that observed in normal subjects. Now, if there is an impaired mechanism in such individuals, for removing triglycerides from the blood, this is exactly what one would expect without any alteration in the normal effect of such a diet on lipid transport. It is also known that many such individuals are hypertriglyceridemic on any isocaloric diet, and also during a prolonged fast, as pointed out by Dr. Nikkila. Thus, the concept that carbohydrate has a different action in hyperlipemic subjects than in normal subjects cannot be supported.

Dr. Bierman: I have a question related to studies, mainly in experimental animals, which have shown that carbohydrate feeding increases hepatic lipogenesis (from nonlipid precursors).

Does Dr. Sailer have any idea why labeling from plasma glucose fails to appear in triglyceride fatty acids which on the basis of the work in experimental animals should be produced by the liver during high carbohydrate feeding?

Dr. Sailer: We did this investigation expecting to find a high incorporation of the glucose label into triglyceride fatty acids, but we did not find it. We can only say that 10% of the esterification accounts for incorporation of plasma glucose into plasma TGFA. Certainly there are fatty acids synthesized, but we have no evidence that the *de novo* synthesized fatty acids may lead to hypertriglyceridemia.

Dr. Ahrens: In reply to Dr. Havel's comment we introduced the term "carbohydrate-induced hyperglyceridemia" in order to distinguish it clearly from the fat-induced form. In both cases we intended the terms to mean "the ingestion of carbohydrate" (or fat as the case may be) that leads to (induces, literally) a high plasma glyceride level. In neither case did we mean to imply causation; indeed, we argued that a defect in lipoprotein-lipase action (not fat itself) probably causes the fat-induced form. We did not know the mechanism underlying the carbohydrate-induced form, but later, when we showed the defect in response to tolbutamide, we reasoned that we were dealing with a defect in removal. Presentations here seem to support this guess of ours with very excellent data. When the mechanisms are clearly understood and agreed upon, I would be delighted to see the terms thrown out; until then, I would argue that they are simple, informative, and give the clinician a clue to treatment.

Dr. Kendall: From Dr. Stein's presentation this morning, it seems to me that we may be involved in a time sequence here. How long does it take the liver to synthesize a molecule of very low density lipoprotein? From the time that free fatty acid is first presented to the liver, how much time does it take to appear in the very low density lipoprotein fraction? Is this time the same for fatty acids synthesized from carbohydrates in the cytoplasm of the liver cell?

Dr. Sailer: If you plot the appearance of tritium labeled triglyceride (e.g. from palmitic acid) and of C^{14}-labeled triglyceride (from glucose) against time, you get an identical curve for both in the same person. That could mean that the pools are identical and incorporation from glucose comes no later than from fatty acid esterification.

Dr. Groen: I would like to return to the question of "carbohydrate-induced hyperlipidemia". Isn't it true that Dr. Ahrens and his coworkers only showed that dextromaltose, sucrose, and glucose induced the hyperlipidemia in these patients? Strictly speaking, does that give us the right to call this a "carbohydrate"-induced hyperlipidemia?

Dr. Ahrens: The carbohydrates that we have fed to our patients at levels of 45–85% of calories included starches, dextromaltose, dextrins, galactose, fructose, sucrose, and dextrose. We have seen no differences between any of them in the induced hyperlipemia. Hence, our use of the word "carbohydrate" seems justified.

Dr. Miettinen: I wish to comment on our sterol balance data collected during the last four years. We have been able to confirm the data presented by Dr. Goodman in his kinetic studies. Overweight patients excreted increased amounts of neutral and acidic fecal sterols. Similarly, patients with Type IV hyperlipidemia excreted more fecal cholesterol and bile acids, but this may be because most subjects were overweight.

Furthermore, when we carried out sterol balance studies in 43 patients with Type II hyperlipoproteinemia, we observed that fecal bile acid excretion was significantly lower than in normocholesteremic subjects; and when patients with Type II hypercholesterolemia were put on cholestryramine, the increment of cholesterol elimination as fecal bile acids was much less than in control subjects. This suggested that there is some defect in bile acid synthesis and/or excretion in Type II hypercholesterolemia.

Discussion Following Dr. Chobanian's Paper

Dr. Adams: Dr. Chobanian, the synthesis of which lipid species fell off in the severe atheromatous lesions?

Dr. Chobanian: The synthesis of all lipid groups appeared to diminish in the severe lesions when related to tissue weight.

Dr. Scott: Did you to observe a different rate of synthesis in normal tissue from different parts of the aorta? It has been shown that there are different metabolic activities for different parts of the aorta.

Dr. Chobanian: The increased synthesis of sterol esters was confined primarily to the fatty acid component. Identification of the individual fatty acids of this fraction was not possible.

Dr. Stein: How long would you say the synthetic enzyme activity is preserved in the material?

Dr. Chobanian: That is a very difficult question to answer. If we study the tissues at 37°, for varying periods of time, we find similar activities if we go for four to six hours. We have had a straight-line relationship in the incorporation rates for as long as 18 hours. However, I don't think we can be sure what post mortem changes are taking place here.

Discussion Following Dr. Boyd's Paper

Dr. Lindstedt: Dr. Boyd expressed activity of the enzyme as a percent conversion of the added isotope, while actually enzyme activity should be expressed as micromoles per hour. This requires that the specific radioactivity of the cholesterol is the same in all experiments, that the added isotope is mixed with exactly the same amount of endogenously present cholesterol. Couldn't some of the observed changes be due to changes in liver cholesterol concentration? It must be difficult to assess an enzymatic activity in a system where one adds water-insoluble substrate to a homogenate.

Dr. BOYD: Yes, I quite agree this is a difficulty. The basic problem is that we are confronted with a situation in which the substrate (cholesterol) is present at all times, and perhaps in varying concentrations. Even the best preparations of cytochrome P450 that we have prepared still have cholesterol present. This is, therefore, rather different from other hydroxylation systems, especially drug hydroxylation systems.

Dr. AHRENS: Dr. Boyd, have you looked to see whether or not cholesterol 7α-hydroxylase is inducible with any of the agents that are known to induce hydroxylations in the endoplasmic reticulum, such as barbital?

Dr. BOYD: Yes. In our hands, phenobarbital does not induce this enzyme. The cholesterol 7-α-hydroxylase activity is not raised in animals previously treated with phenobarbital to a level such that the cytochrome P450 will be raised by a factor of 3. Carcinogenic hydrocarbons can actually raise the 7-α-hydroxylase activity.

Dr. MIETTINEN: Dr. Boyd, are you able to detect any of the 7-α-hydroxy cholesterol in the liver of untreated or cholestrymine treated rats?

Dr. BOYD: No, we have not been able to do so.

Dr. CONNOR: If you fed dietary cholesterol to the rat would the activity of this enzyme system change?

Dr. BOYD: When animals are fed 1% cholesterol for five days, the activity of the enzyme was almost doubled.

Discussion Following Dr. Dempsey's Paper

Dr. HOWARD: How much of the triol is normally absorbed?

Dr. DEMPSEY: I believe that Dr. Connor can answer that better than I.

Dr. CONNOR: In the rabbit, it seems to be about 6% of the ^{14}C-labelled triol determined by stool recovery and then checked with the intake.

Dr. HOWARD: Do you think that the effect of the compound is on absorption of cholesterol or on the metabolic effects you have shown here?

Dr. DEMPSEY: One effect is definitely on absorption; another effect, *in vivo*, may also be on cholesterol synthesis. Six percent of the dose, depending upon the dose level, could cause inhibition because *in vitro* the triol is effective at micromolar levels.

The fact that these intestinal slices are inhibited by the triol indicates that the triol can somehow reach the enzyme system in whole cells.

Dr. SCALEN: What are the effects of these inhibitors on kinetic constants such as K_m or V_{max} for the substrates studied?

Dr. DEMPSEY: They would be classed as competitive inhibitors of the Δ^5-dehydrogenase. The type of inhibition seen in the case of the Δ^7-reductase is not so easily classified. It is difficult, with these water insoluble substrates, to do the kinds of experiments required to obtain true kinetic constants. However, we noted that increasing substrate ($\Delta^{5,7}$-cholestadienol) concentration doesn't completely overcome the inhibition. Therefore, I would have to say that the cholestane derivatives are non-competitive inhibitors of the reductase or are causing some kind of mixed inhibition.

Dr. Fumagalli: I wonder if you have seen an accumulation *in vivo* of lathosterol after treatment with the cholestadienol?

Dr. Dempsey: What we see is a compound that migrates slightly more polar than lanosterol, but I can not say that there is not some lanosterol present in association with the unknown compound.

Discussion Following Dr. Moore's Paper

Dr. Miettinen: During the last two years we have carried out ileal bypass operations on 15 patients with Type II hypercholesteremia and carried out sterol balance studies before and after operation.

Neutral sterol excretion was not consistently changed, though in some patients it was significantly reduced, particularly late, several months after operation. Increase of cholesterol elimination from the body, primarily as fecal bile acids, ranged from 1.9 to fivefold, the total increment being about 2.0 g/day. As in Dr. Moore's series, serum cholesterol decreased by about 40%.

As an index of compensatory cholesterol synthesis, we have been using determination of plasma methyl sterols. Their concentration increases from fourfold to sixfold after ileal bypass which is more than one could expect on the basis of fecal steroid elimination. This suggests that cholesterol synthesis increase in some tissues more than can be accounted for in fecal steroid loss. It is possible that the liver, which normally contributes relatively little to serum cholesterol and fecal steroids is now increasing cholesterol synthesis many times, resulting in an increased concentration of plasma methyl sterols.

Dr. Moore: I believe that your studies confirm the changes that we have observed. I think there may be some differences in the methods used for measuring the fecal steroid excretion.

I did not mention any correction made for possible loss of neutral sterols. We have not done this. However, in our studies of 25 patients, we have found that the proportion of the total fecal steroids made up of bile acids is 45%. We believe that if we were losing a significant amount of neutral sterols we would see a change in the percentage of bile acids, unless all of our patients were losing the same amounts of neutral sterols.

The second is that we have found a very high positive correlation between the calculated cholesterol turnover rate and the measured fecal steroid excretion rate in these 25 patients. There is only about 100 mg/day difference between calculated turnover rate and fecal steroid excretion rate. The correlation coefficient is +0.96. So, even though we haven't proven the absence of a loss of neutral sterols, I think that at least we are fairly certain of the magnitudes of our values for fecal steroid excretion.

Dr. Ahrens: Dr. Moore, have you measured turnover by more than one method n any one patient?

Dr. Moore: We have measured turnover rate in some of the patients who had cholesterol synthesis studies and also fecal steroid excretion studies. We have found that the three parameters are generally fairly close together. The calculated turnover rate is a little higher usually than the fecal steroid excretion rate. The estimated synthesis rate before surgery is a little lower than the fecal steroid excretion rate or the turnover rate, but becomes similar to them in the studies after surgery.

Dr. Ahrens: Is it true that the correlation is good between results obtained by all three methods, but, more important, that the absolute data are very similar?

Dr. Moore: Yes, that is correct.

Dr. Ahrens: My second question is directed at choice of therapy. If patients respond favorably to cholestyramine, why perform an ileal bypass? If they do not respond to cholestyramine, when would you decide to perform ileal bypass?

Dr. Moore: Dr. Buchwald has done a study in a few of these patients who have not responded to cholestyramine, but then later did respond to the ileal bypass procedure.

In choosing the patient for therapy, the patient should have the benefit of diet therapy, and perhaps cholestyramine (if they can handle and afford it) or Atromid. If the patient does not respond satisfactorily to any of this therapy, then I believe the ileal bypass procedure should be done.

Our experience in the Type II patients, who make up probably 50% of our group, has been that they have not responded satisfactorily to diet or drug therapy, but they have responded to the ileal bypass procedure. We may be approaching the point where we can say that a Type II patient probably should have the benefit of the operative procedure without wasting a long period of time with present drug therapy.

Section X

ENVIRONMENTAL AND HOST FACTORS IN CORONARY HEART DISEASE, INCLUDING RISK FACTORS: AN EPIDEMIOLOGICAL VIEW

INTRODUCTION

Frederick H. Epstein

A large part of present knowledge about coronary heart disease, from the practical point of view of prediction, prevention, and control, has come from epidemiological studies. Coronary heart disease epidemiology, a discipline virtually unknown twenty years ago, has appeared with a speed and decisive impact which has few parallels in medical science. Indeed, thanks to epidemiological studies, there are now no other chronic diseases, excluding those like tuberculosis which are clearly infectious in origin, which can be predicted with such a high degree of accuracy and none in which so much has been learned about possible causes and the potential for prevention. In fact, progress has been so great that in the view of some a point has been reached where little further advance can be expected; pending new etiological hypotheses, emphasis should be directed toward controlled, preventive trials to establish the causal nature of the associations which have been demonstrated. The first part of this view is open to much argument, but the need for preventive trials is unquestioned; these are covered in another part of this symposium.

Under the circumstances, it was not easy to decide on a topic within the whole field of coronary heart disease epidemiology which would be most suitable for this international symposium. Epidemiologists should be pleased that they might tire an audience so easily with repetitive reports, because this implies good communication of findings and results, though not necessarily their all-important documentation. Yet, a long session devoted to careful, scientific, and critical documentation would not have been very stimulating or transmitted the sense of excitement and new venture which continues to surround the epidemiological approach. Alternatively, emphasis could have been placed on the aspects of epidemiological data which have the most immediate practical applicability, the development of powerful predictive indices and functions to identify high risk groups, or on the epidemiological counterparts of the search for new mechanisms of atheroma formation, for example the interrelationships between carbohydrate and lipid metabolism. Or, a theme could have been chosen to illustrate how epidemiology builds a scientific bridge between clinical and laboratory investigation and what is now so properly called community medicine.

Brief mention has been made of alternative topics to indicate that the one chosen does not span the whole breadth and depth of the discipline. The decision to present a global view in terms of geographic areas was based on several considerations. The belief that the consequences of premature atherosclerosis are preventable comes largely from the demonstration of geographic variations in disease frequency which must be due mostly to the environment which some populations have created for themselves. Identification of the detrimental ingredients of such environments would point one way toward prevention. Yet, despite the obvious scientific and practical importance of geographic variation, no systematic and deliberate attempt has been made, since the very beginnings of such studies, to bring all the information together in one place. In fact, the chairman of this session must confess to a rather selfish interest in the theme proposed to his colleagues on the program committee: to gain for himself a more comprehensive view of a very complex field in which the multitude of accumulating data has made it more and more difficult to see common features and unifying concepts among a great array of detail. Hopefully, then, the presentations comprising this session, given as they are by men of outstanding stature in their own parts of the world, will convey an encompassing picture of the current state of international epidemiological research in coronary heart disease and, by inference, atherosclerosis. Hopefully also, some trends will emerge, on comparison of the findings, which will shed new light on etiological influences, strengthen the evidence regarding existing hypotheses and, perhaps, cast a shadow or two on some treasured notions.

There was an awareness from the beginning that it was possibly overly ambitious to attempt so much in so little time. To the extent that the speakers for their respective areas have had inadequate time to do full justice to all the important work in progress, have had to omit investigations worth reporting or have had to forego critical evaluation of certain findings, the blame should fall upon the chairman who took more than a calculated risk. Still, it would seem that the chance was worth taking, even if nothing were to be gained other than opening and reopening an essential and exciting field of research with immediate practical implications. If more questions are raised than answered, this will be all to the good and set the stage for further work, further collaborative efforts and, eventually, another meeting with a richer harvest.

In order to enhance understanding and comparability of the data to be presented and to ensure coverage of the key issues, there was a great temptation to ask speakers to make their presentations under preassigned subheadings. However desirable in theory, this would probably have been difficult to carry out in practice, dulled individual style, and been rightly resented as pedantic. Nevertheless, the reader will wish to reassemble some of the data according to his own observations and ask certain questions, such as whether nutritional habits have the same importance in all ecological settings or whether the predictive value of serum cholesterol and blood pressure level is similar under different conditions of life.

Finally, due to time limitations, we are acutely aware of gaps in scientific coverage. For instance, little mention will be made of work in Central and South America even though this is a fertile area for research in cardiovascular disease epidemiology. A good deal of epidemiological work is going on in the Soviet Union, partly in collaboration with other countries under the auspices of the World Health Organization. There are networks linking the territorial United States with studies in Puerto Rico and Hawaii and Japan. Small countries may make large contributions; Yugoslavia is one example. Lastly, variations in coronary heart disease frequency commonly occur within the same country, and such intranational differences are sometimes easier to interpret in terms of causative factors than international comparisons.

As this great cavalcade rides past, it should be remembered that it is not engaged in an exercise or a show but headed for a region not included in these reports, where countries will not develop into breeding grounds for atherosclerosis and where the good life in all its aspects has yet to be created.

CURRENT DEVELOPMENTS IN EUROPE

Geoffrey Rose

CHANGING INCIDENCE OF DISEASE

There are large international differences within Europe in coronary heart disease (CHD), both in mortality [1575] and in prevalence [793]. The pattern, however, is capable of swift change. Some countries with a previously low mortality have shown a rapid rise (Table 1). In Norway the rise affects both sexes, but in West Germany it affects only men. In Czechoslovakia, on the other hand, there has been little change in either sex. Among middle-aged men working in offices in various European cities, as far apart as Moscow and Naples, the prevalence of ECG evidence of ischemia is now remarkably uniform (Table 2, based on a W.H.O. cooperative survey, Rose et al., 1968).

Preliminary results from the U.S./U.K./Norwegian Migrants Study show that immigrants from Norway and Britain to the United States aquire the higher CHD mortality of their new country (Reid, personal communication); changes in smoking habit account for only a part of the effect. Similarly, migrants from Italy to Australia show a large increase in CHD mortality occurring progressively over the next 20 years (Table 3, Stenhouse and McCall, 1969). All the evidence suggests that the incidence of this disease can be profoundly altered within a few years by a change in personal or cultural habits, that such changes are still continuing, and that some of the striking current differences within Europe remain unexplained.

GENETIC FACTORS

Familial aggregation of CHD has been recognized for some time. In two recent twin studies in Europe it has been shown to be due, in part at least, to true genetic factors. In a Swedish inquiry into angina prevalence [296] based on mail questionnaires, it was shown that concordance was significantly greater for monozygotic than for dizygotic twins. In the Danish Twin Study (Hauge and Harvald, personal communication) mortality from coronary occlusion was also shown to exhibit significantly greater concordance in monozygotic than in same-sex dizygotic pairs; the genetic effect showed up more clearly in women.

An interesting interaction between genetic and environmental factors has emerged from work on oral contraceptives and their relation to thrombosis.

Table 1. *Patterns of changing mortality from arteriosclerotic and degenerative heart disease (I.S.C. 420–2) in certain European countries, at ages 55–64*

Country	Sex	Deaths/100,000/year										
		1956	1957	1958	1959	1960	1961	1962	1963	1964	1965	1966
Czechoslovakia	M	413	449	403	417	385	396	383	409	428	454	458
	F	164	172	157	153	120	117	120	121	129	130	141
West Germany	M	450	463	448	450	481	500	557	530	525	549	540
	F	177	178	169	165	172	173	186	175	164	175	176
Norway	M	398	420	449	445	478	520	526	588	544	583	599
	F	104	128	115	137	133	143	149	153	146	138	152

Table 2. *Age-adjusted prevalence of S-T depression among middle-aged municipal clerks in various European cities*

	Brussels	The Hague	Milan	Moscow	Naples	Odense
Prevalence percentage	2.5	2.6	3.4	2.8	3.6	2.9

χ^2, 10 d.f. $= 6.04$, $P > 0.8$.

Table 3. *Mortality from arteriosclerotic and degenerative heart disease (I.S.C. 420–2) among male Italian migrants to Australia, compared with native-born Australians, and home-based Italian population*

Country of birth	Years of residence	Deaths/100,000/year		
		age 40–49	age 50–59	age 60–69
Italy	0–6	16	123	260
Italy	7–19	51	170	376
Italy	> 20	130	344	758
Australia	(life-long)	169	592	1,472
Italy	(resident in Italy)	80	240	680

These drugs are known to increase the risk of thrombosis, both in veins and in the cerebral arteries. An effect on coronary thrombosis has not been proven. A cooperative study in Sweden, England and the U.S.A. [749] demonstrated that venous thromboembolism is more likely to occur among women who are not blood group 0, and that this effect is enhanced among women taking oral contraceptives; the relative risk was increased by 60% for women who were not group 0 among medical patients, but by 250% among "pill" takers. This fits in with the observation that CHD is apparently more prevalent among persons who are not group 0 (Allan and Dawson [38], and various earlier studies).

A clue to a possible mechanism of the action of these effects comes from the recent work of Langman et al.[1], Oliver et al. [1123], who report significant

1 Langman, M. J. S., Elwood, P. C., Foote, J., Ryrie, D. R.: AB0 and Lewis blood-groups and serum cholesterol. Lancet **1969 II**, 607.

associations between blood group (both Landsteiner and Lewis), serum cholesterol, and serum intestinal alkaline phosphatase activity. They suggest that there may be genetically determined differences in lipid absorption from the intestine.

HABITS AND ENVIRONMENT

Hardness of Drinking Water. "The water story" continues to unfold. Studies in various countries confirm an inverse relation between water hardness and mortality, particularly, but not exclusively, from cardiovascular diseases. Crawford et al. [339] measured the association in large towns in England and Wales between calcium content of water supply and cardiovascular mortality and obtained a correlation coefficient at ages 45–64 as large as −0.72. The association could not be accounted for in terms of any of a large number of other socioeconomic variables. Necropsy studies by the same group have shown: (a) no general association between water hardness and atherosclerosis [341], although calcification of arteries was much commoner in a hard water area; (b) a higher lead content of bones in a soft water area [342]; (c) a tendency in a soft water area for sudden deaths from CHD to occur in men with less atherosclerosis than corresponding cases in a hard water area.

A recent report from a medical officer of health in East Anglia [1242] describes local changes in mortality following the introduction of artificial water-softening. Two neighboring towns were compared (Table 4). Each was supplied by a different water authority, one of which introduced water-softening in 1958. Six years later this town's cardiovascular and total mortality rates (previously lower than its neighbor's) had become substantially higher.

Diet. Earlier reports by Yudkin [1586] led a number of investigators to attempt to confirm their belief in an association between sugar intake and CHD. These further studies have been generally negative (e.g., Howell and Wilson [723]).

A survey of elderly men in Prague [446] revealed a higher prevalence of CHD among those whose eating was concentrated into a smaller number of meals each day (Table 5). An eating pattern of less frequent meals also tended to be associated with overweight, impaired glucose tolerance, and hypercholesterolemia.

Carbon Disulphide. Following preliminary reports of an association between CHD mortality and prolonged exposure to carbon disulphide, a study was carried out in a viscose rayon factory in Wales (Tiller et al., 1968). A large significant excess of CHD deaths was observed among spinners (exposed to carbon disulphide) as compared with other nonexposed workers. The report points out that this rather special industrial hazard might give a clue of more general importance in the etiology of CHD; cigarette smoke, for example, contains hydrogen sulphide.

Physical Activity. The tendency for an inverse association between occupational activity and CHD is well known. A study among British civil servants (Reid et al., unpublished data) has also shown a strong association between the prevalence of "ischemic-type" ECG findings and the duration of the walk to work each morning (Table 6, Rose [1252]). The association could not be accounted for in terms of differences in age, smoking habit, grade of employment, blood pressure, serum cholesterol or glucose tolerance; those who walked less tended

Table 4. *Mortality changes in Scunthorpe following introduction of water-softening in 1958, compared with the neighboring town of Grimsby where water remained hard*

	1950–53		1964–67	
	Scunthorpe	Grimsby	Scunthorpe	Grimsby
Water hardness (calcium carbonate ppm)	488	224–250	100	224–250
Cardiovascular deaths per 100,000/yr	568	634	704 (+24%)	549(−13%)
Other deaths/100,000/yr	702	926	766 (+9%)	761(−18%)

Table 5. *Association between meal frequency and prevalence of CHD in 1133 men aged 60–64 in Prague*

Meals per day	No. of men	Prevalence percentage of CHD		
		"possible"	"probable"	Total
<4	568	20	30	*50*
4	409	22	24	*46*
>4	156	22	20	*42*

"Probable" only: χ^2 for trend 9.00, $P<0.02$.
"Probable" + "possible": do. 3.75, $P<0.2$.

Table 6. *Relation between duration of daily walk to work and prevalence of "ischemic-type" ECG findings, blood pressure, blood sugar (2 hrs. after 50 g of glucose) and relative ponderal index, among 8,948 male British civil servants aged 40–64 (excluding men with dyspnea or angina, and messengers)*

	Duration of walk to work (min)			
	0	1–9	10–19	≥20
No. of men	389	1,185	4,073	3,301
Percentage with "ischemic-type" ECG	6.33	5.14	4.64	4.18
Mean systolic B.P.	135.5	134.1	134.8	134.5
Mean blood sugar (mg%)	76.4	76.8	77.0	76.7
Mean rel. ponderal index	1.019	0.997	0.994	0.990

Table 7. *Time trends in CHD mortality rates (age-adjusted, per 100,000 per yr.) among British male doctors, 1954–1965, compared with rates for all men in England and Wales*

	Doctors (age)			Rest of country (age)		
	35–64	65–74	75–84	35–64	65–74	75–84
1954–57	294	1,284	2,020	219	1,119	1,821
1958–61	273	1,556	2,496	252	1,274	2,148
1962–65	276	1,492	2,512	290	1,461	2,471

to be a little more overweight. It remains to be seen whether the duration of the walk to work is merely an indicator of some other etiological characteristic (e.g., a generally greater level of physical activity). Alternatively it would be encouraging if further studies were to show that as little as 20 minutes walking each day might help to protect a man from CHD. A controlled trial will be needed to test this hypothesis.

Cigarettes. Despite the overwhelming evidence of an association between cigarettes and mortality, there has, as yet, been no general abandonment of the habit. Doctors, however, have often heeded the warning, and in various countries their smoking rates have declined considerably. In Britain it is reported (Doll and Hill, personal communication) that CHD mortality among doctors is now showing a more favorable time trend than in the country as a whole (Table 7). It is not, of course, certain that this is due entirely to the change in smoking habits, although this is the most likely explanation; but it is at least encouraging evidence that the epidemic of CHD is reversible.

Epidemiologists concerned with CHD are increasingly turning to controlled trials as the only means of testing the nature of observed associations, identifying those risk factors that are actual causes, and evaluating the possibilities of prevention. Various trials are in progress in Europe as well as in America. Among these is a controlled trial being conducted at the London School of Hygiene and Tropical Medicine into the effects of antismoking advice in high-risk subjects. It is already clear that most of these coronary-prone men can be persuaded to give up cigarettes completely. The effect on CHD incidence in this and other preventive trials will be awaited with interest.

CURRENT DEVELOPMENTS IN ATHEROSCLEROSIS STUDIES IN AFRICA

A. G. SHAPER

Developments in Africa were not covered in the First International Symposium on Atherosclerosis in 1966, so this survey of atherosclerosis studies carried out in Africa will summarize what has been done and will review current developments.

The presentation is somewhat factual and nonspeculative, because I am attempting to see whether any significant contribution has indeed come from the African continent and whether the "unique opportunities" for atherosclerosis research, which we so often claim, are in fact present. Whenever possible studies are cited in which direct and matching comparisons have been made between African material and European or North American material.

There can be no doubt that there is a truly low incidence of myocardial infarction and thromboembolic phenomena in virtually all indigenous African peoples and that the incidence of myocardial infarction in those of European and Indian origin permanently settled in Africa is similar to that in Europe and North America [1461]. Over the past decade there has been no apparent increase in myocardial infarction rates in African subjects although the incidence of thromboembolic phenomena, particularly pulmonary embolism, in hospital patients coming to autopsy has more than doubled [896]. It is important to emphasize that African coronary arteries, aortas, and cerebral vessels are not immune to atherosclerosis, and myocardial infarction does occur in African subjects, albeit very infrequently. When found, it is usually seen in an autopsy of an elderly person and is usually associated with significant atherosclerosis and often with hypertension [845].

MORPHOLOGY AND BIOCHEMISTRY

Direct comparison of coronary arteriosclerosis has been made between matched African (East and West) and white American groups, using a method based on the premise that thickening of the coronary arteries provides a reasonably good estimate of the amount of arteriosclerosis present [361]. The Africans have significantly less coronary arteriosclerosis and less foci of lipid deposition and calcification than the white Americans [1326]. Differences in coronary artery thickness between the two groups are apparent by the age of 20 and are more pronounced between males from the two areas than between females [467]. Histologically, American whites aged 20–40 years have significantly more atheromatous lesions than Africans, and the majority of the coronary artery lesions in Africans are of the preatheroma type [362] without necrosis and with very little lipid. Comparative studies of aorta, coronary, and cerebral vessels in white and black South Africans show a low atherosclerosis index in all subjects until the third decade; then there is a progressive rise, most dramatic in the aorta and coronaries of white men. The cerebral vessels are about equally affected in the two racial groups, and cerebrovascular disease as a cause of death is as common in the African male and female as in the white male and female. No coronary occlusions occur in the Africans [977].

In general, the more advanced coronary arteriosclerosis in white Americans and white South Africans is accompanied by considerably more biochemically demonstrable lipid than is seen in African subjects and by a high cholesterol-triglyceride ratio in the coronary artery [976, 1330]. White Americans also have more oleic acid and less palmitic and stearic acid in their coronaries. They show considerable individual variation in the amount of lipid present, particularly cholesterol, in keeping with the considerable individual variation in their amount of arteriosclerosis and in contrast to the uniformly low amounts of lipids and uniformly small amount of arteriosclerosis in African coronary arteries.

In more detailed pathological and biochemical studies [1327] it is seen that below 30 years of age the cholesterol content of African and American white coronary arteries is not significantly different, despite very clear differences in the blood cholesterol levels from childhood. Furthermore, the kinds of fatty acids and the relative proportion of each one are similar in East African and American whites. From 30–39 years onwards, the cholesterol and lipid phosphorus levels are markedly higher in white American coronaries. The only real qualitative difference in the kinds of lipids in the arteries of white Americans and Africans is seen in the fourth decade.

The general qualitative similarity of the coronaries in the two groups suggests that coronary atherosclerosis is not a different disease in the two groups but is only present to a different degree. Thus, African males in the third and fourth decades have less coronary atherosclerosis because they have less of the same kind of lipids than American whites, not because Africans have unusual classes of lipids or fatty acids in their coronaries. In children, the only difference seen was that American white children had more "fatty streaks" than African children, suggesting a possible relationship between fatty patches and atheroma.

Studies in South Africa [976] show that quantitative chemical differences between corresponding arteries of European and African children are slight in the first six months of life. The chemical changes associated with atherosclerosis develop earlier and progress faster in the aortas and coronary arteries of Europeans than the corresponding arteries of Africans. Male subjects show increasing interracial differences in total lipid content of these vessels from the third decade onwards; no interracial differences are seen in the coronary arteries of females or in the cerebral vessels of males or females. The same pattern is followed by cholesterol, phospholipids and calcium concentrations; triglyceride levels only showed an interracial difference in the aortas.

The differences between Africans and Americans (white or black) in the blood levels of cholesterol, triglycerides, lipid phosphorus, and total esterified fatty acids have been repeatedly demonstrated [851]. When relatively wealthy East Africans were compared with poor East Africans and with white Americans, the poor East Africans showed the expected low levels of serum cholesterol while the levels in wealthy East Africans did not differ from their American white counterparts. Despite this similarity, the serum fatty acid patterns were quite different in the two groups, with the wealthy Africans showing a significantly lower proportion of polyunsaturated fatty acids and lower levels of cholesterol lineolate [1329]. This useful study emphasizes the qualitative differences which may be present despite similar total or esterified cholesterol levels in groups and these differences may be of biological and pathogenetic significance.

Studies in the composition of the adipose tissue of African and non-African groups has not yielded information of obvious significance. Despite striking differences in diet, comparison of African, Indian, and European subjects (communities differing significantly in their incidence of atherosclerosis) showed no marked differences except for lower concentrations of lauric and myristic acid in African subjects [957]. Comparison of East African subjects with North American white and black groups confirmed the well-known differences in blood lipid levels between Americans and Africans, but there were only very small differences in the relative values for fatty acids. Oleic acid levels were lower in the African subjects and palmitic and palmitoleic were significantly higher. All groups had adequate reserves of linoleic acid [851]. A similar study in East African and North American diabetics showed that the fatty acid pattern of adipose tissue was not strikingly different from their nondiabetic counterparts with oleic acid again being lowest in East Africans [1346].

In South Africa, comparisons of adipose tissue fatty acids were carried out on white, colored and African males and females [831]. Interracial differences were confined to myristate which showed a progressive fall from white through colored to African subjects, which was strikingly correlated with the total fat intake of these groups. For no clear reasons, linoleate levels were higher in the colored group.

Thus, despite marked differences in the dietary habits of the various racial groups studied, the depot fat composition was very similar among them.

BLOOD COAGULATION AND LYSIS

There has been an intermittent interest over the past decade in the possibility that African subjects might be protected from thromboembolic phenomena and also perhaps from severe atherosclerosis by having a different pattern of blood coagulation. Comparative studies in white and African subjects in South Africa [973] indicated lower plasma prothrombin levels and serum factor VII levels in Africans but better prothrombin consumption and increased levels of antihemophilic globulin. There was clearly no evidence to suggest that the African's freedom from severe atherosclerosis or myocardial infarction is due to a lesser coagulability of his blood.

On the other hand, fibrinolytic activity was much greater in the African subjects. In a comparison of coagulation and clot-lysis in East African and American white subjects matched for age and sex, using material preserved in liquid nitrogen, the African subjects were found to have shorter euglobulin lysis times than the Americans and shorter clot-lysis times on urokinase stimulation [849]. In a more comprehensive study on fresh material [1345] indigenous East Africans were compared with Indian subjects living in Uganda, the latter group having a high incidence of myocardial infarction. Fibrinolytic activity was significantly greater in African than Indian subjects, and in Indians with an abnormal glucose tolerance test the lysis time was even longer than in Indian nondiabetic subjects. The Indian subjects also had a greater clot-binding power than the African subjects. No differences were observed in platelet adhesiveness between African and Indian subjects, but a striking difference in venous flow rate was seen (very slow flow rates in African subjects), possibly related to differences in blood viscosity. In the Indian subjects, there was a significant interrelationship of lysis time with both skinfold thickness and with serum cholesterol level, but not with the serum triglyceride level.

In a further study in which Africans, Indian, and European subject in Uganda were studied, these fibrinolysis findings were confirmed, and platelet adhesiveness, measured by the rotating bulb technique and by the glass-bead filter technique, was exactly the same in all three racial groups (Shaper et al., unpublished data).

In African and Indian young men (about 20 years old) fibrinolytic activity is brisk and is the same in both groups. In middle-aged and elderly Africans, the fibrinolytic activity remains unchanged and is as brisk as that seen in the young Africans and Indians. Only in the Indian and European subjects studied is there a striking decrease in fibrinolytic activity with increasing age.

RISK FACTORS

A great deal of concern focuses on the "risk" factors in atherosclerosis, i.e. hypertension, diabetes mellitus, cigarette smoking and possibly obesity, sedentary occupation and mental stress. Diabetes mellitus is a common disease in most African countries, and hypertension is probably the commonest of all cardiovascular disorders in the continent. While there are small, often isolated groups in whom blood pressure levels are low and do not rise with increasing age, these groups represent the exceptional and not the usual finding. The concurrence of diabetes mellitus, obesity and hypertension is also common, and yet despite the presence of all these conditions in middle-aged or elderly subjects for periods of 10–20 years, myocardial infarction is as rare in the African diabetic or hypertensive subject as it is in the rest of the African populations. Cigarette smoking is not a common habit, and its importance cannot be assessed.

A high degree of physical activity is assumed to be present in most communities in the underdeveloped parts of the world that are usually free from myocardial infarction. It might be wise to temper this assumption with fact; detailed ergonomic studies in agricultural communities in Africa indicate that because of limiting environmental factors very modest amounts of work (2 to 3.5 hours per day) are possible and are indeed carried out [222].

There are still a few cardiovascular philosophers who enthuse over the uncomplicated, non-competitive life of the noble savage. Those more familiar with the stresses of poverty and violence and the problems of traditional societies will cite factual testimony to the frequency of emotional stress factors in developing societies.

In brief, it would appear that the so-called risk factors are really aggravating factors which accelerate the development of atherosclerosis and increase the risk of myocardial infarction in communities already prone to atherosclerosis and its complications, but will not do so in communities not prone to develop complicated atherosclerosis.

"EXCEPTIONAL" GROUPS

In Africa there are several isolated groups of particular interest to those concerned with atherosclerosis. These are the nomadic peoples of Somalia, Kenya, and Tanzania whose diets consist mainly of milk, meat and blood. They are lean, active people in whom blood pressure levels are low and do not rise with increasing age and in whom there is apparently no clinical or electrocardiographic evidence of ischemic heart disease (IHD). Despite the reported dietary background, these groups usually have low blood cholesterol levels, although in one group, the camel-herding Rendille nomads of Northern Kenya, Western patterns of cholesterol levels are seen [842, 917, 1344]. It has been claimed that these groups are exceptional in that they constantly live on high fat diets without showing hypercholesterolemia or complicated atherosclerosis. It is also suggested that "freedom from emotional stress or abundance of physical exercise may be present as overriding protective mechanisms despite a long continued diet of milk and meat" [917]. Stamler (1968) has critically reviewed these "exceptional" groups and emphasizes that serious doubts must be raised as to the validity of the very high food intake estimates in a population engaged in moderate physical activity who are generally very lean. There seems good evidence that nutritional trends, i.e. irregularity of food supply on a seasonal basis, are of major importance in accounting for the pattern of cholesterolemia in these population groups, as indeed in other groups throughout the world. Certainly, "western" psychological stresses are not essential for the development of hypercholesterolemia, and the capacity of habitual physical activity to prevent hypercholesterolemia is at best limited. Until further reliable data on the habitual diets throughout the year of these nomadic peoples are forthcoming, the exceptional status of these groups must remain in doubt.

ANIMALS IN AFRICA—WITH EMPHASIS ON ELEPHANTS

The animals of Africa have attracted almost as much attention as the so-called "exceptional" human groups, and, perhaps, one should make comment on the much-publicized statement that elephants suffer from atherosclerotic heart disease. Fibrous intimal plaques have been described in the aorta and coronary arteries of wild East African elephants, but lipid deposition was not a constant or conspicuous feature of the lesions and ulceration, hemorrhage and thrombosis were never seen. Most of the plaque lipid was cholesterol with a mean value by weight of 3%. Medial sclerosis was a much more prominent lesion, and these medial lesions increased in number, size, and severity with age much more rapidly than the intimal lesions. Both medial and intimal lesions were more common in female elephants at all ages than in male elephants. The mean plasma cholesterol level in the elephants was 80 mg/100 ml and triglycerides were 35 mg/100 ml. There was a correlation observed between the level of plasma cholesterol and the severity of atherosclerosis in the elephant population (McCullagh, 1969) [948]. It seems widely accepted that aortic fatty streaks and fibrous plaques in ruminants are not necessarily a consequence of a diet rich in saturated fatty acids or of a high cholesterol level in the plasma, and the significance of these comparative arterial studies to the understanding of human atherosclerosis is probably limited.

Probably of greater importance are the findings of Crawford [337] who has compared the tissue fatty acid patterns in domestic British cattle with those obtained in wild buffalo from Uganda. The British beef contained 10 times as much lipid as the wild buffalo meat and even more striking was the difference in the proportion of fatty acids containing more than one double bond. In wild buffalo of woodland habitats 30% of the fatty acids were polyunsaturated; in wild buffalo of grassland areas, 10% were polyunsaturated while domestic British beef contained only 2% polyunsaturated fatty acids.

Analysis of the fatty acids from other East African wild animals showed that those living on oil rich woodland and bushland vegetation also had the higher percentage (23–29%) of polyunsaturated fatty acids. Animals living on water rich grassland resembled domestic animals, man, and zoo animals in having 2–8% of poylunsaturated fatty acids, with the exception of domestic chicken which had 17% polyunsaturated fatty acids. Preliminary analysis of the lipids of hearts and aortas showed that the fatty acids of these tissues also differed in wild and domesticated animals.

Since man's tissue lipids approximate the domestic pattern on which he is dependent, the question is raised as to whether the total domestic development of water-rich vegetation is nutritionally detrimental to man and whether the resultant low balance of polyunsaturated to saturated and monounsaturated fatty acids may be related to arterial disesae.

MAJOR OPPORTUNITIES IN AFRICA FOR RESEARCH INTO ATHEROSCLEROSIS

In attempting to define these major opportunities, I will focus on those situations which are possibly unique. In the economically advanced countries of the world, virtually everyone in the population is at risk insofar as the development of severe atherosclerosis and myocardial infarction is concerned. Factors of age and sex, and certain atherosclerosis-accelerating factors further determine which individuals among the prone community will suffer death or incapacity. In studies of the basic underlying process of atherosclerosis and in the study of those factors which lead to the complications of atherosclerosis, there are virtually no control groups available which can be matched by age and sex with those manifestly ill with the disease. In the African scene, situations exist in which control populations virtually free from severe atherosclerosis and its complications live in close proximity to communities in which the problem is severe. Furthermore, rapid and progressive changes in socioeconomic circumstances are providing even better control groups, racially identical but differing significantly in dietary patterns and other socioeconomic circumstances. These situations provide an opportunity for the testing of hypotheses concerning the mechanisms of atherosclerosis and of thrombus formation and dissolution. It seems not unreasonable (to the simple mind) to assume that those parameters which are truly fundamental to the development of severe atherosclerosis and its complications should be manifestly different when measured in communities prone to the disease as compared directly with those communities which are not. Thus, blood lipid and arterial lipid values do show this difference. Fibrinolytic activity does also and relates to blood cholesterol, body fatness, and reduced glucose tolerance; while platelet adhesiveness does not show the difference that the simple mind requires for a parameter to be regarded as fundamental to the problem. It is in this field of clot formation and dissolution that Africa offers a particularly useful research opportunity, if not a unique one.

If a particular pattern of diet is the major determinant among the multiple factors involved in the etiology and pathogenesis of atherosclerotic disease, then the work of Crawford on the fat content and composition of animal products is of extreme interest. I would suggest this field as, perhaps, a truly unique one in which Africa may make a major contribution to the story of atherosclerosis and possibly to the primary prevention of the severe disease and its complications. The comparative studies of various animals for vascular lesions, interesting and useful though this approach may be, is not the correct one; rather by the improved knowledge of how the feeding of domestic animals may affect their tissues and their by-products and how these may ultimately affect man and his blood vessels, a major contribution may develop.

CURRENT DEVELOPMENTS IN THE EPIDEMIOLOGY OF ATHEROSCLEROSIS IN ISRAEL

JACK H. MEDALIE

The Middle East continues to be a cauldron of seething upheavals, and in recent decades the interplay of political, military, social, and economic forces has led to two streams of immigration. One comes from Europe following World War II and the Nazi atrocities and the second from the Middle-Eastern and North African countries with the opening of Israel's borders to any Jew. Within the country too, we have witnessed large movements of population.

The new environment thus created has demanded processes of adjustment from the immigrants and the "hosts" which almost defy the imagination. With this adjustment, the morbidity and mortality patterns of the hosts and of the migratory groups, (which resembled those from their countries of origin) are changing rapidly. Even Beduin have developed myocardial infarction. The present pleuralistic population of Israel consists of nearly three million 86% of whom are professed Jews. Of the latter 2.4 million, 43% are locally born, 30% from Europe, and 27% from Asia or Africa.

Unique opportunities in this area exist. Whether they have been utilized is an open question. I shall try to review briefly some of the recent developments related to atherosclerosis.

Pathology. The work of Sacks and Vlodower [1277] on 904 autopsies of adults aged 40 and over as well as of an eleven-year analysis of death certificates and an investigation of 400 medico-legal autopsies [1014] have confirmed the preponderance of European-born males as compared to those born in other countries in possessing myocardial infarction or coronary thrombosis. There is also a higher proportion of males at all ages dying with this condition than females.

It seems to be agree, that while the atherosclerotic changes found in the arteries are structurally similar among all the different cultural groups, there are fewer (as evidenced by narrowing) among the Eastern-born adults. The prevalence of macroscopically visible scars in the myocardium is no different between European-born males and Asian-African born. These scars are called "old infarcts" by the pathologists. I wonder whether this is the correct term and, if so, what is the explanation of their equal occurrence among the preceding groups?

Investigating 211 consecutive autopsies among Ashkenazi, Yemenite, and Beduin infants and fetuses, Neufeld, Vlodower et al. [1504] found that while the developmental structural pattern of the coronary arteries were similar in all three groups, quantitative differences in the thickness of the walls were already apparent at this tender age.

The Ashkenazi male infants had more intima and musculoelastic tissue than their female counterparts as well as having more than the Yemenites or Beduin males. The females interestingly showed no ethnic differences, and there were no sex differences between the Yemenites and Beduin. Let us then accept the fact that the atherosclerotic process is structurally the same in all groups studied and begins at a very early stage in life. To explain the rest of these early findings we have to postulate that the cultural behavior patterns of Ashkenazi women start influencing the arteries of male offspring *in utero* or shortly after birth

Table 1. *Ischemic heart disease prevalence. (Age-adjusted rates/100)*

	Eastern Europe	Central Europe	Southern Europe	Israel	Middle East	North Africa	Total	Regional differences (*p*)
Number examined	1,928	1,374	1,735	1,431	2,372	1,219	10,059	—
Angina pectoris (definite)	4.0	3.7	4.0	3.3	2.4	2.2	3.3	<0.01
Verified previous myocardial inf.	2.8	2.6	1.5	2.0	0.7	0.9	1.8	<0.01
ECG: probable possible infarct and LBBB	2.7	3.1	1.8	2.0	1.2	1.7	2.1	<0.01
IHD Group I	3.2	3.1	1.9	2.4	1.0	1.8	2.3	<0.01
Rank order (1-highest, 3-lowest)	1		2		3			

Table 2. *Vascular lesions of the central nervous system* [a, b]

Age groups	Born in Africa/Asia		Born in Europe/America	
	male	female	male	female
45–54	47.4	60.2	31.4	31.3
55–64	227.0	277.2	144.5	145.7
65–74	701.0	769.0	611.1	638.6

[a] Mortality rates (per 100,00) in Israel (1950–1960) as reported in death certificates (ICD: 330–334).
[b] Modified from Kall and Groen.

but for some reason the female fetuses are immune to this process; or is this due to "gene" transmission?

Biochemistry. Besides the work on arterial wall metabolism, reported on at this conference by Stein, Zehavi and Dreyfus [1587] might have found a laboratory method for differentiating "thrombotic states" from other conditions, e.g. cerebral hemorrhage, by utilizing a platelet aggregation method.

Ischemic Heart Disease. Dreyfus et al. in 1953 first observed the ethnic differences in the prevalence of myocardial infarcts among hospitalized patients in Israel. Recently gross differences between the Beduins, Arab villagers, and Jewish port workers were reported by Groen et al. [574, 575] with the Beduins having the lowest prevalence rates of myocardial infarction and lowest cholesterol values, followed by Arab villagers with the port workers having the highest rates and values.

These differences were further confirmed by Medalie, Neufeld, Riss et al. [964] reporting on the first stage of a long-term prospective population study of ischemic heart disease among a stratified-random sample of over 10,000 adult male civil employees who found significant variations between areas of birth for the prevalence of angina pectoris, myocardial infarction and ischemic heart disease (IHD) (Table 1). The six areas of birth grouped themselves into a rank order with Eastern and Central Europeans having the highest rates while the Middle Easterners and North Africans the lowest. Israeli born and those from South-Eastern Europe tended to lie somewhere between these extremes for all diagnoses (Table 1).

Emphasizing the difficulties and pitfalls of prevalence data, Medalie, Kahn et al. [963, 964] continued testing the association of Group I, severest ischemic heart disease group, with selected variables while adjusting both for age and area of birth. The associations found resemble those found in similar studies, and the results and associations of the five-year incidence study should be available shortly.

Cerebrovascular Accidents (CVA). A true deficiency in this area has been the absence of a population study of cerebrovascular events, because the biases inherent in studies of mortality and morbidity based on death certificates for hospitalized patients are difficult to measure and interpret. However, certain tendencies or patterns which emerge from the recently reported studies are:

1. Equal mortality rates between the sexes with a tendency for higher female rates irrespective of area of birth or age groups (over 45).

2. Unlike ischemic heart disease, cerebrovascular mortality rates are higher in those born in Asia or Africa (Table 2).

3. The cerebrovascular events of the European-born tend to be occlusive processes, e.g. thrombosis [23, 846, 847].

4. The interplay of cerebral and cardiovascular pathology is an unclear field. Lavy, Carmon et al. [846] found a significant increase in ECG abnormalities among CVA patients in all age decades as compared to controls. They suggest that these arrhythmias, conduction disorders, and any condition reducing cardiac output may facilitate cerebral ischemic episodes.

On the other hand, Blum et al. experimenting on cats found that stimulation of certain cerebral and hypothalamic areas led not only to the production of epileptic attacks but also to ischemic changes and arrhythmias on the ECG. Thus, some of the ECG changes reported by Lavy et al. [846, 847] may have their origin in the stimulation of cerebral areas during cerebrovascular events. Also, Cahana et al. stressed the relationship of generalized systemic disorders such as polycythemia, subacute bacterial endocarditis etc. among 33 patients under 40 years of age with a cerebrovascular accident.

ASSOCIATED CONDITIONS

Diabetes Mellitus. Contradicting the impression of clinicians, the prevalence and two-year incidence of diabetes mellitus among 10,000 adult males aged 40 and over (Herman et al.) shows (Table 3) high rates among the Middle East and North African males as compared to the European-born.

If the North Africans and Middle Easterners have such high rates of diabetes mellitus and the latter is a definite risk factor in the production of ischemic heart disease, why do these groups of people have so little IHD? Is diabetes only a recent phenomenon and, therefore, in a decade or two they will have high rates of IHD, or are other factors at work, e.g. physical activity, which counterbalance this increased amount of diabetes? Can it be that diabetes is a somewhat different condition among the Asians? Before dismissing this thought, it is interesting to note that Brunner and Altman [254] found greatly reduced rates of complications among 76 long-standing adult Yemenite diabetics (except for retinopathy) when compared to matched case-controlled nondiabetics.

Table 3. *Prevalence and incidence of diabetes mellitus. Age-adjusted rates per 1,000 males aged 40 and over*

	Eastern Europe	Central Europe	South-East-Europe	Israel	Middle East	North Africa	Total
Prevalence	40.5	37.8	42.5	62.5	56.5	59.5	49.5[a]
Two-year incidence	8.5	16.2	15.2	14.3	20.3	17.1	15.5[b]

[a] 498 out of 10,059.
[b] 144 out of 9,079.

Advancing to a multivariate analysis of 15 variables with the two-year development of diabetes [767] revealed that the three variables age, weight/height ratio and peripheral vascular disease were strongly related to the incidence. The association of peripheral vascular disease with the development of diabetes mellitus was an unexpected finding which raises many important questions. Is diabetes mellitus in obese, middle and old age adults primarily due to generalized peripheral vascular changes which among other things lead to disturbed carbohydrate metabolism and increased blood glucose levels? Have these people normal insulin levels? As diastolic blood pressure is related to age and height-weight index and is dependent on increased peripheral resistance, why is it not strongly associated with the development of diabetes? If we could unravel some of these mysteries we might advance considerably in our understanding of ischemic heart changes as well.

One further point about diabetes is this interesting epidemiological finding: there is a significant inverse relationship between diabetes and serum uric acid [672], which is thought to be due to differential and competitive reabsorption in the proximal tubules of the kidneys.

Blood Pressure. The distribution of casual blood pressure readings among 10,000 adult males revealed the expected rise with age but no bimodality in the distribution curves. It also revealed a remarkable uniformity and lack of variation among the larger areas of birth as well as between four individual countries (Iraq, Yemen, Poland and Germany). Two interesting findings of the same study were: (a) that the correlation between systolic pressure and overweight (weight/height ratio) is simply a reflection of the more basic association of diastolic pressure with overweight, and (b) an inverse relationship between blood pressure readings and the diameter of the major and minor arterioles in the fundus of the eye (Michaelson et al.).

Continuing the blood pressure analyses on the 10,000 adult males, Kahn carried out a multiple regression analysis and found that the total proportion of variance in systolic pressure associated with a linear combination of the eighteen independent variables investigated was 21.6% for the entire study group and ranged from 16.6% in East Europeans to 29.0% for North-African born. The four variables which were significantly associated by multiple regression analysis with variance in systolic pressure in all areas of birth were age, pulse rate, ECG ischemic changes (interesting new feature), and weight/height ratio.

One of the fascinating findings of this analysis is a point about which epidemiologists have been dreaming and talking for a long time. This is the fact that there is varying significance of some of the variables in different areas of birth. Some variables (e.g. age and pulse rate) are significantly related to the systolic pressure right across the board (while others, e.g. smoking, diabetes, and number of children in family, are significantly related to systolic pressure in some areas of birth but not in others. Are some of these statistical coincidences? More likely they show that in the multifactorial constellation of systolic pressure, the same variables have differing degrees of importance in the different areas of birth. The implications of these findings for more specific preventive activities are extremely important.

Physical Activity and Fitness. Although no definitive study has been done in this area, a few reports all point to a pattern of an inverse relationship between physical activity or fitness and various parameters of ischemic heart disease. Some of these studies are the following: (a) A group of "low-risk" adults were found to be distinctly more fit than a "high-risk" ischemic heart group. (b) Captive monkeys with little opportunity for physical activity gained weight and showed marked structural changes in their coronary arteries and increase of pericardial fat, as compared to monkeys on the same diet but with much more freedom of activity [1504]. Interestingly, both groups showed a steady rise in serum cholesterol and phospholipids. Could this be related to the stress of captivity more than to diet and/or physical activity? (c) There were gross ischemic heart morbidity differences between sedentary (seated at least 80% of their working time) and non-sedentary workers among 5,279 males and 5,229 females followed retrospectively by Manelis, Brunner et al. [915] over a 15-year period on the Kibbutzim (collective cooperative settlements). These differences were of the magnitude that would be hard to explain away on the basis of selection factors, personality, other illnesses etc., that are inherent in this type of study. A subsample of these workers showed no differences in their average serum total cholesterol, the percentage alpha cholesterol or their triglycerides, leading the authors to suggest that the effect of physical activity is "not mediated via serum lipoprotein levels".

Psycho-social Aspects. Every serious clinician is convinced of the importance of psycho-social aspects in the production and precipitation of myocardial infarction and yet the proof of this still eludes us. This failure has many facets, including the inability to measure stressful factors in a valid and reliable way as well as the fact that some recent Israeli studies suffer from having been carried out on controls and patients after the infarct [403]. An attempt has been made to measure some of the social aspects of living such as the different forms of social mobility in a long-term prospective study on 10,000 adult males, and it will be interesting to see whether Shamgar, Laslou et al. come up with some of the answers that we need.

Cholesterol and Dietary Factors. Total serum cholesterol levels range widely between the different ethnic groups with the nomadic Beduins having the lowest. Even, however, at the other extreme, the highest values, among the Central and Eastern European born Israeli Jews, are distinctly lower than those recorded by the large American population studies.

The distribution of cholesterol among the 10,000 over 40 male government employees rose with age till the 50–54 age group, after which it plateaued off [767]. The distribution curves were "normal" and those of each of the six areas of birth resembled each other closely. The age-adjusted mean ranged from a low of 195 mg-% among the North African born to a high of 219 mg-% of the Central Europeans. Although in absolute figures this range is not a large one, the variation between the areas of birth was significant ($p<0.01$).

The dietary patterns of the 10,000 government males have been recorded (Medalie [964], *Physician's Fact Book*) as well as those of special groups such as Beduins and Yemenites (Groen et al.). The North Africans (and Middle East born) have a larger intake of calories mainly from carbohydrates derived from bread, which accounts for about one-third of their daily calories and their large intake of vegetable proteins. Their total and saturated fat intake, however, is lower than the Central Europeans (Table 4). Groen mentions a low content of sugar and cholesterol intake among the Beduins and Yemenites. This was not characteristic in the large survey of the North Africans or those from the Middle East.

A multiple regression analysis of 18 selected independent variables as related to cholesterol [767] shows that the proportion of cholesterol variance associated with a linear combination of these variables was 10.3% for the total study population. This reflected a range from a low of 6.6% for East Europeans to a high of 12.3% for those born in the Middle East. After allowing for those on diet, there was only a small increase, and the range was from 7.4% to 13.4%. In no area, however, did all dietary variables explain as much as 3% of the cholesterol variance. These percentages are dismally small in terms of ability to estimate or predict an individual's cholesterol value having knowledge of his status with respect to the dietary and all other independent variables examined (Table 5). Turning to the individual variables we note again (cf. under blood pressure) that while one variable, hematocrit, shows a significant association in all areas of birth, other variables such as weight/height ratio, blood pressure, smoking, bread etc. are significant in some areas of birth but not in others (Table 6).

The only items of diet significantly associated with cholesterol are total carbohydrate and bread, among those born in Central Europe. Bread is the only variable to show a negative relationship; it does this in some other areas of birth too, although the association was not significant. This poses a problem.

Table 4. *Distribution of dietary variables by area of birth. Average age-adjusted values/day*

		North Africa 1,191	Central Europe 1,363	Units
Calories:	Total	2,928	2,645	cals.
Fat:	Total	88	97	g
	Saturated	26	33	g
	Oleic acid (mono-unsat)	30	33	g
	Linol. acid (poly-unsat)	22	20	g
CHO:	Total	421	341	g
	from starch	300	215	g
	from sugar	121	126	g.
Protein:	Total	110	100	g
	Animal	49	45	g
	Vegetable	61	46	g
Calories from bread		1,026	690	cals.
Weight		73	73	kg
Wt/ht ratio		4.44	0.43	kg/cm
Total serum cholesterol		195	219	mg%

Table 5. *Cholesterol multiple regression analysis. Cholesterol percentage variance associated with variables*

Variable		Percentage of variance[a] ($n = 9{,}902$)
Fat:	Total	
	Saturated F.A.	
	Oleic A (M-U)	
	Linoleic A (P-U)	
Chol:	Total	
	Starch	
	Eggs	
	Bread	
Total calories		
Education		2.3
Wt/ht		1.7
Systolic B.P.		1.0
"Problems"		
Hematocrit		2.4
Age		0.8
Smoking		0.7
Uric acid		1.2
All fats[b]		0.8
All diet items[b]		1.9
All items (= 100 R^2)		10.3

[a] Not shown unless significantly diff. from zero.
[b] After allowance for all nondietary variables.

Is bread important *per se* in relation to low cholesterol levels, or is the consumption of bread part of a pattern of life which includes a large amount of physical activity etc., all of which together reduce the cholesterol level? The question is partly answered by Groen's finding that by substituting bread for the saturated

Table 6. *Cholesterol multiple regression analysis. Selected variables significantly associated with cholesterol by area of birth*

	Total	Israel	East Europe	Central Europe	South Europe	Middle East	North Africa
Hematocrit	+	+	+	+	+	+	+
Wt/ht	+		+			+	+
Age	+			+		+	
Smoking	+		+	+	+		
Bread				—			
"Problems"							
Sat. fat acid							

fat in the diet, he obtained a decrease in average serum cholesterol of volunteer groups to levels as low as when the saturated fat was replaced by polyunsaturated fat, suggesting that bread *per se* is important.

The absence of a significant association between cholesterol and diet in a "free-living" population group contrasts strikingly with the results of human experimental dietary studies, where groups of Europeans were put on Yemenite-type diets [573, 574, 575] and Yemenites were put on Western-type diets [254]. The former groups showed a decrease in their average cholesterol values, while those of the latter groups increased markedly. In other words, on an experimental short-term basis there does not seem to be any doubt that a marked change of diet can produce an alteration in the average total serum cholesterol in a relatively short time. Possible explanations for the difference between the volunteer and population studies follow:

(a) The methods of dietary evaluation in population studies are insufficiently accurate.

(b) The changes in volunteer groups are a short-term effect and might not be sustained over a long follow-up period.

(c) There is no major relationship between diet and cholesterol in free-living population groups. Together with this there is perhaps a sufficient relationship so that, if all other factors are kept constant and the diet is changed, the cholesterol level can and evidently does respond.

CURRENT DEVELOPMENTS IN INDIA*

Ivan J. Pinto, Peter Thomas, F. Colaco and K. K. Datey**

Western researchers have shown that high levels of certain biological variables like serum cholesterol, serum triglycerides, blood pressure, weight and glucose

* The authors wish to thank the Dean of the K.E.M. Hospital for permission to publish this work.

** Pinto, I. J., Vahia, N. S., Vengsarkar, A. S., De Souza, A.: Report to the Indian Council of Medical Research (1968).

tolerance are associated with coronary heart disease. However, it is quite apparent from the reports of several Indian workers that Indians develop ischemic heart disease (IHD) at serum lipid and blood pressure levels much below those generally seen in western countries. In the present report an attempt is made to assess the role of various factors in the causation of ischemic heart disease with the help of a review of the recent literature from Indians and the personal experience of the authors.

Prevalence of IHD. Most of the studies on the prevalence of coronary heart disease in India have been based on hospital admissions, and it has been expressed as a proportion of coronary heart disease among cardiac cases. This proportion varies from 11% to 23% in most hospitals (see Table 1). A few studies have

Table 1. *Incidence of IHD in different parts of India*

Author	State	Percentage of IHD	Source	Duration of study
K. S. Mathur et al. [940]	UP, North India	23.3	Hospital, private	1947–1961
Bhargwa et al. [151]	Rajasthan, North India	13.57	Hospital admissions	1945–1964
Padmavati [1143]	Delhi, North India	11.29	Hospital admissions	1951–1955
Samani [1286]	Maharashtra, South-West India	12.1	Hospital admissions	1941–1956
Warrier [1524]	Kerala, South India	21.7	Hospital admissions	1966

compared the proportion of coronary heart disease admitted to the hospital over the years and have shown an increase in incidence. In Indian hospitals, admissions are restricted to serious cases needing urgent admission and this leads to erroneous results.

Few epidemiological studies of IHD (see Table 2) have been carried out in India using strict clinical and electrocardiographic criteria for diagnosis. Among these the report of Sarvotham [1296] requires special mention. They surveyed 2,030 persons, which constituted about 7% of the total urban population of Chandigarh (North India), with 100% response. The prevalence among 1,233 males in Chandigarh from 30 to 60 years comes to 65.4 per thousand which is nearly the same as in Tucumseh, U.S.A. [439]. This is lower than in Kagan's [766] series at Framingham (96 per thousand) and the Rhondda Fach Valley [679] with a prevalence of 106 per thousand. The prevalence in a study of people over 30 years of age conducted in a sector of the city of Bombay composed of semi-skilled workers showed a prevalence of 29 cases per thousand. The total sample studied which was 569, constituted 25% of the people residing in that area.

Age. The peak prevalence of coronary heart disease in the Chandigarh group [1296] was in the age group over 70 years, while the peak prevalence in the Bombay group was in the age group 50–60 years, the same as European and

American studies [679, 766]. The prevalence of ischemic heart disease in the age group below 40 is 24 per thousand in the Chandigarh series [1296].

The proportion of young patients with IHD is also quite high in the series reported from Bombay; 36% of our cases were below 40 years and 17% of cases of Shah [1342] were below 40 years.

Table 2. *Prevalence of ischemic heart disease among men of all ages*

Area	Total No.	IHD patients	Prevalence No./1,000 population
Chandigarh Sarvotham [1296]	1,361	84	65.4
Agra Mathur [940]	901	48	53.0
Bombay Datey [364]	569	16	29
Tecumseh Epstein [439]	1,782	66	66
Framingham Kagan [766]	2,282	219	96
Rhondda Fach group	537	57	106.0

Table 3. *Proportion of IHD in men and women below 40 years*

Author	Epidemiological studies			Author	Cases studied		
	No. of IHD	No. of pts.	percentage		No. of IHD	No. of pts.	percentage
Datey [364]	16	2	12.5	Bhargwa [151]	505	76	15.2
Sarvotham [1296]	134	38	26.1	Mukherjee [1053]	306	81	26.0
Mathur [939]	48	7	14	Pinto [1177]	270	98	36.2
				Shah [1342]	100	17	17
				Warrier [1524]	155	34	22.5

Body Weight and Body Structure and IHD. In a series of 202 patients with ischemic heart disease from Bombay, only 21% of the patients were overweight. No patient was excessively obese. Similar results were obtained by Shah [1342].

Somatotyping was done by a modified Seldon technique by Shah [1342]; the majority of their patients were ectomorphs. Our results were similar. The findings of both these workers are at variance with Gertler [526] who concluded that the endomorphic mesomorph was most prone to suffer from coronary heart disease.

Datey reported that their cases with ischemic heart disease were not shorter than the normals. In their series the average height of the normals was 160 cm and of the diseased, 159 cm.

Tobacco Smoking in IHD. No correlation was found between smoking and coronary heart disease by Sarvotham and Datey in their epidemiological studies. On the other hand, Pinto et al. [1177] analyzed the smoking habits of control and ischemic heart disease patients and found that the majority of patients with ischemic heart disease were heavy smokers, and this relationship was highest and statistically significant in the age group below 40 years.

Heredity and IHD. Datey reported an incidence of positive family history in 12.5% of cases in their series. Pinto et al. [1177] reported that 6% of their ischemic heart disease patients gave a positive family history of coronary heart disease. This figure is lower than that given by Gertler [526], who reported a positive family history in 15% of IHD cases, making allowances for the reliability and comparability of family history.

Personality and IHD. In a controlled study of cases of ischemic heart disease in the lower socioeconomic group, Pinto et al. [1177] found that the percentage of patients with an obsessive, compulsive trait were significantly high in ischemic heart disease. The percentage of depressives was also high. The cases of IHD were under stress, and the stress was mostly internal or as the result of interaction between the external and internal environments. Their results were similar to those reported in the higher socioeconomic group of western workers [1258]. They concluded, that irrespective of class, race or creed, personality and the environment with the stress and tensions that they generate were responsible for and closely related to IHD.

Hypertension and IHD. Hypertension is a known high risk factor in the development of IHD. This relationship has been well brought out by the prospective Framingham studies [766]. In North India, Sarvotham [1296] found that 43.8% of the men and 46.1% of the women with IHD were hypertensive. In Bombay Datey found that seven of their patients (37.5%) were hypertensive, and four of these had enlarged hearts. Pinto[1], however, found that the average blood pressure level of IHD patients was 122/81 mm of Hg. Hence, it appears that in his series, at least, patients developed IHD at lower blood pressure levels.

Serum Cholesterol and IHD. The serum cholesterol values in normal Indians ranged from 152 to 174 mg/100 cc according to the age. These values are significantly lower than normals reported by western workers but are similar to the various populations from different parts of India, irrespective of their diet and ethnic background (see Table 4).

We found that the serum cholesterol values were significantly raised in coronary heart disease patients both in the age group 21–40 years and 41–60 years. Similar results have also been reported by other western workers in the higher socioeconomic group and by Gertler [525] in a mixed population consisting of the higher and lower socioeconomic groups. It is interesting to note that the mean serum cholesterol values in coronary heart disease patients in our series were lower than the mean cholesterol values of the normals in western countries. However, it is possible that as atherosclerosis is so widespread in the west, these reported normal western values are high and really represent predisease levels

---

1 See footnote p. 328.

Table 4. *Showing mean normal values of serum cholesterol in mg/100 cc of blood according to different authors*

	Age							
	21–30		31–40		41–50		51 and above	
	M	S.D.	M	S.D.	M	S.D.	M	S.D.
Mathur [940]	159 ± 25		170 ± 42.6		178 ± 42.4		188 ± 17.4	
Padmavati [1143]	164 ± 25		174 ± 40		172 ± 22.5		150 ± 30	
Srikantia [1402]	161 ± 9.6 (21–30)		173 ± 5.3 (31–40)		175 ± 5.1 (41–50)		174 ± 16.0 (above 50)	
Vengsarkar [1497]	151.8 ± 44.3 (21–40)		—		167.5 ± 36.3 (41–60)			
Gertler [526]	195 ± 41		224 ± 42		236 ± 41		—	
Kannel [772]	—		219 ± 45 (30–34) 222 ± 42 (35–39)		229 ± 46 (40–44) 231 ± 37 (45–49)		—	
Keys [794]	209 ± 38.7 (20–34) 224.6 ± 38.4 (27–40)		228.3 ± 40.8 (30–40) 228.7 ± 38.5 (30–48)		230.0 ± 40.4 (40–54) 231.3 ± 38.2 (35–54)		—	

M = Mean serum cholesterol.
S.D. = Standard deviation.

Table 5. *Serum cholesterol, uric acid and triglyceride levels in normals and IHD* (Pinto[a])

Age group	Group	Cholesterol percentage of (mg)	Uric acid percentage of (mg)	Triglyceride percentage of (mg)
<40	Control	176 ± 43	3.0 ± 0.8	46 ± 16
	IHD	199 ± 49	4.1 ± 1.1	74 ± 60
	P value	<0.001	<0.001	<0.05
>40	Control	182.8 ± 45.2	3.0 ± 0.6	48 ± 32
	IHD	203 ± 45	4.5 ± 1.3	78 ± 40
	P value	n.s.	<0.001	<0.001

[a] Pinto, I. J., Vahia, N. S., Vengsarkar, A. S., De Souza, A.: Report to the Indian Council of Medical Research (1968).

in clinically asymptomatic people with atherosclerosis and do not really present normal serum cholesterol levels [796].

Pinto et al. [1177] broke up their results in five-year period to see if any rise in serum cholesterol levels occurred over the years (see Table 6). They found shat the level of serum cholesterol is increasing in the total population, and in the age group below 40 years the rise in serum cholesterol values is statistically significant. They concluded that this finding may be responsible for the increased incidence of coronary heart disease in the younger age group.

Triglycerides and IHD. Hypertriglyceridemia has also been cited as an important index of altered lipid metabolism in coronary heart disease. Albrink [35] and Carlson [281] considered that the presence of higher serum triglyceride level makes individuals more prone to IHD. On studying Table 7 it appears that the levels of serum triglyceride vary in Indian reports but are much lower than in western works. Pinto et al. [1177] encountered low serum triglyceride levels in IHD patients and have made a pointed reference to the difference in their

Table 6. *Rise of normal values of serum cholesterol over period of five-year study* (Pinto, [1177])

Years	Age group	
	below 40	above 40
	Case Material 1960–1965	
Vengsarkar [1497] (Bombay)	151.8 ± 44.3 (45)	167.5 ± 36.3 (37)
	Case Material 1965–1969	
Pinto [1177] (Bombay)	176 ± 43.5 (34)	182.8 ± 45.2 (33)
t Test	2.430	1.550
P value	$P<0.05$	n.s.

Table 7. *Serum triglyceride levels in normal Indians and Indians with IHD compared to western values*

Authors	Location	Normal	IHD	*p* value
Bandopadhyay [91]	Rajasthan	125 ± 16 (S.E.)	177 ± 15 (S.E.)	not reported
Mukherjee [1053]	Bengal	110 ± 3.5 (S.E.)	115.5 ± 4.75 (S.E.)	not significant
Vaishwanam [1490]	Nagpur	63.4	105.3	not reported
Kroman [830]	U.S.A.	109 ± 19.05 (S.D.)	178 ± 64.18 (S.D.)	<0.001
Carlson [281]	Scandinavia	100.9	202	<0.001
Pinto [1177]	Bombay	46 ± 16 (S.D.)	74 (S.D.)	<0.05

S.D. = Standard deviation.
S.E. = Standard error.

findings as compared to Albrink [35]. As most of their IHD cases had serum triglyceride levels below 160 mg%, they did not consider hypertriglyceridemia as a high risk factor in their cases of IHD.

Serum Uric Acid and IHD (see Table 5). Pinto and Calaco [1177] have also found that, though the mean serum uric acid level is significantly raised in IHD patients, the levels were much lower than those reported by western workers [526]. They, therefore, did not consider hyperuricemia as a high risk factor.

Hyperglycemia and IHD. In the epidemiological studies Datey et al. found that only two of the 16 cases of IHD had hyperglycemia. His findings in the

IHD group were different. Glucose tolerance tests were carried out in 145 out of 167 consecutive cases of myocardial infarction at repeated intervals up to two years [364]. He found that the incidence of hyperglycemia was 70% at the onset of attack and in 36% of these cases the hyperglycemia was transient. According to their criteria, 17% of their cases had hyperglycemic curves but were not diabetic. Hyperglycemia was considered an important risk factor in their cases of IHD.

Diet and IHD. There is much evidence that among the environmental factors diet influences serum cholesterol levels and the incidence of IHD. In Bombay, these are much lower than in the Indians residing in East Africa. The diet of Indians in Bombay contains less than 40 g of fat while the Indians who reside in East Africa consume more than 100 g of fat [1341]. Malhotra [908], on the other hand, found that the incidence of IHD in a selected group of the All-India Railway employees was seven times higher in South Indians as compared to North Indians; even though the latter consume nine times more fat, most of which is animal in origin, and their serum cholesterol levels are about the same. The North Indians consume 47.46 g of fat [908] which is still less than North Americans (A.R.S., U.S.A. 1965) who consume 147 g of fat. He suggested that the presence of the deficiency of bile in the intestinal lumen of North Indians resulted in less fat absorption. He relates the difference in incidence of ischemic heart disease to possible differences in chain lengths of plasma triglyceride acids in the fats consumed. The South Indians eat one-tenth as much fat composed of long-chain fatty acids, in contrast to North Indians whose dietary fats consist mostly of short-chain fatty acid triglycerides. He suggests that thrombosis is enhanced by long-chain acids of not less than 16 carbon atoms, whereas short-chain acids produce hardly any enhancement.

The findings of Datey are different. The total caloric intake in their sample was 1,980 calories made up of 37.8 g of fat mostly in the form of seed oil containing long-chain fatty acids, 52.9 g of proteins, and the remainder of carbohydrate in the form of cereals. Nevertheless, the prevalence of IHD in Bombay (29 per thousand) is less than half that of Chandigarh (65.4 per thousand) [1296]. The results do not seem to support the contention of Malhotra [908] that IHD is less common in North India or that the populations consuming fats in the form of long-chain fatty acids are more prone to IHD than those who consume fats in the form of short-chain fatty acids.

Physical Activity and IHD. Coronary heart disease tends to be more frequent among persons with sedentary habits. Sarvotham [1296] did not find a single case of it in their sample among the heavy manual workers. Shah [1342] found it more frequently among the sedentary workers. Thus physical activity has played a significant role in preventing the development of coronary heart disease in those series reported by Indian researchers.

SUMMARY AND CONCLUSIONS

An analysis of the reports of ischemic heart disease seems to indicate that in India, the subject who suffers from myocardial infarction is not short or overweight, but is an ectomorph with a negative family history. He possesses an obsessive compulsive or depressive personality which is susceptible to stress.

The values of serum triglycerides, serum cholesterol, and uric acid are much lower in these patients with ischemic heart disease than in comparable series done in the West; nevertheless, these values are significantly higher in patients with ischemic heart disease as compared to normal controls. The majority of these patients are hyperglycemic.

The question, then, arises as to why Indians develop the disease at lower lipid and blood pressure levels. One possible explanation could be that in India the threshold for lipid infiltration and accumulation is lower, but this again is begging the question because one would have to answer why this is so! Is it possible that there may be some tissue factor (rather than a humoral one) which causes this hyperactivity? Obviously there is some mechanism operating in these patients which produces the disease and which we have not measured. Possibly family studies of first-degree relatives of patients with coronary heart disease may give us the answer.

CURRENT DEVELOPMENTS IN THE PACIFIC

I. A. M. Prior and J. Grimley Evans

From the time of Captain Cook to the twentieth century the Pacific area has offered unique opportunities for scientific endeavor and discovery. It is fitting to pay our respects to Captain James Cook at this bicentenary of his first voyage in the Pacific.

Within this area there are people of the same ethnic groups, such as Polynesians, living at differing stages of material development and in differing environmental situations; some are undergoing rapid social and environmental change through migration and economic development; at the same time people of different ethnic origin are merging and living within the same environment. In some of the groups there exists the opportunity to study subjects before and after migration, and also to have groups remaining in their more primitive and unsophisticated communities to act as controls.

The groups under study in prospective surveys within the area include Caucasians in Western Australia—the Busselton Study, where 91% of a total population of 3,700 adults were examined, including glucose tolerance tests (GTT) and cardiovascular assessment [350]. Australian aboriginals are being studied, as well as a group of 780 New Guinea highlanders, by Whyte, Sinnett and their group [1367]. A further Melanesian group in a coastal situation in New Guinea are being studied by Maddox, and he has recently carried out a follow-up study on the Island of Gau among Fijian Melanesians (I. Maddox, personal communication). Damon and his group have carried out a survey in the Solomons also Melanesians [353].

In New Zealand, Maori and European groups are being studied, and the high risk status of the N.Z. Maori adult suggested by mortality data was confirmed [1196]. This led to studies among further groups of Polynesians in the Cook Islands, in the more developed area of Rarotonga, and on the atoll of Pukapuka in an endeavor to disentangle the environmental and genetic factors contributing to the metabolic maladies of the Polynesians [1198].

More recently, in 1966, the Tokelau Islands were involved in a hurricane, and a decision was made to resettle a major section of the total population of this group in New Zealand. This represents a very acute change of social and environmental factors, and offers a valuable opportunity to study the influence this may have on cardiovascular function.

In Hawaii different groups have been studied in a variety of ways, and the Polynesians have emerged with a higher coronary heart disease (CHD) rate than the Japanese [136], the principal factors distinguishing the two races being greater degrees of hypertension, overweight, and history of diabetes in the Hawaiians [97]. A major prospective survey of Japanese in Japan, Hawaii, and on the West Coast of America is now established with large numbers in the samples, which will seek to explore further the influence of changing environment and social conditions on CHD and hypertension (A. Kagan, personal communication).

In Japan major studies are underway seeking reasons for the high death rate from hypertension in some areas and low rates of CHD mortality.

Studies in Taiwan, the Taiwan Cardiovascular Study, have been concerned with the prevalence of postexercise, S-T depression, and factors relating physical characteristics and exercise responses. Discriminant function analysis showed that major discrimination factors separating the group with positive response were age, blood pressure, and certain ECG abnormalities at rest [304].

The pattern of these Pacific studies highlights the "experiments of nature" that are in progress which must be studied if important opportunities are not to be missed.

CHD Risk Factor Distributions. The findings in the New Guinea group show a virtual absence of many of the risk factors [1367], and a similar picture is suggested in the preliminary report from the Solomons [353]. The constellation of risk factors in relationship to known CHD is clearly important, and differences found may give clues to the contributing causes of the disorder. The distribution of risk factors in groups allows comparisons to be made between populations, providing similar standards are used.

Groups studied in New Zealand, Maori and European (Carterton), and in the Cook Islands, Rarotonga (a developed high Island) and Pukapuka (a low atoll) illustrate the wide differences in risk factors from these samples that may be found in males (Table 1). The lowest rate is on Pukapuka, where 26% (17 of 65) had one or more risk factors, while the highest rate was found in Carterton European men, 81% (59 of 73). The contribution of weight is greatest in the N.Z. Maori, where 30% (47 of 157) were greater than 120% relative weight, and lowest in the Pukapukans, 8% (5 of 65). A wide variation is seen in cholesterols, with 44% of the Europeans (32 of 73) having levels >260 mg, as compared to 16% N.Z. Maori (25 of 157), 8% Rarotongans (6 of 80) and 2% Puka-

Table 1. *Males 40–59 years*

	Risk factors									
	One or more	Percent-age	R.Wt.[a]		B.P.[b]		Chol.[c]		Smoking[d]	
Maori	114	73	47	30%	61	39%	25	16%	55	35%
Total	157									
Rarotonga	54	68	11	14%	39	49%	6	8%	14	18%
Total	80									
Pukapuka	17	26	5	8%	3	5%	1	2%	11	17%
Total	65									
Carterton	59	81	8	11%	31	42%	32	44%	26	36%
Total	73									

[a] Relative weight (R.Wt.) 120% and over (1913 Actuarial Study used as standard).
[b] Blood pressure (B.P.): diastolic 95 mm and over.
[c] Cholesterol: 260 mg and over.
[d] Smoking: 10 and more cigarettes per day.

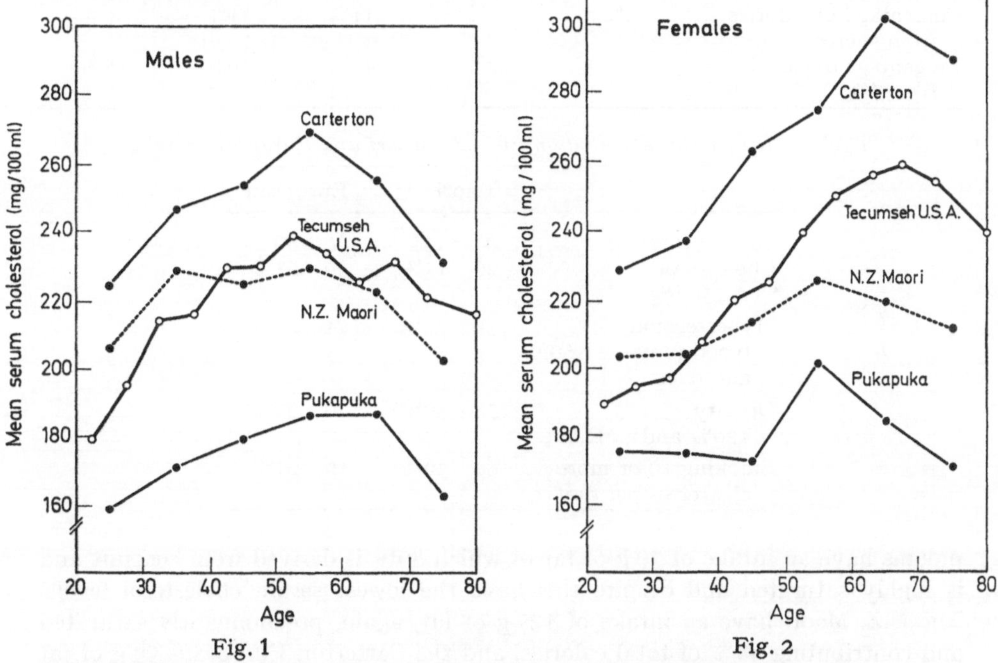

Fig. 1. Males: mean serum cholesterol mg/100 ml in four population studies by age

Fig. 2. Females: mean serum cholesterol mg/100 ml in four population studies by age

pukans (1 of 65). The extent of hypertension is greatest in the Rarotongans (49%), Carterton Europeans (42%), N.Z. Maoris (39%) and then Pukapukans (5%).

Serum Cholesterol. The serum cholesterol is accepted as one of the most significant predictors for CHD, and the differences observed in manifestations of atheroma may be expected to follow this. The striking differences in cholesterol levels between the Pukapukans, New Zealand Maori, and Carterton Europeans are seen in Fig. 1 and Fig. 2. The inclusion of the Tecumseh findings confirms the notably higher rates in the Carterton Europeans as compared to those in Tecumseh. The considerable difference between the N.Z. Maori and Carterton subjects raises a number of questions and certainly suggests some genetic difference in addition to an environmental or dietary one where, on average, the Maori fat intake would be as high as, or higher than, in the N.Z. European.

The diet pattern of the groups under study does show important differences that could play a part in the different cholesterol levels (Table 2). The Pukapukans have an intake of 70 g of fat of which 80% is derived from coconut and is highly saturated and despite this have the lowest serum cholesterol levels. The N.Z. Maori have an intake of 125 g of fat, again, predominantly saturated and contributing 44% of total calories, and the Carterton Europeans 99 g of fat and contributing 39% of total calories. The sucrose intake also shows considerable variation: 9 g in Pukapuka, 71 g in N.Z. Maori and 61 g in Carterton Europeans. The diet pattern of atoll-dwelling Polynesians varies in relationship to available resources and custom, and it is, therefore, interesting to record the higher calorie and fat intake found among Tokelauans than among Pukapukans: total calories 1,930, 119 g fat contributing 56% of total calories, a lower carbohydrate intake, 167 g, and only 7 g of sucrose.

Table 2. *Diet: comparison of daily food intake*

	Pukapuka	Rarotonga	N.Z.Maori	Carterton European	Tokelauans
Total calories	1,800	2,100	2,560	2,270	1,930
Protein g	60	60	73	73	55
Fat g	70	63	125	99	119
Carbohydrate g	225	320	284	272	167
Sucrose g	9	35	71	61	7
Percentage of calories from sucrose	2%	7%	11%	11%	1.5%
Percentage of calories from fat	35%	27%	44%	39%	56%

Table 3. *Risk factor distribution in N.Z. Maori and European females*

	Maori		European	
40–59 years	$N=155$		$N=80$	
Cholesterol >250 mg	26	17%	50	63%
Hypertension blood pressure 160/95 and over	39	25%	21	26%
Obesity 120% and > R.Wt.	78	50%	20	25%
Smoking 10 or more cigarettes per day	60	39%	19	24%

Risk Factors in N.Z. Maori and European Females. The distribution of certain risk factors in N.Z. Maori and European females are set out in Table 3 for subjects aged 40–59 years. The greater degree of obesity, defined as 120% r.wt. or greater, in the Maori, 50% (78 of 155) as compared to 25% (20 of 80); the notably higher cholesterol levels in the Carterton European females, 63% (50 of 80) 250 mg or greater, as compared to 17% (26 of 155) in the Maori females, are the striking differences between the groups. Analysis of risk factors in females in the 30–59 age group with positive histories of angina shows a similar pattern. In addition, 50% of the Maori women had serum uric acid greater than 6 mg, as compared to only 14% of the European women.

The mortality statistics in New Zealand indicate a death rate from coronary heart disease in Maori women that is three to four times greater than in the Europeans. The factors contributing to this high risk status have yet to be properly determined, but obesity, a high rate of hypertension, and of diabetic abnormality may be key factors.

Table 4. *Prevalence of angina in N.Z. Maori and European studies*

	Carterton European	New Zealand Maori
	Males	
30–59	3.2/100	3.0/100
60 and over	8.2/100	12.0/100
	Females	
30–59	4.9/100	8.2/100
60 and over	21.2/100	12.3/100

Angina Rates. The age-adjusted angina rates among the N.Z. Maori groups and Carterton Europeans show an interesting pattern, with the rate among the Maori females being higher in the 30–59 age groups, while the European females reach a particularly high rate of 21.2/100 in the 60 and over group.

ECG Patterns. The Blackburn Code has allowed adequate comparison between groups and represents an important milestone. The ECG codings of the New Guinea natives by Whyte and Sinnett are compared to those of Tecumseh in Table 5. The complete absence of large Q-waves and a low overall Q-wave rate suggests virtual absence of CHD; the high rate of T-inversion, particularly in New Guinea women, raises problems of interpretation. The ECG findings comparing Carterton Europeans, Rarotongans, and Pukapukans with Tecumseh are shown in Table 6, age-standardized on to the Tecumseh population. The lowest Q-rate is in Pukapukans. The high T-inversion rate in Rarotongan and Pukapukan females is of interest.

Risk Factors in Busselton Study. Age and sex specific rates for CHD in the Busselton Study were very similar to those in Tecumseh, U.S.A. Risk factors were analyzed using age and sex specific eightieth percentile values to simplify the data into upper and lower ranges. In both sexes, upper range serum cholesterol, blood pressure and blood sugar levels after a glucose load were each significantly and independently associated with coronary heart disease; the risk ratio for each being approximately twofold. In males only, upper range serum uric

Table 5. *Comparison of New Guinea and Tecumseh ECG coding*

ECG item	Minn. Code		New Guinea	Tecumseh
Males 40–59 yrs.				
			$N = 139$	$N = 98$
Q-waves	I	1	0	1.3
		2	0.7	1.4
		3	0	0.5
	Total		0.7	3.1
L.A.D.	II	1	2.9	6.8
Tall R	III	1	3.6	3.8
S-T depression	IV		0.7	3.3
T-wave inversion	V		5.8	14.8
I-V cond. defects	VII		0.7	3.4
Females				
			$N = 121$	$N = 801$
Q-waves	I	1	0	0
		2	0	0.4
		3	0	0.5
	Total		0	0.9
L.A.D.	II	1	3.3	3.6
Tall R	III	1	0	1.7
S-T depression	IV		0.8	8.0
T-wave inversion	V		25.6	15.6
I-V cond. defects	VII		0	1.2

Table 6. *ECG coding*

Minn. Code	Males				Females			
	Tec.	Cart.	Raro.	Puk.	Tec.	Cart.	Raro.	Puk.
I (1)	0.8	0.2	—	—	0.8	0.5	0.4	—
I (2, 3)	1.4	0.5	3.9	0.4	1.4	0.5	0.6	—
II	6.0	3.2	3.4	1.0	4.9	2.5	3.4	2.1
III (1)	6.0	2.7	8.5	1.5	4.1	1.7	1.7	—
IV	2.5	0.7	1.3	—	4.0	4.0	2.9	3.2
V	11.6	4.6	5.4	5.6	12.4	3.6	14.1	15.6

Frequency (as a percentage) of ECG abnormalities age-standardized on to Tecumseh population by direct method in decadal age groups.

acid levels showed a strong relationship of similar magnitude to and independent from the association of upper range blood pressures. In this prevalence study they did not find any significant association with obesity, nor with current cigarette smoking and coronary heart disease [1533].

Carbohydrate Metabolism. The earlier studies in N.Z. Maoris showed a high rate of diabetes, often combined with obesity, hyperuricemia and clinical gout; 9% of men aged 20 and over and 7% of women [1197]. Bassett [99] showed a similar pattern of obesity and diabetes in Hawaiian Polynesians, but with normal uric acid. The prevalence rate of diabetes showed a gradient related to weight and to certain dietary factors. The establishment of the one-hour plasma glucose level as a variable contributing to risk factor status at Tecumseh was the stimulus to include this measurement in studies carried out in the Tokelau Islands in 1968 and in N.Z. Maori groups in 1968 and 1969. The percentile distributions of one-hour plasma glucose in three Polynesian groups, Tokelauans, and two N.Z. Maori groups show a change in glucose handling with age: these are set out in males and females aged 20–39, 40–59 and 60 and over for atoll-dwelling Tokelauans and town-living N.Z. Maoris in Rotorua in Table 7 (males) and Table 8 (females) and do not show any remarkable differences.

Defining diabetic abnormality as a one-hour plasma glucose of 250 mg or more following a 100 g glucose load, or blood glucose 120 mg and over fasting

Table 7. *Distribution of one hour plasma glucose after 100 g glucose load*

Males		25th percentile	50th percentile	90th percentile
Fakaofa Tokelaus	20–39 $N=41$	106 mg	126 mg	164 mg
	40–59 $N=41$	125 mg	146 mg	167 mg
	60 and over $N=19$	150 mg	167 mg	224 mg
Rotorua N.Z. Maori	20–39 $N=51$	98 mg	112 mg	181 mg
	40–59 $N=56$	118 mg	138 mg	248 mg
	60 and over $N=22$	112 mg	175 mg	250 mg

and 130 mg or over two hours after the 100 g glucose load, the prevalence of diabetic abnormality in the Tokelauans and in the two Maori samples from Tiki Tiki and Rotorua showed a lower rate in the Tokelauan males but was essentially the same in the females. The results in the 30–59 age groups are set out in Table 8 for males and Table 9 for females. The selection of subjects for glucose tolerance tests varied in the different areas: an increase of 1/10th in the blood sugar or more at one hour after a glucose load in the Tokelaus; a one hour plasma glucose >160 mg in Tiki Tiki or >200 mg in Rotorua, and this will influence the prevalence data. These findings, however, indicate a strong predisposition to diabetes in Polynesians, and the notably higher rate in the Tokelauans as compared to that found in Pukapukans in 1964 may relate to their greater degree of obesity, particularly in the females, as well as to the more refined screening methods adopted. The fact that, in the Rotorua sample of 97 females and 82 males in the 30–59 age group, ten new female cases and seven new male cases were picked up at the six-year re-examination, gives an idea of the extent of the problem in Polynesians. This gives an incidence rate of around 1.6 per year per 100 females and 1 per year per 100 males in this age group.

Work in progress includes the assessment of lipoproteins by paper electrophoresis and by nephelometry using the method and equipment developed by Thorpe. It is hoped that this will throw some light on the family and group distribution of lipoproteins that, in conjunction with the cholesterol and triglyceride levels, will give a clearer picture of these important components and their relationships.

Table 8. *Distribution of one hour plasma glucose after 100 g glucose load*

Females		25th percentile	50th percentile	90th percentile
Fakaofa Tokelaus	20–39 $N=70$	114 mg	130 mg	193 mg
	40–59 $N=56$	115 mg	150 mg	230 mg
	60 and over $N=51$	126 mg	156 mg	212 mg
Rotorua N.Z. Maori	20–39 $N=36$	110 mg	129 mg	202 mg
	40–59 $N=67$	123 mg	150 mg	250 mg
	60 and over $N=26$	123 mg	188 mg	285 mg

Table 9. *Diabetic abnormality in three Polynesian groups*

	No.	Diabetic abnormality	Percentage
Males 30–59 years			
Fakaofa	67	3	4.5
Tiki Tiki	87	8	9.0
Rotorua	82	11	13.2
Females 30–59 years			
Fakaofa	97	10	9.7
Tiki Tiki	94	14	14.8
Rotorua	97	12	12.0

SUMMARY

The pattern emerging from these studies highlights the complex metabolic problems associated with atherosclerosis and yet, at the same time, it gives an indication of ways and means whereby some beneficial changes might be introduced. The Pacific basin, with its scattered populations, poses problems of travel and communication. Despite this there are great changes taking place that involve movement of people into new environs with considerable change in living habits and customs. It is here that a major contribution may be made, providing that the trained personnel and funds for such studies can be found.

CURRENT DEVELOPMENTS IN SOUTH AND CENTRAL AMERICA AND THE CARIBBEAN

W. E. Miall

The epidemic of ischemic heart disease which has developed in the indus trialized countries during this century has not yet reached its peak, and yet the disease is already the leading cause of death in every European country, clinically afflicts one man in five by age 60 in the U.S.A., and is estimated to cost Britain 1% of its gross national product [1037]. Although knowledge of risk factors has increased, largely from epidemiological observations, there is still no evidence that changing the environment with respect to these risk factors has any influence on the incidence of the disease. We are, therefore, not yet in a position to prevent a similar epidemic in the developing countries as they in turn reap some of the doubtful benefits of increasing affluence.

In some industrialized countries the risk factors are widespread. In such circumstances it may be more difficult to determine the real etiological factors involved, because many subjects who have not yet experienced clinical coronary heart disease are nevertheless already potential candidates for future attacks. Where the disease is still relatively infrequent it may be expected that the critical environmental factors would be more easily revealed in clear cut differences between affected and unaffected subjects. This is one of many reasons why epidemiological studies in low-incidence areas may be rewarding.

South and Central America and the Caribbean together form a vast and geographically scattered area inhabited by peoples of different ethnic origin at various stages of so-called development. The epidemic of ischemic heart disease has probably only just started in the Caribbean and in parts of South America. The diversity of the populations and their environments, together with the rapid changes in living standards which are now taking place in parts of this region provide natural opportunities for epidemiological exploitation. Unfortunately the number of cardiovascular studies which meet the criteria of modern epidemiology is still small. W.H.O., P.A.H.O., the International Epidemiological Association, the Medical Research Council and the Division of Collaborative Studies of the U.S. National Heart Institute have recently stimulated much interest in epidemiological techniques in the region, and a number of prospective studies are now in progress.

Two large scale mortality studies, the International Atherosclerosis Project (I.A.P.) (see Dr. Strong's contribution, this volume) and the Inter-American Investigation of Mortality have between them given firmer foundations for the previously-held beliefs that large differences exist in the prevalence of atherosclerosis within the area, and that these are reflected by corresponding differences in mortality from arteriosclerotic heart disease. Ten of the 14 countries cooperating in the I.A.P. were Central or South American, or Caribbean, and within these territories marked differences were found between populations of the same ethnic origin [952]. This is illustrated (Fig. 1) using data from the I.A.P. for three ethnic groups, Caucasians, peoples of African origin, and those of American Indian-Caucasian blood. The prevalence of coronary artery stenosis, and the mean percentage of intima involved with raised atherosclerotic lesions are plotted for males aged 45–54 years. The differences within ethnic groups are as great as those between ethnic groups, suggesting that geographical differences in atheroma are largely of environmental origin. Ethnic factors possibly influence the quantity but there is no evidence that they affect the quality of atherosclerotic lesions [1457].

What was already known of the relative economic status, living standards and mortality statistics of the region had predicted that such differences would

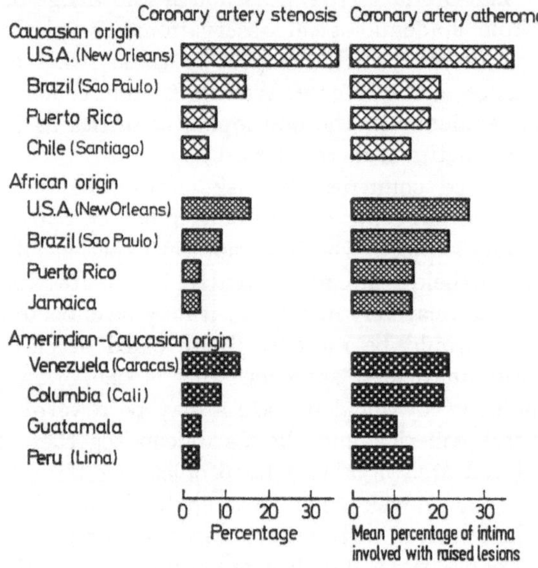

Fig. 1. Percentage of males aged 45–54 years with coronary stenosis, and mean percentage intimal surface involved with atherosclerotic lesions (in left anterior descending coronary artery) by ethnic group and geographic location. (Adapted from International Atherosclerosis Project, McGill et al. [952]

be found, but they are now scientifically established and can be used as a basis for the design of specific epidemiological investigations to elucidate their causes.

What is Known of the Risk Factors in These Regions? Scrimshaw and Guzman analyzed the results of dietary surveys and of serum lipid levels in the populations from which the autopsies of the International Atherosclerosis Project were derived, ranking the populations according to the percentage of calories derived from fat, the percentage of total fat of animal origin, serum cholesterol levels and the consumption of sucrose. The rank order correlation coefficients for these and that for advanced atherosclertoic lesions were highly significant in the case of serum cholesterol (0.755) and for the percentage of calories derived from fat (0.668). Countries with high fat consumption, high total caloric intake, and high serum cholesterol levels had higher prevalences of atherosclerosis. The correlations with sucrose consumption and other variables were insignificant. No relationship was found in the International Atherosclerosis Project between the extent or severity of atherosclerosis in either the coronary arteries or the aorta and any measure of body weight, height or obesity [1018]. This is an interesting and potentially important negative finding, because there is considerable evidence that obesity is a risk factor for myocardial infarction.

Robertson and Strong [1243] showed that in both sexes, at all ages, and in each geographical region covered by the I.A.P., hypertension was a potent factor in causing raised atherosclerotic lesions in the coronary arteries and the aorta but that the magnitude of the differences in atheroma between hypertensive and nonhypertensive subjects still varied according to geographical region and ethnic group. They also showed that atherosclerosis was greater in diabetics than in nondiabetics even when diabetics with hypertension and atheroma attributable to other causes were removed before making the comparison. These workers concluded that both hypertension and diabetes are not primary causes of atheroma, which may be severe in persons with neither disease, but when present they accelerate the natural progression of atherosclerosis in all populations.

The Inter-American Investigation of Mortality [1201], originally designed to give reliable mortality data from cities collaborating in the I.A.P., revealed unusually high mortality from diabetes mellitus in Mexico City, which had an age-adjusted death rate (37.6 per 100,000) twice that of its nearest rival, Caracas (19.7 per 100,000). The lowest rate among these Central and South American cities was found in Cali, Colombia with a rate of 8.1. These very large differences in diabetes mortality do not correlate closely either with the prevalence of atherosclerosis found in the I.A.P. or with the reported mortality from arteriosclerotic heart disease, and clearly warrant further study.

In the 14 countries participating in the I.A.P. no attempt was made to assess the influence of two other major risk factors, physical inactivity and smoking, but this important study has shown that factors which are known to increase risk in the industrialized countries are also risk factors in South and Central America. A great deal more needs to be known about the prevalence of these risk factors in the region but some recent unpublished findings are of interest, and show where further studies may lead to advances in knowledge.

High Altitude Studies. Several studies have reported low systolic blood pressures in people living at high altitude. The World Health Organization has supported population studies of arterial pressure and ischemic heart disease in Peru, where investigations are being conducted by Pénaloza and his colleagues in the High Altitude Research Institute of the Peruvian University "Cayetano Heredia" in Lima.

Studies carried out at Milpo, a town at El. 13,500 and at Colquijirca at El. 14,000 have recently been completed. In both populations systolic pressures were low and showed little increase with age; diastolic pressures were not markedly below those found in many other surveys, so that pulse pressure values in these high altitude dwellers were much reduced. Cholesterol levels in males, averaging 170–190 mg/100 ml, showed little increase with age.

Despite the high altitude and the clinical and electrocardiographic signs of chronic hypoxia, angina pectoris was found in only two of 1,450 adult males and in none of the 300 females in these studies. No case of myocardial infarction was found using clinical criteria and no major Q-wave abnormalities (Minnesota Code 11) were found in the electrocardiographs [1269]. The hypothesis that chronic hypoxia causes increases in coronary blood flow and in the myocardial collateral circulation, for which there is some evidence, is being investigated by studies of cardiac metabolism at high altitudes.

These Peruvian studies included an analysis of the blood pressure levels of 100 expatriate Europeans and Americans who had been living at high altitude for from 2 to 15 years. A fall in systolic and diastolic pressure occurred in half these men, a definite rise in only 10%. After a prolonged stay at high altitude such men are believed to have arterial pressure levels resembling those of the indigent population [934].

Population studies of Peruvians living at lower altitudes are needed to confirm whether prolonged hypoxia really exerts protective effects against arterial hypertension and ischemic heart disease. It is perhaps worth noting in this context that serum uric acid levels have recently been shown to be highly significantly and positively correlated with altitude in Colombia [10], a finding which, together with the Peruvian data, would suggest that serum uric acid levels are not directly related with coronary artery disease and atheroma.

Coincident Myocardial Disease. Epidemiological research into cardiovascular disease in parts of South America, particularly Venezuela and Brazil, is partly determined by the high prevalence of Chagas' disease, human infection resulting from *Trypanosoma cruzi*. In Venezuela it is believed that 20% of the rural population have evidence of *T. cruzi* infection, and of these approximately 50% show signs of myocardial damage. It is estimated that in Venezuela there are 250,000 cases of Chagas' cardiopathy; the problem is even greater in Brazil where it is said that 50% of the population of some rural areas are infected.

Prospective population studies are currently being carried out in Venezuela [1203] to compare the pattern of cardiovascular disease in areas selected as having different prevalences of Chagas' infection. The presence of the cardiopathy is diagnosed on the basis of cardiac lesions and positive complement fixation tests. The cardiac lesions, in life, are nonspecific, cardiomegaly with electrocardiographic abnormalities of which conduction defects are characteristic. The serological test is always of low titre and once positive does not revert spontaneously or following treatment. Furthermore, different laboratories in South America have been found to produce totally different results when provided with split samples of the same sera [63]. It is clearly an area where more specific diagnostic procedures would greatly facilitate research. Reliable population data concerning atherosclerotic heart disease will certainly accrue as a by-product of these studies.

Ethnic Differences. The Caribbean is a region where subjects of different ethnic origin living in similar environments can be directly compared. Poon-King et al. [1186] carried out a large population study of diabetes mellitus in Trinidad and showed that subjects of Indian origin have a higher prevalence than do those of African origin, a finding which accords with similar results obtained in South Africa. It is believed on clinical evidence that ischemic heart disease in general, and myocardial infarction in particular, are more common in Trinidadians of Indian origin and studies have recently been initiated to put this impression on a firmer foundation.

Ashcroft et al. [63] have recently completed a survey of characteristics relevant to cardiovascular disease in men and women aged 35–54 of African and Indian origin in Guyana. Africans were found to have arterial pressures higher than Indians in each age and sex group, and blood pressure was significantly correlated with factors associated with obesity. Blood pressure distributions in Africans were similar to those found in Jamaica and were appreciably lower than those reported in population surveys of St. Kitts [1310], the Bahamas [750] and Georgia [950]; in Indians they were similar to those reported in Fiji

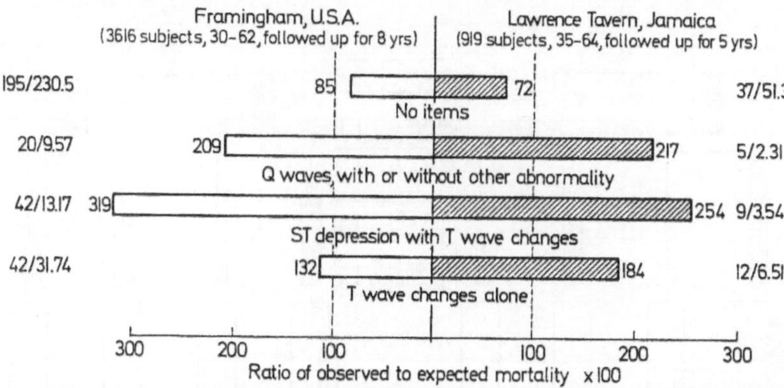

Fig. 2. The ratio of observed to expected deaths according to initial ECG in the follow-up surveys of Framingham, U.S.A. and Lawrence Tavern, Jamaica-both sexes

[893]. Cholesterol levels averaged about 200 mg/100 ml and were 10 mg lower than those reported in St. Kitts [1434]. Coconut oil with its high proportion of saturated fatty acids is the main source of dietary fat in Jamaica and Guyana; cotton-seed oil with a high proportion of unsaturated fatty acids is the main source of fat in St. Kitts. Cholesterol levels in Guyana were also positively correlated with obesity and with arterial pressures.

A high prevalence of S–T and T-wave changes in the electrocardiograms in these Guyanese adults, with a greater prevalence in women than in men, suggested hypertension as an important primary cause. On the other hand, such changes were also more common in those with obesity, in those with high cholesterol levels, with low physical activity and with high socioeconomic status, factors which are known to be associated with coronary artery disease but which in Guyana also are associated with hypertension. Ashcroft and his colleagues state that their preliminary analysis neither confirmed nor disproved an expectation, based on clinical evidence, of a high prevalence of hypertension and a low prevalence of coronary artery disease.

In Jamaica epidemiological studies have shown that myocardial disorders are more prevalent than was previously suspected from clinical experience or unselected autopsy series [1442]. Age specific rates for abnormal Q and QS items, S–T depression and T-wave changes in the electrocardiogram were closely comparable or slightly higher in Jamaica than was reported in the original study undertaken in Framingham where coronary artery disease and myocardial infarction are believed to be much commoner [979]. Few of these abnormalities could be attributed to primary valvular heart disease which was rarely encountered; many were associated with hypertension, some with diabetes; half the ECG abnormalities which elsewhere would be classified as due to probable or possible ischemia were not associated with hypertension.

These Jamaica surveys have been used as baselines for prospective studies and the first five-year follow-up survey of a rural community has recently been

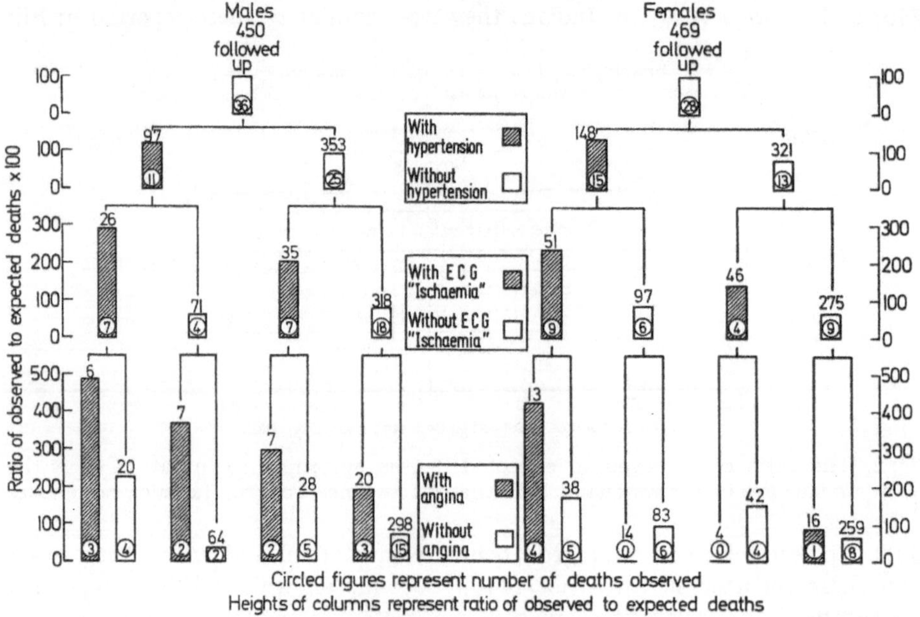

Fig. 3. The ratio of observed to expected deaths in subjects with an without hypertension, ECG "ischemia" and angina. Five-year follow-up of males and females (35–64 years), Lawrence Tavern, Jamaica

completed (Miall et al., unpublished data). Fig. 2 shows the age adjusted mortality ratios of observed to expected deaths for those with and without hypertension (160 and/or 95 mm Hg), with or without ECG ischemia (Minnesota code 1_{1-3}, 4_{1-3}, 5_{1-3} and 7_1) and with or without angina. It is clear that each of these characteristics defines groups with markedly different five-year mortality ratios. (The overall mortality was closely similar to that found in a recent five-year follow-up survey of subjects of the same age range in Wales.) Furthermore, the ratios of observed to expected mortality for four groups of ECG characteristics (Fig. 3) bear a striking similarity to those reported in the first eight years of follow-up at Framingham [680].

Three conditions together probably account for the majority of these cardiac abnormalities, hypertension, coronary artery disease, and the cardiomyopathy first described from Jamaica by Stuart and Hayes [1433], but present cardiovascular survey techniques seem inadequate for specifying with any accuracy the prevalence of coronary heart disease in populations such as that in Jamaica where myocardial damage due to hypertension is common and cardiomyopathies also exist. Recommended cardiovascular survey techniques have not revealed the differences in atherosclerosis which have been shown to exist by such studies as the International Atherosclerosis Project. Rose et al. [1254] have also found in samples of European populations that neither the prevalence rates of symptoms nor those for ECG findings were recognizably correlated with corresponding national mortality rates for ischemic heart disease.

Current Investigations. Diabetes and hypertension are major risk factors for atherosclerosis in the Caribbean. The Medical Research Council's Epidemiology Unit in Jamaica is currently investigating, on a population basis, the association between blood sugar and blood lipid levels and their relationship with hypertension, ECG abnormalities, and prognosis. Preliminary results suggest that 15% of a sample of Jamaican adults aged 25–54 years in a rural area may show blood sugar levels exceeding 170 mg/100 ml one hour after a glucose load. Stuart and McIver, also in Jamaica, are undertaking a controlled therapeutic trial for mild hypertension to determine whether early treatment can prevent subsequent progression of the disease and diminish its cardiac complications.

In Puerto Rico, Garcia Palmieri and his collaegues have started a large scale prospective study of coronary heart disease in urban and rural samples which together include 10,000 males aged 45–64 years. This study should provide valuable data from a country in which coronary heart disease mortality in males has been shown to run at only half the rate for the U.S. mainland [511]. Preliminary results from Puerto Rico have shown urban males to have prevalences of hypertension and diabetes, higher serum triglyceride and cholesterol levels, higher intakes of protein, total calories and fat, a higher consumption of cigarettes, and less physical activity than those in the rural areas. Despite all these differences the prevalence of coronary heart disease, using criteria similar to those of the Framingham study, was reported to be the same in the two populations [510].

In many developing countries there are no reliable vital statistics; death rates for specific causes are too inaccurate for research use and morbidity data are virtually non-existent. In such countries epidemiology should be a major method for obtaining measurements of public health and for indicating areas in which research effort should be directed. The knowledge which should come from further cardiovascular research in many of the countries showing rapid socioeconomic development is likely to be particularly appreciated by those populations which have previously experienced greater economic progress and which are now, especially in terms of atherosclerosis, suffering from its effects.

CURRENT DEVELOPMENTS IN NORTH AMERICA

THE POOLING PROJECT REPORT, COUNCIL ON EPIDEMIOLOGY, AMERICAN HEART ASSOCIATION

HENRY BLACKBURN*

Three major contributions have been made to the general problem of atherosclerosis in man by epidemiological studies among living populations. One is the demonstration of large differences between regions in the frequency of atherosclerotic complications, and between individuals in the risk of coronary heart disease (CHD). Another is the identification and measurement of the importance of predisease personal characteristics associated with these regional and individual differences. A third is the demonstration that risk factors for CHD can be safely modified and that this may, in turn, reduce the risk of CHD. These contributions from cardiovascular epidemiology owe their origins to prior clinical and laboratory observations, as do the principal etiological hypotheses tested so far in population studies.

Differences in CHD Frequency. The evidence is now clear that the burden of clinical CHD at any age is virtually absent in many populations of the world while being a heavy one in others. There are, for example, tenfold differences and more in CHD incidence among middle-aged men between parts of northern Europe and the Mediterranean Basin. The distribution of risk factors in these contrasting areas indicate that elevated blood lipids are probably a *necessary* cause, and other factors *contributing* causes for CHD differences between populations. These and other considerations of cultural differences will be taken up in a report by Keys later in this symposium.

There are several practical by-products of these epidemiological observations of CHD in natural populations. One is that manifestations of CHD and the personal characteristics associated with it are found to be different from those seen by the physician in select clinic and hospital groups. Another is that comparisons of disease rates are found not to be valid without standard protocols, shared personnel, and central classification.

RISK FACTORS

The second major contribution of cardiovascular epidemiology to the understanding of atherosclerosis is the concept and measurement of CHD risk factors.

* Presented on behalf of the following collaborating principal investigators: Dr. J. T. Doyle (Albany Study); Dr. O. Paul (Western Electric Study, Chicago); Dr. J. Stamler (People's Gas, Light and Coke Co., Chicago); Drs. T. R. Dawber and W. B. Kannel (Framingham Study); Dr. J. M. Chapman (Los Angeles Study); Drs. A. Keys and H. Blackburn (Minnesota Study); Statistical Coordinating Center (Dr. F. H. Epstein and Prof. F. E. Moore, principal investigators, University of Michigan, School of Public Health). The "Pooling Project" is supported by grant HE 13107–01 from the NHI, NIH, USPHS, Bethesda, Md. and has received staff assistance from the Heart Disease and Stroke Control Program (Dr. S. M. Fox, III, Chief), USPHS, Arlington, Virginia.

True, there is little new about gluttony, sloth and "excess humors", which have been characteristic of mortality risk since antiquity. However, there is a great deal of new knowledge about the distribution of the CHD risk characteristics in the free-living population outside hospitals, about the association of risk characteristics with one another, and about the CHD risk related to various combinations of characteristics.

With several exceptions, most of the current information on predisease characteristics associated with subsequent CHD risk comes from North American studies, and much of it from the six which have collaborated in the Pooling Project of the American Heart Association, Council on Epidemiology. These studies and their principal investigators are: the Framingham community (W. B. Kannel), Albany civil servants (J. T. Doyle), Chicago Gas Company employees (J. Stamler), Chicago Western Electric employees (O. Paul), Los Angeles civil servants (J. M. Chapman) and Minnesota business and professional men (A. Keys, H. L. Taylor and H. Blackburn). The current efforts are to extract and apply the maximum amount of the risk information from these studies, involving 8,663 men free of CHD at entry, and 73,000 person years of experience. The chief purposes of the several manipulations of these data are: (1) to learn more about the relative contributions of the factors to risk, and (2) to find the most efficient discriminants or predictors of future risk. The data from the Pooling Project have not yet been reviewed by the collaborating groups, prior to release for publication. Therefore, only a descriptive summary of some of the key findings can be given in this published report, even though the actual, supporting data were presented at the time of the Symposium. This would seem preferable to reviewing and summarizing from the literature the reports of the individual, contributing projects since they are already quite well known. It may be stated that, in general, the trends from the separate studies were consistent so that it was justifiable to pool the data. This and the resultant fact that the analyses are based on such large numbers give a firmness to the interpretation of the data which could not be achieved before.

Single Risk Factors. Considering one risk factor at a time, the ratio of the rates for myocardial infarction (MI) and CHD deaths in those men in the upper third of values for the population, to the rates for those men in the lower third can be calculated. Overall, blood pressure levels in the upper third are associated with twice the CHD risk in subsequent follow-up. Overall, systolic blood pressure does as well as diastolic pressure in predicting future CHD among men free of CHD at entry. Serum cholesterol alone is a significant risk predictor, as strong or stronger than blood pressure alone; cigarette smoking is important, and relative weight is a much weaker predictor than the others. The effect is consistently significant in all studies, by different investigators, using different methods.

The predictive power of single risk factors for the same end points (MI and CHD deaths) among men varies with age. Younger men (35–44) are at greater relative risk than older men (45–54 and 55–64), i.e. relative to colleagues of the same age with lower values. Though the younger man is *relatively* worse off, his *absolute* risk of CHD in a given period, say 10 years, is far lower. Five times a very small risk, say 2/1,000 per year in low risk men at age 35, gives an absolute risk of 10/1,000, whereas 1.7 times a large risk, say 20/1,000 in low risk men at age 60, is 34/1,000. Blood pressure seems to be relatively more important at younger (35–44) and older (55–64) ages than in the intermediate age group; most answers seem to produce new questions. Cholesterol level is most predictive in the youngest age group while the highest risk ratio for smoking is in the age range 45–54.

Combinations of Risk Factors. Other data from the Pooling Project deal with combinations of risk factors. Taking men ages 30–49, initially free of CHD, and four risk factors (serum cholesterol above 250, diastolic pressure 90 or over, a pack or more cigarettes per day, relative weight 1.21 or above), the incidence of myocardial infarction and CHD deaths is calculated. In such younger men, the upper third of the distribution is represented by blood pressure levels of 90 diastolic or more, and cholesterol above 250 mg; in terms of that fantasy used in clinical medicine, both cut-off values are well "within the normal range".

The absolute risk of CHD in that analysis is given as the rate of new CHD events per person years of exposure. It shows a stepwise increase from the rate when all four factors are low to the situation where all are high, with an elevenfold gradient in relative risk. Some 13% of the healthy population at this age in the Pooling Project has all three or four factors high, and this 13% of men develop almost one-third of the new events in a given period. Also 70% of these North American men have one or more of the four factors high and develop, in a given period, almost 90% of the CHD cases. When two factors are considered, the combined elevation of serum cholesterol and blood pressure give the greatest excess risk; for the same end points, combined blood pressure and relative weight give the lowest, little more than blood pressure alone. This indicates what we know otherwise, that they are highly interrelated. This sort of information is essential to preventive approaches which are most effectively concentrated among the persons most susceptible.

Life Table Analysis. Another biostatistical approach in the Pooling Project uses the actuarial life table function at five-year intervals and gives the probability of surviving from one five-year period to the next between ages 35 and 65 while remaining free of a CHD event. The advantage of this analysis is that each individual contributes a person-year of experience at each year of age so long as he is in the exposed population and does not withdraw by having a CHD event, or is not lost by dropping out of the study or dying from a competing risk. This is the only way to take into account all the experience for persons entering at various ages and being followed for different durations. When these data are displayed as decrement curves in Fig. 1, clearly, each of the four factors is of value in predicting coronary risk and offers more in combination than separately. The curves show a remarkable, orderly progression so that almost 90% of men aged 35 remain free of CHD by the time they reach age 65, while only half of the men who are "not low" on all four factors are still unaffected over the same time span.

Sensitivity-specificity of Risk Factors. The table presents another approach to the analysis of multiple risks, based on the clinical concept of sensitivity and specificity of a predictive test, and was compiled by Epstein [437] on the Framingham data. The predictive power of the presence of two out of three risk factors is described in terms of CHD experience in eight years of follow-up.

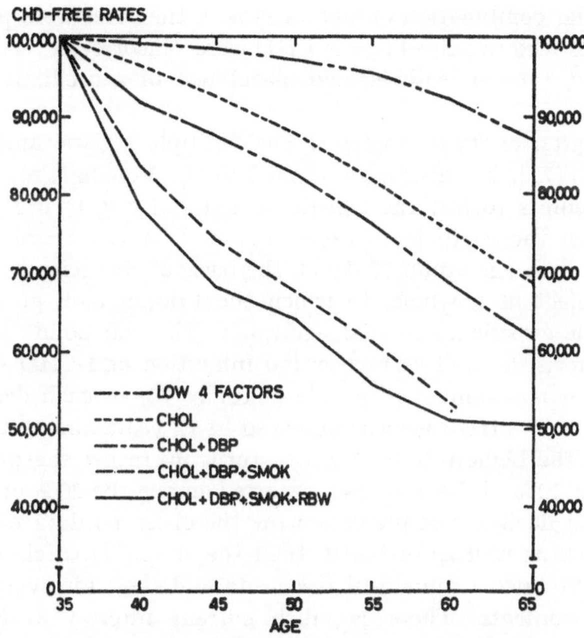

Fig. 1. The actuarial life table function at 5-year intervals and the probability of surviving from one 5-year period to the next while remaining free of a CHD event

Table. *Predicting coronary heart disease (CHD) by means of two of three risk factors*[a] *in men 40 to 59 years of age*[b]

		Test results		Total
		positive	Negative	
New events of CHD in 10 years (estimated)	yes (+)	28	92	120
	no (−)	52	828	880
Total		80	920	1,000
				($N = 1{,}387$)

Sensitivity $= \frac{28}{120} \times 100 = 23\%$ Predictive value (+) $= \frac{28}{80} \times 100 = 35\%$

Specificity $= \frac{828}{880} \times 100 = 94\%$ Predictive value (−) $= \frac{92}{902} \times 100 = 10\%$

Risk ratio $= \frac{35}{10} = 3.5$

[a] Positive test result: Two of the following three: serum cholesterol more than 250 mg/100 cc; blood pressure "abnormal" (W. H. O. Criteria); Left ventricular hypertrophy on electrocardiogram.

[b] Based on eight-year incidence data from the Framingham population. Modified by permission of the author and published by permission of the Journal of the American Medical Association (Epstein, 1967).

By this particular combination of factors 23% of the cases were predicted, while only 6% of cases who remained free of CHD were "incorrectly" labelled positive. This is a severe, though realistic, and useful test of a predictive method in a chronic disease.

Multiple Regression-Type Analyses. The multiple logistic analysis of Truett and Cornfield [1477], has also been applied to the Pooling Project data in one of the first attempts to test the logistic in material largely independent of the data from which the coefficients were computed. A risk score was calculated for the Framingham age group 50–59 on the basis of coefficients computed from the Pooled Project as a whole, to which the Framingham group contributed only 20% of the experience in that age range. The end points in this instance are angina pectoris, as well as myocardial infarction and CHD death.

There is an equal number of people (actually 70) in each decile of the risk score. Only one new CHD case was observed in 12 years among the lowest 10% of scores, 21 in the highest 10%. The risk turns up rather sharply at the upper extreme. Almost 40% of the new cases occurred among the 20% of the population in the two upper deciles. The prediction fits the observed data well, it separates categories of risk as well as or better than the simple cross-classifications seen so far, and it provides a numerical risk score and rank for every individual.

Other Developments. There is much current interest in North America in describing the risk characteristics related to sudden death, and to other individual CHD manifestations. There is also now good evidence that behavioral characteristics are associated with CHD risk in North American men. These, along with the role of physical activity and a number of other possible risk factors, are subjects of continued investigation.

FUTURE NEEDS

This information is a central contribution of the long-term observational studies of North American men, first examined in a state of health. Continuation of these studies at a minimum level of follow-up on death and major disability would be the most economic way to obtain information on the risk characteristics and course of many less frequent but important diseases such as stroke, peripheral vascular disease and noncardiovascular maladies.

Long-term studies are still needed concerning atherosclerosis in women and in children. However, there is no major new hypothesis or methodological advance in North America giving impetus to new observational studies. Rather, attention is currently turned to application of current knowledge in clinical trials and pilot studies attempting to modify elevated factors of CHD risk. These will be detailed later in this symposium by their investigators.

PREVENTION

Suffice it to say here that results of the first generation of trials and pilot studies are now in the hands of the scientific leadership, public health agencies and funding bodies of this country. They provide good evidence that substantial numbers of people can be induced to modify their elevated risk factors, and that substantial reductions in the levels are attainable. The early evidence is favorable that the rate of atherosclerotic complications can be safely reduced by simple hygienic procedures.

Continued pursuit of the pathogenesis and fundamental mechanisms of atherosclerosis in clinic and laboratory is obligatory. But, identification of persons with excess CHD risk is now possible with a confidence unknown for any other major disease. Further, cardiovascular epidemiology provides overwhelming evidence that the bulk of the problem of atherosclerosis is determined by cultural patterns and personal habits and therefore requires a personal and social hygienic approach to prevention.

RISK FACTORS AND ATHEROSCLEROTIC LESIONS*

Jack P. Strong and Douglas A. Eggen

The preceding papers have considered the epidemiologic evidence for environmental and host factors which entail an increased risk of developing coronary heart disease (CHD). The bulk of evidence from many sources indicates overwhelmingly that severity of mural atherosclerosis is closely associated with morbidity and mortality from CHD. Obviously, however, atherosclerosis is not the only condition determining risk of clinical CHD. Conditions predisposing to the occlusive event at a given severity of atherosclerosis also may influence risk of CHD. Thus, CHD is usually the end result of at least two processes, coronary atherosclerosis, and occlusion resulting from thrombosis, hemorrhage, or embolism. The primary roles of the myocardium and conduction system are less well understood in relationship to morbidity and mortality from CHD.

This report will summarize the evidence bearing on the relationship of CHD risk factors to atherosclerotic lesions. Since atherosclerotic lesions cannot be visualized directly during life, autopsy studies are necessary to determine the relationship of risk factors for CHD to atherosclerotic lesions *per se*. Recently published results of the International Atherosclerosis Project (IAP) [952] and other recent autopsy studies will be used to demonstrate these relationships. These studies have provided valuable information concerning lesions and risk factors in spite of the many well-known limitations imposed by the very nature of autopsy studies [958]. Lesions in the coronary arteries will be the principal focus of this report; however, aortic atherosclerosis is related also to many of the risk factors for CHD.

Methods in Autopsy Surveys. Methods used in the IAP have been described in detail [591], and the methods of other surveys referred to are described in

* The work herein has been supported in part by research Grants HE-08974 and HE-07913 from the National Heart Institute, NIH, and the Public Health Service.

the publications cited. Only a brief description of methods in the IAP will be given here. Arterial specimens collected at autopsy following a standard procedure were fixed in a flattened position, packed in plastic bags, and shipped to a central laboratory where they were stained grossly with Sudan IV under standardized conditions. The coded specimens were evaluated by a team of pathologists who estimated visually the percentage of the surface covered by different types of lesions. Periodic checks of reproducibility and reliability of the grading procedure were conducted to control inter- and intra-observer variability. To reduce the

Table 1. *Mean percentage of intimal surface involved with raised atherosclerotic lesions in the combined coronary arteries of males who died of accident, cancer, infection, or selected miscellaneous causes not associated with coronary heart disease (basal group*[a]*)*

Location-race group	Age in years				Unweighted mean
	25–34	35–44	45–54	55–64	
New Orleans white	10.6	16.9	29.8	32.0	22.3
Oslo white	3.5	16.9	27.5	32.8	20.2
Durban Indian (Asian)	5.0	8.4	23.4	32.9	17.4
Manila Filipino	4.3	11.0	18.5	28.3	15.5
New Orleans Negro	3.3	10.2	17.7	26.2	14.4
Caracas I-w[b]	4.6	12.4	13.3	21.5	13.0
São Paulo white	2.2	8.0	14.3	19.8	11.1
Puerto Rico white	2.1	6.7	12.7	17.4	9.7
Santiago white	2.0	6.1	11.5	17.6	9.3
Jamaica Negro	2.5	5.7	10.3	17.8	9.1
Puerto Rico Negro	1.6	7.3	5.3	19.3	8.4
Lima I	1.6	4.2	10.3	17.0	8.3
Cali I-w	0.9	4.9	13.1	13.8	8.2
Costa Rica white	1.9	4.6	10.8	15.4	8.2
Mexico I-w	0.4	4.6	11.8	12.1	7.2
São Paulo Negro	1.6	5.2	6.2	11.0	6.0
Durban Bantu	1.8	3.2	7.0	10.6	5.6
Guatemala I-w	1.8	3.9	5.7	10.5	5.5
Bogotá I-w	0.7	3.4	6.8	11.0	5.5

[a] Men between the ages of 25 to 64 years, by location-race and by 10-year age group. Data from the International Atherosclerosis Project [1457].

[b] I-w: American Indian-white and I: American Indian.

sampling bias inherent in all autopsy surveys, analyses of the data have been performed on cases dying of selected diseases as well as on the total sample. Illustrative results to be presented here will be based on analysis of the percent surface of coronary arteries covered with raised atherosclerotic lesions which include fibrous plaques, calcified lesions, and other complicated lesions (thrombotic, ulcerated, and hemorrhagic). Data on the extent of atherosclerotic lesions obtained by these methods have been examined to determine the association with many of the risk factors for CHD. Results of the examination of differences in extent of lesions with age, sex, race, geographic and ethnic groups, serum lipids and dietary fat, hypertension and diabetes, physical activity, obesity, hardness of water supply, and cigarette smoking will be considered in this report.

Geographic and Ethnic Groups. Geographic and ethnic differences in average extent of coronary atherosclerosis at a given age are large. Data from the IAP (Table 1) illustrate such differences. On the average, cases from populations such as New Orleans (white and Negro), Oslo, and Durban (Indian) have approximately three to five times as many raised lesions in the coronary arteries as do cases from the Durban (Bantu), Guatemala, São Paulo (Negro), and Bogotá populations. Strictly comparable figures are not available for CHD mortality for all of the populations in the IAP. Where such data are available the measures of athero-

Table 2. *Ranking of nine cities based upon mean percentage of intimal surface involved with raised atherosclerotic lesions (RL) in coronary arteries combined, compared with ranking of the locations by mortality rates*[a] *for atherosclerotic heart disease for males by 10-year age group*

Location-race group	Age group							
	45–54				55–64			
	surface involved with raised lesions		mortality		surface involved with raised lesions		mortality	
	mean percentage	rank	rate	rank	mean percentage	rank	rate	rank
North American city[b]	29.8	1	310	1	32.0	1	878	1
Caracas	13.3	3	122	2	21.5	2	474	2
São Paulo[c]	14.3	2	120	3	19.8	3	397	3
Cali	13.1	4	92	6	13.8	6	260	7
Lima	10.3	7	94	5	17.0	5	244	8
Santiago	11.5	6	75	8	17.6	4	370	5
Mexico	11.8	5	83	7	12.1	7	281	6
Bogotá	6.8	8	109	4	11.0	8	381	4
Guatemala	5.7	9	43	9	10.5	9	110	9

[a] Mortality rates per 100,000 from Interamerican Investigation of Mortality [1201].
[b] Arterial lesions for New Orleans whites; mortality rates for San Francisco (all races, predominantly whites).
[c] Arterial lesions for São Paulo whites; mortality rates for São Paulo (all races, but predominantly whites).

sclerotic lesions rank the populations in much the same order as CHD mortality rates [1457]. This is illustrated in Table 2 where ranking of data on coronary artery lesions is compared with ranking by mortality rates for nearly comparable populations in the Interamerican Investigation of Mortality [1201]. The coefficients of rank correlation between lesions and mortality rate for these two age groups are 0.71 and 0.77, both of which are significantly greater than zero ($P<0.05$).

Age. Age has the strongest and most consistent association with lesions of all known risk factors. Fig. 1 shows the variation with age in mean extent of coronary raised lesions in 19 location-race groups of the IAP [422]. The upper left (reference) curve shows the unweighted mean of all means for the 19 location-race groups. The average involvement with raised atherosclerotic lesions increases

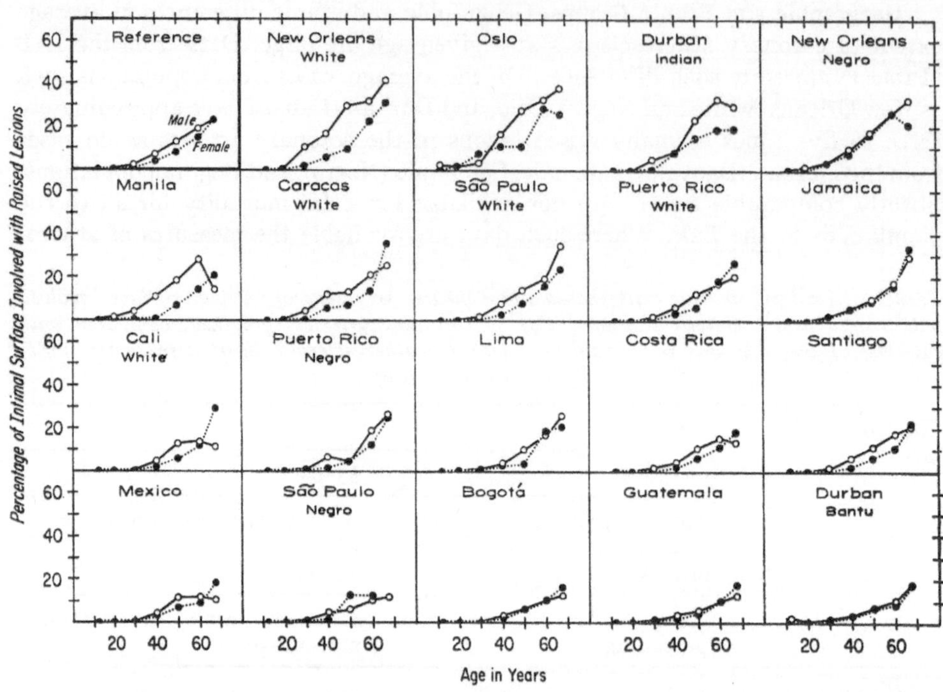

Fig. 1. Mean percentage of intimal surface involved with raised lesions in coronary arteries of the basal group (excluding CHD and diseases associated with atherosclerosis such as hypertension and diabetes) by age and sex. The *reference curve* is based on the unweighted mean of the means for each age group in all 19 location-race groups. (Courtesy of Dr. H. C. McGill, Jr., et al. Permission by Dr. Robert E. Stowell, ed. [952])

Table 3. *Unweighted mean percentage of intimal surface of coronary arteries involved with raised atherosclerotic lesions, and the ratio of mean for males to that for females. Subjects were from four 10-year age groups of each location-race group (25–64 years)*

Location	Mean percentage of intimal surface with raised lesion		Ratio male/female
	male	female	
White			
New Orleans	22.3	10.0	2.23
Oslo	20.2	13.8	1.46
São Paulo	11.1	7.0	1.59
Puerto Rico	9.7	7.3	1.33
Santiago	9.3	5.0	1.86
Costa Rica	8.2	5.3	1.55
Negro			
New Orleans	14.3	13.6	1.05
Jamaica	9.1	8.2	1.11
Puerto Rico	8.4	5.2	1.62
São Paulo	6.0	6.9	0.87
Durban	5.7	5.1	1.12

with age in every population sampled. Sternby [1422] has presented similar results from a sample of autopsies of 66% of all deaths during an 18-month period in Malmö, Sweden.

Sex. Coronary atherosclerosis is considered generally to be more extensive in men than in women. The data of the IAP [1457] and those presented by Sternby [1422] indicate that this is consistently true for the white populations; however, this sex difference either is less or is not detectable in the Negro populations [1457]. A comparison of sex differences in the white and Negro populations sampled in the IAP is shown in Table 3. With the exception of the Puerto Rico Negro (which had the fewest cases of all groups) the sex difference in the Negro is lower than in the white. Thus, the effect on lesions of factors associated with sex are not simple and clear-cut.

Race. In addition to the difference in sex distribution of coronary atherosclerosis between white and Negro, there is some evidence that there is also a generally lower susceptibility to lesions among the Negro. In the three locations where both Negro and white populations were sampled for the IAP, the Negro had less extensive lesions than the white. In Durban, South Africa, the Bantu had less extensive lesions than the Asian Indians. These findings are in keeping with clinical and epidemiological findings concerning CHD. Any genetic or racial effect is undoubtedly confounded to some extent with socioeconomic differences between the groups even though the samples were usually drawn from the lower socioeconomic groups. As shown in Table 3, however, a strong gradient in coronary atherosclerosis exists among the Negro populations and among the white populations of the IAP. Thus, environmental background may be more important than racial background in determining the extent of coronary atherosclerosis.

Serum Lipids and Dietary Fat. Atherosclerotic lesions seem to be related to levels of serum cholesterol and dietary fat when comparing populations, but there are no conclusive data for positive association between atherosclerotic lesions and serum lipids or diet within a population. The few studies that have related serum lipids and lesions have not found a positive relationship. Prospective studies with careful documentation of habitual diets, thorough serum lipid studies, autopsy follow-up, and standardized evaluation of lesions are required to determine the relationship of diet, serum lipids, and lesions in individual persons. Such definitive studies have not been performed.

Fig. 2 compares serum triglyceride levels, serum cholesterol levels and extent of coronary lesions in three populations from the IAP. These data [907] suggest that current triglyceride levels may not parallel population differences in atherosclerotic lesions and that the well-recognized and documented population difference in serum cholesterol levels may be decreasing. If confirmed, these findings may have broad implications regarding pathogenesis of lesions and the expectation of CHD in the previously underdeveloped populations.

Hypertension and Diabetes. Hypertension (or high blood pressure) and diabetes mellitus (or carbohydrate intolerance) are two CHD risk factors of prime importance. Data from the IAP [1243] confirm many previous studies which have reported aggravation or acceleration of atherosclerotic lesions in persons with these disorders. The IAP data indicate that on the average persons with hypertension or diabetes have consistently more coronary and aortic atherosclerosis

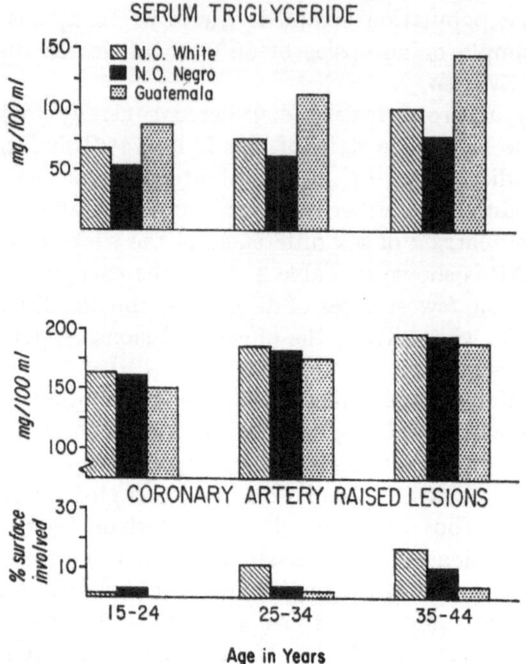

Fig. 2. Serum cholesterol and serum triglyceride levels in samples of male blood donors at hospitals contributing to the autopsy samples in the International Atherosclerosis Project, with extent of atherosclerotic lesions in males for these autopsy samples, by decade of age. Data from Malcom [907]

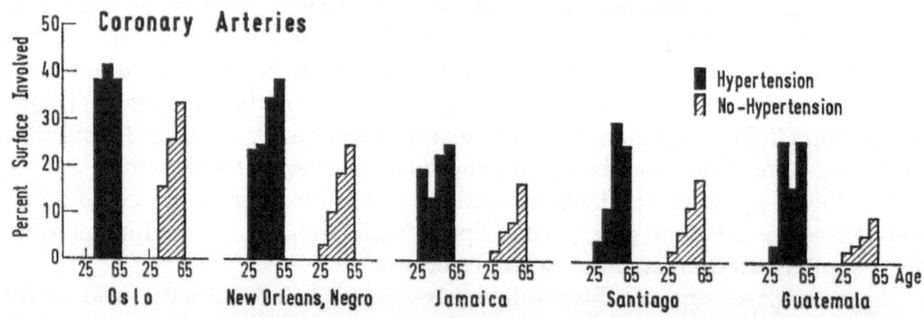

Fig. 3. Mean extent of raised atherosclerotic lesions in coronary arteries of men by presence or absence of hypertension, by age and by location-race group. Data from International Atherosclerosis Project (Robertson [1243])

than persons without hypertension or diabetes for all sex, age, race, or geographic location groups. In Fig. 3 raised lesions in the coronary arteries of men with hypertension and men either with no hypertension or with unknown status with respect to hypertension are compared for five location-race groups. In all groups and at all ages the extent of lesions is greater in the known hypertensives than in the remaining cases.

A comparison of coronary atherosclerosis in men known to have diabetes with that in men either without diabetes or of unknown status with respect to diabetes is given in Table 4. There is a strong indication that men with diabetes have more coronary atherosclerosis than those without. Similar associations between coronary lesions and hypertension or diabetes have been reported recently by Sternby [1422] for an autopsy survey in Malmö, Sweden.

Hypertension and diabetes do not appear to be primary causes of atherosclerosis, however, because atherosclerosis may be severe and extensive in persons without either disease. The findings of these autopsy studies indicate, however, that hypertension and diabetes accelerate the natural progression of atherosclerosis in all populations.

Hypertension is a good example of a risk factor which may influence the process of atherosclerosis and may also add risk of clinical disease. Hypertension

Table 4. *Mean percentage of intimal surface involved with raised atherosclerotic lesions in the coronary arteries of males age 45–64 years*[a]

Location-race	Age in years			
	45–54		55–64	
	diabetes	no diabetes	diabetes	no diabetes
New Orleans white	46	37	46	37
Durban Indian (Asian)	60	29	43	37
New Orleans Negro	35	27	47	30
Caracas I-w[b]	21	20	47	27
Jamaica Negro	8	14	31	20
Santiago white	26	13	35	19
Guatemala I-w	28	7	46	13
Unweighted mean	32	21	42	27

[a] By seven location-race groups, by presence or absence of diabetes, and by 10-year age groups. Data from International Atherosclerosis Project [1243].

[b] I-w: American Indian-white.

almost certainly accelerates atherosclerosis; also, it probably renders a given degree of coronary atherosclerosis more serious by imposing a greater work load on the heart.

On the other hand, hypertension alone in the absence of severe atherosclerosis does not appear to influence greatly the rate of CHD. For example, in Jamaica, hypertension is prevalent but CHD is uncommon. Hypertension aggravates atherosclerosis in this population, but the increase is superimposed upon a relatively low base. The resulting severity of atherosclerosis may not be sufficiently great to produce frequent CHD.

Physical Activity. Most studies of the relationship of physical activity of work and CHD have not examined the association between activity and lesions, although they provide evidence that activity is related to CHD. Those studies that have examined the association between mural lesions and activity have failed to show an association [1035]. Our studies, which are crude in classifying activity but standardized in evaluating lesions, also do not disclose consistent relationships of occupational physical activity and coronary atherosclerosis [1432].

Obesity. Obesity is usually classified as a secondary risk factor in CHD exerting its effect through concomitant hypertension, diabetes, or hyperlipidemia. There is disagreement in the literature on the relationship of lesions and obesity as expressed by various indices of body weight. The results of the IAP indicate that severity of atherosclerosis in the coronary arteries and aorta is not associated strongly or consistently with obesity, body weight, or body height [1018].

Table 5. *Mean of percentage of intimal surface of coronary arteries involved with raised lesions by age and average rate of cigarette smoking last 10 years of life, total sample of white and Negro men*[a]

Age in years	Computations	Average number of cigarettes smoked per day for last 10 years of life		
		0	1–24	25 or more
	White			
25–34	number of cases	8	21	14
	mean	2	8	11
35–44	number of cases	27	21	39
	mean	19	33	40
45–54	number of cases	13	57	82
	mean	31	40	39
55–64	number of cases	33	46	80
	mean	36	47	38
	Negro			
25–34	number of cases	20	63	17
	mean	4	4	15
35–44	number of cases	11	77	44
	mean	7	16	20
45–54	number of cases	22	84	49
	mean	17	32	38
55–64	number of cases	37	73	36
	mean	28	35	29

[a] Data from a current study on the relationship of cigarette smoking to atherosclerosis in New Orleans white and Negro males. Department of Pathology, Louisiana State University Medical Center.

Water Hardness. The work of several investigators, most notably that of Morris [1036] and Schroeder [1317], have shown that there is a negative correlation between the mineral content of drinking water and mortality from CHD. No significant correlations were found between mineral content of water in 14 cities represented in the IAP and either extent of atherosclerotic lesions or percentage of cases with coronary artery stenosis [1430]. Thus, there is little evidence in the IAP data that water hardness or mineral content influences the atherosclerotic process. Any effect on cardiovascular mortality is probably mediated through some other mechanism.

Cigarette Smoking. The propensity for heavy smokers of cigarettes to develop CHD can, at least in part, be attributed to atherosclerotic lesions since lesions are more extensive in heavy smokers than in nonsmokers. Two recent studies of autopsied men have shown consistent trends of more coronary atherosclerosis in heavy smokers when compared to nonsmokers of similar age and race [75, 1432]. Table 5 presents data from the New Orleans sample showing mean extent of raised lesions in coronary arteries by cigarette smoking habits and age in autopsied white and Negro men. In this study smoking habits were determined

Table 6. *Percentage of cases with various degrees of atherosclerosis in sets of men matched according to age and cause of death* [a]

Smoking habit		Total		Degree of coronary atherosclerosis			
		No.	percentage	none (percentage)	slight (percentage)	moderate (percentage)	advanced (percentage)
Never smoked		46	100	4.3	63.0	13.0	19.6
Current rate	<20	46	100	2.2	34.8	34.8	28.3
(cigarettes	20–39	92	100	1.1	27.2	39.1	32.6
per day)	40+	46	100	2.2	8.7	41.3	47.8

[a] Data from Auerbach [75].

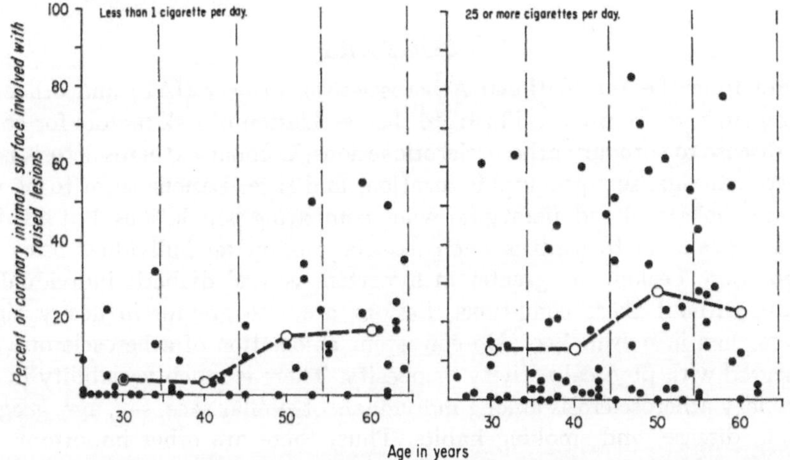

Fig. 4. Scatter plot showing percentage of coronary intimal surface involved with raised atherosclerotic lesions by age for New Orleans Negro males dying from accidents and diseases excluding those that have been associated with atherosclerosis or cigarette smoking, by average rate of smoking over last 10 years of life

by interviewing surviving relatives [1432]. Lesions are consistently more extensive for those averaging 25 or more cigarettes a day for the last 10 years of life than for those averaging less than one cigarette per day. Similar results were obtained when the analyses were limited to a basal group of cases after removing those dying from coronary heart disease, hypertension, diabetes, stroke, and conditions thought to be caused by smoking. Data from an autopsy survey by Auerbach [75] are given in Table 6. Advanced coronary atherosclerosis was much more prevalent in the heaviest smokers than in those men who had never smoked. In addition, there was a regular progression in average severity of lesions with increasing rate of cigarette consumption. Aortic atherosclerosis has also been shown to be greater in the heavy cigarette smokers [1276, 1432].

Unexplained Variability. One intriguing finding in all studies of human atherosclerosis is the wide variation among individuals in extent of lesions which persists in the most homogenous subgroups. This variability is illustrated in Fig. 4 which shows scatter plots of coronary raised lesions in 35- to 64-year-old New Orleans Negro men dying from accidental causes and other causes not known to be associated with cigarette smoking or atherosclerosis and classified according to smoking habits. Even after selecting cases according to race, sex, age, disease, and level of cigarette consumption, there is still much variability to be explained. For the 25- to 34-year age group the surface involvement with raised atherosclerotic lesions ranges from zero to 32% in the nonsmoker or light smoker and from zero to 63% in the heavy smoker. Great variability is also present in subgroups of subsequent decades. Even if other risk factors had been considered, there would still have been much variability remaining. This variability should be investigated intensively by epidemiologic, pathologic, genetic, and other methods. This unexplained variability could be the result of genetic influences which regulate susceptibility to other etiologic agents.

SUMMARY

Data from the International Atherosclerosis Project (IAP) and other recent autopsy surveys are used to illustrate the association of risk factors for coronary heart disease to coronary atherosclerotic lesions. Coronary atherosclerosis is found to vary with age, sex, geographic location, and race. Lesions seem to be related to serum cholesterol and dietary fat when comparing populations, but insufficient data are available to confirm such associations on an individual basis within a population. Lesions are greater in hypertensive and diabetic individuals than in those without these conditions. Lesions are also greater in heavy cigarette smokers than in nonsmokers. No consistent association of atherosclerotic lesions is observed with physical activity or obesity. There is much variability in extent of coronary atherosclerosis among individuals of similar race, sex, age, geographic location, disease, and smoking habits. Thus, there are other important factors involved in development of atherosclerosis that have yet to be determined.

Section XI

SELECTED PAPERS ON EPIDEMIOLOGY OF ATHEROSCLEROSIS

AN ASSESSMENT OF CORONARY HEART DISEASE AND CORONARY RISK FACTORS IN A NEW GUINEA HIGHLAND POPULATION

R. B. Goldrick, P. F. Sinnett and H. M. Whyte

The present study was carried out on 95% of the 1,500 members of a single clan of Enga-speaking people living at Tukisenta in the Western Highlands of New Guinea fifteen miles from Laiagam. These people live in scattered hamlets at an altitude of 8,000 feet. Wild life is scarce so hunting makes slight demands on their energy and contributes little to their nutrition. As land is plentiful and tribal fighting is a thing of the past, their major activities are restricted to preparation of sweet potato gardens, harvesting of the crop, collection of firewood for their homes and occasional house building. We have selected this primitive population for study because the recent introduction of pyrethrum as a cash crop and discoveries of minerals in the area should assure a rapid urbanization.

This investigation has three main objectives. First, to establish the prevalence of coronary heart disease (CHD) in a New Guinea population living in its traditional manner, secondly to correlate this with social, nutritional, anthropometric, medical and biochemical parameters, and thirdly to assess prospectively over the next two or more decades, the effects of urbanization on these parameters and on the prevalence of CHD.

Here, we wish to define the extent to which these people have features which are termed "coronary risk factors". For this purpose we will use only those data which were obtained on the 777 individuals over the age of 15 years.

Diet. A dietary survey was undertaken on a subsample of 90 adults. All items of food consumed by each subject were weighed over a period of seven consecutive days and analyzed. Their diet consisted almost entirely of sweet potato, carbohydrate (mainly starch) providing 94% of the total caloric intake and fat less than 3%. Protein intake was assessed at the remarkably low figure of 25 g/day. The daily caloric intake was 2,300 for males and 1,770 for females.

Nutrition. In spite of the low protein intake the entire group was remarkably healthy. There was no clinical evidence of malnutrition, serum albumin and hemoglobin levels were normal, and only three cases of malaria were identified. By European standards both sexes were close to 100% of their ideal body weights in their early twenties. Thereafter, there was a parallel decline in weight for males and females to 80% of ideal by the age of 60 years. Skinfolds remained uniformly low in males at all ages indicating that the decline in body weight was due to loss of muscle. Skinfold thickness in females was greater than in males until the age of 40 years after which differences between the sexes disappeared. Thus, it appears that New Guinea females lost both muscle and adipose tissue with advancing age.

Physical Fitness. This was assessed by bicycle ergometry and the Harvard Pack Test [325] in 126 New Guineans and was found to be superior to that of Australians.

Blood Pressure. The New Guineas showed no rise in either systolic or diastolic blood pressure with age, and there was little evidence of hypertension. In this connection it is interesting to note that the urinary sodium excretion averaged 10 mEq/24 hr.

Serum Lipids (Fig. 1). The serum total cholesterol was low by European standards and did not rise with age. On the other hand, the serum triglycerides were relatively high at all ages and in both sexes by comparison with U.S. data [489]. The most striking degree of hypertriglyceridemia was observed in females below the age of 20 years. The cause of the hypertriglyceridemia in this population

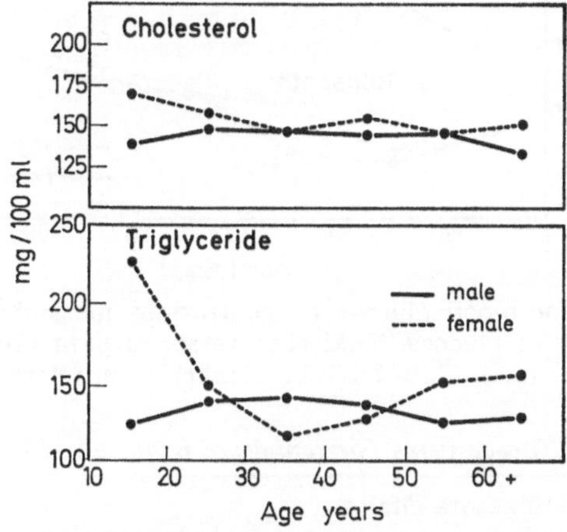

Fig. 1. Mean values for serum total cholesterol and triglyceride concentrations in 777 New Guinea natives

has not been ascertained. However, it seems reasonable to assume that the very high intake of dietary carbohydrate may be a major etiological factor.

Glucose Tolerance. Blood glucose levels one hour following the ingestion of 100 g of glucose (Fig. 2) were considerably lower at all ages than in comparable studies carried out in the U.S.A. [652]. Fasting blood glucose levels showed no tendency to rise with age and no cases of diabetes mellitus were detected in this population.

Coronary Heart Disease. Clinical evidence of atherosclerosis and its complications was minimal, for only two subjects gave a history compatible with the diagnosis of angina pectoris and no one showed evidence of peripheral vascular disease or previous cerebrovascular accident. However, other degenerative diseases such as corneal arcus, cataract and osteoarthritis were present respectively in 43%, 32%, and 15% of natives over the age of 40 years. Analysis of the 777 electrocardiograms classified according to the Minnesota code [1255] confirmed the impression of the rarity of CHD. Electrocardiographic findings on natives aged 40–59 years are shown in table the and have been compared with data from U.S. males and females in the Tecumseh survey [1130]. Our conclusions about the rarity of CHD are based on the complete absence of large Q-waves and a low overall incidence of Q-waves. However, T-wave inversion was common, especially in females in whom the rate exceeded that in Tecumseh. We doubt that this pattern is indicative of CHD, because it has been described as occurring extensively in normal African and Negro populations [239, 585, 885]. It could however, lead to confusion in interracial comparisons of electrocardiograms,

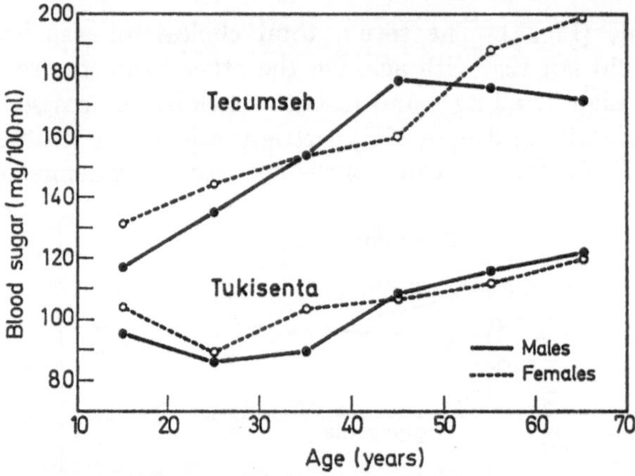

Fig. 2. Mean values for blood glucose concentrations measured one hour following the ingestion of 100 g of glucose. Tukisenta refers to data obtained in the present survey. Tecumseh data have been taken from reference [1255]

Table. *ECG code items (percentage of frequency, 40–59 years)*

ECG items	Minnesota code[a]		Males		Females	
			New Guinea 139	Tecumseh[b] 798	New Guinea 121	Tecumseh[b] 801
Q-waves	I	1	0	1.3	0	0
		2	0.7	1.4	0	0.4
		3	0	0.5	0	0.5
	total		0.7	3.1	0	0.9
Lt. axis deviation	II	1	2.9	6.8	3.3	3.6
Tall R waves	III	1	3.6	3.8	0	1.7
S-T depression	IV		0.7	3.3	0.8	8.0
T-wave inversion	V		5.8	14.8	25.6	15.6
I-V conduct. defect	VII		0.7	3.4	0	1.2

[a] See reference [1255].
[b] See reference [1130].

particularly if the criteria of Higgins et al. [680] are used in which classification is based on the combined occurrence of Q-waves, S-T segment depression, and T-wave inversion.

We conclude that both CHD and the common "coronary risk factors" are rare in this New Guinea population living in its traditional fashion. It is our hope that further study of these people during progressive urbanization will assist in identifying those factors which are most significant in the etiology of CHD.

METABOLIC FACTORS ASSOCIATED WITH CORONARY HEART DISEASE IN BUSSELTON MALES

T. A. Welborn, D. J. A. Jenkins, G. N. Cumpston, D. H. Curnow, D. V. Goff, C. J. Johnstone, N. S. Stenhouse and M. Summers

This presentation explores the possible relevance of "risk-factors" for coronary heart disease (CHD) other than blood pressure and serum cholesterol levels. The term "risk-factor" is used here to denote variables relating to the prevalence of CHD since incidence data is not yet available from the population under study.

Busselton, in Western Australia, is a rural community 150 miles south of the capital city, Perth. In November 1966, the first of a series of surveys of health and disease in this community was conducted. 91% of the target population of adults attended the survey for comprehensive medical screening; and the data for male subjects in the study will be described.

The criteria employed for the survey diagnosis of CHD are summarized in Table 1 and have been described in greater detail elsewhere [1533]. The criteria are those proposed by Epstein et al. [439] and depend on positive histories for angina pectoris (AP) or myocardial infarction (MI) or on positive electrocardiographic findings from 12 lead ECGs classified by the Minnesota Code [1255]. "Probable" CHD was diagnosed on the basis of verified AP or MI and/or positive ECG changes (essentially major Q-wave, S–T segment, or T-wave changes). A diagnosis of "suspect" CHD related to nonverified chest pain histories or to borderline ECG abnormalities. All remaining subjects were classified as having "no CHD".

Table 2 shows the mean values for physiological variables in the several diagnostic groups. In accordance with previous studies, "probable" CHD males were older and had higher mean levels of blood pressure and serum cholesterol than males with no CHD. "Probable" CHD males also showed higher mean serum uric acid levels. At one hour after oral glucose, they had elevated mean blood sugar and serum-insulin levels. There was a small tendency for CHD subjects to be more obese. Almost invariably, the mean values for "suspect" CHD subjects are intermediate to those of the other two groups.

To assess the discriminating ability of these variables, age of course must be taken into account. Thus the age-specific 80th percentile values were taken as the dividing limits between "upper" and "lower" ranges. (If CHD cases were no different from the general population, one would expect 20% of CHD subjects to have "upper range" values.) The right-hand side of Table 2 shows that 33–35% of the "probable" CHD males had high diastolic blood pressure and serum cholesterol levels, and also serum uric acid levels; these trends were highly significant. "Upper range" blood sugar levels and percentage desirable weight showed significant but less powerful associations with CHD, whereas the "one hour" serum insulin had no significant ability to discriminate coronary heart disease cases under the conditions of this study. Various uncontrolled

Table 1. *Diagnostic criteria for coronary heart disease (CHD) on the basis of probable (+) or suspect (?) histories of angina pectoris (AP) or myocardial infarction (MI) or frank (+) or borderline (?) ECG findings*

Busselton population 1966
Respondents in survey (1,638 males, 1,693 females) = 91%

Coronary heart disease (CHD):
Diagnostic categories —

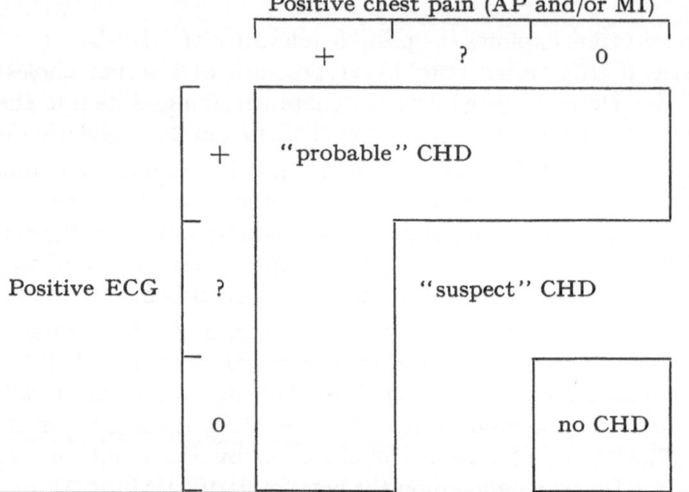

Table 2. *Mean values in 1966 for physiological variables in Busselton males with no CHD, "suspect" and "probable" CHD*[a]

1,638 Busselton males

	Mean values for physiological variables			"Probable" CHD: observed percentage of subjects with values above 80th percentile ("expected" percentage = 20%)
	no CHD (N=1422)	"suspect" CHD (N=105)	"probable" CHD (N=111)	
Age (yrs)	47	51	62	...
Diastolic BP (mm)	79	82	84	35% ($p<0.001$)
S. cholesterol (mg%)	220	225	240	35% ($p<0.001$)
S. uric acid (mg%)	5.5	5.5	6.0	33% ($p<0.001$)
"One hour" blood-sugar (mg%)	101	103	123	29% ($p<0.01$)
Percentage desirable wt.	112	114	115	27% ($p<0.05$)
"One hour" serum-insulin (μU/ml)	41	48	33	25% (n.s.)

[a] The proportion of "probable" CHD subjects with values exceeding the age specific 80th percentile of all males in the population is shown in the right-hand column.

factors undoubtedly contributed to the known variability and wide range of serum insulin values including exercise, and variable intervals between food ingestion, the glucose load, and the time of the blood sample.

A further, more intensive examination of subjects with CHD in Busselton was made in July, 1968, eighteen months after the initial survey. Cases of "probable" or "suspect" CHD under the age of 60 years were recalled together with an age, truly-matched random sample of control subjects with no CHD, from the same community. Subjects were asked to attend fasting, with avoidance of physical activity, in order to provide basal measurements of serum lipids, insulin, and glucose. This investigation was a pilot study to investigate the feasibility and

Table 3. *Mean values in the 1968 follow-up study for physiological variables in males with "probable" CHD compared with approximately age-matched control males*[a]

146 Busselton males (age <60 yrs)	mean values for physiological variables		"probable" CHD: observed percentage of subjects with values above 80th percentile of controls	
	no CHD (N=46)	"probable" CHD (N=44)		
Age (yrs)	44	48	...	
DPB (mm)	82	92	36%	
S. cholesterol (mg%)	237	250	39%	
S. uric acid (mg%)	5.4	5.9	45%	($p<0.05$)
F. blood-sugar (mg%)	83	89	39%	
Percentage desirable weight	110	114	34%	
S. triglycerides (mg%)	127	159	43%	($p<0.05$)
S. insulin (μU/ml)	10	12	34%	
S. free fatty acid (mg%)	363	397	34%	
Blood ketones (mg%)	47	48	11%	

[a] The proportion of "probable" CHD subjects with values exceeding the 80th percentile of the control males is shown in the right hand column.

value of obtaining fasting blood samples and of measuring a more extensive range of possible "risk-factors". The response rates for "probable" and "suspect" CHD groups was 90%, but for the invited control subjects was only 70%.

Table 3 shows the mean values for physiological variables in control males and "probable" CHD males. (The lack of exact age matching in the two groups reflects the poor response rate of the control subjects.) In general, similar trends are observed for mean diastolic blood pressure, serum cholesterol, and serum uric acid levels as in the initial study. Using the 80th percentile levels of the "no CHD" males as the cutting point for upper and lower ranges, it is seen that the proportion of "probable" CHD males with elevated values for these variables is 34–45%, considerably exceeding the expected proportion of 20%. Because of the small numbers of subjects, however, only serum uric acid achieves possible significance ($p<0.05$) as a discriminating factor.

The additional metabolic factors measured in this pilot study (Table 3) were fasting serum triglycerides, serum-insulin, serum free fatty acids, and blood ketones (beta-hydroxy butyrate). Particular care was taken to measure accurately the low levels of fasting serum-insulin, since immuno-assay methods commonly give spuriously high values especially in low concentration ranges. One further practical point is that with regard to the free fatty acid and ketone levels, the time of day (i.e. the duration of overnight-fasting) was found to influence the values obtained. In future studies it is recommended that the time of testing be restricted to between 7:00 and 9:00 a.m., rather than between 7:00 and 11:30 a.m. as in this study.

Table 4. *Linear correlation coefficients (r) between various physiological variables and the CHD score*[a]

Correlation coefficients:

			r	
CHD score	triglycerides 0.23 ($p<0.01$)	insulin	0.38	$p<0.001$
		uric acid	0.34	
		cholesterol	0.35	
		weight	0.33	
		blood sugar	0.24	$p<0.01$
		FFA	0.23	
	blood sugar 0.22 ($p<0.01$)	insulin	0.40	$p<0.001$
		weight	0.34	
		age	0.30	
		FFA	0.26	$p<0.01$
		triglyceride	0.24	
	blood pressure 0.27 ($p<0.001$)	age	0.48	$p<0.001$
		weight	0.27	
		FFA	0.27	
		insulin	0.26	$p<0.01$
		uric acid	0.25	

[a] 146 males: 46 with no CHD ... 0; 56 with "suspect" CHD ... 1; 44 with "probable" CHD ... 2 — "CHD score"

Serum triglyceride levels were moderately elevated in the males with CHD, and their discriminating power was of possible significance ($p<0.05$). The differences in the mean fasting levels of serum insulin and of serum free fatty acids were less marked, but the distribution of these variables was such that suggestive trends emerged for "probable" CHD subjects to exhibit elevated values. Such trends may prove to be significant when larger numbers are studied. With regard to blood ketone levels, the hint that CHD subjects show a diminished proportion of subjects with upper range values is intriguing. If confirmed in a larger study this may suggest a separate metabolic fate for free fatty acids in CHD (possibly incorporation into triglycerides?).

Another way of examining the strength of association of metabolic factors with CHD is by the use of simple correlation analyses. A "coronary heart disease score" is allocated: subjects with no CHD are given a score of zero; those with "suspect" CHD a score of 1; and those with "probable" CHD a score of 2. Linear correlation coefficients between the "CHD score" and the levels of physiological variables are then obtained (Table 4). CHD in males showed significant correlations with blood pressure ($p<0.001$), fasting blood sugar ($p<0.01$) and fasting serum triglycerides ($p<0.01$), but no significant associations with the other variables were obtained. However, a large number of metabolic factors had strong associations with these three major correlates of CHD. Time permits only two points to be made from these data. First, a common trio, serum insulin, serum free fatty acids, and body weight, are positively correlated with each of the three major variables correlating with CHD, namely blood pressure, blood-sugar and serum triglyceride levels. Thus, although not related directly to the survey manifestations of CHD, insulin and free fatty acid levels were closely associated with recognized metabolic concomitants of CHD. If such findings were confirmed in a larger study the possible etiological role of insulin and/or free fatty acids in atherosclerosis will require the more close scrutiny. Next, the strong relationship between serum uric acid and serum triglycerides, and of triglycerides (but not uric acid) with CHD, suggests that the association between uric acid and CHD discerned in males of the initial total population study was mediated by a common link with lipid metabolism. This also requires further pursuit and the delineation of independent relationships of various factors.

In conclusion, the pilot study reported suggests that to obtain fasting blood samples in population studies may prove to be valuable. First, from the practical aspect of discrimination of CHD risk, the data suggest that serum triglycerides may prove to be a superior discriminant. Second, in the search for more direct etiological factors in atherosclerosis, the measurement of serum insulin and free fatty acid levels may provide useful clues as a basis for further research. Finally, the more complete definition of primary biochemical abnormalities in atherosclerosis is clearly important in giving a more rational basis for the application of preventive measures.

SUMMARY

The adult population of Busselton (6,500), a rural town in Western Australia, have been studied since 1966 for cardiovascular disease. In 1966, 91% were screened for evidence of CHD; physical and biochemical measurements were also obtained. In 1968 a more intensive re-examination was made of possible cases of CHD previously diagnosed on the grounds of chest pain and/or ECG record, together with a control group from the same population. In the males attending the follow-up study (total number 146) fasting serum triglycerides appeared to be a better discriminant for prevailing CHD than other factors. Among the men there was a positive correlation between CHD and serum triglyceride, fasting blood sugar, and blood pressure levels. Insulin, free fatty acids, and body weight showed significant correlations with each of the preceding factors, though not directly with CHD.

RELATIONSHIPS BETWEEN ADIPOSE TISSUE CELLULARITY AND CARBOHYDRATE AND LIPID METABOLISM IN A RANDOMLY SELECTED POPULATION

P. Björntorp, A. Gustafson and G. Tibblin

The relationship between obesity and diabetes mellitus, well-known to clinicians, has long been suspected to be due to an unknown influence of adipose tissue on carbohydrate metabolism. The role of adipose tissue was suspected by Ogilvie [1117], who found hyperplasia of the islets of Langerhans in obesity. It has now been shown by a number of laboratories that obese patients often have hyperinsulinemia after a glucose load, and it has been suggested that this is directly related to the amount of adipose tissue [82], particularly the size of the expanded fat cells [1283]. Albrink and Meigs [37] have suggested that the increase in plasma triglyceride, found in patients with acquired obesity, could also in some way be connected to a factor in adipose tissue.

In a recent study from this laboratory it was shown that plasma glycerol correlated positively with body fat [180]. It was suggested that this was a consequence simply of the number of fat cells since, *in vitro*, glycerol release from adipose tissue is apparently dependent only on fat cell number [182]. Furthermore, body fat correlated with fasting plasma insulin, and this could be due to an increased fat cell diameter in obese patients (see preceding). These results indicated two regulatory factors in adipose tissue for carbohydrate and lipid metabolism, viz. fat cell number and fat cell diameter. In order to try to elucidate these complex interactions, determination of all pertinent variables was undertaken in a group of individuals in which age and environmental factors were standardized as much as possible. Therefore, oral glucose tolerance with plasma insulin, triglycerides and cholesterol, as well as free glycerol, were determined and correlated with measurements of body composition, including body fat, fat cell diameter, and total fat cell number.

MATERIAL

The persons investigated consisted of a randomly selected sample of a population of men in the city of Göteborg, born in 1913 [1470]. This population sample was obtained in the following way. From the Revenue Office, which must by law keep a register up to date of all people living in the city, all men born in 1913 on the days which were even multiples of three, were selected for investigation. As described previously the attention to the first investigations by these selected men was high (8% nonparticipants). This population which was originally examined in 1963 is now followed for different purposes, utilizing the special examination resources of a well-equipped hospital. For these purposes different subsamples, again randomly selected, are utilized.

For the present investigation the men born on the 6th of every month during the year of 1913 were investigated in 1968. They comprised a total of 85 men of whom 81 participated in the investigation.

METHODS

The men reported to the laboratory in the morning after having fasted during the preceding 15 hours. They did not smoke on the morning before or during the investigation.

First, venous and capillary blood was drawn for determinations of serum cholesterol [336], triglycerides [280] and blood free glycerol [843]. Thereafter they took 100 g glucose, dissolved in 200 ml water, perorally. Blood glucose and plasma insulin were determined before and 30, 60, 120 and 180 min after glucose ingestion, using a glucoxidase method [859] and a radioimmunochemical method [594], respectively.

In 49 of the men, again randomly selected, fat cell size and number were determined. This was performed with needle biopsy according to Hirsch and Goldrick [686] from the subcutaneous depot to the left and below the umbilicus. In every third of these men a sample was also taken in the gluteal region. Fat cell size was determined according to a method utilizing formalin fixation and freeze-cutting whereafter fat cells were measured microscopically (Björntorp, unpublished data).

In another randomized sample of the population, body composition was determined utilizing the technique of isotope dilution for determination of total exchangeable potassium and total body water [876, 877], and calculations according to Moore et al. [1020] in order to obtain total body fat. These determinations were then also correlated with simple anthropometric measurements such as body weight, length, waist circumference and skinfold measurements. The highest correlation coefficient (r: 0.87) was then obtained for the expression:

$$BF = 0.381 \times WC + 0.019 \times SF - 24.783;$$

where BF = body fat in kilograms; WC = waist circumference in centimeters and SF = sum of skinfold measurements (triceps plus subscapular plus abdominal, in millimeters). This investigation will be published elsewhere (Tibblin, 1969).

In the sample now investigated this formula was utilized in order to obtain the body fat. By calculations according to Hirsch and Gallian [685] the total number of fat cells in the body could be estimated.

RESULTS

Fig. 1 shows the distribution and Table 1 the mean and standard deviations of the measured variables. It may be seen that the distributions of fat cell number, triglycerides, free glycerol and the sum of glucose or insulin were skewed to the right. Therefore, these were recalculated on a logarithmic basis, and the skewness apparently disappeared except for free glycerol, which now apparently was skewed to the left. By recalculation of the square root an apparently normal distribution was obtained.

Table 2 gives the correlations between different body composition data and plasma concentrations of hormones and metabolites. It may be seen that body

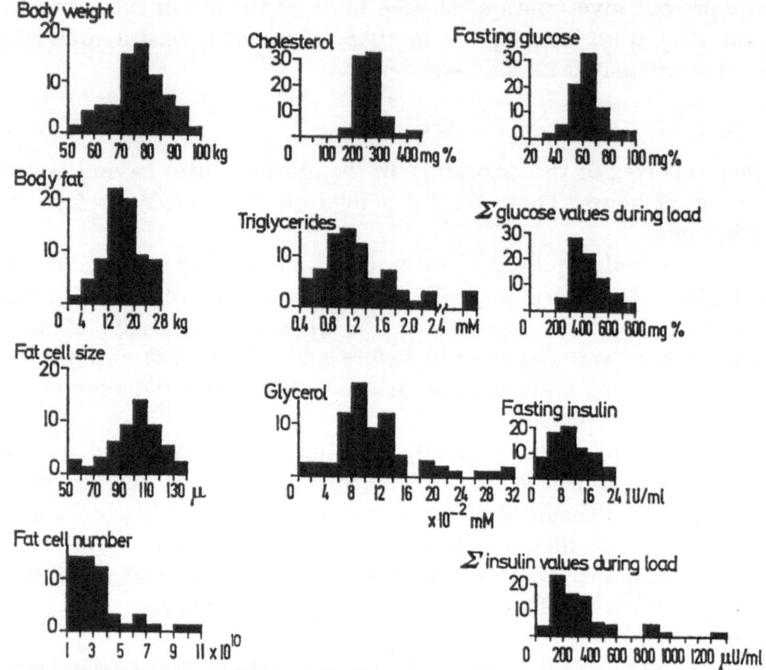

Fig. 1. Frequency distribution of metabolic variables studied in a sample of men born in 1913

Table 1. *Results of metabolic studies in men born 1913*

	Mean ± S.D.	*n*
Body weight	75.6 ± 9.5 kg	81
Estimated body fat	16.3 ± 5.6 kg	81
Estimated fat cell number	$3.3 \times 10^{10} \pm 2.0 \times 10^{10}$	49
Fat cell diameter (abdominal)	102 ± 16 μ	49
Fat cell diameter (gluteal)	110 ± 9 μ	15
Fasting glucose	64 ± 11 mg-%	80
Fasting insulin	10 ± 5 μU	77
Sum of glucose during load	497 ± 122 mg-%	79
Sum of insulin during load	320 ± 232 μU	76
Cholesterol	259 ± 45 mg-%	81
Triglycerides	144 ± 60 mg-%	80
Free glycerol	0.10 ± 0.06 mM	81

fat correlated with fat cell diameter, while body weight did not. Body weight, however, correlated with fat cell number.

Fasting insulin correlated with increasing degree of statistical significance with body weight, body fat and fat cell diameter, while a negative correlation was found with fat cell number. Triglycerides showed no significant correlation with body composition data. Glycerol correlated positively with fat cell number and negatively with fat cell diameter.

Table 2. *Correlation coefficients (r) between selected variables measured in men born in Göteborg in 1913, or their logarithms*

Parameter	Body fat	Body wt.	Fat cell diameter	Estimated fat cell number
Fat cell diameter	0.40[b]	0.14	1.0	−0.77[c]
Estimated fat cell no.	—	0.28[a] (0.38[b])	−0.77[c]	1.0
Fasting insulin	0.35[a]	0.22	0.51[c]	−0.35[a]
Triglyceride	0.08	—	0.18 (0.14)	0.14 (0.06)
Glycerol	0.06	0.02	−0.35[a] (−0.35[a])	0.41[b] (0.33[a])
	Triglycerides	**Glycerol**	**Sum insulin dur. load**	
Fasting insulin	0.30[a] (0.60[c])	−0.33[a]	0.40[b]	
Sum of insulin during load	0.35[b] (0.17)		1.0	
Sum of glucose during load	0.25[a] (0.27[a])			
Glycerol	0.03	1.0		

[a] $p<0.05$. [b] $p<0.01$. [c] $p<0.001$.

Triglycerides showed positive correlations with fasting insulin as well as with the sum of insulin or glucose values during the glucose tolerance test. No correlation was seen with glycerol, which correlated negatively with fasting insulin. Fasting insulin and the sum of insulin values during the glucose tolerance test correlated with a high degree of significance.

DISCUSSION

The calculation of fat cell number is, of course, fairly approximate, because the size of fat cells in all locations of the body is not known. It should, however, give a reasonably good estimate for comparative studies within the group, because there was no difference (and a positive, although weak, correlation) between fat cell size in the gluteal and abdominal region. Furthermore, Hirsch et al. [687] have found no difference between fat cell size at different regions, and Bjurulf [185] found a strong correlation between fat cell size in different parts of the body.

Thus, fat cell number correlated with glycerol concentration in plasma. Glycerol concentration is also strongly correlated with glycerol turnover rate and with plasma free fatty acid turnover rate [180]. Glycerol concentration, therefore, probably gives an estimate of total adipose tissue lipid mobilization. The correlation between this and the number of fat cells indicates that lipid mobilization during short term fasting is dependent upon the number of fat cells in the body as we have earlier suggested [180, 182].

Fat cell diameter, on the other hand, showed correlations with plasma insulin. Fasting insulin correlated also, although considerably less pronounced, with body fat and body weight. The connection between fat cell size and insulin production, previously indicated in obese patients by Salans et al. [1283] is apparently also valid in individuals from a general population.

Plasma triglycerides showed correlations with insulin values and with the sum of glucose values during the peroral glucose tolerance test. This has recently been shown also by Abrams et al. [7]. Reaven et al. [1215] suggested that insulin produces an increased liver synthesis of very low density lipoproteins. An interference of glucose-insulin metabolism with lipoprotein removal mechanisms is another possibility.

It would, of course, be tempting to see a connection between adipose tissue fat cell size, insulin production, and plasma triglycerides. This is, however, hampered by the fact that there was no correlation between fat cell size and plasma triglycerides. An alternative explanation would be that insulin production is the primary event regulating both adipose tissue fat cell size and plasma triglyceride concentration.

CARBOXYHEMOGLOBIN AND SERUM CHOLESTEROL LEVELS IN SMOKERS CORRELATED TO THE INCIDENCE OF OCCLUSIVE ARTERIAL DISEASE

Knud Kjeldsen

The etiology and pathogenesis of human atherosclerosis is not well understood. Many different factors seem important, and from animal experiments a large number of atherogenic compounds have been described [326]. It is well known that certain diseases, e.g. diabetes, hypertension and obesity, are connected with an increased frequency of atherosclerosis, and that physical inactivity, increased blood lipids, and excessive cigarette smoking are important risk factors in patients with atherosclerotic heart disease.

Coronary heart disease (CHD) is perhaps the most common of all diseases in western countries. CHD is not uncommon in nonsmokers. During the last decades, however, several large epidemiological studies have shown, with little contradictory evidence, a significant association between cigarette smoking and the morbidity and mortality of CHD. It is outside the scope of the present paper to review these investigations, and only a few important conclusions should be mentioned: (1) the mortality from myocardial infarction is 1.5 to 2 times higher in cigarette smokers than in nonsmokers; (2) the risk is highest among younger and middle aged men; and (3) the risk increases rapidly with both the number of cigarettes smoked and with inhalation of the smoke. In men smoking more than 20 cigarettes per day the risk of a fatal coronary occlusion is three times the nonsmoker risk [401], with more than 40 cigarettes per day six times the nonsmoker risk, and if these excessive smokers also are physically inactive, nine times the nonsmoker risk [483].

Epidemiological evidence of a connection between smoking and atherosclerosis does not necessarily mean that this connection is a causal one. Autopsy studies, however, strongly suggest that this association has a causal significance [75, 1275]. The precise manner in which smoking induces atherosclerotic changes in the arterial wall continues to evade investigators. Much attention has been focused on the acute cardiovascular effects of nicotine, but so far no evidence has been presented to connect nicotine to the development of atherosclerosis. In animals nicotine is not atherogenic [576, 790, 1460, 1537] and does not induce areas of cardiac necrosis [1536]. It also seems worth noting that exposure of cholesterol-fed rabbits to small concentrations of carbon monoxide (0.02 vol%) for 10 weeks significantly increases the aortic atheromatosis, and in three-quarters of the animals induces cardiac necrosis [70]. Furthermore, carbon monoxide under these circumstances calls forth significant elevations in serum cholesterol and triglyceride values of the exposed animals [806].

Table 1. *Intensity of smoking in normal subjects and in subjects with cardiovascular disease*

Smoking category	Controls		Subjects with atherosclerotic diseases	
	n	percentage	n	percentage
Light	121	16.4	3	5.3
Moderate	463	62.7	34	59.6
Heavy	154	20.9	20	35.1

Astrup [68] first demonstrated that blood from smokers with occlusive arterial diseases contained remarkably high concentrations of carbon monoxide and pointed out the pathophysiological importance of the resulting decrease in oxygen release to the arterial wall. Later investigations confirmed this observation [808, 1055].

A natural extension of the animal studies would be an investigation of carboxyhemoglobin and serum cholesterol levels in a human population and relation of these values to smoking values and clinical signs of cardiovascular disease. A population of about 1,000 industrial workers was chosen, about half of these were tobacco workers. Due to their unlimited access to tobacco, the tobacco workers could be expected to have smoking habits different from a standard population. The volunteers filled out a questionaire concerning personal data, smoking habits, and clinical signs of atherosclerotic vascular diseases. Thereafter blood samples for estimation of carboxyhemoglobin and serum cholesterol estimation were drawn after the subjects had smoked their usual dose of tobacco in their usual manner. All samples were taken at approximately the same time of the day (after lunch).

In 59 subjects a diagnosis of atherosclerotic cardiovascular disease was made: four had earlier myocardial infarction, 12 stenocardia, and 28 atherosclerosis obliterans. Fifteen had more than one diagnosis. Among the 59 diseased subjects only two were nonsmokers; and one of these had, until two years earlier, been a heavy cigarette smoker. Furthermore, a significantly higher number of the diseased subjects were heavy smokers ($p<0.01$; Table 1) and a significantly higher number inhaled the smoke ($p<0.05$; Table 2). The results of carboxyhemoglobin and serum cholesterol analyses in normal subjects and patients with atherosclerotic diseases are shown in Table 3. Average carboxyhemoglobin values were in the controls 3–4% and in the atherosclerotic subjects 6–8%. Highly significant differences were also found in serum cholesterol values of the two groups. Healthy smokers had significantly higher serum cholesterol levels than nonsmokers ($p<0.01$), while no such difference was present in the diseased subjects (Table 4). Both carboxyhemoglobin and serum cholesterol concentrations increased with the intensity of smoking (Table 4), suggesting a positive correlation

Table 2. *Number of normal smokers and smokers with cardiovascular disease inhaling or not inhaling the smoke*

Inhalation	Controls		Subjects with atherosclerotic diseases	
	n	percentage	n	percentage
Yes	584	79.1	51	89.5
No	154	20.2	6	10.5

Table 3. *Results of carboxyhemoglobin and serum cholesterol analyses in normal subjects and in patients with cardiovascular disease*

Group	n	Carboxyhemoglobin (saturation percentage)		Serum cholesterol (mg/100 ml)	
		M ± S.D.	range	M ± S.D.	range
Controls	934	3.4 ± 3.2	0–19.0	245 ± 45	121–478
Patients	59	6.8 ± 3.8	0–17.0	284 ± 55	198–471
		$p<0.001$ ($t=6.58$)		$p<0.001$ ($t=5.38$)	

between carboxyhemoglobin and serum cholesterol values. The pooling of all data gave a highly significant correlation in normal subjects ($r=0.92$, $p<0.001$) as well as in subjects with cardiovascular diseases ($r=0.73$, $p<0.001$).

A remarkably large proportion of the patients were tobacco workers (52 out of 59). Table 5 shows that the tobacco workers had significantly higher carboxyhemoglobin and serum cholesterol values than other workers. It may be concluded from this study that:

1. There is a significant correlation between excessive smoking habits and the presence of clinical symptoms of atherosclerosis, as well as between high carboxyhemoglobin saturations and clinical signs of atherosclerosis.

2. Carboxyhemoglobin saturations of 8–19%, which were found in 40% of the patients with cardiovascular disease are of the same magnitude as those provoking atherosclerosis and cardiac necroses in animals.

3. As in animals, such carboxyhemoglobin concentrations may increase blood cholesterol levels in man.

Table 4. *Average values of carboxyhemoglobin and serum cholesterol in smokers and nonsmokers in control group and group of patients with arteriosclerotic cardiovascular disease*

Smoking category	Carboxyhemoglobin (saturation percentage)			Serum cholesterol (mg/100 ml)		
	controls M ± S.D.	patients M ± S.D.	significance	controls M ± S.D.	patients M ± S.D.	significance
Smokers	4.2 ± 3.1 (738)[a]	7.0 ± 3.7 (57)	$p<0.001$ $t=5.52$	247 ± 44 (738)	290 ± 33 (57)	$p<0.001$ $t=4.89$
Nonsmokers	0.4 ± 0.9 (196)	0.5 ± 0.7 (2)	n.s. $t=0.16$	236 ± 49 (196)	284 ± 56 (2)	$p<0.02$ $t=2.32$
Light smokers	2.5 ± 2.5 (121)	3.7 ± 2.5 (3)	n.s. $t=0.76$	245 ± 38 (121)	279 ± 67 (3)	n.s. $t=1.45$
Moderate smokers	4.1 ± 3.0 (463)	7.3 ± 3.6 (34)	$p<0.001$ $t=4.95$	246 ± 45 (463)	286 ± 50 (34)	$p<0.001$ $t=4.52$
Heavy smokers	5.7 ± 3.0 (154)	7.0 ± 4.0 (20)	n.s. $t=1.45$	253 ± 45 (154)	298 ± 53 (20)	$p<0.05$ $t=2.18$

p = Probability that difference is not due to chance.
t = Student's t calculation.
n.s. = not significant.
[a] The number of subjects in each category is enclosed in parentheses beneath the mean (M) and standard deviation (S.D.).

Table 5. *Results of carboxyhemoglobin and serum cholesterol analyses in tobacco workers and in other workers*

	n	Carboxyhemoglobin (saturation percentage)		Serum cholesterol (mg/100 ml)	
		M ± S.D.	significance	M ± S.D.	significance
Tobacco workers	458	3.9 ± 3.5	$p<0.02$ ($t=2.41$)	252 ± 47	$p<0.01$ ($t=2.68$)
Other workers	535	3.4 ± 3.2		244 ± 47	

4. Among the healthy smokers about 15% had carboxyhemoglobin levels of a magnitude similar to the diseased subjects. As a working hypothesis it may be assumed that these subjects represent a group having a higher than normal risk of developing atherosclerotic cardiovascular disease. There is some early evidence that this hypothesis may be correct. The material is presently being reinvestigated after an interval of three and a half years. Only three subjects had developed clinical signs of cardiovascular disease, and they all belonged in this group.

HEART RATE: AN IMPORTANT RISK FACTOR FOR CORONARY MORTALITY — TEN-YEAR EXPERIENCE OF THE PEOPLES GAS CO.

EPIDEMIOLOGIC STUDY (1958-68) *

D. M. Berkson, J. Stamler, H. A. Lindberg, W. A. Miller, E. L. Stevens, R. Soyugenc, T. J. Tokich and R. Stamler

During the past decade, the concept has emerged concerning the role of risk factors in the genesis of premature clinical coronary heart disease [45, 782, 1403]. In particular, the effects of high serum cholesterol levels, elevated blood pressure, cigarette smoking, and overweight have been delineated, as well as the probable influences of several other factors (e.g. hyperglycemia, hyperuricemia, physical inactivity, certain personality-behavior patterns [45, 142, 144, 370, 400, 435, 770, 782, 1159, 1257, 1403, 1404, 1405, 1406, 1408, 1410, 1412]).

This report presents data indicating that resting heart rate may also be an important, independent risk factor. This conclusion is based on the ten-year mortality findings from the prospective study of middle-aged male employees of the Peoples Gas, Light and Coke Company in Chicago [1406].

METHODS

The cohort under study was originally identified as of January 1, 1958. At this time the total male labor force age 40–59 at the Peoples Gas, Light and Coke Company numbered 1,594 men. Of these, 1,465 (91.9%) underwent complete standardized examination in 1958, and 1,329 were identified as a cohort free of definite clinical coronary heart disease [1406]. These 1,329 men constitute the basis for this report.

The resting heart rate was measured from lead II of a standard electrocardiogram recorded in 1958. The relationship of heart rate to age-adjusted ten-year mortality rates were analyzed independently and in association with four other risk factors also measured in 1958—serum cholesterol, casual diastolic blood pressure (fifth phase), cigarette smoking habit and relative weight (ratio

* The cooperation and support of Eric Oldberg, M.D., President, Chicago Board of Health and Chairman, Chicago Health Research Foundation is gratefully acknowledged. In addition, the authors wish to acknowledge the contributions of Wanda Drake, Celene Epstein, Dana T. King and William McAtee. Thanks are also extended to Paul Meier, Ph.D., Professor, Department of Statistics and Biological Sciences Computation Center, University of Chicago, and to the Medical Department and Executive leadership of the Peoples Gas Light and Coke Company, particularly Remick McDowell, Chairman, and Leslie A. Brandt, President. The research presented herein was made possible by grants from the Chicago Heart Association and the National Heart Institute, National Institutes of Health, United States Public Health Service (HE 04197 and HE 09426).

of observed weight to desirable weight for height, from life insurance tables [53, 55, 1406, 1412].

Attribution of cause of death was based on a detailed review of all obtainable data, evaluated independently of information on risk factors. Findings included death certificates, autopsy reports, hospital records, etc. Sudden death was defined as death occurring within one hour of observed onset of illness.

Mortality rates were age-adjusted by five-year age groups to the U.S. male population, 1960, by the direct method. The comparative distributions by five-year age groups were generally similar for the U.S. male population age 40–59 in 1960, and the 1,329 men in the Gas Company cohort age 40–59 in 1958, free of CHD and followed without systematic intervention. When two rates were compared, the difference between them was tested for significance by the usual t-test. When rates for more than two groups were compared for statistical significance of differences, the chi-square test was employed. In addition, a linear regression method was utilized with calculation of a weighted slope [252]. (While relationships between independent and dependent variables may be curvilinear rather than linear, an assumption of linearity for the purpose of the t-test is under most circumstances reasonable. It is less so when the curvilinear relationship is U-shaped [see below]).

RESULTS

The distribution of resting heart rates and their relationship to ten-year mortality rates from all causes, all cardiovascular-renal (CVR) causes, coronary heart disease (CHD) and sudden death are presented in Table 1. With stratification of the population into six groups (resting heart rate <60, 60–69, 70–79, 80–89, 90–99 and $\geqq 100$ beats per minute, or into four groups (<60, 60–69, 70–79, $\geqq 80$) or into two groups (<80, $\geqq 80$), mortality rates from all causes, CVR diseases, CHD, and sudden death were higher for those with faster, resting heart rates. The higher mortality rates were recorded particularly for men with resting heart rates of 80 or more beats per minute. Death rates were approximately twice as high in the group with rates $\geqq 80$, compared to the group <80. For the six-group analyses, all chi-square values indicate that differences among groups are statistically significant (p values <0.05 or $\leqq 0.01$). The slopes for all causes and for sudden death are significantly different from zero ($p<0.05$). For the four-group comparisons, chi-square values indicate that the differences among groups are statistically significant for all causes ($p<0.01$), CHD ($p=0.05$) and sudden death ($p<0.05$). For the dichotomized two-group analyses, p is <0.05 for all causes, all CVR disease, and CHD.

For sudden death, the six- and four-group analyses suggest a U-shaped curve, i.e. the mortality rate for the group with heart rate less than 60 beats/min is four times that of the group with heart rate 60–69. The mortality rate from sudden death of this latter group is notably lower than the death rates of all other groups (Table 1, see the following).

Although the 1,329 men were all free of definite coronary heart disease at entry examination in 1958, some had suspect CHD, ECG abnormalities or other illnesses which might increase both heart rate and mortality. In order to evaluate this possibility, a subgroup of the 1,329 men was identified, numbering 1,094 men

Table 1. *Relationship between resting heart rate in 1958 and ten-year mortality rates, by cause (cohort of 1,329 men originally age 40–59 and free of definite coronary heart disease) Peoples Gas Co. study, 1958–68*

Resting heart rate, 1958, in beats/min	No. of men	Ten-year mortality, 1958–68							
		all causes		all CVR diseases[a]		coronary heart disease		sudden death	
<60	158	11[b]	72.5[c]	8	52.1	4	26.5	4	26.5
60–69	445	50	108.5	23	50.1	16	35.5	3	6.5
70–79	480	53	98.2	26	49.2	16	31.4	12	23.7
80–89	161	28	159.0	15	84.7	11	61.4	4	25.6
90–99	51	12	198.5	5	75.9	4	61.9	2	29.9
≥100	34	9	228.7	5	143.5	4	124.6	3	91.0
<60	158	11	72.5	8	52.1	4	26.5	4	26.5
60–69	445	50	108.5	23	50.1	16	35.5	3	6.5
70–79	480	53	98.2	26	49.2	16	31.4	12	23.7
≥80	246	49	178.2	25	92.7	19	71.0	9	36.8
<80	1,083	114	98.2	57	49.3	36	32.0	19	16.8
≥80	246	49	178.2	25	92.7	19	71.0	9	36.8
All	1,329	163	113.3	82	57.3	55	39.3	28	20.3

[a] All Cardiovascular-Renal Diseases.

[b] No. of deaths.

[c] Ten-year rate per 1,000, age-adjusted by 5-year age groups to U.S. male population, 1960.

Table 2. *Relationship between resting heart rate in 1958 and ten-year mortality rates, by cause (cohort of 1,094 men originally age 40–59 and free of all cardiovascular-renal diseases, other life-limiting diseases, and ECG abnormalities, except minor T-wave abnormalities), Peoples Gas Co. study, 1958–68*

Resting heart rate, 1958, in beats/min	No. of men	Ten-year mortality, 1958–68[a]							
		all causes		all CVR diseases		coronary heart disease		sudden death	
<60	128	6	50.8	3	24.7	3	24.7	3	24.7
60–69	387	40	103.9	16	42.5	12	32.2	2	4.9
70–79	396	35	80.5	13	30.5	8	19.7	6	15.4
≥80	183	29	151.5	12	62.4	10	52.9	6	32.6
<80	911	81	86.5	32	34.6	23	25.3	11	11.9
≥80	183	29	151.5	12	62.4	10	52.9	6	32.6
All	1,094	110	97.5	44	39.4	33	29.9	17	15.3

[a] See footnotes of Table 1.

free of suspect CHD and life-threatening illness of any type. All men in this cohort had completely normal resting ECGs, except for 187 with minor non-specific T-wave abnormalities (low voltage, diphasic or flat T's).

In this cohort, the proportion of men with heart rates of 80 or greater was slightly lower than in the group of 1,329 men, 16.7% and 18.5% respectively. Thus, there was some association between higher heart rate and abnormal medical findings. The data for this group of 1,094 men also revealed a relationship between 1958 resting heart rates and ten-year mortality rates (Table 2). For the four group analyses, the chi-square test demonstrated that the differences among death rates for all causes are significant ($p<0.05$), and the slope is also significantly different from zero. The chi-square test for sudden death yielded a p value <0.10 but >0.05. For the dichotomized two-group analyses (heart rate <80 and $\geqq 80$), the differences in mortality rates were significant for all causes.

Table 3. *Relationship between resting heart rate in 1958 and ten-year mortality rates, by cause (cohort of 907 men originally age 40–59 and free of all cardiovascular-renal diseases, other life-limiting diseases, and all ECG abnormalities) Peoples Gas Co. study, 1958–68*

Resting heart rate, 1958, in beats/min	No. of men	Ten-year mortality, 1958–68[a]							
		all causes		all CVR diseases		coronary heart disease		sudden death	
<60	116	5	44.8	3	26.5	3	26.5	3	26.5
60–69	338	34	100.9	12	36.3	8	24.4	1	2.7
70–79	323	27	75.2	8	22.7	5	15.0	3	9.4
≥80	130	20	143.8	8	57.3	7	51.7	4	31.4
<80	777	66	82.7	23	29.0	16	20.4	7	19.2
≥80	130	20	143.8	8	57.3	7	51.7	4	31.4
All	907	86	92.3	31	33.7	23	25.2	11	12.1

[a] See footnotes of Table 1.

Once again, the four-group analysis indicated a U-shaped curve for sudden death (Table 2).

The same analysis was also carried out after excluding from the cohort of 1,094 men the 187 with minor T-wave abnormalities. Of the 187, 53 (28.3%) had resting heart rates of 80 or greater in 1958. In contrast, only 130 (14.3%) of the residual 907 men had such heart rates. Thus, there was indeed an association between higher heart rates and minor T-wave abnormalities. And this residual cohort of 907 men had a slightly lower proportion of men with heart rates of 80 or greater than the cohorts of 1,094 and 1,329 men (14.3, 16.7 and 18.5%, respectively). These data, then, support the hypothesis that, to some degree at least, association of heart rate and mortality may reflect underlying pathophysiology responsible for a relatively rapid heart rate.

Nevertheless, for this group of 907 men free of any ECG abnormality, life-threatening illness, or evidence of CHD (definite or suspect), essentially the same association was recorded between resting heart rates and mortality rates (Table 3). By chi-square test, for the four-group analysis, differences among groups in mortality rates were significant for all causes ($p=0.05$) and sudden death ($p<0.05$). The slope was significantly different from zero for all causes

Table 4. *Relationship between heart rate and ten-year mortality rates, by cause, in the absence and presence of one other risk factor in 1958 (cohort of 1,329 men originally age 40–59 and free of definite coronary heart disease) Peoples Gas Co. study, 1958–68*

Risk factor groups	No. of men	Ten-year mortality, 1958–68			
		all causes		coronary heart disease	
Heart rate <80, relative weight <1.15	509	64[a]	116.2[b]	19[a]	36.4[b]
Heart rate ≥80, relative weight <1.15	118	23	165.3	8	55.5
Heart rate <80, relative weight ≥1.15	574	50	82.8	17	28.7
Heart rate ≥80, relative weight ≥1.15	128	26	187.9	11	83.6
Heart rate <80, cholesterol <250	707	67	89.3	20	27.5
Heart rate ≥80, cholesterol <250	143	23	149.3	8	54.9
Heart rate <80, cholesterol ≥250	376	47	114.5	16	40.4
Heart rate ≥80, cholesterol ≥250	103	26	216.3	11	93.5
Heart rate <80, diastolic blood pressure <90	872	78	85.6	24	27.1
Heart rate ≥80, diastolic blood pressure <90	172	28	154.5	11	61.9
Heart rate <80, diastolic blood pressure ≥90	211	36	148.4	12	50.9
Heart rate ≥80, diastolic blood pressure ≥90	74	21	215.5		
Heart rate <80, <10 cigarettes	485	34	61.9	11	19.9
Heart rate ≥80, <10 cigarettes	75	14	146.2	6	63.5
Heart rate <80, ≥10 cigarettes	594	79	130.4	25	42.2
Heart rate ≥80, ≥10 cigarettes	171	35	189.2	13	71.6

[a] Number.
[b] Rate per 1,000.

Table 5. *1958 status with respect to heart rate, blood pressure, cigarette smoking and ten-year mortality rates, by cause (1,329 men originally age 40–59 and free of definite coronary heart disease) Peoples Gas Co. study, 1958–68*

1958 risk factor status			No. of men	Ten-year mortality, 1958–68			
heart rate	cigarette smoking	diastolic pressure		all causes		CHD	
NH	NH	NH	378	20[a]	48.3[b]	5	12.0
H	NH	NH	45	6	114.9	3	70.3
NH	NH	H	107	14	118.3	6	51.8
H	NH	H	30	8	221.6	3	52.0
NH	H	NH	491	57	115.8	19	38.9
H	H	NH	127	22	171.1	8	62.3
NH	H	H	103	22	190.4	6	55.0
H	H	H	44	13	265.4	5	94.9
All			1,325[c]	162	113.2	55	39.4

[a] No. of deaths.
[b] Rate per thousand. All rates are age-adjusted by 5-year age groups to U.S. male population, 1960. High (H): Heart rate >80; >10 cigarettes per day; diastolic blood pressure >90 mm Hg. NH is not high, i.e. below specified cutting points.
[c] No smoking data available on 4 of the 1,329 men.

($p=0.05$). For the dichomotized two-group analyses, the difference between groups was statistically significant ($p=0.05$) only for all causes, although the ten-year cause-specific mortality rates were two or more times greater for the group with heart rates of 80 or greater, as compared with the group of less than 80 beats per minute.

Again, the four-group analysis yielded a U-shaped curve for sudden death (Table 3). The significance of this finding is unclear, in view of the small number of sudden deaths in the entire study to date, and specifically in the group of men with 1958 heart rates less than 60 (four decedents altogether, three of whom were in the cohorts of 1,094 and 907 men; see Tables 1–3).

With regard to the major relationship revealed by the foregoing analysis, i.e. the positive associations between resting heart rates and mortality rates, analyses were also done to assess whether these merely reflected associations between heart rate and other established risk factors, e.g. blood pressure, serum cholesterol, relative weight, and smoking status in 1958. Towards this end, simple correlation coefficients were calculated between heart rate and these factors. The mean value of the continuous variables was also calculated for each heart rate group (<60, 60–69, 70–79, <80, ≧80) as well as their 1958 prevalence rates of hypertension (diastolic blood pressure ≧90 mm Hg), hypercholesterolemia (≧250 mg/dl), overweight (relative weight ≧1.15), and cigarette smoking (≧10 cigarettes per day). Mean serum cholesterol and prevalence rate of hypercholesterolemia were similar for all heart rate groups, and the correlation coefficient between heart rate and serum cholesterol was insignificant (0.09). Therefore, the analysis of the relationships between heart rates and mortality rates was not confounded by serum cholesterol. This was also true for relative weight. Furthermore, the relationship between heart rate and mortality was consistently apparent when the cohort of 1,329 men was stratified into two serum cholesterol groups (<250, ≧250), and into two relative weight groups (<1.15, ≧1.15) (Table 4).

However, mean diastolic blood pressure, prevalence of diastolic hypertension (pressure of 90 mm Hg or greater) and prevalence of cigarette smoking (defined as 10 cigarettes or more per day) increased with resting heart rate. Simple correlation coefficients were also significantly positive between resting heart rate and blood pressure ($r=0.23$), and resting heart rate and cigarette smoking ($r=0.18$).

Therefore, in order to further investigate the confounding effect of these risk factors, the group was also stratified according to the presence or absence of diastolic hypertension or cigarette smoking, and the analysis of the relationship between heart rate and mortality rate was repeated. Mortality rates from coronary heart disease were consistently higher in those resting with heart rates of 80 or greater irrespective of the presence or absence of either of these risk factors considered singly (Table 4).

All three factors (heart rate, blood pressure and smoking) were also evaluated concurrently in relation to ten-year mortality rates (Table 5). For each of the four paired comparisons (none of the three risk factors present versus faster heart rate only; hypertension versus hypertension+faster heart rate; ≧10 cigarettes per day only versus cigarettes+faster heart rate; and hypertension+

cigarettes versus hypertension+cigarettes+faster heart rate) mortality rates for all causes were sizeably greater for the group with faster heart rate versus the matching group with heart rate <80 beats/min. This was true also for CHD mortality rates for three of the four paired comparisons. CHD mortality rates were similar for the pair with hypertension, with and without faster heart rate. For all causes, the ten-year mortality rate for the group with all three risk factors high was more than five times that of the group with none high (265.4 versus 48.3 per 1,000). For CHD, the mortality rate was eight times greater in the former group than the latter (94.9 versus 12.0 per 1,000). The findings were similar for the cohorts of 1,094 and 907 men. Corresponding differentials in mortality were recorded when other three-factor combinations were considered, e.g. faster heart rate, hypertension, hypercholesterolemia, or faster heart rate, cigarette smoking, hypercholesterolemia.

DISCUSSION

The results of this study indicate that for middle-aged men, resting heart rate is another important risk factor for premature mortality from sudden death, coronary heart disease, CVR diseases and all causes. A resting heart rate of 80 or more is related to risk of dying in middle-age, and this association is apparently not attributable to observed low-order correlations between heart rate and presence of other life-limiting diseases, ECG abnormalities, hypertension, or the cigarette smoking habit. The greater risk of CHD death associated with resting heart rates of 80 or greater was recorded for men not manifesting hypercholesterolemia, hypertension, cigarette smoking, or overweight on original examination. In general, faster heart rate appeared to interact with these other traits, when present, with resultant multiplicative effects on risk of mortality. Faster heart rate together with cigarette smoking and elevated blood pressure was associated with marked increases in ten-year mortality rates over those recorded for men with none of these three risk factors, in the order of nine- and four-times for CHD and all causes respectively.

The finding of an association between resting heart rate and risk of CHD is in agreement with observations from the Framingham and Western Electric studies. In the former prospective investigation of over 5,000 adults originally age 30–62, the 12-year mortality CHD rate was almost four times greater for men and women with pulse rates over 92 than for those with pulse rates less than 67 [770]. The study of Western Electric Co. middle-aged male employees in Chicago found that heart rates of 90 or greater were associated with increased incidence of CHD [1159]. Similarly, as reported in the Build and Blood Pressure Study, tachycardia, i.e. heart rate of 90–100 per minute, is apparently one of the so-called minor impairments adding to risk of mortality in persons with obesity or hypertension [53]. The data of the present report are unique, therefore, primarily in indicating that the relationship between faster heart rate and risk of mortality is apparently independent of coexistent diseases, ECG abnormalities, and the cardinal coronary risk factors. Hopefully the pooled data from major U.S. prospective studies will be utilized shortly to reinforce this analysis, thereby making possible a comprehensive assessment of the validity of this tentative conclusion [402, 1021].

At this juncture, the mechanisms of the apparent association between heart rate and CHD mortality remain obscure. Further work is needed to assess whether faster heart rate reflects low level cardiopulmonary fitness and whether this is a significant factor related to the observed greater mortality.

Another hypothesis is that individuals with faster heart rates have them as a result of their emotional reaction to the ECG recording. Presumably, then, this would be a sign of cardiovascular hyperreactivity or lability, in turn related to risk of mortality.

Despite efforts to rule it out, consideration must also be given to the possibility that occult myocardial damage from coronary heart disease may have already been present in the men with faster resting heart rates, and this accounted for their higher subsequent mortality rates. Obviously, this possibility cannot be completely excluded by the data available, even for the cohort of 907 men free of any signs of life-limiting disease and any abnormalities in the resting ECG. Unfortunately, exercise and post-exercise ECG data were not available on these men, to shed further light on this matter [143].

It would be of great value to know whether persons with faster heart rates actually have more severe coronary atherosclerosis than persons with slower heart rates. Everything else being equal in terms of risk (serum cholesterol, blood pressure, smoking habit, etc.) faster heart rate should presumably lead to more infiltration of atherogenic lipoproteins into the coronary arteries, due to more frequent increases of lateral pressure, than slower heart rates. To our knowledge, no autopsy or antemortem angiographic data are available on this matter. Of course, it is also possible that with equal severity of atherosclerosis, persons with faster heart rates have higher risks of myocardial ischemia and necrosis than persons with slower heart rates.

Finally, the suggestive finding that risk of sudden death is also increased for men with the slowest heart rates (less than 60 beats/min) is worthy of note in view of recent similar findings, based on six-hour monitoring of ECGs during ordinary daily activities of 301 randomly selected Bell Telephone System employees [682, 683].

SUMMARY AND CONCLUSION

In middle-aged men of the Peoples Gas Company long-term prospective epidemiologic study, resting heart rates of 80 and greater were associated with sizeable increases in risk of dying over the next ten years from all causes, all CVR diseases, coronary heart disease, and sudden death. These associations were independent of coexistent diseases, ECG abnormalities, and other major coronary risk factors (hypercholesterolemia, hypertension, cigarette smoking, overweight). Therefore, faster heart rate is apparently an independent coronary risk factor.

PROGNOSTIC IMPLICATIONS OF SERUM CHOLESTEROL IN CORONARY HEART DISEASE*

Charles W. Frank, Eve Weinblatt and Sam Shapiro

Although much attention has been given to the relationship of the serum cholesterol level in general populations to the incidence of coronary heart disease (CHD), little information exists concerning the prognostic implications of the serum cholesterol level in men with coronary disease, and none at all has yet been reported in relation to the prognosis of coronary heart disease in women. This report will present new data from the Health Insurance Plan of Greater New York (HIP) study on the incidence and prognosis of coronary heart disease. Detailed descriptions of the study's methodology and criteria for diagnosis have been published [1348]. In a defined population of 110,000 men and women aged 25 to 64, all patients who sustained a first diagnosis of myocardial infarction (MI) or angina pectoris in the four years 1961–1965 were invited to attend a special study baseline examination, at which standardized observations were made including measurement of the serum cholesterol concentration. There were 745 men and 220 women who completed this baseline examination, conducted approximately six months after clinical onset of disease. The prognosis of these patients will be presented for the three and one-half years following the baseline examination.

Table 1 presents some of the pertinent characteristics of the study cohorts as observed at the baseline examination. The male MI cohort consisted of 470 men who survived their initial myocardial infarction and completed the baseline examination. The male angina cohort is composed of 275 men who developed angina pectoris in the absence of historical or ECG evidence of a myocardial infarction or of aortic valve disease. The mean serum cholesterol concentrations were identical in these two cohorts, both among men under and over 55 years of age.

As to be expected, the female coronary population was on the average older than the male. The mean serum cholesterol level among the women with CHD was considerably higher than in the men. In contrast to the findings for men, the mean serum cholesterol levels for women over age 55 was considerably higher than for the younger women in both cohorts.

Table 2 and all of the subsequent tables present the prognosis of the various cohorts over the three and a half years following the baseline examination. The prognosis is expressed in terms of the cumulative probabilities of three end points: death from all causes, death from cardiac causes only, and first or first recurrent myocardial infarction. Life table technics were used in cumulating these probabilities to take into account the varying time periods of observation.

* This study is supported in part by the U.S. Public Health Service, NIH Grant HE-05794 to the Health Insurance Plan of Greater New York (HIP).

Table 1. *Characteristics at baseline examination*

	Males		Females	
	MI	angina	MI	angina
Number	470	275	91	137
Mean age	53.2	54.7	57.4	56.0
	Serum cholesterol level (mg-%)			
All ages	244	244	283	269
55+	242	243	289	276
<55	246	244	261	257

Table 2. *Prognosis within 3.5 yr of baseline*

	No.	Probability percentage of death		
		all	cardiac	first MI
		Males		
MI	470	13.6	11.7	18.9
Angina	275	13.6	9.2	14.6
Total	745	13.6	10.8	17.3
		Females		
MI	91	9.5	9.5	16.2
Angina	137	7.0	4.7	10.1
Total	228	8.0	6.6	12.5

Table 3. *Prognosis within 3.5 yr of baseline for males: depending upon serum cholesterol (mg%)*

	No.	Probability percentage of death		
		all	cardiac	first MI
		Myocardial infarction		
Cholesterol 270+	108	10.7	7.8	11.8
<270	329	12.9	11.5	20.3
		Angina		
Cholesterol 270+	59	12.9	10.9	19.6
<270	204	14.0	8.7	13.4

The top portion of this table presents the prognosis of the male MI and angina cohorts separately and combined. The total mortality experience of the myocardial infarction and angina cohorts among the men was identical, and only small differences are noted in relation to the other end points. Among females the patients beginning with angina appeared to exhibit a somewhat better prognosis than the myocardial infarction patients, but the differences noted are small and could readily have been due to chance.

Table 3 summarizes the prognosis of the male patients and emphasizes a finding which we first reported at the American Heart Association meetings last year [484]. An elevated serum cholesterol concentration has no demonstrable prognostic significance in the three and one half years of observation following the baseline examination. Table 3 contrasts the prognosis of men with baseline cholesterol levels of 270 mg% or greater with that of men who exhibit lower cholesterol levels for each cohort separately. None of the differences indicated is statistically significant ($p>0.10$). The observed differences are in opposite direction in the two cohorts.

In contrast, Table 4 shows a striking disadvantage for hypercholesterolemic women with coronary heart disease. Thus, the probability of death within three and a half years of baseline for women with a cholesterol value of 270 mg%

Table 4. *Prognosis within 3.5 yr of baseline for females: depending upon serum cholesterol level (mg%)*

	No.	Probability percentage of death		
		all	cardiac	first MI
		Myocardial infarction		
Cholesterol 270+	42	17.6	17.6	26.8
<270	36	2.8[b]	2.8[b]	8.7[b]
		Angina		
Cholesterol 270+	56	9.5	9.5	15.7
<270	78	5.3	1.3[a]	6.4

[a] Indicates that the difference between the two rates exceeds confidence limits of 90%.

[b] Exceeds 95%.

or greater, at the baseline examination following the initial myocardial infarction, was 17.6%. For women with lower levels of serum cholesterol, this probability was only 2.8%. This difference exceeds confidence limits of 95%. Similarly, hypercholesterolemic women in the angina cohort were at a disadvantage although only the difference in cardiac death rate was statistically significant.

In order to examine in more detail the prognostic relationships of the serum cholesterol level with respect to other pertinent parameters in women, and in view of the similarities already demonstrated between the angina and MI cohorts, the experience of these two cohorts has been combined in Table 5. This table examines these relationships by age, and the presence or absence of hypertension, diabetes, electrocardiographic abnormality, and overweight. The hypercholesterolemic women are at a disadvantage in both older and younger subsets, when the cohorts are cut at age 55. In contrast with the previously reported findings in our male cohorts [485, 1528, 1529], that the history of, or the finding of elevated blood pressure by the time of the baseline examination carries with it a considerably greater probability of an adverse event in the ensuing few years, a similar classification of the female coronary cohorts does not demonstrate any disadvantage for the hypertensive woman with coronary disease.

Table 5. *Prognosis of women within 3.5 yr of baseline after first MI or onset of angina. Serum cholesterol in relation to other pertinent parameters*

	Serum cholesterol (mg%)	No.	Probability percentage of death all	cardiac	first MI
			Age		
All ages	270+	98	13.0	13.0	20.6
	<270	114	4.5[a]	1.8[b]	7.2[b]
Age 55+	270+	75	12.8	12.8	21.5
	<270	70	5.9	1.5[b]	7.4[a]
Age <55	270+	23	13.1	13.1	17.4
	<270	44	2.3	2.3	6.8
			Blood pressure		
B. P. elevated	all	136	7.8	5.5	9.5
B. P. normal	all	92	8.2	8.2	17.0
B. P. elevated	270+	57	11.0	11.0	15.0
	<270	71	5.9	1.4[a]	6.0
B. P. normal	270+	41	15.9	15.9	28.3
	<270	43	2.3[a]	2.3[a]	9.3[a]
			Diabetes		
Diabetes	all	29	15.8	15.8	11.7
No diabetes	all	199	6.9	5.3	12.7
No diabetes	270+	81	10.2	10.2	21.9
	<270	103	5.0	2.0[a]	7.0[b]
			Electrocardiographic abnormality		
ECG abnormal	all	112	11.5	11.5	18.9
ECG normal	all	116	4.6[a]	1.9[b]	6.5[b]
ECG abnormal	270+	55	19.2	19.2	26.7
	<270	45	4.4[a]	4.4[a]	13.7
ECG normal	270+	43	5.1	5.1	12.6
	<270	69	4.5	0.0	2.9[a]
			Overweight		
Relative wt.	115+	46	6.5	6.5	8.7
	<115	182	8.3	6.6	13.5
Relative wt.	115+				
	270+	21	14.3	14.3	19.0
	<270	23	0.0	0.0	0.0
Relative wt.	<115				
	270+	79	12.1	12.1	20.4
	<270	89	5.8	2.3[b]	9.3[b]

[a] Indicates a difference that meets or exceeds a confidence limit of 90%.
[b] Indicates a difference that meets or exceeds a confidence limit of 95%.

Since hypercholesterolemia is commonly noted in diabetes, the interrelations between these two conditions were examined. Some 13% of the women evaluated at the baseline examination were diabetic. The apparently higher mortality of the diabetic women cannot be demonstrated as statistically significant with the frequencies available. The disadvantage of hypercholesterolemia is demonstrated in non-diabetic women.

As with the male coronary cohorts previously reported [484, 1528], women with coronary disease whose electrocardiogram was shown to reveal certain specified abnormalities at the baseline examination had a significantly worse prognosis than women whose electrocardiogram was found to be normal, or near normal, at the baseline examination. The adverse influence of hypercholesterolemia is well demonstrated in the subset of women with an abnormal electrocardiogram at the baseline examination. Among women with a normal electrocardiogram at the baseline, the disadvantage of an elevated cholesterol level is demonstrable only in terms of the probability of the first recurrence. Mortality among women with a normal ECG is low; however, with the size of these study groups, no judgment can be made about the relation of serum cholesterol to mortality in this subset.

Finally, we see interrelations between the cholesterol level and relative weight. Women who weigh 15% or more above the average of women of the same age and height show no disadvantage in their prognosis. However, within each weight category the hypercholesterolemic women exhibited a higher rate of adverse events. Clearly, the disadvantage of the hypercholesterolemic women was not mediated by overweight.

DISCUSSION

There is considerable uncertainty as to what specific pathogenetic mechanisms immediately precede a recurrent infarction or sudden death in patients with established coronary heart disease. A new event may be induced by a new coronary artery occlusion, but this in turn may be caused by a variety of pathologic processes besides continuing atheroma growth. Furthermore, a recurrent infarction or fatal arrhythmia may be precipitated in patients with established coronary heart disease by mechanisms other than a fresh vascular occlusion. Thus, although coronary atherosclerosis is a prerequisite for the incidence of coronary heart disease, other factors may become dominant in determining the future course of events or the prognosis of patients with established coronary heart disease. The observed patterns of prognosis in relation to the serum cholesterol level in the two sexes may reflect a situation in which the role of these other factors, over a given time interval, is relatively more important in men than in women.

There are well established sex differences in the age trends for the serum cholesterol concentration in the United States [1022]. Between ages 40 and 60 U.S. white males show only a slight increase in the average cholesterol concentration. In contrast, the average cholesterol value for U.S. white women rises sharply, exceeding the male values after age 45. This rapidly rising serum cholesterol level in women may well reflect an increasing rate of atherogenesis, which perhaps exceeds the rate for men at the same age. During these two decades women are probably making giant strides toward catching up with the amount of coronary atherosclerosis already produced by men. Support for this contention can be found in the report of the International Atherosclerosis Project [422].

It is reasonable to suggest that, in a population of patients with coronary heart disease, the rate of continuing atheroma formation is of more relevance to the prognosis of women than of men. Among women with coronary heart disease presumably the rate of atheroma formation is related to the level of serum cholesterol.

SUMMARY

In summary, data have been presented from the Health Insurance Plan of Greater New York study of the incidence and prognosis of coronary heart disease concerning the prognostic significance of the serum cholesterol level in men and women with recent onset of clinical coronary heart disease. The observations are based upon a follow-up of 745 men and 228 women who experienced an initial episode of myocardial infarction or angina pectoris during a four-year period of case finding in a defined population of some 110,000 adults aged 25 to 64. The starting point for the prognostic statements is the study's baseline examination conducted on the average six months after clinical onset of disease.

The serum cholesterol level in men bore no relationship to prognosis over the three and one-half years following baseline examination. By contrast hyper-cholesterolemic women exhibited a significantly higher probability of first or first recurrent infarction and death than women with lower levels of serum cholesterol at the baseline examination. These differences cannot be accounted for by age, blood pressure, overweight, diabetes or ECG findings.

Discussion Following Dr. Welborn's Paper

Dr. Berkson: Dr. Goldrick, were those T-wave inversions, of the so-called "juvenile T-pattern"?

Dr. Goldrick: In pattern, yes, but not in age distribution. They were much more common in middle age than in youth.

Dr. Biss: Dr. Goldrick's paper has pointed out many risk factors. The finding of a low serum cholesterol in his tribe is very important, because it has reconfirmed similar observations among tribes or population groups where the serum cholesterol level was around 150 mg% throughout life. Regardless of any other risk factors, wherever such a study has been undertaken, all such population groups have been proven free of atherosclerotic heart disease.

Dr. Pollock: Dr. Goldrick spoke about the supply of carbohydrates, can he tell us what kind of carbohydrates?

Dr. Goldrick: The carbohydrate was predominantly in the form of starch.

Dr. Bruner: The data from New Guinea reminds us of data we found twelve years ago in Israel with the Yemenites, who at that time showed no increase in serum cholesterol with age. Now an age dependent increase in cholesterol is seen in Yemenites. The conclusion is evident: the age related cholesterol increase is not an obligatory but rather an environmentally dependent phenomenon.

Dr. Boyle: I would like to ask Dr. Welborn if the difference in means he showed, between those with and without coronary heart disease, could be due to age alone. Disease-free men of 47 years were being compared with patients with coronary disease of 62 years.

Dr. WELBORN: Undoubtedly age is a factor contributing to the differences reported. We didn't state any significance levels for comparison of means, but when analyzing the discriminant power of the variables, we took age into account by using the age specific percentile values. I acknowledge the point that the difference of means is partly age dependent, but I also would like to point out that rising blood pressures, serum cholesterol levels, or coronary heart disease itself probably represent pathological aging phenomena in any case. The state of the disease in a community is summarized by showing the mean levels in this way.

Discussion Following Dr. Kjeldsen's Paper

Dr. STAMLER: Recently I had occasion to analyze a set of data possibly related to Dr. Kjeldsen's findings. These were reviewed for a paper on regional differences in coronary mortality, presented last June in Leiden at the Boerhaave Course on Ischemic Heart Disease [1407].

Mortality rates of middle-aged men and women from the economically developed countries are significantly correlated with the average number of cigarettes smoked per year by the population at age 15 and over. In conspicuous contrast to other variables, correlation coefficients between cigarettes smoked and CHD mortality rates are higher for women (0.782) than for men (0.648).

The number of motor cars per 100 persons and CHD mortality rates are also significantly correlated for several age-sex groups (r=0.439–0.583). Does this reflect a relationship between carbon monoxide exposure and CHD risk, per Dr. Kjeldsen's paper, or between sedentary living and CHD risk, or both, or neither!

Time does not permit a review of the nutrient data. Suffice it to note that this analysis updates and extends earlier work [1403–1407]. It again demonstrates significant positive correlations between several nutrients and CHD mortality rates for middle-aged men from the 20 countries, but only a few of the r's are significant for women.

Is it valid to suggest, based on these data, that given an habitual diet, more or less atherogenic due to its saturated fat, cholesterol and calorie content, cigarette smoking plays a particularly crucial role in accounting for the extent of premature coronary disease mortality among women?

Dr. ADAMS: Has Dr. Kjeldsen any information about carboxyhemoglobin levels in pipe and cigar smokers?

Dr. KJELDSEN: Yes, the material was also divided according to which type of tobacco the volunteers smoked. Cigar smokers had rather high values even in healthy subjects, in fact, a little higher than cigarette smokers. It should be stressed, however, that it was only valid for the tobacco workers who had been used to inhaling cigar smoke for many years. Pipe smokers had the lowest values, only about 1% on the average.

Dr. BENDITT: One interesting thing in your figures, Dr. Kjeldsen, was that the carboxyhemoglobin content was much higher in the smoking coronary group than in the smoking noncoronary heart disease group, and this was most dramatic in your 30-year age group. It raises the question of whether or not these people smoke more or whether they have some kind of a hemoglobin aberration. Have you looked at it from that standpoint?

Dr. KJELDSEN: We have done some measurements of carbon monoxide uptake from cigarette and cigar smoke, and it seems to be mainly their exaggerated way of inhaling the smoke which calls forth the very high carbon monoxide concentrations.

Dr. BEAUMONT: In relation to the importance of inhalation which was shown by Dr. Kjeldsen in France, Daniel Schwartz found that people who smoked only 10 cigarettes or less but inhaled deeply had almost the same risk as people who smoked 40 or more and did not inhale. People who smoked 40 usually inhaled also, but they had the same risk, not more.

I was surprised to see that Dr. Kjeldsen found a correlation between smoking and blood cholesterol level. If I remember correctly, cholesterol and smoking were not correlated in Schwartz's study. Finally, is it still true that the risk of smoking falls when one stops smoking?

Dr. STAMLER: The answer is yes, particularly for middle-aged persons, i.e. those who quit at ages 45–54 and 55–64. It is less true for older persons, but even they benefit. Data on this matter are available from several prospective studies, e.g. two American Cancer Society investigations, the U.S. Veterans study, the combined Albany and Framingham study, the British physicians study, our Peoples Gas Co. study. However, no field trial has as yet been completed on this matter, with random allocation to two groups, experimental and control, to assure full comparability. Drs. Reid and Rose are currently carrying out such a trial with British civil servants.

Dr. KJELDSEN: I am familiar with the data of Schwartz and Beaumont and that is one of the few papers where inhalation and cholesterol levels have been correlated. As I remember, in this paper there was also found a positive correlation in the younger age groups between serum cholesterol levels and cigarette smoking. Isn't that correct?

Dr. STAMLER: I think it is also true in most of the American epidemiological studies that there is no sizable or significant correlation between cigarette smoking and cholesterol level. I think your data are a little different from most other studies in that regard.

Dr. KATZ: One of the attractions of Copenhagen are the women and their cigar smoking. I don't know whether they really smoke the cigars or whether they use them as part of their decoration. What is the effect on this particular group?

Dr. KJELDSEN: Most of them really do smoke cigars, and the disease subject with 19% carboxyhemoglobin was a woman.

Discussion Following Dr. Berkson's Paper

Dr. BEAUMONT: In Dr. Berkson's paper the cumulative effect of several associated risk factors was once more pointed out. But he has also shown that some risk factors can associate without enhancing the overall risk: here heart rate and hypertension and, in another paper, cigarette smoking and hypertension. Would he like to comment on the significance of noncumulative risk factors?

Dr. GLAGOV: Several years ago we speculated that the special predilection of atherosclerosis for the coronary arteries was due to special hemodynamic factors occasioned by myocardial contraction. In this connection we hypothesized that persistently elevated heart rates should increase the risk of coronary atherosclerosis by increasing the long-term average tension in the coronary arterial wall. Your paper suggests that heart rate may be related to hypertension as concerns coronary heart disease but is independent of the other risk factors. Could these data also be interpreted as supporting the notion that elevated heart rate and elevated pressure both act to the detriment of the artery in the same way, i.e., by increasing long-term average medial tension? May I also ask you to comment on the possibility that "physical fitness" and "low emotional tension" environments may help to reduce coronary heart disease by lowering long-term heart rates?

Dr. BERKSON: In response to Dr. Beaumont: one of the problems in evaluating the cumulative impact of risk factors (and this has been a key difficulty for all the long-term prospective epidemiologic studies) is that with stratification of the population at risk, the cells become small and the confidence limits of observed rates become large. Therefore, it becomes difficult or impossible really to determine whether risk factors are having a cumulative effect. This problem was one of the stimuli to our national cooperative Pooling Project, about which Dr. Henry Blackburn spoke briefly. By combining the data from multiple studies, it becomes possible to partially overcome or minimize the foregoing difficulty. Hopefully, the kind of analysis we did here to assess resting heart rate as a risk factor, and its possible contribution independent of other factors, as well as its cumulative impact in association with them, will be done for all studies combined in the Pooling Project. It will then become clear as to whether our apparent failure to show a cumulative effect of faster heart rate and hypertension in combination is merely a result of small numbers, or is actually a consistent finding. At present we believe the data are inadequate to make any definitive judgment on this matter. A similar problem of small numbers arises in our Peoples Gas Company study in regard to the combination of hypertension and cigarette smoking. The Pooling Project data on this matter should be available shortly for general review.

We certainly agree with Dr. Glagov's comments that both elevated heart rate and blood pressure may have a detrimental effect on the coronary arteries by increasing average medial tension, i.e. by a direct "wear and tear" effect on the arterial wall. We have considered the additional possibility that both these mechanisms exert their apparent deleterious effect by increasing the exposure of the arterial intima to atherogenic lipoprotein, by the infiltration process.

With respect to Dr. Glagov's last question, it is certainly possible that reduction in heart rates achieved by bettering environmental conditions, both in relation to physical fitness and emotional tension, might lead to reduced incidence and mortality from coronary heart disease. Our group is exploring this matter further in the Peoples Gas Co. study, in terms of occupational physical activity and heart rate, in order to try to get at least a bit better evaluation of the fitness aspect. For the present, I think it is a reasonable "best medical judgment" to infer that measures aimed at slowing pulse—including cessation of cigarette smoking and exercise (properly supervised, safe, regular, moderate, exercise)—might be helpful in an overall regimen of coronary prevention, along with dietary measures and control of hypertension when present.

CONCLUDING REMARKS

Ancel Keys

This symposium comes just fifteen years after the first large-scale international symposium on this subject. Except for old-timers in this field, it is hard to realize what a vast change has occurred since that symposium of the World Congress on Cardiology in 1954 in Washington, D.C. The progress has been enormous, not only in millions of dollars being spent for research and tons of publications accumulated over the years but, more importantly, in facts ascertained and understanding achieved. Yet, there is little reason to be content.

We rejoice in better methods, in the great increase in the number of workers and projects in epidemiological research around the world, and in the more sophisticated analyses of far more data. We are happy to see the start of large-scale trials on secondary prevention, though many of us regret that only drugs are being tested. However, what about meeting the big challenge, the need for primary prevention?

Serious systematic work on the epidemiology of coronary heart disease began in the late 1940s, roughly twenty years ago, and from the outset the goal was recognized to be primary prevention. Every responsible worker today continues to agree about that urgent priority. Except for a few small-scale trials, microscopic in comparison with the need, and a trial of a drug that scarcely qualifies as a public health approach, we have not even started to attempt primary prevention. Nothing is now being done, or is even seriously proposed, to reduce in any important way the incidence and mortality rate of coronary heart disease. Unless there are sudden, completely unexpected developments, the prospect is that the 1970's will pass with no real improvement, with no concrete figures to indicate that the burden of this disease will have been altered by a third of a century of effort.

The coronary picture as a whole is unchanging but there is a bright spot. Coronary care units, now being established everywhere, offer improved immediate prognosis of heart attacks. The patient who lives to be admitted to such a unit has a better chance of leaving the hospital alive. Epidemiology can claim no credit, nor are there epidemiological data to show what, if any, may be the effect of coronary care units on the long-time prognosis of the coronary patient.

Still, perhaps twenty years is not the end of time; conceivably, in another ten years real efforts at coronary prevention could be starting. While we are frustrated now, we may be consoled by dreaming that some day ideal, critical, large-scale experiments to test the idea of prevention by some means may be devised, funded and put into operation. Hopefully, the results would then, perhaps in 1979, as an earliest possibility, allow a start on efforts to control the number one cause of death in the United States and in many other populations. In the meantime, investigators in this field who would not be lost in the routine of operating the big trials could hope to find fascinating but not necessarily relevant research projects concerned with anything but the main issue of prevention.

Is it reasonable to hope that coronary heart disease can be prevented or at least delayed until extreme old age? If some measure of prevention is possible, must that be achieved only at the expense of exchanging coronary heart disease for other, perhaps more disagreeable, disorders, or at an unacceptable economic cost, or of impossible restrictions on the mode of life?

Years ago, when some of us pointed to the lack of coronary heart disease among the Bantu people of Africa as proof that the disease is not an inevitable affliction, the standard response was: "Who wants to be a Bantu?" When we cited the Japanese in Japan in contrast to the Japanese in California, the retort was: "Who would rather have a stroke instead of a heart attack?" Many critics muttered about racial differences and asked: "What about white people?"

But such questions are no longer embarrassing. As will soon be reported in detail, systematic follow-up studies on white populations in Europe show that a very low incidence of coronary heart disease can be associated with a very favorable all-causes death rate and a mode of life that need not be either disagreeable or expensive. Therefore, it is eminently reasonable to expect favorable answers to questions about the possibility and cost of prevention of coronary heart disease.

However, now another question must be asked. What is to be done about prevention? What efforts can be made, while we hopefully (naively) await the results of great controlled experiments and the definitive answers about cause and effect, and how, and how much, that everyone would like? As indicated earlier, with the most optimistic timetable the unveiling of the answers is a decade away, even if the great trials are undertaken and successfully concluded. In the meantime, what advice and help about preventing this disease is to be offered to the public and the health establishment that is supposed to serve that public? The area of universal agreement currently covers only limited situations and segments of society.

It is agreed that treatment, on an individual patient basis, is desirable with disorders that may predispose to coronary heart disease: diabetes, severe hypertension and hypothyroidism are the prime examples. Not many eventual coronary victims qualify in these regards. Moreover, a large proportion of those who are so afflicted are undetected, and of those whose condition is known, a substantial number are not effectively treated. There is no public evidence of any program, or plan to develop a program, to alter this situation.

Obesity is often said to be one of the most common health problems in the United States, and every organization concerned with health advises its correction and control. Yet, as a feature in efforts to prevent coronary heart disease, obesity control offers less than many people think. First, except when extreme or associated with hypertension, all recent studies show that obesity is not a big risk factor for coronary heart disease. Secondly, even with intensive medical efforts obesity of major degree is remarkably refractory to efforts at correction. Also unceasing propaganda for many years does not seem to have reduced the frequency of obesity in the United States.

Cigarette smoking is perhaps the most common of the so-called risk factors and would seem the most obvious and simple target for a prevention program. Unfortunately, no easy way of breaking the habit, or of preventing it at the outset, is in sight. The tobacco interests, and their congressmen friends, are not very helpful. The most hopeful sign is the recent decrease of the habit among physicians; what the general public will do remains to be seen.

Finally, consider the diet and the blood lipids, the area most talked about in connection with the idea of preventing coronary heart disease. It is no longer possible to deny that the diet, notably the fats in it, strongly affects the blood cholesterol concentration and that the risk of developing coronary heart disease tends to be an exponential function of the serum cholesterol level. Follow-up studies in the United States consistently indicate that the incidence of myocardial infarction in middle-aged men is proportional to something like the cube, the third power, of the serum cholesterol concentration. A significant lowering of the serum cholesterol level is quickly, cheaply, and safely produced by dietary changes that are not extreme nor destructive of eating pleasure. A 50% reduction in the saturated fatty acids and cholesterol in the usual American diet (middle-class white), with substitution of vegetable oils for some of the hard fats, is effective.

Still there is great resistance to recommending incorporation of these facts into public advice and preventive programs. Seemingly, the current "official" view is that only the private physician dealing with his private patients may be concerned about blood lipids and the diet and that this restriction must prevail until there is incontrovertible proof that dietary management will causally and predictably prevent coronary heart disease.

In 1960, an Executive Committee on Diet and Heart Disease was established to explore the matter of mass field trials on this approach to the prevention of coronary heart disease. In 1962 research grant awards for a big "feasibility study" were made by the National Heart Institute to six Principal Investigators. The one-year study was stretched to two years, the work-up of the data and the report writing went on thereafter. At the end of 1967, the Principal Investigators and Central Staff reached some unanimous conclusions. They were published with the full Report in 1968:

1. A dietary "mass field trial on a free-living population should be planned and put into operation as soon as possible."

2. Such "a mass field trial on a free-living population can be undertaken with hope of success only with a nondouble-blind design" [384].

In medical trials where patients' reports of sensations and physicians' subjective impressions must be used as end points in the evaluation of treatment, a double-blind design is essential to assure unbiased evaluation of the results.

But, where the end points are specified electrocardiographic changes and death, as most of us insist should be the case with studies on the prevention of coronary heart disease, insistence on the double-blind protocol is nonsense and serves only to prevent efforts at prevention. To demand a double-blind diet program to be followed by free-living people for five years is about as absurd as to insist on double-blind trials of changing smoking habits and physical activity.

The conclusions of the National Diet-Heart Study, the fruit of seven years of work, are apparently unpalatable in some quarters. Yet, time runs on and may be running out. The continued absence of a policy in regard to the prevention and control of our leading cause of death is a confession of bankruptcy that cannot be tolerated indefinitely.

Impatience at the lack of a program aimed at preventing coronary heart disease is reinforced by new epidemiological findings. Bantu and other peoples of peculiar race and culture are not alone in being far less prone to this disease than we are, *we* meaning Americans and other populations so beset by this modern epidemic. A few bits of data will illustrate the point and, hopefully, may engender more impatience. The full material will be published before long.

In 1956, after explorations on the epidemiology of this disease in various parts of the world, the need was apparent for systematic parallel studies on different populations. Properly defined samples of men should be examined and characterized by rigidly standardized methods and then be followed over the years with periodic re-examinations. The aim would be to obtain truly comparable incidence rates and to relate those rates to the characteristics of the populations and of the individuals. Colleagues and former students in Italy, Yugoslavia, Japan, Finland and Greece were interested in joining a cooperative study. We had also previous experience in Spain [797], and South Africa [241] but lack of personnel and financial support in those countries ruled them out. On the other hand, officials in the Netherlands who learned of the project arranged to help a parallel study in that country.

It was agreed to study men aged 40–59 at entry who would comprise substantially all men of the age in geographically defined areas (a 4/9ths sample in the Dutch area). Dr. Henry L. Taylor organized a parallel study on men employed by railroads in a defined area of the United States. Later, a study on a comparable cohort of railroad men in Italy was organized. Methods and the organization of international examining teams were tried out in 1957 in Italy and Greece, and the systematic full-scale program began the next year. Methods and entry characteristics have been reported [793]. In all, 12,770 men made up the 16 cohorts under study. Some of the cohorts have completed their 10 year follow-up examinations, but current analysis covers only the five years of follow-up and re-examination completed by all cohorts.

Table 1 summarizes official vital statistics for the seven countries concerned. The figures are age-standardized death rates for 1965 of men and women aged 35–64 years. All-causes death rates of the women in the seven countries do not differ much and coronary heart disease is not indicated to be a great factor in the total mortality. For men the differences between the countries in all-causes death rates are large, and great differences in the deaths attributed to coronary heart disease seemingly account for much of the variation in total mortality.

At equal age in middle life the all-causes death rate of men in Greece is only 54% that of American white men; the coronary death rate of the Greeks was reported to be only 17% that of the Americans. The Finns are even less fortunate than the Americans, both in all-causes and reported coronary deaths, but without other evidence the differences in coronary heart disease indicated in Table 1 may be questioned.

Table 1. *Death rates, per 100,000 in 1965 of men and women aged 35–64, age-standardized (mean of rates for ages 35–44, 45–54, 55–64)* [a]

Country	Men		Women	
	CHD	total	CHD	total
Greece	78	712	30	436
Netherlands	243	831	55	431
Yugoslavia	116	960	78	618
Italy	187	985	67	519
Japan	79	986	46	585
U.S.A. (white)	461	1,286	134	628
Finland	534	1,432	109	567

[a] "Total" = deaths from all causes; "CHD" = deaths ascribed to coronary heart disease. Calculated from data of the World Health Organization.

Table 2. *Death rates, age-standardized, per 10,000 per year, over a five-year period for men aged 40–59 at the start. All cohorts in each country combined* [a]

Cohorts in	Coronary	All causes
Greece	8	36
Yugoslavia	11	75
Japan	9	91
Italy	7	95
Netherlands	35	111
U.S. railroad	47	94
Finland	47	134

[a] Provisional summary of data to be published in collaboration with Doctors C. Aravanis, H. Blackburn, F. S. P. van Buchem, R. Buzina, B. S. Djordjevic, F. Fidanza, M. J. Karvonen, N. Kimura, A. Menotti, V. Puddu and H. L. Taylor.

In 1957, when this long-term work was started, we had little inkling of the differences indicated in Table 1; we had only the impression that Finland and the U.S. were similar in the incidence of coronary heart disease and that the disease was considerably less common in Italy and Japan. When the areas were chosen it was realized that they were not necessarily representative of the whole countries involved.

The five-year experience of mortality in the International Cooperative Study is summarized by countries in Table 2. Though the pattern is not identical with that of the national vital statistics, there are distinct similarities. The differences between the groups of cohorts proved to be even greater than reported between the countries as a whole. Note that the U.S. railroad men, being selected as fully employed in regular jobs at entry, had, as expected, a more favorable mortality than the general population from which they were drawn. Among those railroad men there were 124 deaths in five years or 81.6% of the 152.0 deaths which would equal the rate for age-matched white Americans.

Therefore, death from coronary heart disease was far less common in the Greek, Yugoslav, Japanese and Italian cohorts than among the Americans, Dutch and Finns, and the advantage of the groups with less coronary mortality was not compensated by other causes of deaths. The differences in susceptibility to coronary heart disease were also clearly shown in the age-adjusted incidence rates of myocardial infarction among men judged to be free from coronary heart disease at entry. Similar differences were indicated for the incidence of angina pectoris and for coronary heart disease diagnosed with less rigid electrocardiographic criteria.

The differences between those populations are not related to differences between the cohorts in relative body weight, body fatness, smoking habits, urbanicity of residence or physical activity. This is not to say that those items are unimportant in etiology; we simply note that they do not explain these observed differences in rate. The incidence rates were closely related to the mean serum cholesterol levels of the cohorts ($r=0.84$ for 16 cohorts), equally closely related to the mean percentages of calories provided by saturated fatty acids in the diets and also, and independently, related to the average blood pressures, or the frequencies of hypertension, in the several cohorts. In this five-year material the incidence rate of coronary heart disease was unrelated to percentage of calories provided by either proteins or polyunsaturated fatty acids in the diet and only weakly related ($r=0.4$) to total fats in the diet.

The findings in this study confirm some relationships strongly suspected previously, but they are also providing some negative surprises. Neither relative body weight nor body fatness (skinfold thickness) prove to be important risk factors for either coronary heart disease or for all-causes deaths. In general, the most favorable mortality tends to occur at relative body weights close to the average for U.S. men according to the actuarial tables, not the "desirable" or "ideal" weights so widely praised in the United States. Another surprise is the relative lack of a major death or coronary incidence penalty associated with smoking in the countries other than the United States. Again, this is not to deny that smoking may not promote coronary heart disease and other life-shortening disorders. The data simply indicate that in these non-U.S. populations smoking by itself is, at most, a minor risk factor. To evaluate the significance of these, and many other, features of the International Cooperative Study, far more detailed exposition is needed than is possible here. In this brief compass, and with what may seem to be disjointed illustrations, I have attempted to stress several points:

1. Coronary heart disease need not be the scourge it presently is in many populations, nor must it be exchanged for other afflictions and causes of death.

2. In all populations and situations, serum cholesterol and blood pressure are major contributors to risk.

3. Relative body weight, body fatness and smoking habits are not universally major risk factors.

4. Great differences between populations in the incidence of this disease are not explained by differences in physical activity.

5. There is still much to be learned from long-term comparisons of populations, but such studies should be considerably larger than those undertaken to date.

Finally, there are now ample bases on which to develop real efforts toward primary prevention of this disease. The time for genuine action is overdue.

Section XII

NUTRITIONAL STUDIES AND ATHEROSCLEROSIS

RECENT ADVANCES IN NUTRITION AND ATHEROSCLEROSIS

ALAN N. HOWARD

Cardiovascular disease, with its final outcome of coronary thrombosis and myocardial infarction, is the end-product of many different factors in which nutrition plays a major role. As shown in Fig. 1, atherosclerosis which results from vascular injury and hyperlipemia leading to stenosis of the blood vessels may give rise to thrombosis, myocardial infarction, and sudden death. Evidence is accumulating that at each stage nutritional factors may be involved and an attempt is made to summarize these in the following review.

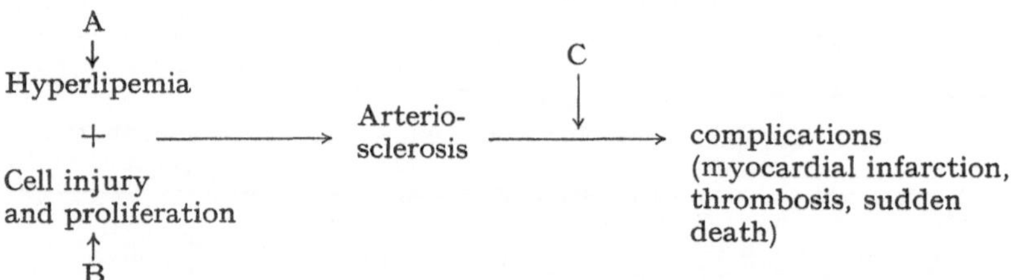

Fig. 1. Possible sites (A, B or C) of involvement of nutritional factors in cardiovascular disease

NUTRIENTS AFFECTING HYPERLIPEMIA

It is now clearly established that unsaturated and saturated fats, dietary sterols, and carbohydrates are all important in determining the level of plasma lipids. It is not my intention to discuss these further since they will be covered by other authors. There are, however, a number of other hypocholesterolemic substances effective in man and animals which are worthy of note. Among them are pectin [461] and unidentified substances in soybean meal [719], alfalfa [329], oats [460], legumes [47, 562] and tea [1585].

Pectin has been extensively studied by Fisher and his colleagues [461] who demonstrated its hypocholesterolemic effect in many species including chickens, rabbits and pigs. Furthermore, Keys et al. [795] observed a decrease with pectin in serum cholesterol in human subjects on an average American diet supplying approximately 600 mg cholesterol per day. A large class of compounds related to pectin such as scleroglucan, carageenin and numerous gums [1225] have a similar effect and these are thought to act by increasing the excretion of fecal cholesterol and its metabolites.

Some of the previously mentioned natural materials are extremely active, and among these alfalfa is of considerable interest. As shown in Fig. 2, rabbits fed a diet composed largely of alfalfa were unaffected by the simultaneous administration by mouth of large doses of cholesterol daily [329]. Such animals showed no elevation of their serum cholesterol values above normal, and at subsequent post-mortem no evidence of experimental atherosclerosis was detected either macroscopically or microscopically. Much if not all of the hypocholesterolemic effect of alfalfa could be attributed to its saponin content. For many years it has been known that alfalfa contains an active growth depressant with hemolytic

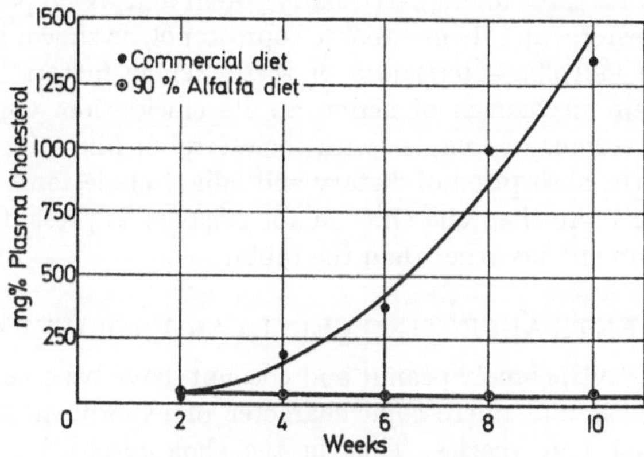

Fig. 2. Effect of alfalfa on cholesterol fed rabbits. Each diet contained 0.6% cholesterol (Cookson et al. [329])

Table 1. *Cholesterol intake and excretion in rabbits given semisynthetic diet containing 20% beef tallow for 16 weeks*[a]

Diet	Source of protein in diet	Dietary cholesterol	Fecal cholesterol and coprostanol
		mg/kg body weight/day	
Semisynthetic 20% beef tallow	Casein 25%	7.35	1.9
Semisynthetic 20% beef tallow	Soybean meal 25%	7.8	8.3

[a] Howard et al. [718]. The figures quoted are the mean daily intake and excretion over a four-day collection period.

properties, identified as a saponin [1168]. It is interesting that the growth depressant effect can be counteracted by feeding cholesterol and that alfalfa saponin can specifically prevent a rise in serum cholesterol in rats fed a lard and cholesterol diet [1548]. Alfalfa saponin probably acts by forming an insoluble complex with cholesterol, thereby increasing its excretion.

Little is known of the mechanism of action of legumes and tea, but they may be similar to alfalfa. The isolation of the active principle in legumes would prove of obvious interest since it has activity in man [47, 562].

The remarkable rise in plasma cholesterol seen in feeding rabbits a semisynthetic diet essentially free of cholesterol [838, 913] has attracted the attention of many investigators. It is quite clear that rabbit chow contains a factor which protects rabbits from hypercholesterolemia and atherosclerosis [719, 828]. Kritchevsky et al. [828] found most of the activity was in the nonlipid part of the chow while Moore [1023] claims that roughage (wheat straw) is involved. It is noteworthy that lignin [417], an indigestible constituent of many cereals, has a bile acid sequestering effect, and this property might explain in part the hypercholesterolemic effect of chow. Most formulations of chow contain soybean meal which Howard et al. [719] found particularly potent and which produces increased excretion of cholesterol and its metabolite coprostanol, as shown in Table 1 [718].

The isolation and characterisation of these "chow factors" are of obvious interest, and their mechanism of action awaits elucidation. One can speculate that they act by forming a complex with cholesterol or bile acids in the intestine or by inhibiting the absorption of dietary and biliary cholesterol at the intestinal mucosa. Whether more than one chow factor exists is at present unknown, as is also their action in species other than the rabbit.

NUTRIENTS AFFECTING CELLULAR PROLIFERATION

Two vegetable oils, namely peanut and coconut, have been shown to dramatically alter the gross and microscopic character of experimental atherosclerotic lesions in at least four species. Thus in the cholesterol-fed rat [568], rabbit

Table 2. *Effect of different dietary fats in rhesus monkeys*

Author	Fat	Percentage diet	Period (weeks)	Plasma cholesterol mg %	Aortic		Atherosclerosis	
					proliferative lesions	atheromatous lesions	diseased percentage	severity
Wissler et al. [1563]	Butter[a]	25	40	1,130	—	—	82	++
	Peanut oil[a]	25	40	550	—	—	93	+++
Scott et al. [1331]	Butter[b]	30	70	1,060	44	56	—	—
	Peanut oil[b]	30	70	724	80	18	—	—

[a] Diet contained 2% cholesterol.

[b] Diet contained 5% cholesterol, 0.4 cholic acid 0.2% propylthiouracil. — not done; ++ severe; +++ very severe.

(Kritchevsky and Wissler, unpublished data), rhesus [1331, 1563] and cebus monkey [1561] these two oils have an atherosclerotic effect which is independent of the level of hypercholesterolemia. Table 2 shows the results obtained by two groups of workers in rhesus monkeys fed butter and peanut oil [1331, 1563]. Although the highest serum cholesterol level was obtained in animals fed butter, the most severe atherosclerotic lesions were produced in monkeys fed peanut oil. These were characterized by thick fatty plaques often with ulceration elevated to the point of occlusion of the ostia of various vessels. It would, thus, appear that peanut and coconut oil must contain some component which has a proliferative action on the arterial intima. It is uncertain whether the fatty acids are to be incriminated or some other contaminant. There is very little similarity between the fatty acid composition of peanut and coconut oil. The former has 7% long chain (>18 carbon atoms) and the latter has 75% short chain (<16 carbon atoms) fatty acids.

In tissue culture, sera from monkeys fed coconut oil or peanut oil increased the rate of proliferation of medial cells compared with control serum [777]. It has been suggested that the mechanism of proliferation and migration of

Table 3. *Esterase activities in the aortas of rats given butter and peanut oil* [a]

Dietary group [b]	Phosphatide acyl hydrolase	Glycerol ester hydrolase	Sterol ester hydrolase
	μequiv/min/g protein		
Control	1,060	630	276
40% butter	840	1,250 [c]	236
40% peanut oil	2,100 [c]	2,880[d]	69[d]

[a] Patelski et al. [1156].
[b] Experimental diets contained 5% cholesterol and 2% cholic acid.
[c] $P < 0.05$.
[d] $P < 0.001$.

medial smooth muscle cells into the intima of the atherosclerotic artery *in vivo* may be related to this stimulatory effect. It is also noteworthy that peanut oil has a very marked affect on aortic lipolytic enzymes and in particular causes a decrease in cholesteryl ester hydrolase (Table 3). If this enzyme is deficient cholesteryl esters may accumulate in the arterial wall, and peanut oil may be acting as an inhibitor of this enzyme [1156]. Cellular proliferation may thus be a consequence of increased lipid deposition.

THE WATER FACTOR

As long ago as 1957, Kobayashi [815] showed that in Japan there appeared to be a direct relationship between deaths from cerebral hemorrhage and the sulphate-bicarbonate ratio of the river water. Throughout Japan the water is soft, yet death rates from coronary heart disease are low. These observations led Schroeder [1317] to examine death rates in the United States in relation to the quality of the drinking water. Rather surprisingly, he found that in 163 larger cities the death rate from atherosclerotic heart disease was highest in those areas with soft water. He, therefore, concluded that some factor in drinking water associated with its hardness or softness was in some way related to deaths from one or both of the two major cardiovascular diseases in the U.S.A. and Japan. His statistical findings have since been confirmed elsewhere in the world, notably in the United Kingdom [339], Holland [161], Sweden [167], and Canada [50]. Two studies which failed to show any relationship between atherosclerotic heart disease and the softness of the water were in Oklahoma [875] and Ireland [1054]. However these can be criticized on the grounds that the difference of the hardness of the water was small in the areas studied and the certification of death subject to some doubt [339].

Analyses of the water supplies in England and Wales showed that the hard water, where the death rate was lower, contained greater quantities of several minerals including calcium, magnesium, and sodium whereas the mean concentration of some other metals such as iron, zinc, lead, tin, nickel and chromium showed no difference [339].

One of the difficulties in interpreting these figures is that the analysis of municipial water at the reservoir can be misleading. Soft water is notoriously acidic and corrosive to metal pipes, and it can be argued that some toxic contaminant is thereby introduced. Evidence in support of this view is the finding that in England the lead content of rib bones was considerably higher in soft

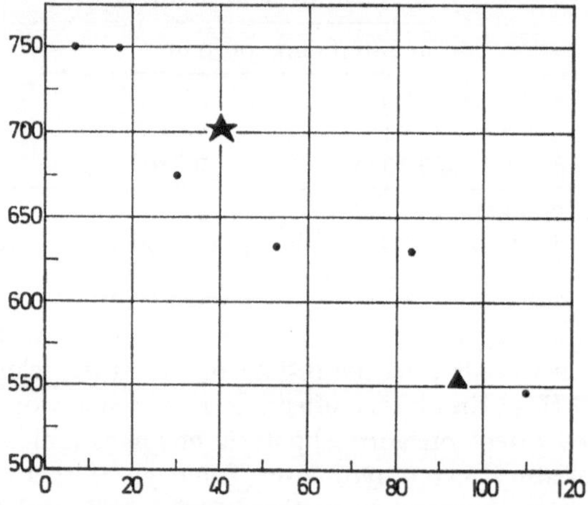

Fig. 3. Deaths from cardiovascular disease in the United Kingdom. (Data from Crawford et al. [339] and from Robertson [1241]). Symbols: ● = from Crawford, ★ = Scunthorpe (softened) and ▲ = Grimsby (hard)

than in hard water areas [342]. Although lead has not been specifically linked with cardiovascular deaths, cadmium, a contaminant of the zinc used for galvanized pipes, has been shown to reproduce the clinical and pathological picture of hypertensive disease in rats. Schroeder et al. [1318] has suggested that cadmium is the most likely mineral responsible for the increase in cardiovascular deaths in soft water areas. This hypothesis is attractive and explains a number of otherwise confusing facts. For instance in Toronto, the higher death rate in soft water areas was found to be due entirely to an excess of sudden deaths [50] in which hypertension might be involved.

Certainly the water factor does not appear to affect the extent and severity of atherosclerosis. In a study in Glasgow, a soft water area, Crawford and Crawford [341] found no greater incidence of stenosis and diseases of the coronaries than in parts of England where the water is hard. They suggested that the water factor did not influence atherosclerosis but rather the susceptibility of the myocardium to infarction.

Indirect evidence of the water factor is also provided by Robertson [1241], who has commented on the rise in death rate from cardiovascular disease in the last seven years in Scunthorpe, Lincs. where the water supply was artificially softened (Fig. 3). In nearby Grimsby supplied with hard water, exactly the same but unsoftened, death rates have been falling. The local water board have taken the unusual step of doubling the calcium content of the towns water supply instead of using a water softener. It remains to be seen if the situation can be dramatically reversed.

Although cadmium is currently implicated, much attention has been directed towards calcium as a protective factor. Increased calcium intake lead to a higher fecal excretion of bile acids because of its bile acid sequestering effect. At a dose of 1.5 g per day calcium will cause a depression of plasma cholesterol in man [1580] but lower amounts are ineffective [1012]. In addition, calcium inhibits the intestinal absorption of several metallic irons notably cadmium and lead [464]. While chromium, a metal which may be deficient in soft water, causes hypocholesterolemia in rats, its effect in man is equivocal [1318].

Apart from the previously mentioned, there is a lack of experimental evidence in animals to conclusively pinpoint any of the proposed factors. Experiments in pigs have given negative results in that no significant difference in the extent of atherosclerosis was found in animals given waters of different hardness [720]. However, the commercial diets used were heavily fortified with minerals which may have obscured any effect. Also it is difficult to reproduce in animals the typical features of human coronary artery disease. Nevertheless the experimental evidence is urgently required to support data which at present mainly relies on epidemiological studies.

CONCLUSIONS AND SUMMARY

Much attention has been directed in the past to the important roles that dietary cholesterol, plant sterols, saturated and unsaturated fats, and carbohydrates play in the production of hypolipemia. However, there are a number of other important, naturally occurring hypocholesterolemic factors in food stuffs which have still to be isolated, and their importance in human nutrition remains to be established. Other nutrients such as peanut and coconut oil may contain a toxic factor having an influence on cellular proliferation in the vessel wall. Its demonstration in several species points to the importance of future research to achieve its isolation and characterization. The increased incidence of cardiovascular disease in areas with soft water is now well documented and suggests a possible protective role of the minerals present in hard water supplies. The so-called water factor may not be involved in atherosclerosis *per se* but may operate either by causing hypertension or making the myocardium more susceptible to injury.

PLASMA LIPIDS AND EXPERIMENTAL ATHEROSCLEROSIS*

W. A. THOMAS, R. A. FLORENTIN, S. C. NAM, A. S. DAOUD, K. T. LEE and E. TIAMSON

Abundant evidence was presented at the first symposium indicating that atherosclerosis similar in many respects to that in man can be produced in a variety of experimental animals by feeding diets that result in elevation of plasma lipids. Recent advances made in the field of plasma lipids and experimental atherosclerosis will be reviewed in this report under the following four headings: (1) relation of dietary lipids to plasma lipids, (2) relation of plasma lipids to arterial wall lipids, (3) changes in arterial wall metabolism of hyperlipemic (HL) diet-fed animals associated with development of gross atherosclerotic lesions, (4) changes in arterial wall metabolism of HL diet-fed animals prior to development of gross atherosclerotic lesions and changes in cultured arterial cells exposed to HL serum.

Relation of Dietary Lipids to Plasma Lipids. Species differences in response to dietary lipids are well known. All that is needed to produce hyperlipemia in rabbits is to add cholesterol to a low-fat commercial pellet diet. Not only are plasma cholesterol levels increased but also triglycerides, phospholipids and all other components of lipoproteins. The degree of hyperlipemia may be altered by manipulating quantity and type of triglycerides but this is of minor importance in atherogenesis in cholesterol-fed rabbits, since levels are very high with cholesterol alone. One recent development is that certain carbohydrates can result in hyperlipemia even in the absence of dietary cholesterol. For example, Kritchevsky et al. [826] have shown in rabbits that when the carbohydrate source is glucose, serum cholesterol levels were 209 mg-% and when starch 640 mg-%. In another recent study Cookson et al. [329] have shown that alfalfa in the diet can prevent hyperlipemia in rabbits even with the addition of as much as 600 mg of cholesterol daily.

With swine recent studies have shown that little or no hyperlipemia is produced when cholesterol is added to a commercial mash diet (unpublished observations from our laboratory). However, when cholesterol is combined with milk powder or with a comparable semisynthetic mixture containing triglycerides at the 40% level by calories, marked hyperlipemia is produced [468].

With rats it is necessary to feed not only cholesterol and triglycerides but also other ingredients such as thiouracil and cholic acid in order to produce hyperlipemia sufficient to induce atherosclerosis and thrombosis. Rats fed such diets with appropriate highly saturated triglycerides develop thrombosis with greater frequency than any other known species. In the past the diets required to produce thrombosis were so toxic that most rats became emaciated and died within a few months. A recent advance has been the development of a much

* The work herein was supported by U.S.P.H.S. Grant HE 07155.

less toxic thrombogenic diet for rats, with cocoa butter as a triglyceride source in which little or no thiouracil is required [1127, 1554]. Another advance made by some of the same investigators with this diet was the demonstration that making rats diabetic by partial pancreatectomy increased the hyperlipemic and atherogenic effect of the diet. Treatment with insulin did not reverse the enhancing effect of diabetes on the incidence and severity of vascular lesions, although it did result in lowering of serum cholesterol values to nondiabetic levels.

Additional studies have been made of several species of subhuman primates since the first symposium, indicating further that they develop hyperlipemia and atherosclerosis readily with diets containing increased cholesterol and triglycerides. In a recent study Wissler et al. [1564] showed that cholesterol-fed Rhesus monkeys kept in expanded confinement developed higher serum cholesterol levels but tended to have less atherosclerosis than cholesterol-fed monkeys kept in traditional cages.

Effects of high lipid diets have been investigated in many other species recently, but these will not be discussed further in this report except to say that Ho and Taylor [690] have made a series of elegant studies on the various ways in which different species attempt to maintain homeostasis when given excessive dietary cholesterol. They suggest that the mechanisms available to cope with excess dietary cholesterol are: (1) limitation of absorption, (2) suppression of synthesis, (3) increase of excretion, and (4) reversible tissue storage. These are discussed in detail in Dr. Ho's report in this symposium. The relation of fatty acids in the diet to plasma lipids has been presented in detail at the first symposium.

Relations of Plasma Lipids to Arterial Wall Lipids. It has been shown in time sequence studies with isotopically labeled plasma lipids that they enter the arterial wall principally through the intima [13]. Apparently only a small portion enters through *vasa vasorum*. Lofland and Clarkson (in press) have shown that nonesterified cholesterol enters the arterial wall of monkeys eight times more rapidly than esterified cholesterol. This latter finding suggests a selective permeability of the arterial wall to these two forms of cholesterol. Phospholipids are synthesized in the arterial wall in amounts that might account for all that is present [529], but undoubtedly some also enters from the plasma. Plasma triglycerides appear to enter at least to some extent, and we can assume that nonesterified fatty acids enter readily.

The studies of Watts [1525] and of Kao and Wissler [776] on low density lipoproteins in the arterial wall were reviewed at the first symposium, but we may be able to extend our interpretation of their results in the light of present knowledge. Kao and Wissler produced in rabbits an antibody to low density (LD) and very low density (VLD) lipoproteins obtained from plasma. This antibody was conjugated with fluorescein and sections of arteries were then exposed to it. In completely normal arteries no fluorescence was demonstrated. In arteries with even slightly thickened intimas fluorescence was found, and much of it appeared by light microscopy to be in smooth muscle cells of the intima. Regions of fluorescence corresponded to regions in which lipid could be demonstrated by oil red O-stains. One possible conclusion to draw is that at least some lipid enters the arterial wall as LD or VLD lipoprotein and that these molecules maintain their integrity for long periods. It is also possible that the apoprotein, which determines the immunological characteristics, is present separated from the lipid components. Another possibility is that LD or VLD lipoprotein with immunological characteristics indistinguishable from plasma lipoproteins is being synthesized in the smooth muscle cells (SMC) of the arterial wall.

If in experimental atherosclerosis plasma lipids enter the arterial wall principally as LD or VLD lipoproteins and remain as such for long periods the percentage distribution of lipids in the arterial wall should resemble that in LD or VLD plasma lipoproteins. We investigated this aspect in swine [468]. Swine fed diets high in cholesterol and triglycerides develop a few atherosclerotic lesions

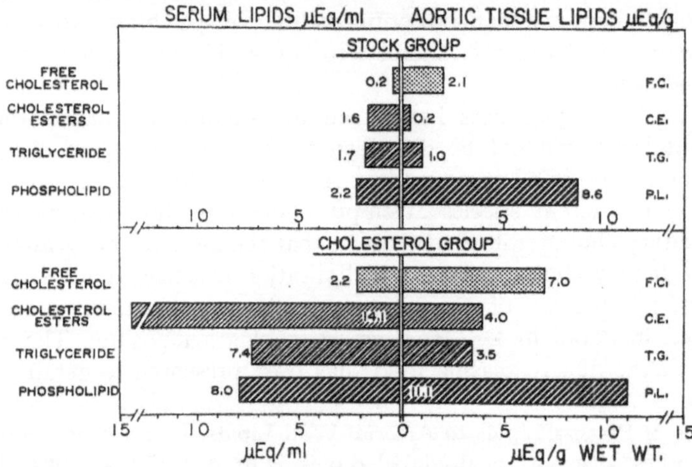

Fig. 1. Comparative quantitative data on lipids in serum and aortic wall of swine fed an atherogenic diet for 160 days. Figures for aortic wall have been calculated as μeq/g and those for serum altered μeq/ml in order to allow direct comparisons. It is apparent that aortic tissue is not acting as a nonselective sponge. With all components except cholesterol ester, the increase in tissue concentration after feeding the atherogenic diet is less than the corresponding increase in serum concentration. This type of analysis does not tell us how the corresponding increase in the aortic tissue is divided between the extracellular and intracellular compartments but morphologic studies on the same swine suggest that most of the lipid is intracellular

in one to two months and fairly extensive lesions by five months. The lesions at five months are mainly proliferative although some have small foci of necrosis. As judged by light and electron microscopy the lipid is principally intracellular with extracellular lipid in the necrotic areas and elsewhere accounting for only a small part of the total. We measured levels of nonesterified cholesterol (NEC), esterified cholesterol (EC), triglyceride (TG), and phospholipid (PL) in the plasma and in intima-inner media portions of aortas of young male swine fed hyperlipemic diets for five months and compared these values with corresponding values in control swine. The results are summarized in Fig. 1.

As shown in the figure the percentage distribution of the four lipid classes in the serum of HL diet-fed swine is approximately that expected when most of the plasma lipid is in LD and VLD lipoproteins. It is obvious that the percentage distribution of the four lipid classes in the aortic wall of the HL diet-fed swine is vastly different from that in the plasma. The aortic tissue values are consistent with the concept that most lipoproteins disintegrate into their component parts either before or after entering the aortic wall and that the parts are either absorbed or eliminated at different rates.

In tissue culture studies it has been shown that NEC passes freely through cell membranes in either direction while EC does not [1263]. EC enters cells with considerable difficulty and in relatively small amounts. Most EC present in cells probably arises from esterification of NEC within the cell and this EC cannot readily escape. If these circumstances apply *in vivo*, we would expect EC from the plasma to flow through the extracellular compartment and out into the lymphatics and bloodstream with relatively little entering smooth muscle cells. We would expect NEC to distribute itself freely in both the intracellular and extracellular compartments of the arterial wall. Some of the NEC in the cells would be esterified to make EC and be trapped. Also, a portion of the NEC is an essential component of cell membranes in both control and HL animals.

Phospholipids are also essential components of cell membranes and are probably largely synthesized within cells. Plasma phospholipids may enter SMC but the results in Fig. 1 would suggest either a low rate of entry or rapid exit and/or degradation; the same statement could also apply to triglycerides.

Thus, when we examine data from multiple approaches, we see that the relation between plasma and aortic tissue lipids is complex and not as yet clearly understood. The immunological data suggest the possibility (although alternative explanations can be made) that at least some plasma lipid enters the arterial wall as LD or VLD lipoprotein. The data from isotope labeling studies suggest that at least two lipid classes (NEC and EC) enter the arterial wall at vastly different rates and that these rates are not related to relative concentrations of NEC and EC in intact plasma lipoproteins. Also, the data from measurements of lipid classes present in early swine atherosclerosis are not consistent with a major portion of lipid being present as intact lipoprotein of plasma origin.

One possible explanation for the preceding immunological observations pertaining to lipoprotein is that lipid present in the arterial wall as LD or VLD lipoprotein is a relatively small part of the total and represents a secondary phenomenon. Permeability at both the endothelial barrier level and the SMC plasma membrane level are probably altered as atherosclerosis progresses. This altered permeability might permit secondary entry of large molecules such as lipoproteins that may be normally excluded, and these molecules might then contribute to further cellular disturbance without having been the primary cause.

Changes in Arterial Wall Metabolism of Hyperlipemic (HL) Diet-Fed Animals Associated with Development of Gross Atherosclerotic Lesions. Many studies of changes in the arterial wall after development of gross lesions were presented at the first symposium. More recent studies are reviewed in the current symposium, especially by Dr. R. F. Scott. Therefore, this portion of the present paper will be limited to a few reports that appear especially pertinent in the context of this paper.

Studies of SMC proliferation in atherosclerosis have been made by Stary and McMillan. Their initial work was presented by McMillan at the first symposium. Since then they have completed a study in which cholesterol-fed rabbits were given an *in vivo* pulse of ^{3}H-thymidine after lesions developed [1414]. Successive groups of rabbits were then sacrificed for periods up to nine days and grain counts made on SMC lesions. Progressive lowering of average grain counts was observed during this period indicating multiple divisions of SMC labeled initially. Sparagen et al. [1394] have also carried out a series of studies of SMC proliferation in atherosclerosis. In one study they labeled cells of rabbits throughout the body with an *in vivo* injection of ^{3}H-thymidine prior to beginning cholesterol feeding. They waited until all labeled cells had disappeared from the blood stream and then began to feed cholesterol. Atherosclerotic lesions that subsequently developed contained labeled cells. Since no cells in the circulating blood were labeled at the time the lesions developed, they concluded that the labeled cells in the lesions must have arisen from cells that were present in the arterial wall at the time the lesions developed. These studies together with those from our laboratory, presented earlier by Dr. R. F. Scott, demonstrate clearly the proliferative nature of the experimental atherosclerotic lesion resulting from HL diets. They also provide a means for quantitating the rate of proliferation at any given time that should be useful in investigating mechanisms and in evaluating therapeutic agents.

A number of studies of lipid synthesizing activities of cells in the arterial wall have been made by Getz et al. [530]. For example, they studied ^{32}P and ^{14}C-acetate uptake into phospholipids of the arterial wall of atherosclerotic monkeys. Results indicated markedly increased phospholipid synthesis in the aorta. Portman [1190] has shown that a major part of the increase in aortic phospholipid synthesis in cholesterol-fed monkeys is of phosphatidyl choline and sphingomyelin with phosphatidyl serine essentially unchanged. St. Clair et al. [1282] demonstrated increased squalene synthesis in aortas of cholesterol-fed pigeons. We demonstrated increased protein synthesis in aortas of cholesterol-fed monkeys at the first symposium; more recently we have shown similar increases in cholesterol-fed swine [468].

Earlier in this symposium Dr. R. F. Scott reviewed studies suggesting increases in oxygen consumption and energy production. All of these studies and many more not summarized here indicate that hyperlipemic diets stimulate increased metabolic activity in the arteries of experimental animals. There have been only a few metabolic studies that clearly show impaired function in early experimental atherosclerosis. Whereat [1543] has presented evidence suggesting some degree of uncoupling of oxidative phosphorylation in aortic mitochondria of cholesterol-fed rabbits. Nonetheless, he demonstrated a great increase in the rate of lipid synthesis of the aorta in similar rabbits.

Several studies of permeability of normal and atherosclerotic arteries of experimental animals have been made recently. Packham et al. [1138] have shown in swine that regions of the aorta around orifices, which are sites of predilection for atherosclerosis, appear to be more permeable to albumin and ^{14}C cholesterol than other regions. Hollander [693] has shown an increased uptake of ^{131}I beta-lipoprotein by arteries of atherosclerotic monkeys. Thus, we have evidence that at least certain lipids, proteins, and oxygen enter the arterial wall more readily in experimental atherosclerosis. These substances could provide the stimulus for (or merely be the result of) increased metabolic activity.

Changes in Arterial Wall Metabolism of HL Diet-Fed Animals Prior to Development of Gross Atherosclerotic Lesions and Changes in Cultured Arterial Cells Exposed to HL Serum. The studies reviewed in the first three sections of this report raise many questions not readily answered by examining arterial tissue after gross atherosclerosis has developed. It is reasonable to assume that one or more molecular species in HL plasma ("x-molecules") are interacting with one or more molecular species in the cells of the arterial wall ("y-molecules") to produce the observed changes.

If there are multiple species of x-molecules interacting independently of each other with multiple species of y-molecules, it will be extremely difficult to elucidate atherogenesis in molecular terms. From an investigative standpoint it would be much more desirable if the primary event were the interaction of one species of x-molecule with one species of y-molecule and if all other interactions were secondary to the primary event. Even if there are multiple different primary events, from a practical investigative standpoint they will probably have to be identified one at a time.

When gross atherosclerosis has developed hundreds of different events are taking place in the cells of arterial tissue that deviate from corresponding events in normal tissue. Moreover, these are not synchronized from cell to cell and in this situation it is practically impossible to distinguish primary from secondary events. This has led to the investigation of specific events that occur in HL animals prior to the development of gross lesions.

Among the most impressive events in gross atherosclerosis is the increase in the number of arterial cells synthesizing DNA and dividing. One hypothesis is that the primary event in atherogenesis is stimulation (or derepression) of DNA synthesis and cell division with classic cell injury occurring as secondary phenomena (as in cancer).

Other prominent events observed even in early gross atherosclerosis are those associated with cell injury and death. Hence, another hypothesis that we may make is that the primary event in atherogenesis is disruption of some vital cell function and that the observed increase in DNA synthesis and cell division is the secondary phenomenon of repair taking place in an excessive fashion.

The preceding two hypotheses are presented in outline form in Fig. 2. Currently available information does not permit us to choose between the two. However, considerable data pertaining to them have been obtained since the first symposium. The remainder of this report will be a review of these new data derived from studies of the arterial wall of HL animals prior to development of gross atherosclerosis and from tissue culture cells exposed to HL serum.

Data Pertaining to DNA Synthesis and Cell Division from HL Animals Without Gross Atherosclerosis and from Tissue Cultures. In our laboratory the preceding aspect has been investigated in young male swine fed the diet shown in Table 1 or some modification. Swine fed this diet begin to develop gross lesions in four to eight weeks [1462]. Emphasis in our studies thus far has been on the first week after beginning the diet. We have investigated mitotic activity by deter-

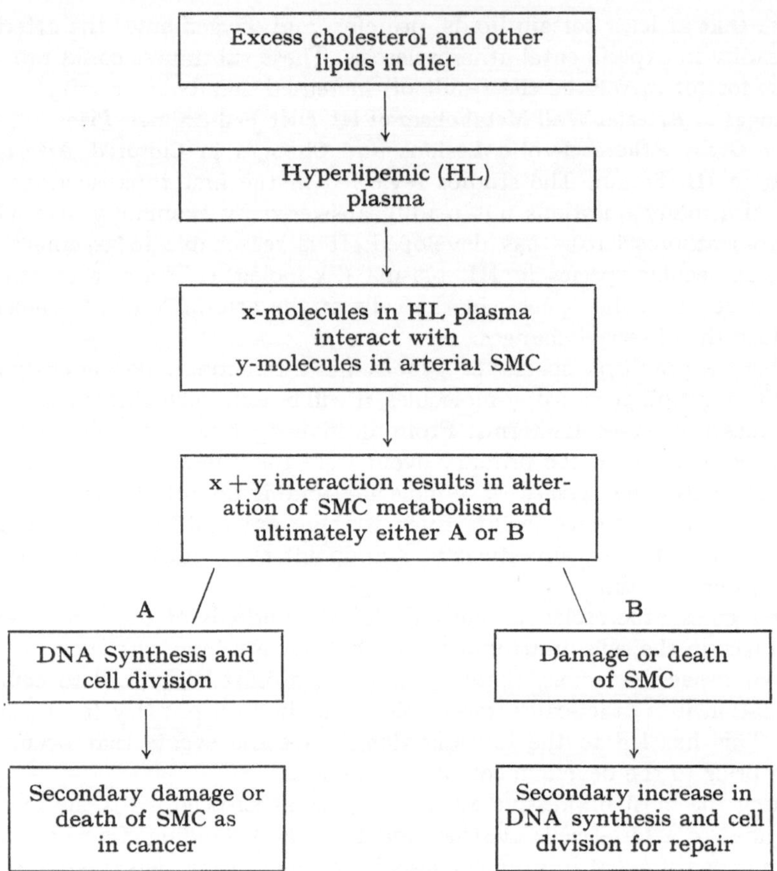

Fig. 2. Flow chart for dietary lipids to hyperlipemic plasma to altered metabolism of arterial smooth muscle cells

Table 1. *The composition of basic diet consumed per day is shown. The HL diet differed only in that crystalline cholesterol was added in varying quantities depending upon the nature of experiments. The calories shown are adequate for normal growth of young swine used in most experiments*

Ingredients	g	Total calories	1704
Peanut oil	38	Fat	40%
Butter	38	Protein	24%
Cholesterol	0	Carbohydrate	36%
Choline chloride	1		
Casein	100		
Salt mix (Wesson)	22		
Vitamin mix (less choline)	11		
Sucrose	155		
Cellulose	35		
Total in g	400		

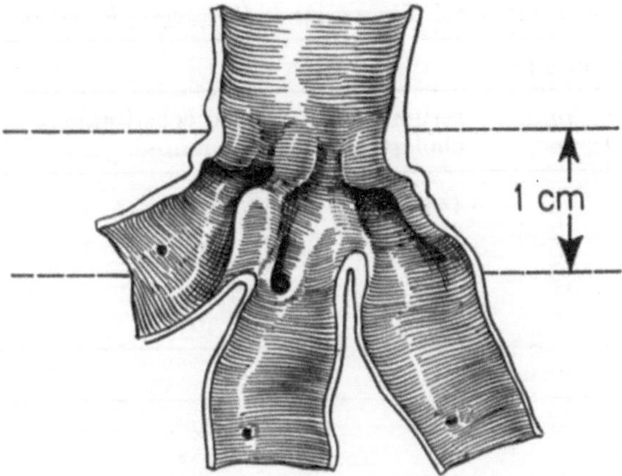

Fig. 3. Trifurcation region of the abdominal aorta of swine, which is a site of predilection for atherosclerosis

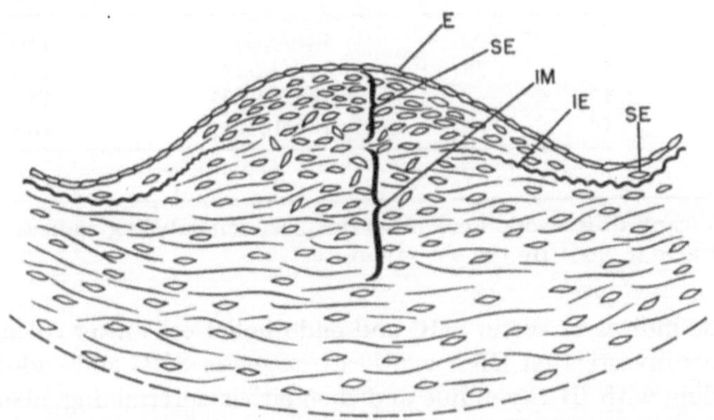

Fig. 4. Cross section of trifurcation region of the abdominal aorta of swine through a cushion. *E* endothelium; *SE* subendothelial intima; *IM* inner media; *IE* internal elastica. It is apparent that the number of smooth muscle cells in the intima is much greater in the center of the cushion than in non-branching areas. In non-branching areas only scattered smooth muscle cells are found in the intima. Internal elasticas are usually discontinuous as shown here. This makes the intima and inner media essentially one unit at the point of discontinuity

Table 2. *Mitotic counts of aortic trifurcation region of swine fed cholesterol for 3 days*

	Cholesterol (12 swine)		Control (12 swine)		p
	mitoses/total cells counted	mitoses/10^4 cells/hr.	mitoses/total cells counted	mitoses/10^4 cells/hr.	
Inner media	457/233,492	4.0	253/248,766	1.9	<0.01
Subendothelial intima	179/104,979	3.2	76/102,741	1.5	<0.01
Endothelium	195/148,432	2.3	82/138,142	1.1	<0.01

Table 3. ^{3}H-*Thymidine radioautography on en face preparations*

Days on diet	Cholesterol groups				
	amount of cholesterol	animal no.	serum cholesterol	labeled cells/total cells counted	labeled cells/ 10^4 cells
1 day	20 g	1	141	53/10,492	51
		2	104	50/8,683	58
		3	99	83/17,351	49
		4	81	98/15,382	64
		5	101	109/17,612	61
		mean	105		57
3 days	20 g	6	158	75/7,276	103
		7	317	63/6,252	100
		8	127	116/10,439	111
		9	147	69/7,425	93
		10	—	107/7,618	140
		mean	187		110
3 days	8 g	11	100	146/9,649	150
		12	78	43/3,027	142
		13	—	141/10,263	137
		14	—	186/10,139	183
		mean	89		156

[a] No significant differences were observed between labeling indices for the two are significant at $p < 0.001$ by the chi-square test.

mining mitotic indices of aortic SMC and endothelial cells after colchicine injections. We have investigated DNA synthesis in aortic SMC and endothelial cells by pulse labeling with ^{3}H-thymidine and then either determining labeling indices by radioautography or specific activities by chemical means [466, 468, 469, 1462] (in press, Florentin).

The region most frequently studied has been the trifurcation region of the abdominal aorta. The anatomy of this region is illustrated in Figs. 3 and 4. Reasons for choosing this region are as follows: (1) it is a site of predilection for gross atherosclerosis that develops later, and (2) more SMC are normally present in the intima in this region than in nonbranching sites.

Results with the two approaches (^{3}H-thymidine labeling indices and mitotic indices) parallel each other and indicate that most cells synthesizing DNA go on to divide. Examples of results from one study of mitoses in swine fed HL diets for three days are presented in Table 2. It is apparent that mitotic indices have increased in all three layers as compared with control values [466]. Results of one study of DNA synthesis in *en face* preparations of endothelial cells at one and three days after initiating HL diets is shown in Table 3. No differences from controls were observed at one day, but at three days differences were established [469]. These studies and others like them show clearly that DNA synthesis and cell diivsion are stimulated by HL diets long before the development of gross lesions. This does not necessarily mean that the primary event in HL *of endothelial cells of swine abdominal aortas* [a]

Control groups				
type of diets	animal no.	serum cholesterol	labeled cells/total cells counted	labeled cells/ 10^4 cells
Mash	1	84	48/10,433	46
	2	82	74/8,036	92
	3	74	21/6,595	32
	4	78	56/8,175	69
	5	78	43/8,967	48
	mean	79		57
Stock	6	72	29/7,775	37
	7	68	32/7,275	44
	8	84	71/11,328	63
	9	70	40/7,766	52
	10	—	42/7,563	56
	mean	74		51
Mash	11	67	75/11,993	63
	12	68	110/18,270	60
	13	—	11/7,045	16
	b			
	mean	68		53

groups at 1 day. At 3 days differences between both cholesterol groups and controls
[b] Specimen inadvertently damaged.

diet-induced atherosclerosis is stimulation of cell division. However, it does indicate that increased cell division is, at least, closely related in time to the primary event.

Perhaps the principal value of these studies is that they define a period in HL diet-fed swine that needs to be intensively studied. If we can map out the metabolic events in aortic walls of HL diet-fed swine that deviate from controls in this early period, we should have a better understanding of atherogenesis in molecular terms.

However, study of the early period in atherogenesis is exceedingly difficult because of the small magnitude of the changes. The ^{3}H-thymidine labeling index as determined by radioautography provides a very sensitive technique that permits us to identify small increases in activity. With techniques used thus far for measuring protein and RNA synthesis in the three-day diet period, we have been unable to detect changes, though they are likely to be present. Measurements of oxygen consumption made recently with the electron probe have shown an increase in consumption by three days (unpublished observations in our laboratory). No other biochemical information is as yet available on this very early period in HL diets.

The difficulties encountered in studying events responsible for increased cell division in the aorta of intact animals has led us and others to explore *in vitro* techniques. We reasoned that if serum from HL animals stimulated DNA syn-

Table 4. *Data on cells growing in 20% hyperlipemic or normal serum and pulse-labeled with ^{3}H-thymidine*

Days after explant	Group	Total cells counted no.	Cells labeled with ^{3}H-thymidine no.	Labeled %	Significance of selected comparisons by chi square
8	N_tN_s	10,183	2,189	21.5	$N_tN_s < N_tH_s$ $p < 0.001$
	N_tH_s	6,607	2,029	30.7	$N_tN_s < H_tH_s$ $p < 0.001$
	H_tN_s	3,315	710	22.5	$H_tN_s < H_tH_s$ $p < 0.001$
	H_tH_s	6,170	1,943	31.4	N_tN_s vs H_tN_s p N.S. N_tH_s vs H_tH_s p N.S.
10	N_tN_s	7,220	681	9.4	$N_tN_s < N_tH_s$ $p < 0.001$
	N_tH_s	5,659	819	14.5	$N_tN_s < H_tH_s$ $p < 0.001$
	H_tN_s	5,066	610	12.0	$H_tN_s < H_tH_s$ $p < 0.001$
	H_tH_s	7,191	1,119	15.6	$N_tN_s < H_tN_s$ $p < 0.001$ N_tH_s vs H_tH_s p N.S.
14	N_tN_s	4,086	473	11.6	$N_tN_s < N_tH_s$ $p < 0.001$
	N_tH_s	3,449	715	17.8	$N_tN_s < H_tH_s$ $p < 0.001$
	H_tN_s	4,476	627	14.0	$H_tN_s < H_tH_s$ $p < 0.001$
	H_tH_s	1,828	336	18.4	$N_tN_s < H_tN_s$ $p < 0.001$ N_tH_s vs H_tH_s p N.S.

thesis and cell division in tissue culture more than serum from controls we would have a technique that might provide information difficult or impossible to obtain *in vivo*.

The first goal was to determine whether or not such an effect of HL serum could be demonstrated *in vitro*. This goal has been achieved with two different approaches in our laboratory [466], with another in Wissler's laboratory [777], and with a fourth in Robertson's laboratory. With one approach in our laboratory ^{3}H-thymidine labeling indices and mitotic indices were determined at intervals in monolayer primary cultures of outgrowths from aortic explants exposed to either HL or normal sera [469]. With the other approach (unpublished observations) aortic media explants were floated in culture media containing HL or control sera. At intervals some of these cultures were pulse labeled with ^{3}H-thymidine and DNA content and specific activities were then determined. In Wissler's laboratory [777] outgrowths from explants were grown on glass and the area covered by cells measured at intervals. With all three approaches HL serum was shown to produce an increase in the parameters being measured as compared to the effect with control sera. Robertson has extended the observations by showing that LD lipoproteins have a similar stimulatory effect on cultured cells (personal communication). For illustration, some of the observations made in one of our experiments are presented in Table 4.

These studies have not as yet been carried further. The obvious next step is to attempt to identify the metabolic reactions that account for the HL serum-induced increase in DNA synthesis and cell division.

Data Pertaining to Cell Damage from HL Animals Prior to Development of Gross Atherosclerosis. Biochemical results clearly indicating damage in arteries of HL diet-fed animals prior to development of gross lesions have not been obtained. Biochemical results reported to date show either no change from controls or increased metabolic activity. In spite of the negative results we reasoned that changes may have occurred that were too small to be detected by available biochemical methods. Therefore, we have carried out an intensive study by electron microscopy of morphologic changes that occur in the aortas of HL diet-fed swine in the first week on diet. SMC and endothelial cells in the aorta die and are replaced (turnover) in control as well as HL diet-fed swine. Thus, we would expect to find a few cells showing changes suggestive of degeneration or death even in controls.

Our studies to date have been directed towards answering two questions. (1) Were there any morphologic changes suggesting cellular damage in the HL diet-fed swine that were not present in controls? (2) Were these morphologic changes suggesting degeneration and death that were seen in both HL diet and control swine more common in one than the other? In studies of the first week on diet in our laboratory the answer to the first question has thus far been no.

We have attempted to answer the second question by making counts using electron microscopy and determining the percentage of total cells observed showing changes suggesting damage (unpublished observations). Comparisons have been made in five pairs of swine, and in all, the percentage of cells classified as degenerating was greater in the HL diet-fed swine than in controls. These results keep open the question of which of the two alternative hypotheses shown in Fig. 2 is correct. Cell injury and cell multiplication are very closely coupled in all tissues, and it is perhaps futile to attempt to separate them until we have more details concerning underlying metabolic events in atherogenesis.

The electron microscopy studies of damaged cells in HL diet-fed swine to date have shown changes in all organelles and have not as yet provided a clue as to the primary intracellular site of damage. In this regard recent studies by Whereat and Orishimo [1544] of mitochondria from aortas of rabbits fed cholesterol for three weeks may be pertinent. None of the rabbits studied had gross atherosclerotic lesions. The phospholipid content of the mitochondria was not greatly changed for any component except for lysolecithin which was decreased. However, when the investigators studied phospholipid synthesis in similar aortic mitochondria they found more than a 100% increase in synthesis rates for all phospholipid components. Values for phosphatidic acid and octadecadienic acid (C 18:2) showed the greatest increase. The significance of these increases is not clear. Whereat and Orishimo [1544] suggest that they may be reflecting some change in activities of electron transport particles and relate to the uncoupling of oxidative phosphorylation that they have observed in rabbit aortic mitochondria after gross lesions develop.

CONCLUSIONS

In this report we have emphasized the role of dietary cholesterol in altering plasma lipids and producing experimental atherosclerosis. We have reviewed studies indicating that excessive dietary cholesterol results in significant changes in arterial wall metabolism even before the development of gross atherosclerosis. The changes are not necessarily due to cholesterol *per se* since excessive dietary cholesterol results in changes in multiple lipid and protein components of the plasma. Information gained thus far on changes in arterial wall metabolism of experimental animals following feeding of hyperlipemic diets shows many altered metabolic activities, but we cannot as yet place them in a meaningful sequential order. However, the scientific tools are probably available and the intellectual climate favorable to permit elucidation in the next few years of the whole series of metabolic events in atherogenesis in cholesterol-fed animals. When this knowledge is available, it will remain to be determined what pertinence the information has for atherogenesis in man.

DIETS THAT LOWER BLOOD CHOLESTEROL IN MAN

HELEN B. BROWN

Information on the relationship between diet, blood lipids, and atherosclerosis was reviewed in 1957 [1145] based on evidence obtained from experimental animals [1193], from epidemiological studies [1406], and from clinical experience. The essential knowledge of the dietary changes required for reducing blood lipid levels in human beings had been available over a decade [26]. These alterations involved total fat, animal fats, and vegetable oils, saturated and unsaturated fatty acids, and cholesterol. Among nonfat dietary constituents were protein, starches and sugar. The question was whether reduction of blood lipids with diet would lower the incidence of atherosclerosis. In 1964 [51], fat was still considered the controlling dietary component. For some investigators, reduction in total fat was of prime importance for reducing serum lipid levels, the amount of polyunsaturated fatty acids was of minor importance. For others, the necessarily high carbohydrate content of low-fat diets was objectionable, and the polyunsaturated fatty acid content was emphasized.

Recent Developments. Further evidence of the close relationship between dietary fat and atherosclerosis comes from a recent epidemiological study of geographic pathology [1333]. An encouraging development is the reduced incidence of coronary artery disease in persons who have maintained a low cholesterol level with fat-controlled diets for five years or more [384, 857, 1227, 1479]. Theoretically, the risk of coronary heart disease drops by 3% for every 1% reduction in serum cholesterol level [330]. Persons in the general population most likely to develop premature coronary disease can now be identified and offered preventive treatment [1406] in which diet plays an important part.

Fat-controlled diets have progressed from the state of being "unappetizing", "impractical" and "bizarre" in 1957 to being palatable and practical for free-living persons. Fat-controlled commercially processed food products can be made [1079] though not presently on the market.

The types of hyperlipoproteinemia (or hyperlipidemia) that are closely associated with atherosclerosis can now be easily recognized by the paper electrophoretic pattern and cholesterol and triglyceride levels [489]. Classification is based on the proportion and amount of three groups of low density lipoproteins: cholesterol-rich beta fraction, triglyceride-rich prebeta fraction and chylomicrons. Dietary requirements for reducing blood lipids of the different types of hyperlipoproteinemia have been determined [863, 866]. This knowledge enables the physician to treat his hyperlipidemic patients with an appropriate diet. Diet remains the principle treatment that can be safely offered to such patients, though drugs may be of additional help in maintaining low blood lipid levels in certain types of hyperlipidemia.

Dietary Fat Components. Results of many quantitative diet studies agree that dietary saturated fatty acids and cholesterol increase the serum cholesterol concentration while polyunsaturated fatty acids reduce it. Monounsaturated fatty acids probably have little or no influence. In these carefully controlled studies, the amount and kind of fat have been altered in a systematic way, using either liquid formula diets [27, 441], single fats and oils [27, 656], specially prepared fats [249, 441] or a variety of fat-containing foods [246, 792]. In all studies, calories were adjusted to maintain constant body weight. Feeding periods usually lasted for 18 days to five weeks, though some studies continued longer. Subjects served as their own controls with a standard or reference diet.

Total Fat. It was originally thought that the amount of fat was critical in a lipid-reducing diet because of the epidemiological evidence that those populations eating low-fat diets (15% or less) had lower blood cholesterol levels and much less cardiovascular disease than those eating high-fat diets (40%). With the demonstration that replacement of saturated with unsaturated fat had a similar effect on serum cholesterol levels [27] emphasis was shifted to quality rather than quantity of fat. At present a moderate fat diet (30%) is often recommended.

Saturated Fatty Acids. Serum cholesterol levels are low with a diet low in saturated fatty acids. Saturated fatty acids are a potent hypercholesteremic component of the diet. According to Keys' formula[1] [792], saturates are twice as effective in increasing serum cholesterol levels as polyunsaturates are in reducing them. The only way of eliminating saturates from the usual American diet is to reduce the use of fat contained in animal products, such as meat, dairy products, eggs, and in certain vegetable products, such as customary shortening and margarine, cocoa butter, coconut oil.

At first all saturated fatty acids were thought to affect serum cholesterol levels in the same way. Now it is known that fatty acids with less than 12 carbon atoms do not influence serum lipid levels [625]. They by-pass the lymphatic system and are absorbed directly into the portal system. Stearic acid (C_{18}), a major component of food fats, has no effect on serum cholesterol levels [656,

[1] Keys' Formula: Δ Serum cholesterol $= 1.35$ ($2\,\Delta$ Saturates — Δ Polyunsaturates).

Table 1. *Influence of monoenes on serum cholesterol reduction*

Reference	Total fat	Sat. F.A.	Mono. F.A.	Poly. F.A.	Serum cholesterol	
	percentage of calories				mg %	difference
Keys et al. [792][a]	18	8	6	4	182	
	36	8	24	4	182	0
Hegsted et al. [656][b]	22	7	7	7	213	
	38	7	26	5	232	19
Brown (unpublished)	15	5	4	6	164	
	25	8	7	10	162	
	38	8	23	7	181	18

[a] Page 751, Table 2, Diets PSO, POO respectively.
[b] Page 285, Table 3, Diets No. 5, No. 36, respectively.

Table 2. *Serum cholesterol levels with 17% and 23% polyunsaturated fatty acids (saturated fatty acid <12% calories)*

Investigator and reference	Polyunsaturates percentage of calories	Serum cholesterol	
		mg %	difference
National Diet-Heart Study [1079][a]	18	175	
	22	171	4
Brown et al. [246][b]	17	172	
	23	167	5
Keys et al. [792][c]	17	159	
	22	161	2
Keys et al. [792][d]	17	162	
	23	157	5
Anderson et al. [48][e]	17	163	
	22	160	3

[a] Diets C and E, respectively, Faribault Hospital Study, compiled from data given in Tables IX.9, XII.3, XII.8.
[b] Diets, standard and III 4, respectively, from Tables 3 and 4.
[c] Diets given Table 1, p. 780, lines 16 and 17, respectively.
[d] Diets given in Table 1, p. 780, lines 18 and 19, respectively.
[e] Diets with corn oil and safflower oil, respectively, Tables 3 and 7.

792]. The three remaining saturated fatty acids, lauric (C_{12}),myristic (C_{14}) and palmitic (C_{16}) account for the entire effect of saturates. Myristic acid, though present in food fat in small amounts, has as strong an effect on blood cholesterol levels [656] as has lauric acid.

Monounsaturated Fatty Acids. Oleic acid is the principal monene. It is present in all food fats and is the main constituent of olive oil. Oleic acid has little or no influence on serum cholesterol levels under usual dietary conditions. Diets using olive oil were the only ones in one study [656] that on repetition did not duplicate their effect on serum cholesterol levels. In two studies [656] (H. B. Brown, unpublished data), serum cholesterol was increased by 20 mg with diets in which the amount of total fat was increased by approximately 18% with the addition of oleic acid. This did not occur in a third study [792] (Table 1).

Polyunsaturated Fatty Acids. All straight chain fatty acids with two or more double bonds are equally effective in reducing serum cholesterol levels. The essential fatty acid, linoleic acid, occurs most frequently in ordinary food products, especially in oils of grains, seeds and nuts. The longer chain, multi-bonded fatty acids present in fish are also effective. Serum cholesterol levels decrease as polyunsaturates increase in the diet. According to Keys' formula, an increase in polyunsaturates is only half as effective in reducing serum cholesterol levels as a commensurate decrease in saturates.

This formula implies a linear relationship between reduction in serum cholesterol and increase in polyunsaturates in the diet over the entire range of possible fatty acid concentrations. A linear relationship was not sustained with diets in which polyunsaturates were increased from 17% to 23% of calories (Table 2).

Cholesterol. Cholesterol is of greater importance in fat-controlled diets than was realized at one time. Cholesterol is present in both animal tissue and animal fat. A linear relationship exists between dietary and serum cholesterol. A reduction of 100 mg dietary cholesterol results in a drop of 5 mg serum cholesterol [656, 792]. This reduction is independent of the fatty acid composition of the diet and occurs whether saturated or polyunsaturated fatty acids predominate. From this point of view, consideration of dietary cholesterol does not appear to be crucial in devising a diet for maintaining a low serum cholesterol level.

The true significance of cholesterol in fat-controlled diets appears when considered in relationship to polyunsaturated fatty acids. To obtain an adequate serum cholesterol reduction, the polyunsaturated fatty acid requirement increases as the dietary cholesterol rises in the diet [245] (Table 3). For a reduction of 18% to 22% in serum cholesterol, a diet with 200 mg cholesterol requires 15% of calories as polyunsaturated fatty acids, and one with 550 mg requires 23%. A maximum effect of dietary cholesterol on the serum level is probably obtained with about 750 mg. Practical fat-controlled diets can be devised with a range of 100 to 350 mg cholesterol.

Although no interaction between cholesterol and other components of the diet were reported in two studies [656, 792], the second institutional study of the National Diet-Heart Study (D-H) reported to the contrary [1079].

Unless cholesterol is dissolved in fat, or eaten with fat, it is not readily absorbed. Additions of crystalline cholesterol to diets low in fat do not have the same hypercholesteremic effect as the same amount eaten with fat or eaten in meat or eggs. For example [1535], ten egg yolks a day were fed to human subjects, resulting in an increase of 40 mg serum cholesterol. When either the fatty acid fraction or the unsaponifiable fraction of ten egg yolks were fed separately, little or no increase in serum cholesterol occurred. When the two fractions were fed six hours apart, there was only a 15 mg increase.

The actual cholesterol content of many food products is probably less than that given in the present food tables. Analyzed values were below calculated values in Hegsted's study [656] and in the second institutional D-H Study [1079]. Fat-controlled diets described in terms of the cholesterol-containing foods they employ may be a more reliable expression of their cholesterol content than the milligrams cholesterol they are supposed to contain.

Hydrogenated Oils. Oils are treated with hydrogen to increase their stability and to give them the plastic properties required for shortenings and margarines. During hydrogenation, unnatural transisomers of fatty acids are formed; they do not affect serum cholesterol levels [48]. Although these are a possible source of harm, there is no indication that trans fatty acids in amounts normally used in practical diets affect human beings adversely [250]. The difficulty in using hydrogenated products in fat-controlled diets is their low polyunsaturated and high saturated fatty acid content.

Interdependence of Dietary Fat Components. The amount and proportion of fatty acids, cholesterol and total fat in the diet are necessarily interdependent. The familiar triangular diagram [27] illustrates how a change in one fatty acid component alters the proportion among all three—saturates, monounsaturates, and polyunsaturates. The proportion of saturates, monoenes, and polyunsaturates in the fat mixture was of greater predictive value for serum cholesterol reduction than was the percent of calories in one study [656].

Although the calories of saturated and polyunsaturated fatty acids remained the same in diets to which oleic acid was added (Table 1) their proportion in the total fat mixture was altered considerably. The change in proportion may have accounted for the unexpected increase in the serum cholesterol level with addition of oleic acid.

The relative importance of these fatty acid components for reducing cholesterol depends upon the amount of dietary cholesterol. As discussed, the difference between 400 and 200 mg cholesterol was of no significance when the diet contained 23% calories of polyunsaturated fatty acids, and was critical when the diet had 15%. In Hegsted's study [656] diets containing 300 mg cholesterol increased serum cholesterol levels 40 mg above control level when saturated coconut oil was the fat; they were unchanged with monounsaturated olive oil and reduced 35 mg with polyunsaturated safflower oil. Undoubtedly this is the reason why the composition of fat-controlled diets is so difficult to understand and why a simple expression of the relationships is so necessary for interpreting the effects of various diets on serum cholesterol levels.

There is a large biologic variation in the serum cholesterol response to the same diet among normal persons. Hegsted estimated the error of estimate was about 10 mg/100 ml with a standard deviation of ± 5 mg. In our experiments, reproducibility with the same or similar diets in one individual was of the order of 10 to 15 mg or 6%. In fact, we obtained only three degrees of reduction in serum cholesterol levels that were statistically significant. In a group of young men with an average serum cholesterol level of 208 mg/100 ml, serum cholesterol reduction of less than 17 mg was not a statistically significant change, a reduction between 17 and 30 mg was significant, but yet less than a 30 mg reduction usually seen with our standard unsaturated fat diet [244]. Any more exact measure of the effect of diet on serum cholesterol levels was impractical when considering small groups of people or an individual response. These results were obtained on subjects who were on a standard diet and one or more variants for 18 days. The relative effectiveness of a particular variant was indicated by the extent of reduction in serum cholesterol levels compared to that obtained with the standard diet in the same subject [246].

The fatty acid composition of the diet at which the change from partial to full effectiveness in serum cholesterol reduction occurred (compared to the standard diet) has been called the critical limit. Critical limits for a diet having 38% fat

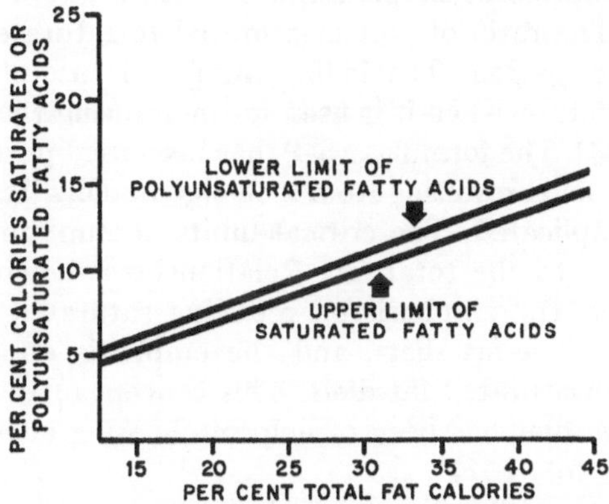

Fig. 1. Critical composition of dietary fat for a serum cholesterol reduction of 200 mg cholesterol. The figure is reprinted from reference [249] with the kind permission of the publisher

Table 3. *Serum cholesterol reduction and dietary polyunsaturates. (Total fat: 38 percent calories, saturates: <12 percent)*

Polyunsaturates in diet	In percent of calories			
	14	15	17	23
Cholesterol in diet (mg)	Serum cholesterol reduction, in percent			
200	—13	—18 [a]	—19 [a]	—21 [a]
450		—10		
550	—7	—8	—8	—22 [a] [b]
700–800	—2	1		—11

[a] Reduction similar to that with standard diet.
[b] The zig-zag line indicates the borderline between the composition of those diets that support 18 percent or more reduction in serum cholesterol and those that support 13 percent or less.

calories and 200 mg cholesterol, were 13% for saturated fatty acids and 14% polyunsaturated fatty acids [246, 249]. Effective diets for serum cholesterol reduction contained from 5% to 12% saturates and 14% to 22% polyunsaturates. The proportion of the fatty acids was 33% or less of fat saturates, 42% or more polyunsaturates, and approximately 25% monounsaturates.

With reduction in total dietary fat, these critical limits, expressed in percent of calories, drops accordingly to 5% saturates and 6% polyunsaturates with 15% total fat, yet the critical fatty acid composition in percent fat remains the same (Fig. 1). With 450 mg cholesterol, the critical amount of polyunsaturates is more than 15% in a diet with 38% total fat; and, with 550 mg cholesterol, is somewhere between 17% and 23% (Table 3). The critical amount of saturates decreases to approximately 7%.

It is difficult to express in simple terms the composition of fat necessary for fat-controlled diets. The ratio of polyunsaturated to saturated fatty acids (P/S) gives inadequate information. The iodine number is useful when a single fat is the only source of fat, or when it is used for monitoring the unsaturation of an experimental diet [384]. The formula, 2 S-P, has been used primarily for predicting the serum cholesterol level resulting from a change in diets. Its use in formulating practical diets is complicated. The critical limits account for the proportion of fatty acids in relation to the total fat. Relationships shown in the figure may explain the reason for the emphasis on reducing saturated fat and cholesterol by the proponents of low-fat diets, and the emphasis on polyunsaturates by proponents of high unsaturated fat diets. This concept of the minimum requirements for an effective diet has been of help in choosing adequate foods for fat-controlled diets [244, 565, 1079].

Other Dietary Factors. This discussion of dietary fat and serum lipid reduction is based on the premise that the diets are nutritionally adequate in all respects, in protein, vitamins, and minerals. Human diets with less than 8% protein calories are associated with an abnormally low serum cholesterol level that is not affected by dietary fat and is the result of the low protein intake [1126]. A protein intake of 8% to 20% of calories does not affect serum lipid levels in human beings, and fat is a principal controlling factor.

There is no evidence that diets rich in polyunsaturates result in a vitamin E deficiency. People who have been on these diets for several years maintain adequate serum alpha tocopherol levels [1079]. There is also no evidence that the ordinary use of oils in cooking and baking develop harmful toxic products during the process, although unsaturated oils develop them more readily than saturated fats [250]. Persons have been cooking with oils in the home for many years with no reported detrimental effects.

The influence of the amount and kind of carbohydrate on serum lipids of normocholesteremic persons is quite limited. Serum cholesterol levels are lower with high starch diets than with high sugar diets [561, 951]. Serum triglyceride levels tend to be higher with high carbohydrate diets, especially with those high in sugar [46]. Yet the change in persons with normal levels is small compared to changes induced in persons with certain types of hyperlipidemia.

Diets for Hyperlipidemia. Diets for treatment of hyperlipidemia follow the basic principles for fat-controlled diets. The particular diet prescription depends on the particular lipoprotein fraction that is elevated [248, 489, 836, 863, 866]. Beta lipoprotein and consequently serum cholesterol, is affected by the fatty acid composition of the dietary fat and the cholesterol content, as discussed. Prebeta lipoprotein and the accompanying triglyceride is affected by the amount of dietary carbohydrate and in many cases, by the starch and sugar content.

The presence of chylomicrons and the associated triglyceride is affected by the amount of fat, regardless of its composition.

For beta lipoprotein reduction with fat-controlled diets, the amount of fat is of relatively little importance compared to the composition of that fat which should be polyunsaturated and low in cholesterol. A low-fat diet of 15% to 25% fat or an unsaturated fat diet of 30% to 38% fat are equally effective in Type II hypercholesteremic patients. For types with high prebeta lipoprotein fraction, Types III, IV and mixed hyperlipemia [247], the unsaturated fat diets with 48% of calories as carbohydrate are most effective. A further limitation of refined sugar may also be required. The presence of chylomicrons requires a low-fat diet, and in extreme hyperchylomicronemia, elimination of all fat-containing foods. Under the latter condition, medium chain fatty acid triglycerides (MCT) that do not form chylomicrons may be of practical help.

Fat-Controlled Diets for Practical Use. An important development in the past decade is the application of the dietary principles of serum lipid reduction to practical everyday eating patterns and foods. No matter how effective formula-type and closely structured diets may be, they are not suited for free-living persons for any length of time. Certain practical realities must be taken into account in developing these eating patterns. Customary food products must form the basis of the eating pattern. Consequently products with saturated fat and cholesterol are included. Even the so-called low-fat foods contain a certain amount of fat which cannot be manipulated. The amount of fruits, vegetables, cereals, grains, bread and coffee eaten during a day contain about 11 grams of fat not usually accounted for in calculating dietary fat [246]. It is difficult to replace all the saturated fat in the usual American diet with polyunsaturated vegetable oil products, so that a palatable unsaturated fat diet contains no more than 38% fat. When more fat is required, as in the diabetic diet, special fat-containing foods without carbohydrate may have to be introduced, such as dry cottage cheese creamed with unsaturated margarine.

The significance for food selection of the effects of individual saturated fatty acids on serum cholesterol levels has not been explored. Our diets from which were excluded butter fat (4% lauric and 8–14% myristic acids), fatty meats and lard (2–4% myristic acid), coconut and palm oils (45–55% lauric and 15–20% myristic acids) provided a trace (0.1% of calories) of lauric acid and less than 1% of calories as myristic acid. It is not known how freely cocoa butter can be used. Although it contains 35% of inactive stearic acid, it also has 24% palmitic acid. However, in the broader context of coronary disease prevention, these saturated fatty acids may influence formation of thrombi. At present it would be well to retain the kind of diets already used successfully for prevention and treatment of atherosclerosis. The composition of the practical diets used in studies for one to six years is shown in Table 4. They vary in total fat from 39% to 64% fat, 6% to 11% saturates with avoidance of fats rich in myristic acid, and polyunsaturates from 7% to 22%, respectively, and cholesterol below 400 mg.

It is easier to describe the nature of fat-controlled diets in terms of the kinds of foods than in terms of fatty acid and cholesterol content, and may be just as accurate. Our quantitative diets [246] were devised to answer such questions as: How much meat and meat fat can be included in the diet? What kind and how much oil? How many whole eggs? An effective unsaturated fat diet has the following ingredients: Two, 3.5 ounce portions of lean meat, fish or poultry, and fat-free dairy products insure 15 g animal fat and less than 300 mg dietary cholesterol. The use of margarine with 40% of fat as polyunsaturated fatty acids and an oil with 50%, insure sufficient unsaturation [244]. A broad selection of fruit, vegetables, cereals and grains fulfill nutritional needs and give satisfaction without weight gain.

Table 4. *Fat-controlled diets used in long-term studies*

Reference	Diet designation	Total fat percentage of calories	Saturates percentage of calories	Poly-unsaturates percentage of calories	Cholesterol mg per day
National Diet-Heart Study [1079]	B[a]	29	6	12	229
	B	30	7	10	282
Stamler [1406]	"CPEP"[b]	30	10	7	307
Turpeinen et al. [1479][c]	—	31	8	11	229
Rinzler [1227][c]	"Prudent"[d]	32	8	10	400
National Diet-Heart Study [1079]	BC	32	7	12	266
National Diet-Heart Study [1079]	C	34	7	13	256
National Diet-Heart Study [1079]	E[a]	37	5	22	117
National Diet-Heart Study [1079]	C[a]	38	7	18	237
Green et al. [565]	—	38	11	16	300
Dayton et al. [384][c]	—	39	9	16	365
Leren [857][c]	—	39	8	21	264
Medical Research Committee [967][e]	—	46	10	20	258

[a] Faribault Hospital Study.
[b] Coronary Prevention Evaluation Program, Chicago Health Department.
[c] With evidence of reduced incidence of coronary heart disease.
[d] New York City Health Department Program.
[e] With no evidence of reduced incidence of coronary heart disease. Fatty acid composition of diet estimated from data given in text.

The significance of the National Diet-Heart Study for this discussion is the use of fat-controlled, commercially processed foods to implement the diets. This study consisted of 2,000 free-living, healthy, middle-aged men, living in five different cities, and 400 state hospital inmates. They were equally divided into three groups and placed on one of three diets for a maximum of two years. By supplying foods of different fat composition, the three diets were successfully administered in a double blind fashion. Foods for the saturated fat diet were made with butter and hydrogenated shortening, foods for the low-fat diet had less polyunsaturated oil than those for the unsaturated fat diet. The Diet-Heart Study demonstrated that lower serum cholesterol levels could be maintained by changing the composition of the foods and that a diet need not be rigidly structured [243], just as a previous study had done [565]. It also demonstrated the hazards encountered by participants when surrounded with the customary saturated fat products. No commercial food products prepared according to the study's specifications, with the exception of oils and margarine, are available on the market today.

DISCUSSION

The composition of diets for reducing blood cholesterol and for maintaining it at a low level is now fairly well established. Dietary fat has to be low in myristic and palmitic acids, contain less than 350 mg cholesterol, and be relatively rich in polyunsaturated fatty acids. There is a certain maximum amount of saturates and a minimum amount of polyunsaturates necessary for effective reduction in serum cholesterol. These critical limits depend upon the amount of total fat and cholesterol in the diet. These fat-controlled diets are a versatile group, adaptable to requirements not only of various types of hyperlipidemia but also to control normal blood lipid levels.

Recently reported studies have shown that fat-controlled diets have reduced the incidence of coronary disease. Since it is possible to identify those persons in the general population in whom coronary disease is likely to develop, there is need to adapt fat-controlled diets for free-living people. Commercially prepared fat-controlled food products for reducing blood cholesterol have been effective when used with little regard to a rigid eating pattern. While further evidence is being accumulated to show the value of fat-controlled diets for treatment and prevention of coronary disease, individuals in the general population who are at high risk should be identified and treatment should be begun. Appropriate fat-controlled commercial products should be developed along with appropriate changes in legal and regulatory requirements. Improvement in the quality of food products has been of benefit nutritionally to peoples in many countries. Coronary disease is another public health problem that could be approached effectively in this way.

THE EFFECT OF CARBOHYDRATE TOLERANCE ON PLASMA LIPIDS AND ATHEROSCLEROSIS IN MAN*

H. Keen and R. J. Jarrett

Although the clinical association of diabetes mellitus and arterial disease has been accepted for generations, it is only recently that a more general relationship

* The borderline diabetes follow-up study, originally supported by grants from the Research Fund of the British Diabetic Association, is now financed by the Department of Health and Social Security, London. Our many co-workers, noted in the bibliography, are thanked for their contribution of time and effort, as are our secretarial and technical assistants. We especially acknowledge the enduring support and interest of Prof. W. J. H. Butterfield and the subjects themselves.

between hyperglycemia and atherosclerosis has attracted attention. This development is largely due to a change in our concept of diabetes itself which, in the case of the non-insulin-requiring variety at any rate, is now increasingly regarded as the extreme of a spectrum of degrees of glucose intolerance, the resultant of many influences, and differing quantitatively rather than qualitatively from "normal" carbohydrate metabolism [785]. The analogy with high blood pressure is attractive and obvious.

The aim of this communication will be to review briefly the basis and strength of the association between raised blood sugar and atherosclerosis; to consider some of the possible mechanisms involved; and to report on the incidence of vascular disease in a seven-year follow-up of a group of moderately hyperglycemic people.

Though time-honored, the assumption of increased atherosclerosis in the clinical diabetic does not go unchallenged, as the following three statements of authoritative workers prove. "The mass of evidence demonstrating a markedly increased incidence and severity of atherosclerosis in diabetes is incontrovertible" [781]. "... the generally accepted association between diabetes mellitus and enhanced human 'atherogenesis' does not withstand critical examination" [1010]. "The relationship between diabetes and disease of arteries is confused. The subject is surrounded by conjecture and assumption. The facts are few" [1205]. Although bias, selection and artifact may confound interpretation of the seemingly clear association of the two diseases, it is difficult entirely to reject the great weight of evidence that coronary and peripheral artery disease, measured either by clinical manifestation or by post-mortem appearances, show a two to threefold excess in the clinical diabetic over the nondiabetic [236, 909]. The Framingham study [771] indicates a similar influence of diabetes on incidence. On one count there is no controversy—that there is a greatly enhanced risk of arterial disease in the diabetic woman compared with her nondiabetic counterpart [1205].

Approaching the association from the other limb, studies of both oral and intravenous glucose tolerance show that subjects with clinical atherosclerosis have hyperglycemic responses far more frequently than matched normals. This is most clearly shown by the studies of Wahlberg [1512] but many similar observations, well summarized by Epstein [436], further strengthen the association.

A special kind of support comes from epidemiological surveys which set some index of glucose tolerance against the manifestations of atherosclerosis, both assessed by the application of standard objective procedures in population samples. In comparatively few studies has the blood sugar/arterial disease relationship been given special attention. In the four of epidemiological proportions, the Tecumseh community study [1131], a similar survey in Busselton, Australia [1533], a survey restricted to male workers in Paris [520], and in our own Bedford Survey [787], the conclusions are essentially similar. After excluding known diabetics, about two to three times as much arterial disease is found among people in the top 10% to 20% of the total range of blood sugar values than in the rest of the population. This association is largely independent of age, of arterial blood pressure, of blood cholesterol level and of cigarette smoking. In common with other statistical "risk factors", the link between atherosclerosis and high blood sugar is least apparent in the oldest people.

Following our Bedford Survey in 1962 [1349], we looked for evidence of arterial disease in three groups of the townsfolk, characterized only by their levels of blood sugar measured two hours after 50 g oral glucose. The 124 people with two-hour blood sugars of 200 mg/100 ml or more were designated newly-found "diabetics"; 229 people had blood sugars between 120 and 200 mg/100 ml and these constituted a "borderline diabetic" group. They were matched as closely as possible by age and sex with a control group taken at random from

Table 1. *Prevalence of "arterial disease" by age in three groups of Bedford population characterized by level of blood sugar two hours after 50 g glucose*

Age (yr.)	Prevalence (percentage)		
	control	borderline diabetic	diabetic
< 50	17	23	41
50–59	20	29	37
60–69	33	40	39
70 +	45	56	76
Total	27	36	49

Table 2. *Incidence of individuals with cardiovascular events between 1962 and 1967 in three Bedford groups characterized by their blood sugar level* [a]

Diagnostic group	Number of individuals		Coronary death		Angina or infarct		Claudication		Stroke		All events	
	M	F	M percentage	F	M percentage	F	M percentage	F	M percentage	F	M percentage	F
Controls	63	56	4.8	—	4.8	5.4	1.6	1.8	—	—	11.2	7.2
Borderline diabetics	105	103	9.5	4.9	9.5	15.5	0.9	—	2.9	2.9	22.9	23.3
Diabetics	38	48	13.2	8.3	7.9	27.1	10.5	2.1	—	2.1	31.6	39.6

[a] Each individual counts for only one event, coronary disease taking precedence; thusec "claudication" and "stroke" refer to that symptom alone.

those people whose two-hour blood sugar values lay below 120 mg/100 ml. Estimates of arterial disease prevalence in these three blood sugar groups were formed by applying the World Health Organization questionnaire and performing, and Minnesota coding, electrocardiograms [1255]. Table 1 shows the relative prevalence by age groups when all these manifestations of arterial disease were counted. The overall gradient was statistically significant although the totals relied heavily on lesser ECG items such as T-wave and ST-segment abnormalities.

Cross-sectional prevalence studies such as this have their limitations in indicating the true force of an association. Those dead and disabled with the disease are not represented. It is the prospective *incidence* study which gives confidence in the reality of the association and here data are very sparse. Epstein [438] reports on the Tecumseh population, restudied after four years. There is a clear link between prior hyperglycemia and subsequent coronary disease morbidity in women and mortality in men. In the Framingham follow-up [771], diabetes doubled coronary mortality in men and increased it by more than fivefold in women. We are just completing the analysis of a five-year follow-up of our three blood sugar groups in Bedford. Table 2 shows preliminary data indicating the profound effect of raised blood sugar on both morbidity and mortality from arterial disease, the former based upon a repeat questionnaire and the latter upon death information and certification.

A common opening move from an opponent in this discussion is to assert that hyperglycemia is not responsible for the vascular disease, but vascular

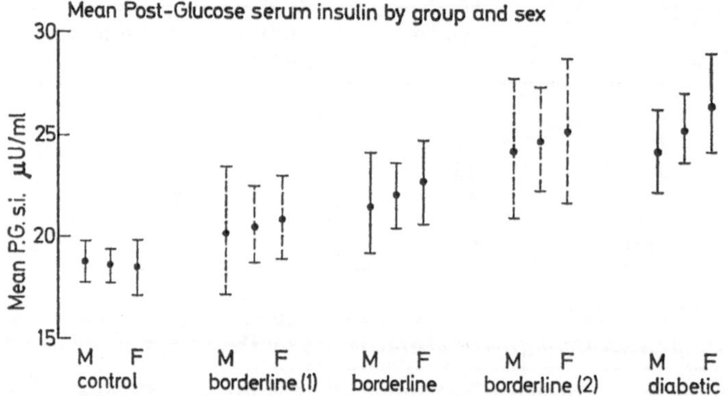

Fig. 1. The level of the serum immuno-reactive insulin (μV/ml) two hours after 50 g glucose in the three Bedford blood sugar groups (see text). In the Borderline Diabetic group, the results are shown for the whole borderline group (two hour blood sugar 120–199 mg/100 ml; see text), and for the subdivisions 120–149 mg/100 ml (borderline 1) and 150–199 mg/100 ml (borderline 2). In each set of three points, these represent the mean for Males (*M*), all of the group and Females (*F*) in the group, with the bar indicating one standard deviation

disease for the hyperglycemia [901]. Against this reversed view, there is autopsy evidence that women with diabetes (but without cardiac infarction) have no more aortic atherosclerosis than an unselected group; furthermore, it is possible to demonstrate severe visceral atherosclerosis without evidence of sustained hyperglycemia [1010]. Also, diabetes in the young is not associated with atherosclerosis at onset, but appears to provide conditions for its accelerated development. However, it is possible that general arterial disease may have extra-pancreatic effects and restrict the tissue access of circulating glucose and insulin, an effect overcome, perhaps, by a compensatory increase in insulin production. The blood sugar may then be lowered only by consequent insulin overaction in the more accessible regions [305].

In fact, hyperinsulinemia is a commonly reported accompaniment of atherosclerosis [312, 1100, 1167, 1486, 1532]. The raised hormone concentration seems to occur independently of obesity which is also very closely associated with hyperinsulinemia [81, 779, 1165], but which, it must not be forgotten, may itself also be associated with atherosclerosis [771]. Hyperinsulinemia holds a central role in many of the metabolic hypotheses of atherogenesis. It was operating in our three Bedford blood sugar groups in whom, when measured two hours after 50 g oral glucose, insulinemia showed a stepwise increase with rising blood sugar categories (see Fig. 1).

Insulin is no less a lipogenic than a carbohydrate hormone and it may be by way of effects upon lipid metabolism that an atherogenic role is played. Mahler [901] and others have shown *in vitro* that insulin favors triglyceride accumulation in aortic endothelium, probably both by stimulation of synthesis locally, and by inhibition of lipolysis. The role of *in situ* lipogenesis in atheroma induction is contested [12] but not disproved. Perhaps of greater importance is the association between insulin levels and circulating triglyceride concentrations. The studies of Farquhar et al. [449] in people with premature atherosclerotic disease would link this insulin-triglyceride relationship to carbohydrate intake, without regard to the type of carbohydrate ingested, itself the subject of controversy and discussion. They suggest that hyperlipidemia is a consequence of enhanced hepatic triglyceride production [1215], a conclusion that differs from that of Sandhofer et al. [1292] and Boberg et al. [199], who favor the view that hypertriglyceridemia results from diminished fractional removal rather than increased synthesis. It is suggested [1278] that hyperinsulinemia may be a consequence rather than a cause of the hyperlipidemia. Nevertheless, carbohydrate intolerance may relate to hypertriglyceridemia via the degree of hyperinsulinemia it evokes, though Bierman and Porte [160] consider the link to be much less direct, perhaps only operating through the common factor of obesity. By contrast, Ford et al. [478] provide statistical evidence, in a predominantly hypertriglyceridemic group, of an independent effect of blood sugar level on plasma triglycerides.

All of these relationships have been observed in highly selected groups—in people with arterial disease, with hyperlipidemias, with obesity or with diabetes. We examined the interaction of some of these metabolic variables in a normal population sample [7, 235]. The 220 members of the staff of a large British pharmaceutical firm were selected by an age/sex/ponderal-index stratifying, but otherwise random, procedure. Physical measurements were made and oral glucose tolerance tests performed after an overnight fast. Venous sugar and insulin levels were estimated on all blood samples and total glycerides and cholesterol on the fasting sample only. The sugar and insulin responses to the load were expressed as areas under the respective curves and their various interrelations are shown in Fig. 2. The very close link between "sugar area" and fasting glyceride in men is evident. Both also correlate with "insulin area", but only at low levels with the various indicators of obesity. The diminished level of correlation between "sugar area" and fasting glyceride level in women, compared with men, is explained in Table 3, which shows a complete absence of correlation in the premenopausal women, but an association as strong as that for men in the postmenopausal. It is tempting to link this finding with the comparative immunity of the nondiabetic, premenopausal woman to atherosclerotic disease, but at present one can only speculate upon its mechanism and significance.

Further evidence of a metabolic component involving carbohydrate metabolism in arterial disease comes from our long-term intervention study in Bedford. Since 1962, we have carried out a double-blind controlled therapeutic trial on

Insulin area	Log. fat fold	Arm circum.	Ponderal index	Glycerides	Cholesterol	Age	
0.322[c] 0.315[c]	0.078 −0.068	0.171 −0.016	−0.310[a] −0.130	0.734[c] 0.376[c]	0.475[c] 0.184	0.475[c] 0.226[a]	Blood sugar area
	0.353[c] 0.163	0.319[b] 0.200[a]	−0.396[c] −0.283[b]	0.296[b] 0.214[a]	0.255[a] 0.067	0.099 −0.078	Insulin area
		0.742[c] 0.752[c]	−0.603[c] −0.683[c]	0.046 0.111	0.160 0.227[a]	−0.033 0.171	Log. fat fold
			−0.758[c] −0.709[c]	0.186 −0.106	0.222[a] 0.186	0.093 0.339[c]	Arm circum.
				−0.364[c] −0.131	−0.341[c] −0.245[a]	−0.328[c] −0.285[b]	Ponderal index
					0.573[c] 0.320[b]	0.418[c] 0.205[a]	Glycerides
						0.555[c] 0.527[c]	Cholesterol

Fig. 2. Multiple correlation analysis of data derived from examination of a normal population sample. Areas calculated from glucose response curves. Ponderal index = height/$\sqrt{\text{weight}}$. This figure is taken from the paper by M. E. Abrams, R. J. Jarrett, H. Keen, D. R. Boyns, and J. N. Crossley. ([7] by kind permission of the Editor)
[a] $P<0.05$.
[b] $P<0.01$.
[c] $P<0.001$.

Table 3. *Correlation*[a] *of fasting plasma glycerides and the area under the blood sugar curve (50 g oral glucose tolerance test) in men and women separately*

Age	Men		Women	
	R	*n*	R	*n*
< 29	0.395	32	0.030	36
30 +	0.726	68	0.515	60
< 34	0.403	40	0.087	42
35 +	0.746	60	0.483	54
< 39	0.517	49	−0.002	53
40 +	0.750	51	0.697	43
< 44	0.465	58	0.088	59
45 +	0.815	42	0.712	37
< 49	0.497	65	0.256	67
50 +	0.802	35	0.655	29
All[b]	0.713	100	0.375	96

[a] Correlations have been calculated for the groups above and below the ages 30, 35, 40, 45 and 50 years.
[b] 24 people omitted from correlation because of incomplete data.

Table 4. *Trial of tolbutamide in "borderline hyperglycemic" group. Characteristics of the population studied*

	Men	Women	Total
Starting No.	129	119	248
Mean age	55.4	58.9	57.1
No. with arterial disease at entry	20	11	31
No. with significant hypertension at entry	15	38	53
No. "attacked" over 7 years	44	37	81
New "events" over 7 years	52	44	96

Table 5. *Age and sex composition of the 248 borderline diabetic subjects enrolled in the therapeutic trial of tolbutamide and diet*

Group No.	1		2		3		4	
TOL CHO	0 0		0 +		+ 0		+ +	
Age group	M	F	M	F	M	F	M	F
20−39	8	4	2	0	4	2	4	8
40−59	14	9	15	7	13	16	19	10
60+	14	16	14	19	11	16	11	12

Group 1: 3 mg tolbutamide twice daily + sucrose "restraint".
Group 2: 3 mg tolbutamide twice daily + 120 g carbohydrate diet.
Group 3: 0.5 g tolbutamide twice daily + sucrose "restraint".
Group 4: 0.5 g tolbutamide twice daily + 120 g carbohydrate diet.

Table 6. *Trial of tolbutamide in "borderline hyperglycemic" group. Number and type of arterial events occurring in seven years of follow-up*

Event	Men	Women	Total
Cardiovascular death	13	8	21
Cardiac infarction	7	5	12
Onset of angina	10	13	23
E.C.G. worsening (M.C.) [a]	14	6	20
Onset of claudication	5	9	14
Stroke	3	3	6
Events in total group ($n = 248$)	52	44	96
Events in high-risk group ($n = 75$)	25	22	47

[a] M.C. = worsening by 1 or 2 grades in Minnesota Code classification.

248[1] "borderline hyperglycemic" people found in the population survey. A randomly allocated half has been treated with tolbutamide, 0.5 g twice daily, and the other half with indistinguishable placebo tablets containing 3 mg of tolbutamide. In addition, one-half of each of these two groups was recommended to limit carbohydrate intake to 120 g daily and the other half simply to "cut down on table sugar". At regular six-month re-examinations, all have been subjected to repeated re-evaluation, the cardiovascular component of which includes the

[1] This total includes a further 19 subjects recruited shortly after the main survey.

Table 7. *Percentage of individuals by sex, who experienced an arterial event during the seven years 1962–1969*[a]

Group No.		1		2		3		4	
		total	% +	total	% +	total	% +	total	% +
All	M	36	33.3	33	39.4	28	32.2	34	29.4
Entrants	F	29	41.5	25	36.0	33	27.3	30	20.0
	All	65	37.0	58	38.0	61	29.5	64	25.0
High Risk	M	4	100.0	10	60.0	8	75.0	6	83.3
	F	8	50.0	12	41.6	16	43.7	11	27.2
Entrants	All	12	66.6	22	50.0	24	54.2	17	47.0
Low Risk	M	32	25.0	23	30.4	20	15.0	28	17.8
	F	21	38.1	13	30.8	17	11.7	19	15.8
Entrants	All	53	30.2	36	30.6	37	13.5	47	17.0

Stastical treatment of combined placebo and tolbutamide groups

	All entrants		High risk		Low risk	
	total	% +	total	% +	total	% +
Groups 1 + 2 (Placebo)	123	37.4	34	55.9	89	30.3
Groups 3 + 4 (Tolbutamide)	125	27.2	41	51.2	84	15.5
Difference	10.2		4.7		14.8	
SE of diff.	5.91		11.55		6.27	
$t =$	1.73		0.41		2.36	
$p =$	<0.1	>0.05	>0.1		$=0.02$	

[a] Figures show total number in each group followed by percentage experiencing an event, in the whole group and the high- and low-risk entry subgroups (see text) successively. The effect of tolbutamide and its statistical significance is shown for the whole group and the two subgroups.

Table 8. *Trial of tolbutamide in "borderline hyperglycemic" group. Blood sugar measurements on "random" samples taken between 4:00 and 6:00 p.m. and without special preparation of the participants*

	Placebo (groups 1 and 2)		Tolbutamide (groups 3 and 4)
11th visit	diff. 4.56	90.77 mg/100 ml S.E. diff. 2.5	86.21 mg/100 ml "t" = 1.8
13th visit	diff. 6.26	86.09 mg/100 ml S.E. diff. 3.2	79.83 mg/100 ml "t" = 1.9
Both visits	diff. 5.35	88.23 mg/100 ml S.E. diff. 2.0	82.88 mg/100 ml "t" = 2.6[a]

[a] $P < 0.02 > 0.01$.

standard questionnaire and an electrocardiogram. A preliminary analysis of the results of treatment after five years [786] suggested a protective effect of tolbutamide against the mixed bag of cardiovascular incidents occurring since 1962, and this analysis has been brought up to the seven-year point for this communication. The composition and characteristics of the group are shown in Table 4 and Table 5 and the nature of the events in the follow-up period in Table 6. Subjects have been divided into low and high risk groups, the latter coming into the trial either with clear clinical or ECG evidence of cardiovascular disease or with clinically significant hypertension. As Table 7 shows, the frequency of cardio-

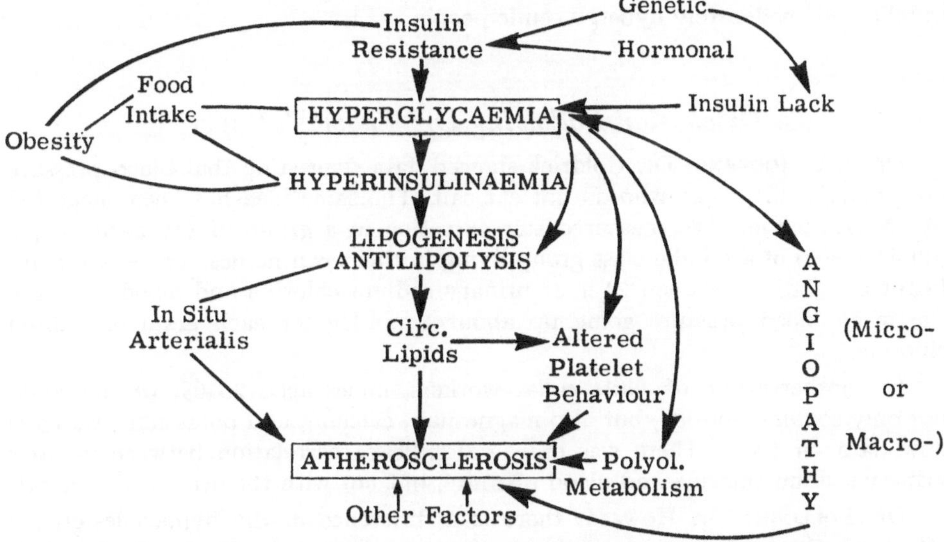

Fig. 3. A hypothetical scheme of metabolic interrelations in atherogenesis

vascular events during the follow-up period is considerably higher in the high, than in the low risk groups, and there is no indication of an effect of treatment. In the low risk individuals, however, the rate of events in the tolbutamide treated group is about half that in the placebo group, a difference significant at the 2% level.

When we tried to explain the protection at five years, we were unable to show a systematic difference between placebo and tolbutamide groups in the blood sugar measured two hours after glucose. However, Table 8 shows the blood sugar comparison when, on two occasions, it was measured without special preparation on a day when the subjects took meals and tablets as usual. On each occasion the mean "random blood sugar" was lower in the treated than the placebo group, the difference not quite attaining conventional levels of statistical significance. If the two sets are pooled, however, the statistical significance of the difference approaches the 1% level.

In conclusion, a statistical link between raised blood sugar levels and both the prevalence and incidence of atherosclerotic arterial disease appears to be established beyond reasonable doubt. The nature of the association is less clear.

The evidence suggests that the blood sugar/arterial disease link may be by way of changes in circulating insulin levels and lipid metabolism in blood and/or tissue, including the arterial wall itself. These associations may encompass and partly explain the dietary and obesity factors in atherogenesis and even provide some explanation for altered platelet behavior in the disease. A direct effect of raised blood sugar may involve localized osmotic damage to the arterial intima due to accumulation of nondiffusible sorbitol (Morrison, this volume). A tentative interlinking scheme is proposed in Fig. 3. Finally, the results of a long-term therapeutic trial are presented suggesting that a significant degree of primary protection against cardiovascular events can be conferred by tolbutamide in mildly and moderately hyperglycemic people.

Discussion Following Dr. Thomas' Paper

Dr. J. V. Joosens: Dr. Goldrick showed data suggesting that blood pressure does not rise in people who do not eat salt. The same idea has been suggested by Dr. I. A. Prior. We measured salt excretion in a group of 511 aged people (60–85 years) of a middle class group living in their own homes. There is a significant correlation between 24-hour urinary sodium chloride and blood pressure, the mean blood pressure going up about 1 mm Hg for each gram of sodium chloride.

In another group of white collar workers, males aged 20–65, we measured not only sodium chloride, but also magnesium, calcium, and potassium; we have now data on 1,100. There was only a significant correlation between 24-hour urinary sodium chloride and blood pressure, but not with the other constituents.

Dr. Pollock: Dr. Howard, there is a difference in the hypocholesteremic effect whether one uses chromium sulfate or chromium chloride, magnesium sulfate or magnesium chloride, at least at the cellular level. The inorganic chemical composition of alfalfa reflects the composition of the soil, which varies with the use of inorganic versus organic fertilizers.

Incidently, there is a fairly good correlation between organic farming and a low incidence of atherosclerosis.

Dr. Zilversmit: I have a question for Dr. Thomas. It seemed from his data on the composition of lipids in the atheromatous lesions of swine fed cholesterol for six months, that there was a rather large increase in free cholesterol compared to ester cholesterol of the artery. This is different from findings in the rabbit lesions: what is the case for lesions of other species?

Dr. Thomas: Your observation is correct, and this puzzled us, too. My own opinion is that it has to do with the stage of the disease in these pigs at six months. We are dealing with a relatively early stage of the disease, with most of the tissue in the proliferative phase. I think with the passage of time the cholesteryl ester component would overtake the free cholesterol.

In our studies in the human, we find in childhood that the free cholesterol predominates, but that in early adult life the situation changes and the cholesteryl ester predominates. The rabbit develops large lesions much more rapidly than the pig with many cells filled with fat. I suspect that we are dealing with a matter of staging there in comparing our results with those of Dr. Zilversmit.

Dr. SMITH: Certainly these observations do not agree with my observations on fatty streaks in young children. In the normal intima of young children, the cholesterol is predominantly free; but if you dissect out the fatty streak containing the fat-filled cells, then, in that area the cholesterol is predominantly esterified. I wonder whether these high free cholesterol levels reflect the fact that most of the tissue being examined is, in fact, not fat-filled cell lesion material, but is the surrounding predominantly normal intima, and, perhaps, mixed up with media as well? The media, of course, is almost entirely free cholesterol in young humans, and I would expect the same finding in young animals.

Dr. THOMAS: That would not be the correct explanation for what we have found because the free cholesterol is tremendously elevated, three to fourfold over the normal values. These were intima plus inner media preparations, incidentally.

Since you are dissecting lesions, you are getting into a comparatively advanced stage when you pick out what I consider a big bag of fat for analysis, and I am not entirely sure what your results mean in relation to developing experimental lesions. Eventually, in any species, the cholesteryl ester will predominate.

Dr. JORGENSEN: Were the lesions which were studied visible? If so, were the other areas of the aorta examined where you should not expect atherosclerotic plaques to develop?

Dr. THOMAS: With the DNA synthesis studies, prior to the development of lesions, we looked into other portions of the aorta as well, in particular, the midportion of the abdominal aorta. To our disappointment, the results were much the same as in the trifurcation area.

When we counted the number of cells that were labeled with ^{3}H-thymidine or were in mitosis in the outer media, we found about the same increase as with the inner media. Thus, the stimulation which appears early on the diet seems to affect all cells of the artery.

Dr. PAUL DUDLEY WHITE: I thought it would be interesting to continue the discussion on risk factors in atherosclerosis by a progress report on my own many years of experience as a practicing cardiologist.

This is based first on a study made in 1937 of 100 cases of coronary heart disease under the age of 40, secondly on a more completely studied series of 100 more such cases in 1950 (published in 1954), thirdly on the follow-up of those cases by Dr. Gertler, and finally on my own experience with some hundreds more in the last few years. It is evident that I am now emphasizing the early recognition of the candidate for atherosclerosis and working more intensely on the sons of my patients before they get into trouble from the teenagers on up.

There are several risk factors to be considered under heredity. We know nothing about the relative proportion of responsibility between heredity and the environment: that still remains to be determined. It may vary in different individuals, and of course this explains the differences between individuals in any given population. Some of us, at least those under the age of 40, are almost immune, and really, in my own experience, under the age of 80.

As a final item under "heredity" there is the very important point of family history. Sometimes it is difficult to obtain, because the patient doesn't know it very well; but this is one more reason for us to begin to instruct the public to keep better records of their own health.

Under "environment" I have little comment to make. The role of hypertension in my young cases, under the age of 40, was but slight. I regard hypertension as a complicating factor, a different disease when superimposed; it does become an important risk factor later, but in my youngest cases it was rare. One final point, the environment may begin even in fetal life. We haven't made an adequate study of what happens to the fetus during the exposure of the mother to all sorts of factors which we regard as important after birth; life, however, begins nine months before birth.

Dr. BIERENBAUM: A comment for Dr. Howard; in 1967 we reported on a six-month study on rats fed saturated and polyunsaturated fats with calcium supplementation. The calcium was very effective in lowering the blood cholesterol level on the saturated diet. It was less on the polyunsaturated diet, but still definitely effective.

Dr. HOWARD: Yes, I think those results agree with those obtained by Dr. Keys recently.

Dr. KEYS: Yes, except that we have no definite indication that there is any substantial effect in the presence of the highly unsaturated fat. We can only really show it with the saturates in man.

Dr. THOMAS: Dr. Howard quoted from our work in comparing the effects of butter plus cholesterol and peanut oil plus cholesterol in the Rhesus monkey, and his interpretation of our results was that the peanut oil was worse than butter. Our own conclusions were actually the opposite. We thought the butter was worse because it produced more necrotic lesions, i.e. more advanced atheromata. We felt that this was the reason for the smaller number of proliferative lesions.

Dr. HOWARD: My interpretation was that with peanut oil you got more proliferation of cells in your monkeys, a finding which did agree with the results obtained by Dr. Wissler.

Discussion Following Dr. Keen's Paper

Dr. KLIMT: Dr. Keen has ended with a very optimistic note on the possibility of preventing cardiovascular complications in diabetics by treating them with tolbutamide. I regret to say that we have contrary information on diabetics. The University Group Diabetes Program, a large-scale, 1,000-patient cooperative trial of hypoglycemic drugs and their effect on vascular complications in diabetics, has, after eight years of continued operation, discontinued the tolbutamide treatment group because of complete absence of beneficial effects and the possible presence of harmful side effects. These were manifested by a threefold excess in cardiovascular mortality in the tolbutamide group when compared with either placebo or any one of the two insulin-treated groups. Thus, in the established diabetic, in contrast to prediabetics, tolbutamide does not appear to play a useful therapeutic role (in press, *Journal of Diabetes*).

Dr. KEEN: I think the emphatic thing here is that we are dealing with two very different starting populations. Dr. Klimt is dealing with a much more grossly hyperglycemic group than we are. In fact, his group starts virtually where ours leaves off, and I think that everybody would agree that there are very gross differences in people with lesser and greater degrees of hyperglycemia especially in relation to cardiovascular disease, as I showed. So I think his contribution bears only on the group that he describes, just as our findings bear only on the group we describe.

Dr. BRUNNER: I would suggest that the association of vascular disease with serum cholesterol in diabetics is dependent on environment rather than an obligatory genetic peripheral effect. A recent review in "Diabetes" of a survey of long-standing diabetics included 79 people between the ages of 40 and 56 years. In none of these patients was there a known case of peripheral disease. There was no case of cerebral vascular disease. There was one man with a myocardial infarction, but no others with even electrocardiographic abnormalities. Only 13% showed x-ray evidence of vascular calcification.

Dr. GROEN: In regard to the paper by Dr. Brown, I wish to comment on the terms in which we should now express our knowledge about the influence of different kinds of dietary fats on serum cholesterol.

In the early years, when we discovered this peculiar antagonistic effect of saturated versus polyunsaturated fat, we were so impressed with it that we didn't look carefully enough at our protocols for the right type of controls. Actually, if you test the effects of polyunsaturated fat on serum cholesterol and compare it with the effect of carbohydrate or protein, there is hardly any difference. Would Dr. Brown be willing to formulate the present status of our knowledge in this way: serum cholesterol is raised by dietary cholesterol, by saturated fat, especially that containing palmitic and myristic acid and, although to a smaller degree, also by oleic acid and possibly sucrose. All other dietary ingredients whether they are polyunsaturated fats or carbohydrates (excepting sucrose) or protein have no effect on serum cholesterol, so that when they are substituted for one of the first named nutrients, the serum cholesterol drops to a low normal level. This is the reason why so-called primitive or Eastern populations have low serum cholesterols. It is not that they eat large amounts of sunflower or any other polyunsaturated oils but that they just eat very small amounts of saturated fats. Their diets consist mainly of starch and protein. This insight into the absence of specificity in the effect of polyunsaturated fats is of great importance in advising people who want to lower their blood cholesterol. It is true that in this country, where people are so accustomed to eating fat, one may counsel them to replace saturated by unsaturated fat, as The American Heart Association has done. However for other countries where the fat contained in the diet is not high the only advice needed is to keep the content of saturated fat and cholesterol in the diet low.

Dr. BROWN: I think that is very true, except that, when considering the relationship between the polyunsaturated fats and dietary cholesterol in these people, it must be remembered that in these populations, the people eat a lot of starches, have a very low cholesterol intake, and also have a very low animal fat intake. Consequently, their serum cholesterol is low. In our population, where we cannot get much below the 200 to 300 mg level of daily cholesterol intake, the polyunsaturated fats are important for maintaining low blood cholesterol levels.

Dr. GROEN: My second remark concerns the paper by Dr. Keen. From the practical point of view, we should not forget that the main reason for the increased serum cholesterol in diabetic patients is the diet which most western physicians still prescribe for their diabetic patients. Diabetic patients, as a rule, eat large amounts of fat meat, butter, cream and eggs. In short, they eat super-atherogenic diets! The possibility that one of the major complications of diabetes is, at least partly, the result of the "therapeutic" diets applied against the disease is an uneasy thought. It should make us all the more interested in the fact that the Trappist monks I studied in Holland and the Yemenites studied by Brunner and Cohen in Israel, both have a high incidence of diabetes. Since these patients are not accustomed to large amounts of fat, they stick to a low fat diet even though they have diabetes. As a result their serum cholesterol is just as low as in nondiabetic Trappists or Yemenites and they have no cardiovascular complications. Years ago Porges and Adlersberg advocated low fat diets for the treatment of diabetes and the excellent results of such diets during the Second World War convinced me that they were right. I hope that the prevention of cardiovascular atherosclerotic complications may rouse the interest of the medical profession in the treatment of diabetics by low fat low cholesterol diets.

Dr. FURMAN: I would like to ask Dr. Keen a question relative to the very interesting age-sex differential he showed in relating the blood glucose level after glucose load to the serum triglyceride level. Perhaps in women, in whom diabetes is very prevalent, there might be in the younger group a higher incidence of insulin deficient diabetes. Since these women were lost due to premature deaths while there was an accompanying rise in adult-onset, insulin-resistant diabetics, might this explain the age-sex difference?

In respect to Dr. Groen's comments, protein deficient (or borderline) nutrition is associated with a lowering of serum lipids. This may be of some relevance to serum lipid levels in those populations in which protein nutrition may be borderline.

Dr. KEEN: In the normal population sample that we examined, no juvenile diabetics have been included. The numbers so excluded must be extremely small. The incidence of diabetes in women under 40 is a fraction of one percent; therefore I don't think their exclusion distorted the behavior of the triglycerides and blood sugar area relationship in that group. I think this represents the operation of some factor in the women under 40 which is overriding the factors which create the relationship in men. Whether this is hormonal or not, we really have no idea.

Dr. KEYS: I wanted to point out that Dr. Brown somehow left lauric acid out of the story. I think it is now well established that lauric acid has certainly as strong an effect on raising the serum cholesterol level, both in man and in animals, as any other fatty acid. This was beautifully shown recently, not only in experiments on dogs and on several species of birds but also in men by Dr. Grande of our group and by many others.

Dr. MEDALIE: I agree with Dr. Keen that the diabetes is certainly a factor in the production of ischemic heart disease, even though there are groups in Africa and the Middle East with high rates of diabetes and low rates of ischemic heart disease. However, the converse is not true. In our incidence of diabetes, we found that whereas peripheral vascular disease contributed significantly to diabetes, myocardial infarction did not. There is, therefore, some difference between these processes.

Concerning the diet, the only negative relationship we found in the multiple regression analysis of cholesterol in the blood was with bread, i.e. the more bread eaten in a free-living 10,000 population, the lower the cholesterol.

Dr. STEINBERG: Dr. Keen, when all of the subjects are pooled, is there a significant protective effect of tolbutamide? Did you look at the blood lipid levels in these people over the years?

Dr. KEEN: The answer to the first question is that it depends slightly on when you make the comparison. We analyzed our figures at five years of trial and, without the division into high and low risk groups, we found an effect of tolbutamide significant at the 5% level of confidence. When we made the same comparison on this occasion, we just fell short of formal statistical significance, with a P value of <0.1 but >0.05. We think it is valid to make this sort of division in looking for primary protection, rather than to blur it with unsuccessful secondary protection.

As to the other question, we didn't, unfortunately, look at the serum lipids.

Dr. DAYTON: Dr. Keen, the literature on diabetes as a risk factor contains the suggestion, at least, that the effect of diabetes on coronary heart disease risk is manifested only in the hypertensive. Do the data from prospective studies bear this out?

Dr. KEEN: There are remarkably few prospective studies on which one can really base an opinion here. So far as our study was concerned, certainly the existence of hypertension greatly increased the risk of a vascular event. Whether there was a special interaction between high blood pressure and high blood sugar, I can't say. I hope we will be in a position to answer this when we have completed our follow-up analysis of vascular events in the control group and in the grossly diabetic group.

Section XIII

SELECTED PAPERS ON NUTRITIONAL STUDIES

INFLUENCE OF THREE DIETARY FATS GIVEN AT THREE CALORIC LEVELS ON SERUM LIPIDS IN MAN

A. J. VERGROESEN, J. DE BOER and H. J. THOMASSON

In a previous experiment THOMASSON et al. [1465] investigated the influence on blood lipids concentration of ten dietary fats with a widely divergent fatty acid composition. Glyceryl trilaurate, olive oil (containing about 70% oleic acid) and safflower oil (containing about 70% linoleic acid) and mixtures of these fats were given as liquid formula diets (LFD) (containing 50 cal% of fat) to Trappists and Trappistines for six weeks. The experimental fats appeared to have a clear influence on free cholesterol, esterified cholesterol, and phospholipid concentrations in the blood, the ratios of these three lipid classes being constant.

The question arose whether and, if so, to what extent dietary fats can influence blood lipid values if given in dietary fat concentrations below 50 cal%. This question is clearly related to the often preached advice to reduce the fat content of the diet to obtain lower blood lipid values.

In the present experiment, therefore, the LFD's contained 20, 35 or 50 cal% of one of the three fats mentioned .The experiment lasted again six weeks and the participants were Trappist monks.

METHODS

The 84 participants were male members of three closed monastic communities of the Trappist order. They normally use a low-fat lactovegetarian diet. Manifest diabetics were not present in this group. The volunteers exclusively consumed the LFD and, in addition, daily 50 g of bread, tea or coffee without sugar or milk, two apples or other fresh fruit, small amounts of raw vegetables (carrots, chicory, black radish). The use of beer or lemonade was restricted. Moreover, three multivitamin tablets (Davitamon 10) and 60 mg iron fumarate were taken daily.

The diets were of the liquid formula type [27] and issued as a dry powder. By mixing the powder with water at 70° C, a palatable emulsion is obtained. The composition of the powder is given in Table 1. The fats used in these diets were: (a) 90% glyceryl trilaurate + 10% safflower oil; the latter oil was added to meet essential fatty acid requirement and counteract the unpleasant character of trilaurate; (b) olive oil; and (c) safflower oil. To each kilogram of fat, 10 grams soy lecithin, 50,000 I.U. vitamin A and 750 milligrams alpha tocopherol were added. After canning, bacteriological checks revealed no important contamination.

The fatty acid composition of the fats is given in Table 2. Each fat was given at 20, 35 and 50 cal%, resulting in nine different diets. The amount of food consumed by each volunteer was recorded and the body weight determined at weekly intervals.

Fasting blood was taken by venipuncture before breakfast on three occasions: one week prior to the experiment and on the first and on the last day of the six weeks' experimental period.

In view of the constancy of the mutual ratios of the blood lipid classes, as found in the previous study, only the concentrations of total cholesterol (TC)

Table 1. *Composition of diets in percentage dry weight*

Ingredient	20 cal % fat	35 cal % fat	50 cal % fat
Ca-caseinate	12.15	13.33	14.77
Skim milk powder	30.44	33.40	36.99
Dextrose	19.43	19.43	19.43
Maltodextrine	28.52	15.65	—
Fat	9.46	18.19	28.81

Table 2. *Fatty acid composition (as a percentage) of fats*

Fatty acid	Glyceryl trilaurate	Olive oil	Safflower oil
C 12:0	98.5	—	—
C 14:0	1.5	—	—
C 16:0	—	14.0	6.5
C 18:0	—	2.5	2.5
C 20:0	—	0.5	—
Total saturated	100.0	17.0	9.0
C 16:1	—	1.5	—
C 18:1	—	68.5	11.5
C 19:1	—	0.5	—
Total mono-unsaturated	—	70.5	11.5
C 18:2	—	12.5	75.5
Total di-unsaturated	—	12.5	79.5

and phospholipids (PL) were measured. TC was determined on an Auto-Analyzer with a modification of the technique described by Abell et al. [6]. PL was determined as lipid phosphorus according to Zilversmit and Davis [1595]. All determinations were done in duplicate.

After clotting, the blood was centrifuged; the serum was stored in a deep freeze until chemically analysed. The TC values of the first venipuncture and the age of the participants were used as criterion for the division of the men into nine groups. Each group consisted of 9–10 volunteers with an average age of 52–53 years and an average TC level of 199–201 mg/100 ml serum. The second and third blood samples are indicated as "initial" and "final".

RESULTS AND DISCUSSION

General. Thirteen volunteers did not complete the experiment. Particularly in the group consuming the 50 cal% trilaurate diet (7 out of 10) and, to a lesser extent, in the 35 cal% trilaurate groups, severe diarrhea occurred, necessitating five volunteers to finish the experiment prematurely. There were no complaints regarding the 20 cal% trilaurate diet. The olive and safflower oil diets were well tolerated. The reasons for eight others dropping out were unrelated to the experiment.

Table 3. *Influence of dietary fat content and dietary fatty acid composition on total cholesterol and lipid phosphorus values* [a]

Dietary fat	90% glycerol trilaurate and 10% safflower oil			Olive oil			Safflower oil		
Cal%	20	35	50	20	35	50	20	35	50
Dietary fatty acids (cal%)									
Sat.	18.2	31.8	45.3	3.4	5.9	8.5	1.8	3.2	4.5
18:1	0.2	0.4	0.6	14.1	24.7	35.2	2.3	4.0	5.7
18:2	1.6	2.8	4.0	2.5	4.4	6.3	15.9	27.8	39.8
n	8	7	6	8	8	9	8	9	8
Serum total cholesterol									
initial (mg/100 ml)	202	203	195	198	194	195	198	204	205
final (mg/100 ml)	202	201	205	175	172	186	164	160	164
change (mg/100 ml)	0	−2	+10	−23	−22	−9	−34	−44	−41
change (%)	+1	−1	+ 7	−12	−12	−3	−16	−22	−20
Serum lipid phosphorus									
initial (mg/100 ml)	8.5	8.5	8.7	8.9	7.8	8.2	8.2	8.8	8.8
final (mg/100 ml)	8.8	9.3	10.0	8.4	7.4	8.0	7.5	7.0	7.0
change (mg/100 ml)	+0.3	+0.8	+1.3	−0.5	−0.4	−0.2	−0.7	−1.8	−1.8
change (%)	+4	+12	+16	−6	−4	−2	−7	−20	−21
Ratio TC/LP	23.0	21.6	20.5	20.8	23.2	23.2	21.9	22.9	23.4

[a] Changes in these values are the individual final values expressed as the percentage of the individual initial values.

Ultimately, the number of participants in each group was 6–9, with an average initial TC and lipid *P* values of 194–205 and 7.8–8.9 mg/100 ml respectively and an average age of 48–51 years.

During the LFD period the average food intake was 2,445 cal/day. This value was lower for the trilaurate groups (av. 2,170 cal/day) than for the olive oil (av. 2,510 cal/day) and safflower oil groups (av. 2,590 cal/day).

The body weight of the participants (mean initial weight 83 kg) decreased during the first experimental week the LFD period (av. 3 kg/6 weeks). This decrease, which was also found in other LFD experiments, is supposedly due to loss of body fluid, caused by the low sodium chloride content of the diets. The greatest loss in weight was found in the 50 cal% trilaurate group (av. 5 kg).

The phenomena concerning body weight, caloric intake and gastrointestinal disorders as described have also been observed in the previous experiment [1465].

Serum Lipids. The serum lipid data are summarized in Table 3. The trilaurate diets (high saturated fatty acid contents) induced the highest TC and LP levels (av. 203 and 9.4 mg/100 ml); the olive oil diets (high monounsaturated fatty acid contents) moderate levels (av. 178 and 7.9 mg/100 ml) and the safflower oil diets (high di-unsaturated fatty acid contents) the lowest levels (av. 163 and 7.2 mg/100 ml). The differences between the three types of dietary fat are significant. The serum lipid levels decrease, therefore, with increasing degree of unsaturation of the dietary fatty acids.

Not only the type but also the amount of dietary fat caused a certain change in the serum lipid levels. With increasing trilaurate and (probably to a lesser extent) olive oil contents in the diets, the serum lipid levels tend to increase. However, an increased safflower oil content in the diets did not induce any increase but even caused a significant decrease in serum lipid levels. In the case of trilaurate or olive oil decrease in serum lipid levels can therefore be obtained by reducing the amount of fat in the diet. However, this advice would have an opposite effect in the case of safflower oil.

The preceding data indicate that the lowest serum lipid levels are obtained if the diet contains 20–25 cal% or more linoleic acid (and very small amounts of saturated and monounsaturated fatty acids). This corresponds with a daily intake of 60–70 g or more linoleic acid. Although the trilaurate groups consumed fewer (ca. 15%) calories than the olive and safflower oil groups, the serum lipid levels of the trilaurate groups were higher. This fact demonstrates that a reduction of the number of calories does not necessarily result in a low serum lipid level. The type of dietary fat seems to be of paramount importance with respect to the magnitude of change in the serum lipid level.

As was found in the previous investigation [1465] the TC/LP ratios of the dietary groups appear to be fairly constant. This means that both the type and amount of the dietary fat changes not only the serum cholesterol values but also equally the lipid *P* values.

LINOLEIC ACID DEFICIENCY IN MAN

F. D. Collins, A. J. Sinclair, J. P. Royle, D. A. Coats,
A. T. Maynard and R. F. Leonard

An association between atherosclerosis in man and linoleic acid intake has been postulated on the basis of epidemiological and nutritional evidence, the latter being correlated with the fact that the level of blood cholesterol can be lowered by the incorporation of polyunsaturated fatty acids in the diet. Most of the experimental evidence has been obtained from studies of communities or groups of subjects who, by social custom or experimental design, consumed diets either low or high in polyunsaturated fatty acids, but the effects of the total absence of linoleic acid in the diet of adult man are unknown. Much information is available from animal experiments and a little from studies on infants [699]. The present report concerns a 44-year-old man who was maintained exclusively on intravenous therapy for 240 days following extensive resection of the small intestine. For the first 100 days his intravenous therapy involved the daily infusion of approximately 4 litres of fluid containing 3,000 calories and 100–125 g of synthetic amino acids. His nutrition, however, was entirely fat-free for that period. Because of the appearance of a scaly skin lesion involving the face, trunk and one thigh, and a failure of erythropoiesis not due to deficiencies of iron, cyanocobalamin or folic acid and because of the nature of his nutritional intake, the possibility of essential fatty acid deficiency was considered.

Table 1. *Composition of infusion mixture* [a]

	Average daily intakes			
	A	B	C	D
Intake/24 hours (litres)	4.0	3.75	3.87	3.91
Calories	3,050	3,170	3,110	3,090
Synthetic amino acids (g)	125	109	117	120
Fats (g)	—	53	26.5	17.7
Linoleic acid (g)	—	22.8	11.4	7.6

[a] The patient was maintained by the intravenous infusion of nutrients in different proportions at the following times:
A: The four weeks before and 43 days after the first fat infusion.
B: The two periods in which fat was administered at a rate of 53 g/day.
C: Fat was administered at a rate of 26.5 g/day.
D: Fat was administered at a rate of 17.7 g/day.

Following an analysis of total plasma phospholipids which revealed the presence of 5,8,11 eicosatrienoic acid, it was concluded that linoleic acid deficiency was present and the intravenous therapy was modified to include the infusion of a soybean fat emulsion [1319]. During a 12-day period fat was infused at a rate of 53 g/day (see Table 1) and coincidentally the skin lesions healed, and the patient thereafter was able to maintain his hemoglobin concentration practically within normal levels. Following the administration of fat the patient was returned to a fat-free regime for 43 days. Fat therapy was then resumed and the skin rash, which had reappeared during the fat-free interval, healed again and did not recur. Following 12 days at an infusion rate of 53 g fat per day, the fat intake was progressively reduced to 26.5 g and 17.7 g per day in an attempt to establish levels of fat intake which would maintain the 5,8,11 eicosatrienoic acid at a minimal level.

Fig. 1 shows that the plasma triglyceride level was high before fat infusion but fell substantially on the administration of fat. It is known that a high carbohydrate-low fat diet can cause a triglyceridemia in man [57] and the infusion mixture was equivalent to a fat-free, high carbohydrate diet. This diet was also cholesterol free and this may explain the low cholesterol levels of 135 ± 5 mg/100ml during the whole period of observation.

The administration of fat caused marked changes in the fatty acid composition of the plasma triglycerides, phospholipids and cholesteryl esters (Table 2), and these were very similar to the changes seen in animals deficient in essential fatty acids. In particular, the percentage of 5,8,11 eicosatrienoic acid decreased and arachidonic acid increased.

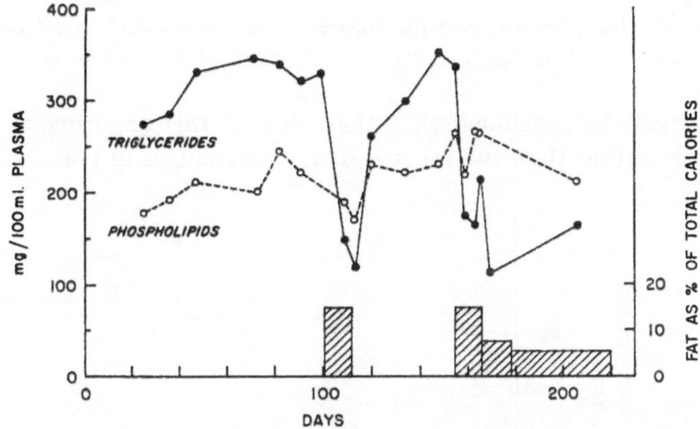

Fig. 1. The concentration of triglycerides and phospholipids in the plasma during intravenous therapy. The patient, who was placed exclusively on intravenous therapy on day 1, was maintained without fat except as shown by the histogram. At the times shown samples of plasma were obtained, the lipids extracted and separated by thin layer chromatography

Table 2. *Changes in fatty acid composition on administrating fat* [a]

Diet fatty acid	Triglycerides		Phospholipids		Cholesterol esters	
	fat-free	fat 53 g/day	fat-free	fat 53 g/day	fat-free	fat 53 g/day
Palmitic	28.3	32.4	32.3	31.3	14.2	12.8
Palmitoleic	8.0	5.9	2.3	1.0	16.8	6.4
Stearic	6.1	6.5	15.8	20.3	0.7	0.8
Oleic	52.2	42.0	29.8	16.5	51.4	35.0
Linoleic	1.1	7.5	1.6	10.9	6.0	26.8
5,8,11 eicosatrienoic	1.9	2.1	9.9	1.2	4.7	2.1
Arachidonic	0.0	2.1	7.1	15.2	5.0	9.1

[a] The figures represent each individual fatty acid as a percentage of the total fatty acids present in the three plasma lipid fractions. In each case a fat-free diet is compared with a diet when fat was administered at a rate of 53 g/day.

Examination of the plasma by paper electrophoresis before fat infusion had commenced showed a pronounced prebeta band. Separation of the plasma lipoproteins by centrifugation showed that the very low density lipoproteins contained 44.5 mg/100 ml of triglyceride while the high density lipoproteins had 220 mg/100 ml of triglyceride. A normal value for the triglyceride content of the high density lipoproteins would be less than 4 mg/100 ml [633]. As both the total triglycerides and the prebeta lipoprotein fraction were high it would seem that there is an abnormal lipoprotein fraction with an electrophoretic mobility corresponding to prebeta but with a density of 1.08 to 1.12. The very low density lipoproteins have a density of 0.93 to 1.01, and thus the abnormal fraction must be associated with a higher proportion of protein. In Fig. 2 is shown the correlation between the amount of triglycerides not in the very low-density lipoproteins and the percentage of 5,8,11 eicosatrienoic acid in the C_{20} fatty acids in the plasma phospholipids. The correlation coefficient is 0.96 ($P<0.001$), but the correlation with the amount of fat in the diet is only 0.18 ($P<0.1$).

Hence, it can be concluded that the cause of this abnormality is the lack of linoleic acid rather than the fat-free diet. The changes in plasma lipids in the

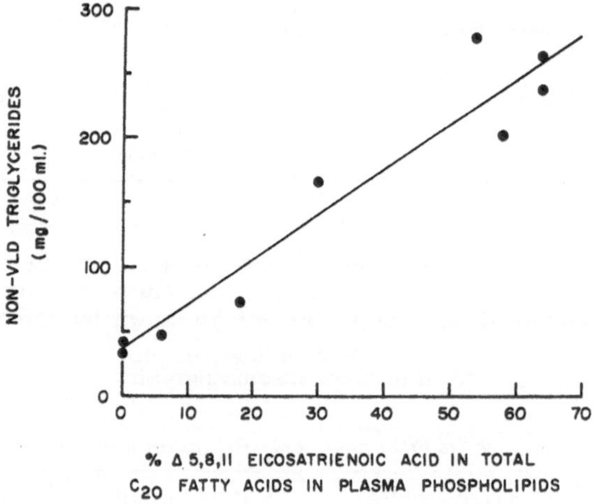

Fig. 2. Relationship between the triglycerides not in the very low density lipoprotein and the 5,8,11 eicosatrienoic acid in the plasma phospholipids. The concentration of the total triglycerides, less the amount in the very low density lipoproteins, is plotted against the percentage of the C_{20} fatty acids in the phospholipids in the form of 5,8,11 eicosatrienoic acid. The slope of the regression line is 3.5 ± 0.37 ($P<0.001$)

patient resemble those in the rat with respect to the alterations in fatty acid composition but differ in other respects. A rat deficient in essential fatty acids and on a diet that is either fat-free or with 5% saturated fat has low plasma triglycerides, and the amount of triglycerides not in the very low-density lipoproteins is within the normal range [1366]. These authors present some evidence that the amount of triglyceride in the high density lipoproteins is elevated but the possible significance of this finding only becomes apparent in the light of the present investigation. Three main conclusions can be drwan from this report:

1. On a cholesterol-free diet lasting for eight months the plasma cholesterol remained at 135 ± 5 mg/100 ml (standard error for 22 separate samples) and this must correspond to his endogenous production.

2. The principal abnormality in the plasma lipids that can be ascribed to the deficiency of linoleic acid is the low proportion of the plasma triglycerides carried by the very low density lipoproteins. This is in spite of the triglyceridemia

that may have been caused by the fat-free diet but which does not occur in rats also on a fat-free diet.

3. When the amount of linoleic acid administered to the patient was decreased from 6.4% cal to 2.2% cal the proportion of 5,8,11 eicosatrienoic acid in the plasma phospholipids rose from 2.4 to 3.6%. This suggests that the optimum requirement for linoleic acid is greater than 2.2% calories, and this conclusion agrees with Adam, Hansen and Wiese [11] who suggested 4% calories for optimum needs.

DIURNAL PATTERNS OF PLASMA TRIGLYCERIDE, FREE FATTY ACID, BLOOD SUGAR AND INSULIN LEVELS ON HIGH-FAT AND HIGH-CARBOHYDRATE DIETS IN NORMALS AND IN PATIENTS WITH PRIMARY ENDOGENOUS HYPERGLYCERIDEMIA

GUENTER SCHLIERF and VEIT STOSSBERG

The change from a high-fat to a high-carbohydrate diet results in most individuals in a transient or persistent elevation of fasting triglyceride levels. Marked hyperglyceridemia may develop in some patients with endogenous hyperlipidemia [28]. In these, a high rate of gross or occult carbohydrate intolerance is observed, the pathogenesis of which is as undetermined as that of carbohydrate-induced hyperlipemia.

Since only few attempts have been made to accurately describe, in terms of plasma levels, what happens to triglyceride (TG) [835], free fatty acid (FFA), blood sugar (BS) and insulin levels [449] during a 24-hour period of high-carbohydrate intake as compared to one of high-fat intake, we have studied diurnal patterns of these parameters in normals and in patients with endogenous ("Type IV") hyperglyceridemias.

MATERIALS AND METHODS

Five patients with endogenous hypertriglyceridemia and five normal subjects were studied twice after they had been stabilized on high-fat and high-carbohydrate diets, respectively. A first 24-hour profile was obtained while the subjects were consuming an isocaloric high-fat formula diet (65% fat) in six divided portions. The second study was performed after the subjects had been stabilized on a high-carbohydrate diet. The formula during the loading period was now high-carbohydrate (>80%), fat-free. Free fatty acid (FFA) and triglyceride (TG)

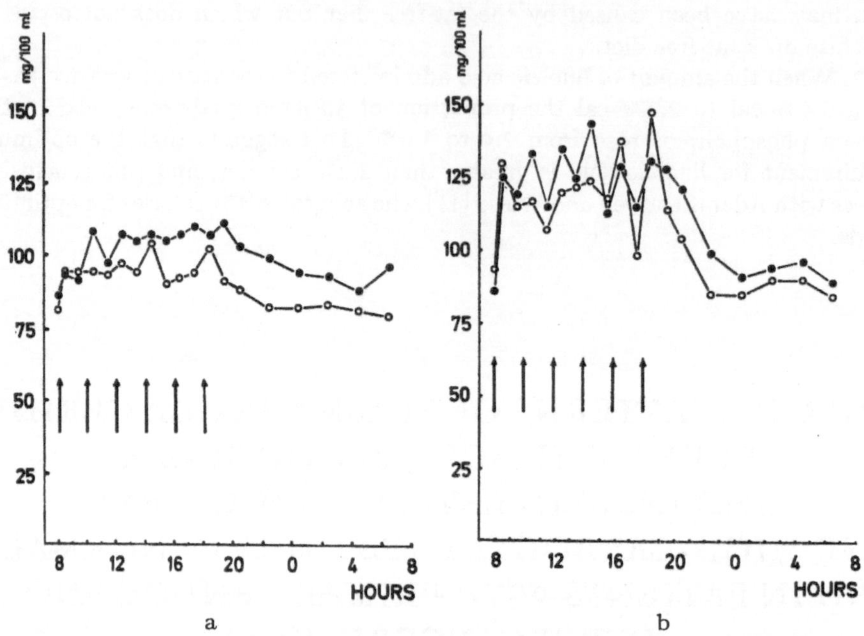

Fig. 1a and b. Mean diurnal blood sugar levels on high-fat (a) and high-carbohydrate (b) formula diets in normals (open circles) and in patients with endogenous (Type IV) hyperglyceridemia (closed circles). Arrows indicate times when portions of formula diet were consumed

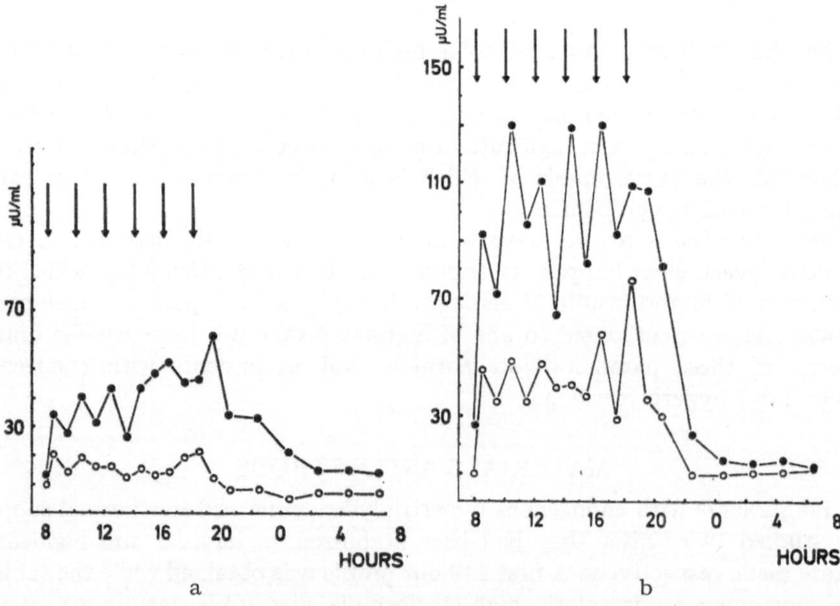

Fig. 2a and b. Mean diurnal plasma insulin levels on high-fat (a) and high-carbohydrate (b) formula diets in normals (open circles) and in patients with endogenous (Type IV) hypertriglyceridemia (closed circles). Arrows indicate times when portions of formula diet were consumed

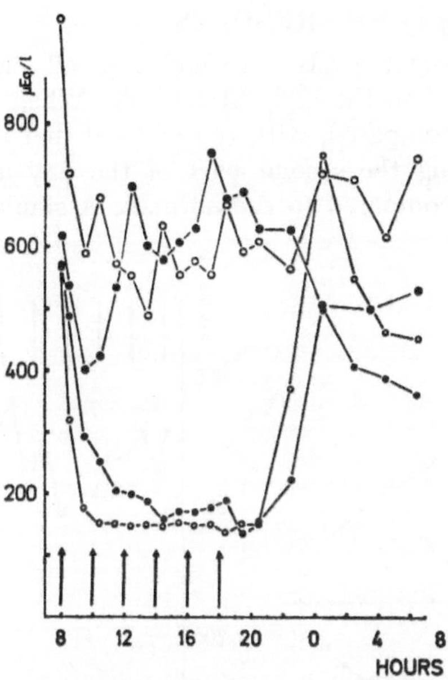

Fig. 3. Mean diurnal free fatty acid levels on high-fat (upper curves) and high-carbohydrate (lower curves) formula diets in normals (open circles) and in patients with endogenous (Type IV) hypertriglyceridemia (closed circles). Arrows indicate times when portions of formula diet were consumed

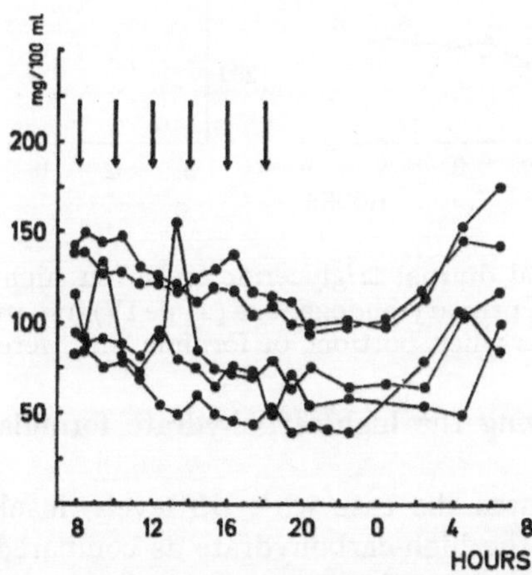

Fig. 4. Individual diurnal triglyceride levels on high-carbohydrate formula diets in 5 normal subjects. Arrows indicate times when portions of formula diet were consumed

levels were determined on the autoanalyzer, blood sugar (BS) was measured enzymatically, and plasma insulin was estimated according to a modification of the radioimmuno-assay of Yalow and Berson [1582]. Evaluation of results was done by analysis of variance after the data had been transformed logarithmically.

RESULTS

Blood Sugar. Blood sugar levels were higher in all subjects with the high-carbohydrate as compared to the high-fat formula. When the diurnal responses of the two groups were compared, with the high-fat diet the blood sugars were significantly higher during the second part of the day and during the night in the hyperlipemics as compared to the normals. A similar difference emerged

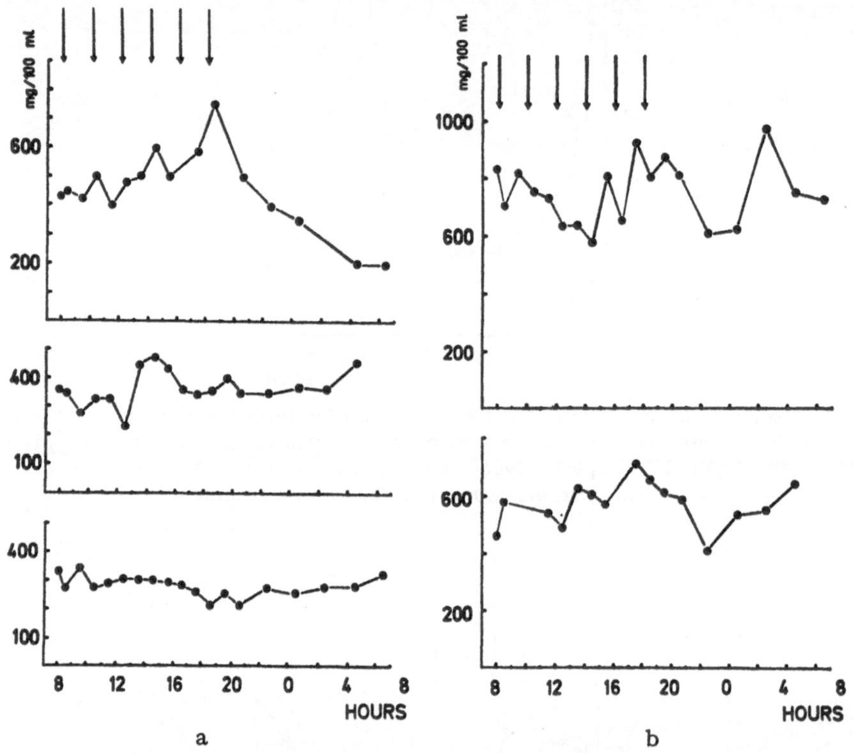

Fig. 5a and b. Individual diurnal triglyceride levels on high-carbohydrate formula diets in five patients with primary endogenous (Type IV) hypertriglyceridemia. Arrows indicate times when portions of formula diet were consumed

during the night following the high-carbohydrate formula. The results are depicted in Fig. 1.

Plasma Insulin. As was the case with BS levels, insulin levels were higher in each subject during the high-carbohydrate as compared to the high-fat diet. Comparison of the response of the two groups of subjects on the high-fat and the high-carbohydrate diets showed that average insulin levels in the hyperlipemics were twice those of the normals on either diet (Fig. 2).

Free Fatty Acids. In each subject, FFA were higher on the high-fat than on the high-carbohydrate diet. Between the two groups, there was no significant difference of diurnal FFA with either diet (Fig. 3).

Triglycerides. With the high-fat diet, there was a sustained elevation of plasma TG during the day in both normals and hyperlipemics, as an expression of the integrated peaks of postprandial lipemia following the intake of each portion of the formula diet. With the high-carbohydrate (fat-free) diet, in all of the normals there was a continued fall of triglycerides during the feeding period with a rebound rise during the night (Fig. 4). Patterns in the hyperlipemics were more variable. While a similar time course of TG was observed in one, TG showed little net change in two while in two others they rose during the day resembling the patterns seen during fat loading (Fig. 5).

DISCUSSION

The time course of the blood sugar levels (Fig. 1) in the five patients of the present study is in agreement with reports [449] of a high rate of glucose intolerance following various carbohydrate loading procedures. Hyperglycemia in the patients was apparent during the later part of the high-fat and high-carbohydrate studies, respectively and occurred in spite of plasma insulin levels which on the average were twice as high as in the normals. Of the alternate explanations commonly given for a decreased glucose tolerance, diminished insulin secretion on the one hand, and some kind of insulin resistance or secretion of a form of insulin which is not fully effective on the other, the time course of blood sugar and insulin levels in our study would be compatible with the latter concept.

Two parameters of lipid metabolism have been considered in the past to be related to the development of insulin resistance, namely elevated FFA levels [1210] and elevated TG [367]. Since there is no difference in FFA levels on either diet at any time interval between the groups (Fig. 3), elevated levels of FFA would not appear to be the cause of a postulated insulin resistance. A strong argument against the concept of insulin insensitivity resulting from high plasma triglycerides is the lack of glucose intolerance in fat-induced hyperlipemia which is characterized by very high triglyceride levels for a lifetime.

We would like to offer as still another explanation for the hyperinsulinemia that of exaggerated protein-stimulated insulin secretion, as has been reported by Estrich and coworkers[1] in mild, adult-onset diabetes. Our main argument in favor of this assumption is a lack of hyperinsulinemia in our patients following mere carbohydrate loading (unpublished data). Hyperinsulinemia might then potentiate hyperlipemia by increased triglyceride production in the liver [1215].

Finally, with regard to the thesis of an insufficiently active kind of insulin in patients with hyperlipemia, recent reports on the occurrence in plasma of a proinsulin, which is measured in the immuno-assay but which may not have much biological activity [547] may be pertinent.

The evaluation of all day TG levels shows that in most normals and in all hyperlipemics, in spite of lower fasting values, diurnal TG are higher during the high-fat than during the high-carbohydrate diet. It has been suggested [488] but not proven that chylomicron triglycerides are less atherogenic than VLDL or LDL lipids. Pending the proof of this suggestion, one might be cautious in prescribing extremely high-fat diets, on a long-term basis, in endogenous hyperlipemia.

1 Estrich, D. L., Fukayama, G., Kinsell, L. W.: Diagnostic implications of plasma insulin, free fatty acid and glucose responses to protein and carbohydrate loads in normal and diabetic subjects. Diabetes **16**, 522 (1967).

CLINICAL EXPERIENCE WITH PARTIAL ILEAL BYPASS IN TREATMENT OF THE HYPERLIPIDEMIAS*

HENRY BUCHWALD, RICHARD B. MOORE, IVAN D. FRANTZ, JR., and RICHARD L. VARCO

In May of 1969, our clinical bypass program at the University of Minnesota entered into the seventh year of study. At present we have documented the preoperative, operative, and postoperative course, with 100% follow-up, of 70 consecutive patients. This paper will attempt to summarize clinical findings in these patients; our concomitant metabolic studies are outlined elsewhere (see p. 295). In order not to duplicate previous reports, referral will be made to past publications. There are several other groups currently engaged in performing partial ileal bypass operations for hypercholesterolemia and their publications show cholesterol reductions in the same range as those found in our series [866, 1428, 1445].

Patient Selection. We have selected patients for partial ileal bypass in the presence of a hyperlipidemia and evidence of atherosclerotic disease and/or a family history of early and severe manifestations of the atherosclerotic process. Of the 70 patients in this series, 61 had evidence of atherosclerosis; whereas nine patients were operated upon prophylactically, i.e. no clinical symptoms, normal electrocardiograms and vectorcardiograms, normal exercise electrocardiograms, and coronary arteriograms free of all plaque deposition. The operation was not offered to patients in heart failure, since an attack on the origin of the arterial process of a patient in end-stage myocardial disease seemed to be of doubtful value. Patients with a secondary hyperlipidemia have not been considered.

To date the patients have been less than 60 years of age, with an average age of 40. Eight of the patients have been under the age of 21, three prepubertal, and the youngest was seven years old.

For at least three months prior to operation, all the patients were on a moderately stringent low cholesterol, low saturated fat diet (less than 30% of total calories from fat, less than 300 mg cholesterol per day, and a polyunsaturated: saturated ratio of approximately 1.5); the Type III and Type IV patients were on carbohydrate restriction as well. The average postdietary cholesterol and triglyceride concentrations are used as the preoperative baselines to which that patient's postoperative values are compared. The same diet is maintained after the operation. The response of 24 patients to dietary management alone over a three-month period and then to diet and bypass has been studied [258].

* The work herein has been supported in part by U.S.P.H. Grant No. HE 11901-01, U.S.P.H. Grant No. H-1875, American Heart Association Grant No. 64G168, and a special legislative grant of the State of Minnesota.

Operative Technique. Partial ileal bypass is carried out from a point 200 cm proximal to the ileocecal valve or at a distance one-third the entire small intestinal length from the ileocecal valve, whichever is longer. For operative technique details see Buchwald [260].

Serum Lipids. All patients have had cholesterol reduction after partial ileal bypass over and above the reduction engendered by diet alone. Table 1 provides the average values for serum cholesterol (in mg%) and the percentage reduction from baseline over a five-year period. The average cholesterol reduction at three months was 40%, and this figure did not change significantly for the next five years. When the patients of the five-year group, four-year group, etc., are separated out and recalculated (Table 2) the figures are essentially unchanged and show that the average three months postoperative cholesterol reduction is

Table 1. *Summary of follow-up on serum cholesterols and percentage reduction from baseline* [a]

	Baseline	3 months	1 year	2 years	3 years	4 years	5 years
Number of patients	70	59	44	31	18	14	8
Average mg%	374	217	236	242	206	234	238
Range mg%	208–908	110–762	144–865	129–766	120–448	135–452	111–486
Average %↓		40	35	36	39	33	37
Range %↓		16–72	5–57	10–54	17–54	21–46	16–53
± S.D. %↓		12.97	13.97	13.89	12.09	9.04	13.42
± S.E. %↓		1.69	2.13	2.54	2.85	2.42	4.75

[a] The abbreviations in this and subsequent tables are: n = number; ↓ = reduction in serum level; $\bar{x}$ = mean; S.D. = standard deviation; S.E. = standard error; and mg% = milligrams per 100 ml.

maintained. Analysis of the degree of cholesterol reduction as a function of the type of hyperlipidemia [489] three months following bypass is presented in Table 3; the percentage reductions for the Type II, Type III, and Type IV patients are not significantly different.

Triglyceride concentrations have only been accurately calculated over a three-year period, and only at three months following bypass do we have a sufficient number of patients to offer significant follow-up data for Type III and Type IV patients (Table 4). The average triglyceride reductions in these two groups are equal to, or slightly greater than, the cholesterol reductions found in these groups. The Type II patients with elevated triglyceride levels generally had a reduction subsequent to ileal bypass, whereas, those with values in the normal range showed a variable response. The triglyceride response of the Type II patients is summarized in Table 5; the average triglyceride concentration remained unchanged over a three-year period.

The total serum lipids and lipoprotein ultracentrifugation fractions were also reduced after bypass and reflect the reductions in the cholesterol and triglyceride values. Since the summer of 1965 we have obtained preoperative serum lipoprotein electrophoretic patterns to aid in typing the patients. A uniform decrease in the beta and prebeta bands after operation has been observed when the staining

Table 2. *Mean serum cholesterol and percentage reduction from baseline as a function of years followed*

	Base-line	3 months	1 year	2 years	3 years	4 years	5 years
5-Year Group n = 8							
$\bar{x}$ mg%	368	234	244	257	233	249	238
$\bar{x}$ %↓		38	34	31	37	34	37
± S.D. (S.E.) %↓		13.47	9.97	11.39	12.36	8.73	13.42
		(4.76)	(3.53)	(4.03)	(4.37)	(3.09)	(4.75)
4-Year Group n = 14							
$\bar{x}$ mg%	348	215	232	237	219	234	
$\bar{x}$ %↓		39	33	31	37	33	
± S.D. (S.E.) %↓		10.30	12.52	12.90	12.82	9.04	
		(2.75)	(3.47)	(3.58)	(3.43)	(2.42)	
3-Year Group n = 18							
$\bar{x}$ mg%	337	207	219	222	206		
$\bar{x}$ %↓		39	35	34	39		
± S.D. (S.E.) %↓		10.07	12.05	12.11	12.09		
		(2.37)	(2.92)	(2.94)	(2.85)		
2-Year Group n = 31							
$\bar{x}$ mg%	376	231	250	242			
$\bar{x}$ %↓		40	36	36			
± S.D. (S.E.) %↓		10.89	11.57	13.89			
		(1.96)	(2.15)	(2.54)			
1-Year Group n = 44							
$\bar{x}$ mg%	360	221	236				
$\bar{x}$ %↓		39	35				
± S.D. (S.E.) %↓		11.91	13.97				
		(1.81)	(2.13)				

Table 3. *Cholesterols and percentage decrease from baseline at three months as a function of the type of hyperlipidemia*

Type [a]	n	Baseline cholesterol mg%	3 months follow-up			
			$\bar{x}$ mg%	$\bar{x}$ %↓	± S.D. %↓	± S.E. %↓
II	44	370	226	39	10.67	1.80
III	4	403	198	46	21.17	10.58
IV	7	411	182	40	23.28	9.50

[a] Classification of Fredrickson, Levy and Lees [489].

Table 4. *Triglyceride reductions in Type III and Type IV patients three months following bypass*

Type	n	Baseline mg%	3 months mg%	%↓
III	4	837	410	50
IV	6	1,998	670	42

intensity of these bands was abnormal before surgery; in several patients, phenotype group changes and reversal of an abnormal electrophoretic pattern to a normal one have been noted.

Clinical Findings. In the high risk population considered for surgery, there have been three coronary deaths in patients prior to being selected for operation. There has been one early postoperative death (four days following operation, from myocardial infarction), for an in-hospital mortality of 1.4%. There have been three late deaths, all from myocardial infarction, occurring three, five, and 26 months after operation. Excluding patients operated upon prophylactically and including the one immediate postoperative death, the survival time in the therapeutic bypass series to date is 1,680 out of a possible 1,886 patient-months, for a cumulative survival of 88%. Ninety-eight percent (44 of 45) of this group who survived at least one year after bypass are alive. These figures compare quite favorably with published data [319, 763, 1226, 1531] on survival of patients with disease of comparable severity. In these other series the five-year survival of patients having sustained myocardial infarction was between 49% to 66%, and the survival of patients free of overt manifestations of atherosclerosis [763] was 92.4% at three years and 86.4% at five years. Thus, the ileal bypass survival statistics seem to parallel survival of a relatively healthy population group.

Table 5. *Triglyceride response: Type II patients*

	Baseline	3 months	1 year	2 years	3 years
n total	44	35	23	13	4
n with reductions		18	10	7	2
n with elevations		17	13	6	2
$\bar{x}$ mg% total group	187	171	168	170	195

Postoperative morbidity is limited to diarrhea; in all but two patients this has been transient. The ability to absorb vitamin B_{12} is essentially lost following the bypass [256], and all patients are placed on 1,000 µg of vitamin B_{12} intramuscularly every two months. Following this precaution, evolvement of a macrocytosis, anemia, or neurological manifestations have not been seen. Sustained weight loss has not occurred after partial ileal bypass, in distinction to the jejunal-ileal bypass procedure utilized in the management of obesity.

Patients with angina pectoris, symptoms of cerebral vascular insufficiency, or intermittent claudications have, almost uniformly, offered testimony to a decrease of these manifestations. The symptomatic improvement has been associated with an increase in work capacity, exercise tolerance, and sense of well being. Regression of xanthomata and xanthelasma following bypass has been observed and pictorially documented [260]. In four patients, exercise electrocardiograms positive in the preoperative period have converted to negative tracings one year or later following operation [257]. Sequential analysis of selective coronary and peripheral arteriograms, performed preoperatively and every two years thereafter, have shown no visible progression of the disease process, defined as the appearance of new plaques or the enlargement of existing plaques [90]. These findings are encouraging in the light of other patient series where definite progression of the atherosclerotic process over comparable lengths of time has been noted in half or more of the patients [419, 1523].

SUMMARY AND COMMENT

Detailed cholesterol and triglyceride statistics in our 70 patient partial ileal bypass series have been presented. Reference has been made to patient mortality and long-term survival, postoperative morbidity, changes in symptomatology, and electrocardiographic and arteriographic data. The average cholesterol reduction from the preoperative baseline (obtained only after at least three months on an appropriate cholesterol lowering diet) is 40% three months following bypass and 37% five years following bypass. We believe that partial ileal bypass is the most effective method currently available to achieve maximal cholesterol reduction.

VITAMIN D AND HYPERCHOLESTEROLEMIA IN ADULT HUMANS

ALAN I. FLEISCHMAN, MARVIN L. BIERENBAUM, ROBERT RAICHELSON, THOMAS HAYTON and PORTIA WATSON

In 1957, Donath and De Langen [398] reported on vitamin-D induced arteriosclerosis and the possible dangers of feeding extra vitamin D to older people. Feenstra and Wilkens [453] found that serum cholesterol increased with increased vitamin D intake when margarine was the main source of dietary fat. Similar results were noted by Pfleiderer [1169] in rats, while Lee and Herrmann [848] showed increased deposition of tissue cholesterol in rats in the presence of vitamin D.

Since vitamin D supplementation in food is fairly widespread, a study of the effect of vitamin D upon serum lipids in adult humans was needed. The results are presented here.

METHODS AND MATERIALS

The study was divided into two phases: in Phase I this was the effect of 50,000 IU and 1,000 IU of vitamin D daily for 21 days upon the serum cholesterol and triglyceride levels of eight adults (four males and four females). After a sample of serum had been taken, each volunteer ingested 50,000 IU of supplemental vitamin D daily for 21 days. A second serum sample was taken, and supplemental vitamin D withdrawn. After 21 days a third serum sample was obtained to study the degree of recovery from the vitamin D treatment. The subjects continued on their normal diets for a further five months so as to obtain maximum clearance, and a fourth serum sample was obtained. These same subjects then ingested 1,000 IU of supplemental vitamin D daily for 21 days, and the serum was again sampled. Finally after 21 days of normal dietary pattern, the last serum sample was obtained.

In Phase II, the experimental protocol of Phase I was repeated on three males and four females, employing only a 21-day recovery period in order to determine the effect upon serum lipids of the two levels of vitamin D without prolonged clearance.

All blood samples were taken after a 14-hour fast, permitted to clot, the serum removed, and immediately assayed for cholesterol and triglycerides by procedures previously described by Fleischman et al. [462]. The standard errors for serum cholesterol and triglycerides were 2.22 mg/100 ml and 2.53 mg/100 ml, respectively. Statistical analysis was performed by the signed-rank test.

RESULTS

Cholesterol. The effect of vitamin D for Phase I of the study is shown in Table 1. After 21 days on 50,000 IU of vitamin D, seven of the eight subjects had increases in serum cholesterol ranging from 24 mg/100 ml to 41 mg/100 ml,

Table 1. *The independent effect of two levels of vitamin D upon serum cholesterol (mg/100 ml) in human adults*

Subject	Pre-experimental	After 21 days 50,000 IU daily	dc/dt	After 21 days recovery	After 6 months	After 21 days 1,000 IU daily	dc/dt	After 21 days recovery
1	244	285	+41	264	225	290	+65	270
2	334	365	+31	328	258	339	+81	312
3	212	234	+22	210	200	210	+10	210
4	165	189	+24	186	165	163	−2	147
5	280	305	+25	297	230	243	+13	244
6	168	199	+31	163	—	—	—	—
7	259	295	+34	243	236	237	+1	235
8	170	171	+1	157	198	193	−5	179
Median			+28				+10	

with a median increase of 28 mg/100 ml, $P<0.01$. The serum cholesterol concentration in the eighth subject remained essentially unchanged. Three weeks after termination of supplemental vitamin D, the serum cholesterol level decreased toward the pre-experimental level, although in at least three of the subjects the serum cholesterol was still relatively elevated, compared to the pre-experimental level.

After six months on an *ad libitum* diet, a further serum sample was obtained from seven of the eight subjects, and 1,000 IU daily of supplemental vitamin D taken for 21 days. In four of the seven subjects, serum cholesterol rose from 10 to 81 mg/100 ml, while in three subjects, it remained essentially unchanged. The median rise for all subjects was 10 mg/100 ml, $P<0.05$. Three weeks after

Table 2. *Serum cholesterol*[a] *changes due to two levels of vitamin D taken without permitting complete clearance by adult humans*

Subject	Pre-experimental	After 21 days 50,000 IU daily	dc/dt	After 21 days recovery	After 21 days 1,000 IU daily	dc/dt
9	173	194	+21	172	206	+34
10	198	235	+37	230	324	+96
11	223	226	+3	193	340	+147
12	260	242	−18	230	462	+232
13	225	241	+16	258	600	+342
14	170	189	+19	180	200	+20
15	236	253	+27	240	474	+234
Median			+19			+147

[a] mg/100 ml.

Table 3. *The independent effect of two levels of vitamin D upon serum triglyceride (mg/100 ml) in human adults*

Subject	Pre-experimental	After 21 days 50,000 IU daily	dc/dt	After 21 days recovery	After 6 months	After 1,000 IU daily	dc/dt	After 21 days recovery
1	240	230	−10	127	183	147	−36	136
2	432	346	−86	356	315	450	+135	315
3	90	103	+13	73	113	155	+42	143
4	51	57	+7	74	60	64	+4	110
5	85	97	+12	76	175	140	−35	119
6	56	46	−10	73	—	—	—	—
7	160	173	+13	182	179	147	−32	—
8	147	149	+2	100	100	94	−6	109
Median			+4.5				−6	

Table 4. *Serum triglyceride*[a] *changes due to two levels of vitamin D taken without permitting complete clearance by adult humans*

Subject	Pre-experimental	After 21 days 50,000 IU daily	dc/dt	After 21 days recovery	After 21 days 1,000 IU daily	dc/dt
9	184	191	+7	234	234	0
10	150	130	−20	120	150	+30
11	161	140	−20	158	226	+68
12	196	156	−40	162	390	+228
13	130	111	−19	138	246	+108
14	80	85	+5	112	100	−12
15	227	417	+190	286	390	+104
Median			−19			+68

[a] mg/100 ml.

terminating the supplemental vitamin D, serum cholesterol levels in subjects exhibiting a rise on supplementation failed to decrease to the level found prior to this later supplementation, suggesting a higher degree of sensitivity to vitamin D and a concomitantly slower clearance in some individuals.

The effect of supplemental vitamin D upon the serum cholesterol levels of the seven volunteers in Phase II is shown in Table 2. After 21 days on 50,000 IU five subjects exhibited serum cholesterol elevations ranging from 16 to 37 mg/100 ml, while one individual remained essentially unchanged, and one showed an 18 mg/100 ml decrease. The median increase for all subjects was 19 mg/100 ml, $P<0.01$. After three weeks without supplementation, these volunteers were given 1,000 IU for 21 days. All seven subjects showed a serum cholesterol increase ranging from 20 to 342 mg/100 ml. The median increase was 147 mg/100 ml, $P<0.01$.

Triglycerides. The effect of supplemental vitamin D on the serum triglyceride levels for the subjects in Phase I (Table 3) showed a highly variable response to 50,000 IU daily. After a six-month rest followed by 21 days on 1,000 IU daily, a similarly variable response was noted.

For the subjects in the Phase II experiment (Table 4), again a variable response was noted after 50,000 IU daily for 21 days. With a three-week rest period, and then three weeks on 1,000 IU daily, five of the seven subjects showed an elevation in serum triglycerides ranging from 30 to 228 mg/100 ml, with a median increase of 68 mg/100 ml, $P<0.05$.

DISCUSSION

The data indicates that ingestion of supplemental vitamin D significantly increases serum cholesterol in adult humans. These findings are in agreement with the results of Donath and De Langen [398], Feenstra and Wilkens [453], and Pfleiderer [1169]. When the two levels, 50,000 IU and 1,000 IU daily, were tested as independent entities in the same individuals by permitting sufficient time for the higher level of vitamin D to clear the body prior to testing the lower level, the median cholesterol rise in these subjects was approximately proportional to the supplemental vitamin D level ingested. When complete clearance of the higher level was prevented before the ingestion of the lower concentration of vitamin D (Table 2), there was a serum cholesterol response which was completely out of proportion to the level of supplemental vitamin D ingested. Thus vitamin D appears to be cumulative in its cholesterol elevating effect. The ability of vitamin D to increase serum cholesterol in an additive manner when coupled with other hypercholesterolemic agents has been reported by Lee and Herrmann [848].

It is interesting to attempt to explain the hyperlipemic action of supplemental vitamin D. One possible mechanism could be through the intervention of calcium metabolism. Yacowitz et al. [1580] found that supplementary dietary calcium significantly lowers serum lipids in man. Fleischman et al. [463] noted that the calcium acted largely by complexing with the polar portions of the ingested fat micellae in the intestine, and possibly prevented lipid absorption. If appreciable amounts of calcium are absorbed before it can complex with the polar portion of the ingested fat micellae, more of the ingested fat will be absorbed, including the exogenous cholesterol. Lipids are absorbed by active transport in the distal portion of the ileum. Kodicek [816] reported that calcium is primarily absorbed in the proximal portion of the small intestine during the first few hours after ingestion. He noted that vitamin D enhanced the activity of the translocase enzyme system of active transport by an allosteric distortion of the lipoprotein macromolecule. Thus, vitamin D could effectively decrease the amount of calcium to complex with the fat. However, no ready explanation appears available for the apparent hysteresis effect noted in the second part of the Phase II experiment, and more detailed study in this most critical area will have to be done.

Thus, in spite of the need for additional studies on the hyperlipemic action of vitamin D, it would seem that caution should be exercised in the use of supplemental vitamin D in adult humans.

ATHEROGENESIS IN MINIPIGS: EFFECT OF DIETARY FAT UNSATURATION AND OF COPPER

DENHAM HARMAN

Atherogenesis is enhanced by substances capable of irritating the arterial wall [613]. A possible constant source of irritative compounds may be the reaction of molecular oxygen with serum and arterial wall lipids [611]. The readily oxidized polyunsaturates comprise about 30% of the total fatty acids, present mainly as esters, in the lipids of both serum [1158] and atherosclerotic plaques [225]. Hence, the oxidation products, including peroxides and compounds of higher molecular weight formed through oxidative-polymerization, as well as substances arising from the reaction of the intermediate lipid free radicals with proteins and other substances, may be produced in amounts large enough to make a significant contribution to atherogenesis. The foregoing suggests that the long-term ingestion of increased amounts of polyunsaturates, increasing the unsaturation of serum and tissue lipids, might actually enhance atherosclerosis [611, 612] even though they tend to lower serum cholesterol levels [656, 791].

In an attempt to evaluate the possibility that lipid peroxidation is significantly involved in atherogenesis, two experiments have been carried out with uncastrated male pigs. Pigs were employed for this study, for under normal living conditions they spontaneously develop atherosclerotic lesions which are very similar, both grossly and microscopically, to those of humans [527, 895, 1030, 1601]. On the assumption that the morphologic similarity of the lesions in swine and man is a result of similar pathogenic processes, the pig should be a good animal for evaluating factors presumed to be involved in human atherogenesis. In the first experiment pigs were fed diets containing 30% by weight of either lard or safflower oil while in the second, pigs were given diets containing 15% by weight of either lard or safflower to which was added 0.0, 0.05, or 0.10% by weight of cupric acetate, a good catalyst for the reaction of molecular oxygen with organic compounds [1487].

METHODS

Genetically small male uncastrated pigs, "Nebraska Miniature Swine" [1534], were ear marked and then allocated at random to form groups of 10 pigs each. Each group was placed in a concrete block pig house (10 × 10 ft) with an outside run (10 × 16 ft); both areas have concrete floors. The pigs were weighed and bled (superior *vena cava*) at intervals of about six months. The serum samples were analyzed for total cholesterol [854, 1334].

The aortas, removed with the first part of their major branches, except for the coronary arteries in the first experiment, were stained with Sudan IV [698] and graded for atherosclerosis on a scale of 0–4+, [405, 825]; in the second experiment, the coronary arteries were also graded. Grading was done blind by three individuals on two occasions one week apart and the average of the six gradings for each area determined. In grading, no distinction was made between fatty and fibrous lesions.

Autopsy serum samples were analyzed for cholesterol and phospholipids (2nd Experiment).

First Experiment. The two groups of pigs were started at age of about three months, shortly after being placed in the pens, on one of the following diets: Group 1—Basal diet (70%w, i.e., by weight) + antioxidant free lard (30%w); Group 2—Basal diet + safflower oil (30%w).

The base diet was a high protein, high vitamin diet such that with the addition of the 30%w fat the final diet was considered to be nutritionally satisfactory for young, rapidly growing pigs. The final diet contained 13.8%w protein, 31.0%w lipid, 11.5% fiber, 6.0%w ash, 8.4 mg of vitamin E per pound (not counting that present in the added lipid) and 516 mg choline per pound; the final diets contained 1,530 cal/pound, 83.0% of the calories from lipid.

The diets were prepared weekly and kept stored in a cool area prior to use; the pigs were fed once a day from a common food trough in each pen. The edible grade safflower[1] oil was shipped in drums and was reported to be stable; i.e., peroxide value below 1.0 mg/kg, for the approximately six-week period required to utilize the contents of a drum. The lard was antioxidant free.

At age 24 months, having been on the special diets for 21 months, the pigs (fasting) were electrocuted, exsanguinated, and complete autopsies performed.

Second Experiment. Six groups were started at age five months on the following diets: (1) Basal diet (85%w) + antioxidant free lard (15%w); (2) Diet 1 plus 0.05%w cupric acetate; (3) Diet 1 plus 0.10%w cupric acetate; (4) Basal diet (85%w) + safflower oil (15%w); (5) Diet 4 plus 0.05%w cupric acetate; and (6) Diet 4 plus 0.10%w cupric acetate.

Cupric acetate powder was mixed in diets (2), (3), (5) and (6) just prior to feeding. The diets contained 16.4%w protein, 16.3%w lipid, 13.9%w fiber and

1 We wish to thank the Pacific Vegetable Oil Corporation, Richmond, California, for the safflower oil used in this study.

Table. *Pig atherogenesis*

Experiment number and diet	Wt. lbs.	Serum		Atherosclerosis [b]		
		cholesterol mg/100 ml	phospholipid mg/100 ml	aorta arch	aorta abd.	coronary art.
Experiment 1						
1. 30 %w Lard	312.5 ± 71.7 [a]	76.4 ± 14.3	—	0.34 ± 0.32	0.40 ± 42	—
2. 30 %w Safflower oil	261.1 ± 51.9	85.5 ± 18.4 [d]	—	0.24 ± 0.26	0.65 ± 0.81	—
Experiment 2						
1. 15 %w Lard + 0.00 %w Cu [c]	200.5 ± 35.2	113.5 ± 15.2	126.8 ± 25.6	0.33 ± 0.23	0.37 ± 0.29	0.48 ± 0.32
2. 15 %w Lard + 0.05 %w Cu	213.0 ± 33.6	102.3 ± 36.1	127.6 ± 24.2	0.46 ± 0.54	0.44 ± 0.51	0.63 ± 0.70
3. 15 %w Lard + 0.10 %w Cu	216.3 ± 28.3	101.3 ± 17.1	119.1 ± 15.4	0.32 ± 0.24	0.37 ± 0.40	0.39 ± 0.15
4. 15 %w Safflower oil + 0.00 % Cu	202.5 ± 55.8	85.0 ± 14.0	88.7 ± 23.8	0.21 ± 0.20	0.35 ± 0.29	0.39 ± 0.20
5. 15 %w Safflower oil + 0.05 % Cu	214.4 ± 21.0	88.7 ± 11.0	92.2 ± 16.2	0.22 ± 0.18	0.19 ± 0.24	0.11 ± 0.18
6. 15 %w Safflower oil + 0.10 % Cu	211.8 ± 44.0	69.5 ± 7.6	74.3 ± 12.8	0.38 ± 0.43	0.41 ± 0.53	0.42 ± 0.15

[a] Mean ± standard deviation.

[b] Atherosclerosis graded on basis of 0–4 +; 0 indicating no atherosclerosis and 4 involvement of the entire intimal surface by atherosclerotic lesions.

[c] Cu = Cupric acetate.

[d] The three average serum cholesterol values obtained for the safflower oil groups during life were all lower than those for the lard group; there is no explanation as to why the autopsy average serum cholesterol value for the safflower oil group is higher than for the lard group.

7.3%w ash; 800 mg choline, 7 mg of copper and vitamin E (25 mg + that present in the added lipid) per pound. In the final diet, 56.7% of the total calories were derived from fat. The animals were fed an average of 2.5 lb of food per day per pig.

After 21 months on the diets, at age 26 months, the animals were killed and autopsied as in Experiment 1.

RESULTS

Autopsy data for Experiments 1 and 2 are given in the Table.

In Experiment 1, six of the ten pigs in the safflower oil group were found to have multiple hard yellowish masses, ranging in size from a few millimeters to 10 cm in diameter, embedded in the omental and peritoneal fat; these masses were composed of varying amounts of adipose tissue, fat-like droplets, giant cells, cellular debris and collagenous tissue. The kidney of a pig receiving safflower oil had significant tubular dilation and interstitial fibrosis associated with a few inflammatory cells while a second pig in the group had a slight degree of kidney fibrosis.

In Experiment 2 the incidence of the yellowish abdominal masses in the pigs on safflower oil was about 30%. The average size and number were markedly decreased, and there were no kidney lesions.

Aortic atherosclerosis in both experiments was small and variable, averaging about 0.3 in the arch and around 0.4 in the abdominal aortic area. Although some trends can be discerned in comparing the various atherosclerosis gradings in the two experiments, the differences are not statistically significant.

DISCUSSION

Feeding male uncastrated minipigs for 21 months on diets expected to result in differing rates of peroxidation of serum and vessel wall lipids did not produce statistically significant differences in aortic and coronary artery atherosclerosis. Some trends were seen which may be real. In both experiments the aortic arch atherosclerosis tended to parallel the serum cholesterol levels, being lower with the safflower oil diets as compared to lard. In contrast, abdominal aortic and coronary artery atherosclerosis was about the same in the pigs on either the lard or safflower oil diets. Addition of cupric acetate tended to enhance both aortic and coronary artery atherosclerosis; the effect appeared somewhat greater with the safflower oil diets. The results with cupric acetate support the possibility that the elevated levels of serum copper found in employed males with a history of myocardial infarction [614] were also present prior to infarction.

Thus the data are compatible with the possibility that lipid peroxidation contributes to atherogenesis, the enhancement being partially or completely nullified by the lowered serum cholesterol levels produced by the dietary alterations. Further, lipid peroxidation may be involved in regulation of serum lipid levels; for dietary copper, like polyunsaturates, tended to lower both serum cholesterol and phospholipid concentrations.

INFLUENCE OF ZINC AND COPPER ON THE DEVELOPMENT OF EXPERIMENTAL ATHEROSCLEROSIS

RONALD S. FILO, CHARLES H. SLOAN, LEE WEATHERBEE and WILLIAM J. FRY

During the past decade increased interest in the investigation of trace element metabolism has been shown in many areas of medicine. A long list of trace metals has been implicated in the pathogenesis of atherosclerosis; however, to date there is no conclusive evidence that such is the case. Pories [1187], Volkov [1509] and Wacker [1510] have all reported specific zinc deficiencies associated with atherosclerosis. Henzel et al. [669] reported that oral administration of zinc sulfate has been beneficial in the treatment of a significant percentage of inoperable and severely symptomatic atherosclerotic patients. Copper has been reported to be antagonistic to zinc in many respects [1494], as well as to enhance experimental atherosclerosis [615]. The present study was designed to investigate the influence of oral zinc or copper administration on the development of experimental atherosclerosis.

METHODS

Forty-five male New Zealand rabbits were divided into six groups. Groups 1, 2, and 3 contained ten rabbits, each. They were on an atherogenic regimen of regular rabbit chow, intermittently supplemented for two-month periods with 2% cholesterol [326]. These three groups were given distilled water, 1.7 mM $ZnSO_4$ or 1.7 mM $CuSO_4$ drinking solutions, respectively. This dosage resulted in an average oral intake of elemental zinc or copper of 35–50 mg/day, which is comparable on a weight basis to the dosages administered in the clinical studies [669]. Groups 4, 5, and 6 contained five rabbits, each, to serve as controls. They received comparable drinking solutions, but remained on a regular chow diet throughout the experiment.

All zinc and copper determinations were made using atomic absorption spectrophotometry. Throughout the experiment, serum cholesterol, zinc and copper were serially determined.

At the termination of the six-month period all the remaining rabbits were scarificed and autopsied. Zinc and copper levels of aortic and liver tissue were determined. The degree of aortic atherosclerosis was graded on a scale of 0 to 4+ by separately grading the aortic arch and thoraco-abdominal aorta, and then averaging the two values.

RESULTS

In the three groups on cholesterol supplementation, there had been a 50% (5/10) mortality in the copper group, a 20% (2/10) mortality in the distilled water group, and zero mortality in the zinc group by the end of the six-month experimental period. All animals in the three control groups survived. In general

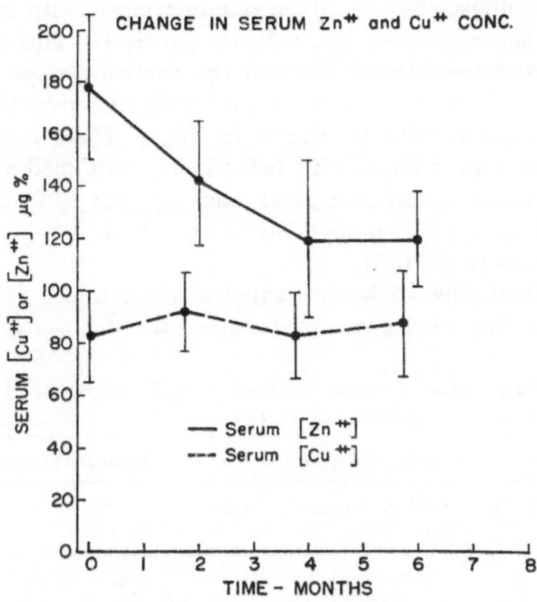

Fig. 1. Serum copper and zinc concentration of 15 control rabbits. Vertical bars indicate one standard deviation

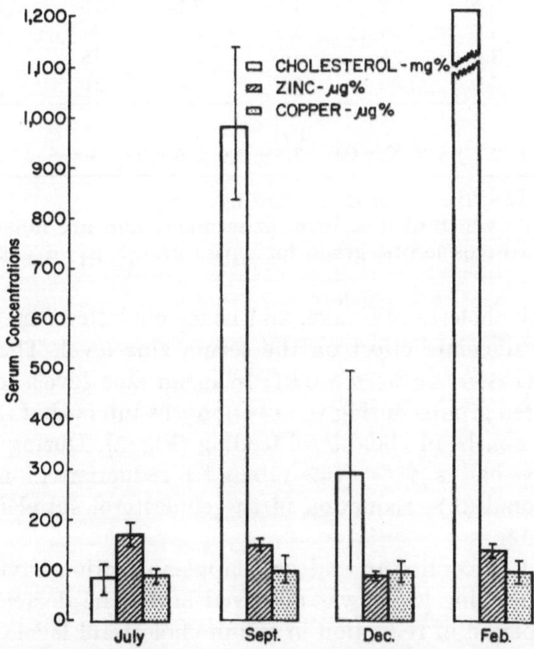

Fig. 2. Effect of dietary cholesterol on serum cholesterol, zinc and copper. July: baseline values; September and February: vallues following two months of dietary cholesterol supplementation; December: values following two months of regular diet

we found that oral administration of either zinc or copper, with one exception, had little effect on their respective serum levels during the entire experiment. No inter-group difference was found between the control groups (groups 4, 5, and 6); changes in mean serum zinc and copper concentration over the six-months period for the 15 control rabbits are shown in Fig. 1. There is no significant change in mean serum copper levels with time; it is maintained at about 82 ± 18 μg%. The initial mean serum zinc level was 177 ± 28 μg%, and over the six-month period fell to 120 ± 18 μg%. This represents a 30% decrease which is statistically significant ($p < 0.015$).

Rabbits on the atherogenic cholesterol supplementation also demonstrated a gradual decrease in serum zinc concentration, as did the controls. However,

Table. *Grading of atherosclerosis of aortas obtained from three groups of rabbits on an atherogenic regimen*

Group I distilled water			Group II zinc			Group III copper		
rabbit No.	gross	micro	rabbit No.	gross	micro	rabbit No.	gross	micro
1	3.5	2.0	14	4.0	2.5	27[a]	1.5	0.5
2	2.5	3.0	16	3.0	2.5	28[a]	2.0	2.0
3	2.5	1.0	18	4.0	3.0	29	2.0	2.0
4	1.5	0.5	19	3.0	3.0	30[a]	1.5	2.5
5[a]	0.5	1.0	20	3.0	3.0	31[a]	1.5	1.0
6	2.5	2.5	21	3.5	2.0	32	1.5	1.0
7[a]	0.5	0.5	22	4.0	2.5	33	2.5	2.0
9	2.5	3.0	24	2.5	2.0	34[a]	1.5	0.5
12	3.0	3.0	25	4.0	2.5	35	2.0	2.0
13	2.0	2.0	26	4.0	3.0	36	3.0	3.0
Mean $N=8$	$\mu_I =$ 2.5 ± 0.6	2.1 ± 1.0	$N=10$	$\mu_{II} =$ 3.5 ± 0.6	2.6 ± 0.4	$N=5$	$\mu_{III} =$ 2.2 ± 0.6	2.0 ± 0.7

$\mu_{II} > \mu_I$ or μ_{III} ($p < 0.005$) for gross grading.

[a] Denotes rabbits which died early in experiment and are not included in determination of mean atherosclerotic grade for entire group; μ_I, μ_{II} or μ_{III}.

the state of dietary cholesterol intake, and hence cholesterol metabolism, seemed to have a more immediate effect on the serum zinc level. There is an average decrease of 38% (145–91 μg%; $p < 0.01$) in mean zinc levels for all three cholesterol supplemented groups during the two-months interval of regular diet which followed the two months of cholesterol feeding (Fig. 2). During this same period the control groups had a 15% (142–120 μg%) reduction in mean serum zinc levels. The additional 23% reduction in the cholesterol supplement groups was significant ($p < 0.02$).

The one possible exception to oral zinc supplementation having some measurable effect on serum zinc levels was observed here. The decrease in serum zinc levels during the period of reduction in serum cholesterol levels was not as great in the zinc supplemented animals, only 29% (145–103 μg%; $p < 0.02$), as compared to 42% (149–86 μg%; $p < 0.01$) for the distilled water and copper supplemented groups. However, this difference was not statistically significant.

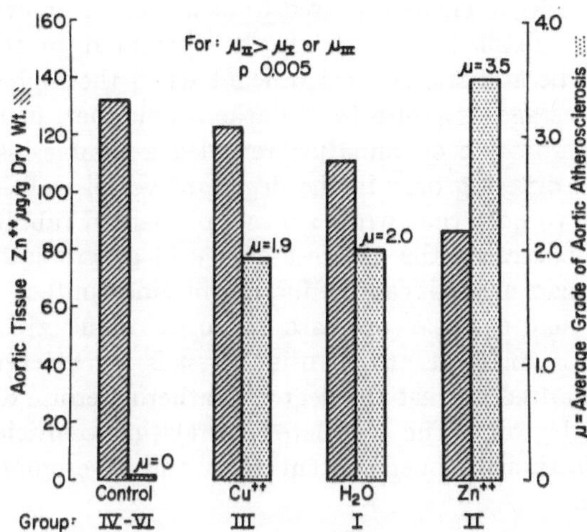

Fig. 3. Relationship of aortic atherosclerosis by group to aortic zinc content

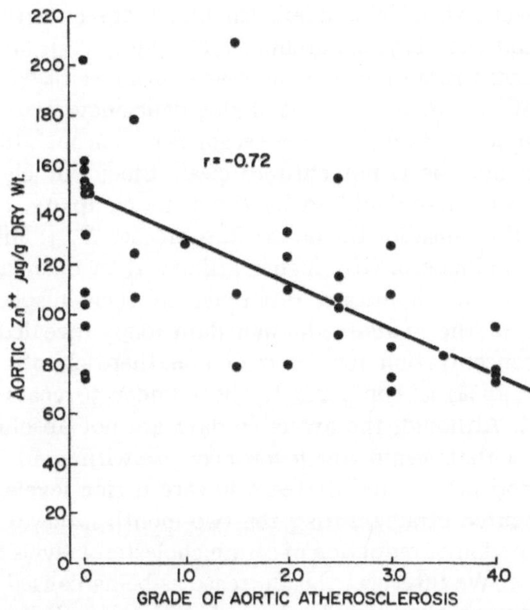

Fig. 4. Relationship of aortic tissue zinc content and atherosclerosis

The results shown in Fig. 2 indicate that the cholesterol metabolism has no apparent effect on serum copper levels since the serum copper concentration does not change significantly during any two-month interval.

The Table shows the gross and microscopic grading of atheromatous involvement for all rabbits on the atherogenic diet. All of these rabbits developed a comparable hypercholesterolemia. The zinc supplemented rabbits had significantly greater atherosclerosis than their counterparts on distilled water or copper supplemented water ($p < 0.005$). There appeared to be a slightly greater atherosclerotic involvement in the distilled water group, as compared to the copper group, but this proved to be statistically insignificant when the higher mortality, and therefore shorter average exposure to the atherogenic diet, in the copper group was considered. Microscopic examination revealed a similar histological picture in all three groups, differing only in the degree of vessel wall involvement.

It is interesting to note that while zinc supplemented rabbits on the atherogenic regimen demonstrated the greatest degree of atheromatous involvement, their aortic tissue had a significant reduction in zinc content (Fig. 3). Further analysis revealed that a linear decrease in aortic tissue zinc correlates with increased severity of aortic atherosclerosis. Fig. 4 is a scattergram of all aortic tissue zinc values plotted against the degree of atherosclerotic disease, regardless of the experimental group. The calculated correlation coefficient is significant ($r = -0.72$). Aortic tissue copper concentration and atheromatous involvement show no correlation.

DISCUSSION

Our finding that oral zinc supplementation does not significantly influence the serum zinc concentration in nondeficient states agrees with the reports by J. K. Miller [999] and Ott [1132]. Furchner [506], and W. J. Miller et al. [1002] demonstrated decreased retention and increased turnover of ^{65}Zn in animals on oral zinc supplementation in the absence of zinc deficiency.

The cause of the 30% decrease in the serum zinc concentration of all control groups over the six months is not entirely clear. Since our chow, and that of our rabbit supplier was manufactured by the same company, a change in diet can be ruled out as the cause for the observed decrease. W. J. Miller et al. [1002] found that younger animals have a higher affinity than older animals for zinc, even though there is no significant difference in their respective absorptive capacities. Analysis of the available human data [669] revealed a significantly lower serum zinc concentration for "normal nonatherosclerotic" patients over 40 years (107.5 ± 14 µg%) as compared to those under 40 years of age (124.3 ± 14.4 µg%; $p < 0.02$). Although the available data are not absolutely conclusive, they strongly suggest that serum zinc levels decrease with age.

An additional and more rapid decrease in serum zinc levels occurred in the cholesterol supplemented groups during the two-month interval on regular diet, i.e. during the time period of reduction of serum cholesterol levels from an extreme hypercholesterolemia. We interpret this decrease as being caused by an increased demand for zinc during the period when cholesterol is being mobilized and excreted from the body, a process accomplished primarily by the liver. This increased demand for zinc is not observed during cholesterol storage.

The absence of any significant difference in aortic copper concentrations between normal and even severely atherosclerotic aortas supports the fact that the correlation between decreased aortic tissue zinc levels and increased atherosclerosis is not purely a matter of dilution of the zinc content by lipid infiltration of the vessel wall. If that were the case, one would expect to find a similar dilutional effect on tissue copper content, unless there was an exactly offsetting increase in tissue copper, which is highly unlikely.

Our data show that dietary zinc supplementation of an highcholesterol diet enhances the atherogenic action of this diet while decreasing the zinc content of the aortic tissue. Regarding these findings, we postulate that while zinc may be directly involved in hepatic cholesterol metabolism, the decrease in aortic tissue zinc content reflects the diminished metabolic activity of this tissue resulting from the atherosclerotic involvement of the blood vessel.

SUMMARY

In summary, we have shown that: (1) in our hands, copper has no apparent relationship with atherogenesis; (2) in an experimental animal model, as well as in man, there appears to be a decrease in serum zinc concentration with increasing age; (3) serum zinc levels, but not copper levels, are affected by the state of cholesterol metabolism; (4) increased atherosclerosis is associated with decreased aortic tissue zinc concentrations; and (5) in contrast to clinical studies reporting beneficial effects of oral $ZnSO_4$ treatment in human atherosclerotic subjects, we found zinc supplementation of an atherogenic diet resulted in the enhancement of aortic atheromatous involvement.

Discussion Following Dr. Vergroesen's Paper

Dr. Wissler: I would like to relate this very valuable study to the extreme atherogenic effect of coconut oil, which Dr. Malmros in Sweden and our group have observed in several species. Coconut oil, which contains abundant lauric acid, seems to be capable of stimulating medial cell proliferation and, apparently, hepatic cholesterol synthesis. Did you test coconut oil in comparison with the trilaurate that you used in these diets?

Dr. Vergroesen: The well-known effect of coconut oil, inducing high blood-cholesterol levels, might explain its atherogenic influence. In the present experiment feeding glyceryl trilaurate induced increased serum cholesterol and phospholipid values. The atherogenic effect of coconut oil might be explained by its high lauric acid content (ca. 50%).

Dr. Hashim: I wonder if the diarrhea is in fact steatorrhea? How much lower did the melting point of dietary fat become with incorporation of 10% safflower oil with trilaurin?

Dr. Vergroesen: The diarrhea was not caused by steatorrhea. The body weight was maintained as constant after the first experimental week, even though the trilaurate group consumed less calories than the other groups.

Dr. Thomasson: I would like to comment on the remarks by Dr. Keys (p. 399).

In the present investigation two experimental factors have been tested: (1) the type, and (2), the dosage level of dietary fat. The three types of fat, i.e. trilaurate, olive oil, and safflower oil have been extensively studied previously [1465]. Replacement of these fats by one another does indeed mean interchange of saturated monounsaturated and diunsaturated fatty acids; thus an increase of one of these fatty acids implies a decrease of one or both of the others. However, the main purpose of the present study was to learn the effect of the replacement of carbohydrates by one of these fats in the diet. This does not involve an interchange of the type of fatty acids, but a substitution of fatty acids for carbohydrates. The replacement of carbohydrates by saturated fatty acids induced an increase and by diunsaturated, a decrease of blood lipids, while replacement of carbohydrates by monounsaturated fatty acids gave scarcely any change in the blood lipid level.

Dr. HOWARD: Dr. Collins, did you actually characterize the HDL by ultracentrifugation or paper electrophoresis?

Dr. COLLINS: It was done by paper electrophoresis and ultracentrifugation of density fractions.

Dr. THOMASSON: Dr. Collins saw skin lesions in this patient. Did he see any reaction when he applied the linoleic acid therapy? Was the skin lesion cured?

Dr. COLLINS: Yes, when we gave the fat transfusion the skin lesions on his forehead, face, one arm and thigh disappeared, and they returned when the fat was stopped, only to disappear again when the fat was resumed.

Dr. BIERMAN: Was the addition of linoleic acid and fat to the diet an isocaloric substitution? Thus, can the effect on plasma triglyceride concentration be explained simply by a reduction in the proportion of calories from dietary carbohydrate?

Dr. COLLINS: This was an isocaloric substitution of a fat-free diet for one with fat in it.

Dr. HASHIM: How much linoleic acid did the patient have, for example, in his adipose tissue, prior to his surgical calamity?

Dr. COLLINS: He had been without fat for 100 days when he developed these lesions. We don't have any idea as to the proportion of linoleic acid in his body. I will say that the arachidonic acid was low. We suspect that if we had examined his body tissue we would have found quite a lot of linoleic acid; it was just the uneven distribution within his tissues.

Dr. FURMAN: In view of the high proportion of serum triglyceride ascribable to the HDL, do you have any information relative to the protein/lipid ratio, cholesterol/phospholipid ratio or any immunologic verification of lipoprotein A in the HDL fraction?

Dr. COLLINS: No, it took us very much by surprise. We knew from the paper electrophoresis and total triglycerides that he was high in triglycerides. When we found very little VLDL we could not believe it. The serum was reasonably clear, but beyond doing a separation of the VLDL, LDL, and HDL, we did no further fractionations.

Discussion Following Dr. Schlierf's Paper

Dr. BIERMAN: Dr. Schlierf, we and others have found that there is a direct relationship between the degree or adiposity and insulin levels, and that the basal insulin level in man is as close an index of adiposity as any other measurement. Thus, one cannot compare two groups of patients with regard to metabolic parameters unless they are grossly matched with regard to both body weight and basal insulin levels. The marked difference in basal insulin levels between your two groups of patients suggests that they were not matched with regard to weight. I wonder if you would comment on that point?

Dr. SCHLIERF: Your point is well taken, Dr. Bierman. The mean weight indices of the two groups were 0.93 (normals) and 0.77 (hyperlipemics) respectively. Nevertheless, our thinking that hyperinsulinism under the experimental conditions used may not solely be related to obesity, can be supported on two counts.

1. By covariate analysis, which estimates that portion of excessive postprandial insulin increase which is related to obesity and then feeds this data into the analysis of variance, a significant difference of insulin areas between the two experimental groups still persists.

2. By eliminating the effect of obesity on postglucose plasma insulin levels, according to your proposal [Bierman et al., Amer. J. clin. Nutr. *21*, 1434 (1968)] through the expression of plasma insulin values as a percentage of the fasting values, it can also be supported. When this is done in the subjects of the present study, hyperinsulinism is still apparent.

In contrast, when either procedure is performed with plasma insulin profiles following glucose loading, we find no evidence of hyperinsulinism in the same subjects. This is in agreement with findings published by your group, by Levy and Glueck and by Dr. Nikkila. Given, therefore, the findings of normal insulin response to glucose, on the one hand, and of an excessive response to a mixed formula diet, on the other, we would like to advance the concept of other dietary constituents being responsible for the hyperinsulinemia.

Dr. BIERMAN: This seems unnecessarily complicated. It might be easier to get weight and age-matched controls.

Dr. SCHLIERF: In order to find volunteers willing to go through the two 24-hour procedures and two 5-day periods of dietary preparation, we had to rely on medical students, whose weight indices were slightly below those of the patients, as mentioned.

Dr. AHRENS: Dr. Schlierf, you showed us some very interesting data in which you questioned whether it was not preferable to suffer a low grade hyperglyceridemia day in and day out than to risk the higher rises in glycerides that are seen after the ingestion of high-fat diets. We cannot forget that the hyperglyceridemia of the high-fat diet is a chylomicronemia, whereas the hyperglyceridemia induced by the carbohydrate diet is characterized by an elevation of prebeta lipoproteins. These are very different kinds of molecular aggregates, and it is as yet unknown which type is the more atherogenic. However, I know of no evidence for any of the complications of ischemic heart disease in any patient with the chylomicronemia caused by lipoprotein lipase deficiency. On the other hand, the increased incidence of ischemic heart disease in patients with any form of carbohydrate-induced hyperglyceridemia is now widely recognized. At first glance, this argues that persistent chylomicronemia poses no increased risk to life, while persistent hyper-pre-beta lipoproteinemia does.

Dr. SCHLIERF: It may not be valid to compare chylomicronemia in Type I disease with that in Type IV or for that matter in normal subjects. In the first group of people, the basic defect is related to an inability to properly metabolize chylomicrons due to lipoprotein lipase deficiency. Dr. Kuo and coworkers [Circulat. Res. *16*, 221 (1965)] have suggested that this very defect which results in delayed uptake of chylomicrons by adipose tissue may also be pertinent to the uptake of chylomicron lipids by the vessel wall. It is, therefore, possible that the same chylomicrons which do not hurt a Type I patient, may very well be harmful to others.

Discussion Following Dr. Buchwald's Paper

Dr. Blankenhorn: Would Dr. Buchwald comment on the weight loss that is seen; and could he specify the sort of anesthesia he is using and the average length of the procedure? This may be important because the operation is now being done in other parts of the country, from time to time, and the results are not always as consistent as his. It is possible that other surgeons using other sorts of anesthesia and, possibly, different technical procedures, might account for some of the different results which are occasionally obtained.

Dr. Buchwald: These patients do not have any sustained weight loss. They have the immediate weight loss of any person following surgery; they rapidly regain this weight. This operation is a one-third bypass. It should not be confused with the 90% bypass practiced by many people for obese patient therapy. In regard to our operative time and selection of anesthesia, all of our patients have had general induction anesthesia because our anesthesiologists believe this is safer than the regional type of anesthesia. The operation takes roughly about two hours skin to skin.

Concerning operative mortality, we have had one death four days post-operation from a myocardial infarction. That gives us a current operative mortality in this high risk group of 1.4%.

Dr. Kachidurian: I would like to ask two questions. First, did the xanthomatous lesions decrease in the homozygous patient? Secondly, was the diagnosis of Type II hyperlipoproteinemia based on phenotype alone, or does it include genetic studies?

Dr. Buchwald: In our homozygous patient, the xanthomata did not decrease. I think I would have to say the diagnosis was made on the basis of electrophoretic staining and the serum cholesterol and triglyceride levels.

Dr. Furman: I am very interested in the application of this procedure to children and would like to know if you have had sufficient experience to date to tell us whether the growth curves of these children are influenced in any way.

Dr. Buchwald: I cannot tell you specifically in the children upon whom we have operated. We hesitated to do children for the first five years. Only this past year have we actually launched into a pediatric study. However, if you can make any translation of data from the rabbit, the lipid lowering effect is comparable to these people in the adult rabbit; yet there is absolutely no interference with growth and development. We have also reviewed records of children who were born with omphaloceles and have long segments of the small intestine resected at birth. These children, if they get over their initial trial, survive with a normal growth curve.

Discussion Following Dr. Fleischman's Paper

Dr. Taylor: Dr. George M. Haas, has been doing some work with vitamin D plus the injection of nicotine. With the induction of a principally calcific arteriopathy in rabbits by a combination of nicotine and vitamin D administration, it could be shown that only one-twentieth as much vitamin D was required when in combination with nicotine, as when vitamin D was given alone, to get comparable calcific lesions. In addition, these rabbits developed arteritis and thrombosis. We have obtained similar results with comparable treatment of macaca mulatta Rhesus monkeys (Amer. J. Path.).

Dr. Kummerow: There may be another explanation for your observations. It has recently been suggested that the fat soluble vitamins may be involved in the arrangement or the positional specificity of the lipid components in cell membranes. Norman et al. [Amer. J. clin. Nutr. **22**, 396 (1969)] have suspected vitamin D of acting or stimulating "the biochemical expression of genetic information" and evidence has been obtained for the binding through hydrophobic linkage of beta-carotene to membrane proteins [Biochim. biophys. Acta **150**, 676 (1968)]. Furthermore, Van Deenen and coworkers [J. Colloid and Interface Sci. **29**, 381 (1969)] have shown that a difference in the degree of unsaturation and the position of saturated fatty acids in phospholipids influence their interfacial characteristics. It is possible that the assembly of lipoproteins is influenced by vitamin D and that your methods may be useful in the study of the assembly of the serum lipoproteins.

The diffusion of lipids through the intima cells in the arteries may occur after a subtle change in the orientation of the lipids in these cell membranes has occurred. This change in orientation may allow lipids to diffuse across the cell membrane and infiltrate the cell. Dr. Levy has suggested that positively-charged lipoproteins may combine with negatively charged mucopolysaccharides. However, the combination between the lipoproteins and mucopolysaccharides may involve subtle changes in interfacial characteristics rather than the combination of charges. Furthermore, fat analyses indicate that the lipid rather than the total beta lipoprotein seems to diffuse into the cell. This observation seems to rule out the concept of lipid precipitation or combination with the mucopolysaccharides in aortic tissue. On the other hand, such a combination may change the character of the cell membrane sufficiently to allow for the diffusion of lipid into the cell.

Dr. Fleischman: Dr. Kodicek in a review article reported that many have now found a distortion in the arrangement of the lipoprotein macromolecule in the presence of vitamin D (i.e. its shape is changed), and this may have some influence on hypercholesteremia, atherogenesis, or adsorption.

Dr. Dempsey: We have seen that vitamin D, depending upon the concentration, can accelerate cholesterol synthesis by liver homogenates. This is a direct effect, and could be what is happening in your studies, *in vivo*.

Discussion Following Dr. Harman's Paper and Dr. Filo's Paper

Dr. Hirsch: Dr. Harman, ceroid is thought to be the end-product of lipid peroxidation, and ceroid is found in mature atherosclerotic lesions. Have you stained your aortas and looked for ceroid? Also, do you have any idea of the antioxidant content of the pigs' sera or of the safflower oil which was fed them? This might also bear on your results.

Dr. Harman: We did not stain specifically for ceroid, just for fat. The serum vitamin E level in the lard groups was about 0.3 mg/100 ml, and in the safflower groups about 0.5 mg/100 ml. Microscopic examination of testicular tissue did not show evidence of vitamin E deficiency.

We have done a fair number of experiments in regard to copper in rabbits. Our experimental design was different from Dr. Filo's in that we used higher dietary copper levels. We have studied the effect of different lipids in the diet along with the copper. By and large, we can say that the rabbit data is consistent with the possibility, as indicated in the pigs, that the lipid peroxidation does enhance atherosclerosis to some extent.

Dr. Wissler: There is one other possible explanation for the differing results between the pig and rabbit that ought to be considered. We have published some of the evidence that there may be quite a difference in pathogenesis of the atheromatous lesions in these two species, and I think this always has to be kept in mind when one sees this kind of difference between the two species.

Dr. Pfeiffer: Dr. Harman mentioned that he kept pigs on the diet for two years. Has he done any analysis of the data after two years?

Dr. Harman: The data I showed here was after the animals were autopsied, after they had been on the diets for 21 months. In other words, at this time the pigs were about 26 months of age.

Dr. Pfeiffer: I asked this because I kept animals between 5 and 6.5 years on such a diet, and the cholesterol levels did not stay up. I noticed your higher cholesterol levels were 120, and they later went down. I found that they will continue to go down to the 50 mg level. I did not see a progressive increase of atheromata. At least I am encouraged to hear that you are not getting massive atherosclerosis in 6 months, which several investigators have reported.

Dr. Howard: Dr. Filo, do you think your data on dietary zinc would fit in with the water factor, because there will be more zinc in soft water if it is in contact with zinc vessels?

Dr. Filo: I can't answer the question because we don't know what the zinc content of soft water is. There is considerable data from previous zinc studies to indicate that none of our animals were in a zinc deficient state. On the other hand, the amount of zinc added was not at a toxic level. This was an intermediate level of zinc, according to data in other animals.

The fact is that we got a rather paradoxical result; increased supplementation gave enhancement of atherosclerosis, yet the tissues showed a decrease in the amount of zinc present. This we can't really explain.

Dr. Howard: This was independent of an effect on cholesterol, presumably?

Dr. Filo: Yes, it was completely independent. Furthermore, we found that with copper and zinc (and this has been reported by other investigators also) the serum levels were not good indicators as to what was going on in the tissues, either in the liver or the aorta.

Dr. Howard: Might the increased zinc content be explained by the great increase in fat in the vessel wall?

Dr. Filo: This was our first thought, but we had a built-in control. We were doing simultaneous zinc and copper determinations on the same vessel, and if this was indeed a dilutional effect, we should have seen similar changes in copper levels but we did not.

Dr. WOLF: Dr. Filo reported a high mortality in the animals fed copper. Would he comment on the cause of death?

Dr. FILO: The animals that died in the group with copper supplementation had far advanced hepatic cirrhosis in four out of the five animals. One of the animals developed a middle ear infection.

Dr. FEIGENBAUM: I wanted to question the need for a 2% cholesterol diet in rabbits. It has been shown a number of times, especially by Prior a number of years ago, that a high cholesterol diet in the rabbit will cause deterioration in almost all tissues of the body. We have found in feeding graded levels of cholesterol that by the time we reached 1% cholesterol in the diet, we could no longer establish any kind of relationship between serum cholesterol and atheromata. At a quarter percent or a half percent, we had very good correlation.

Dr. FILO: I would agree that this is a valid criticism. The only comment that I would make is that we were trying to cause marked atherosclerosis in a relatively short period of time, e.g. six months.

Section XIV

PANEL DISCUSSION ON PATHOGENESIS AS IT MAY INFLUENCE PREVENTION AND THERAPY

PANEL DISCUSSION ON PATHOGENESIS AS IT MAY INFLUENCE PREVENTION AND THERAPY

Dr. WOLF: Drs. McMillan, Kritchevsky, and Groen, if we assume from our experiences in the last few days that we have now the quintessence of available information about the pathogenesis of atherosclerosis, what do you need to do next?

Dr. McMILLAN: Well, it seemed to me that two large issues in pathogenesis particularly rich in critical content and unknown information still remain. One of these is the question as to whether childhood and adolescent fatty flecks or streaks go on to become fibrous plaques and atheromas of clinical significance. The question is generated by world wide observations in geographic pathology which indicate that the child and young adolescent have about the same amount of fatty flecking and streaking of the aorta. Yet, the adult populations of which the young people are antecedent may develop significant atherosclerosis to very different degrees.

For example, in New Orleans both Caucasian and black populations develop significant clinical disease. In some other parts of the world, the progression is slight and clinical disease is minor. Now, it appears that there exists here a pathogenetic model in man which contains the germ of critical knowledge as to what leads to progressive atheroma. Even if it should transpire that the fatty flecks and streaks are not related to the adult lesion, I think one will obtain pediatric and nutritional information of importance to public health.

It is traditional in the teaching of pathology of arteriosclerosis that the fatty fleck or streak is, indeed, the precursor of the adult lesions. This an idea which has much circumstantial evidence to support it. Somewhere in this period of life, perhaps in the chemistry and biology of the vessel wall or perhaps in the transport of lipids, there may lie a critical key as to what does, indeed, lead to significant atheroma.

The second point, while of little interest if one is concerned with the biology of prevention, is of great public health and clinical interest. It is the question of whether arteriosclerotic lesions regress. There is some evidence that this may be true, but it is not conclusive. I believe intuitively that atheromas can regress, but evidence for this is such that I can't defend my position very well. It is important to determine whether arteriosclerosis can regress, and if it does regress, to learn the manner of its regression.

What one means by regression in this context is merely a failure to further initiate clinical disease. It may also be that what one means is an absolute disappearance. The distinction between these two choices is not exclusive and there are others. I suggest that there exists an opportunity to bring forward new pathogenetic information that could have a critical influence on public health and therapy attitudes towards arteriosclerotic disease.

Dr. KRITCHEVSKY: I think that one area which has been somewhat neglected in the past but is now receiving considerable attention is the metabolism of the arterial wall. The site of the lesion must have our attention. I would like to know, for instance, what signal causes the initial proliferation in the artery. If it is an injury, what type of injury? Is it due to a metabolic change caused by a psychological signal?

When we study the chemistry of the artery, we find that one great difference between the young, normal artery and the aging and/or atheromatous artery is the large amount of ester cholesterol present in the latter. We have heard these last few days that the perifibrous lesion exhibits a cholesteryl ester fatty acid spectrum similar to that in the serum. This might correspond to initial deposition of lipid from the serum. With time, the ratio of oleic to linoleic acids becomes reversed, and there is more cholesteryl oleate than linoleate. This, then, may be an expression of cholesterol esterification. We know the artery can synthesize fatty acids, but it can not synthesize linoleic acid, an essential fatty acid.

The question, then, is this. How does the ester get into the arterial wall; why does it remain there; and, if this increase is indeed an expression of the development of the lesion, how can we get rid of the ester cholesterol? There are not many studies which focus on this point. The work of Zemplényi suggests differences in rates of hydrolysis among species. The work of Bowyer and his colleagues also suggests differences in rates of hydrolysis of different cholesteryl esters. There are probably differences in rates of synthesis, as well. Dr. Rothblat's work on the uptake of cholesterol by cells in tissue culture indicates that free cholesterol can be taken up and discharged readily. Ester cholesterol is not taken up readily, and the cell does not excrete cholesteryl esters *per se* at all. In order for the cell to excrete this cholesterol, the ester must first be hydrolyzed. Consequently, perhaps we should find out more about the possibility of inducing aortic cholesteryl ester hydrolase, by use of drugs, diet, or other means. Even if hydrolase activity is increased, it may be necessary to have low serum cholesterol levels so that the cell does not have to work against the gradient to excrete cholesterol easily.

Now, as to the question of the role of phospholipid in the arterial wall, Zilversmit and his associates have shown that the artery synthesizes phospholipid. Our work on the uptake of cholesterol by cells shows that addition of phospholipid to a medium containing just cholesterol and protein inhibits cholesterol uptake, with each phospholipid appearing to have its own index of inhibition.

As to the question of connective tissue, Drs. Kramsch and Robert have shown that lipids of the right size may be trapped by elastin. Is there a way to prevent this trapping, or to spring the trap? Very little has been done in this direction. I think that if we first have a better idea of the aspects of arterial metabolism, we will be able to follow the biblical path and proceed from atherogenesis to atheroexodus.

Dr. WOLF: Now, I turn to the clinical epidemiologist, Dr. Groen, and ask the same question.

Dr. GROEN: I have learned many interesting details about the role of platelet aggregation in lipidemia and about the metabolism of the arterial wall during this Symposium. I have also learned the accuracy by which epidemiologists can now measure the weight of certain risk factors and with what degree of probability they can predict the occurrence of coronary heart disease. However, what has impressed me most is that the more these risk factors are defined quantitatively, the more it becomes obvious that they are insufficient for a satisfactory prediction.

Especially puzzling, as we have heard, is the fact that diet, although so obviously an important causative factor, when applied to the comparison between different population groups, appears to be a poor predictive factor for the individual's risk of acquiring coronary heart disease within his group. It is especially this puzzling discrepancy which makes us hesitate to promise the public that if people would only go on a diet, they would remain free of the disease. It is therefore obvious, as Dr. Strong has formulated it, that there must be still other risk factors at present unknown to us. In what direction can we look for them?

It seems to me that the answer is given in the study of the disease in different populations. The most important result of all comparative epidemiological studies is that there are population groups who hardly have this disease. Anyone who has lived close to such a group can not fail to know the reason for the scarcity of the disease. These different populations differ not only in their diet but also in smoking habits and way of life. Living within a culture in a population means much more than just eating, smoking, and physical activity; it entails interhuman communication. The next task, therefore, is to introduce in our epidemiological studies measurements of these different forms of interhuman communications and the specific frustrations and conflicts which occur as a result of them. The way to do this is to engage the help of people who study people. That is, it is time to cooperate with and benefit from the work of sociologists and social psychologists, just as medicine has derived so much benefit from cooperation with biochemists and experimental pathologists.

I would like to illustrate this thesis by showing some results we obtained with the cooperation of sociologists and social psychologists in our epidemiological studies in Israel.

The basic data of the sociological study showed that the disease among 744 workers in the Port of Haifa is not only distributed differently according to age, sex, region of birth, serum cholesterol content and physical activity, but also by occupation. Skilled and unskilled workers, which makes little difference nowadays, have a very low frequency of myocardial infarct in this prevalence study, and the total prevalence of coronary heart disease, adding together infarcts and angina pectoris, was about 3%. In contrast, the white collar workers had 4% myocardial infarcts, almost ten times as many, and four times as many with coronary heart disease. The customs police, and so on, were in between. This difference was not explicable by age distribution, but there was also no difference in the cholesterol content of these groups. We inquired further into this finding, just as sociologists do, by use of other items in the questionaire by which they measure "job responsibility". We found a very good correlation between myocardial infarction and the way people fill out questionaires about job responsibility. Among those with a high job responsibility, myocardial infarct occurred in 7.9% (many more than the number expected). The prevalence was much less among those with jobs of moderate and low levels of responsibility, and the same was true for total coronary heart disease.

Next, let us look at the answer of the study population to a simple question: "Did you have any work problems in the past?" This was to test the hypothesis which my Dutch colleagues and I had developed from previous studies, that is, the specific frustrations that play a role in the etiology of coronary heart disease are associated with the dominance-submission conflict between the male and the female and between father and children in the family situation and with similar dominance-submission conflicts in work situations. Those who said they had very many or many work problems in the past had 5.8% myocardial infarcts in this prevalence study. Those with only some or no work problems had 1.4%, and the same difference held for total coronary heart disease.

Among the many other questions was: "Do your coworkers like you?" This was asked to see not only if the subjects had conflicts with their coworkers, but above all, whether they subjectively experienced those conflicts and could acknowledge them. Of those who said, "My coworkers like me very much or fairly much", 2.2% had had a myocardial infarct. Those who felt that their coworkers were either indifferent to them or did not like them had a rate of 4.1%, and the same was true for total coronary heart disease.

When we combine the situation of having work problems with the feeling of not being liked by coworkers, we get more data. In the group of people with work problems who said they were not liked, there was no less than 24.4% who had some sign of coronary disease, and 7.3% had had a myocardial infarct. At the other extreme, among those who said there were no work problems and who felt they were liked, 2.7% had coronary heart disease and 0.8% had evidence of a previous myocardial infarct. Now, 0.8% of myocardial infarct in a group is a very low prevalence. It almost approaches the figure for Yemenites and Bedouin. Yet, there were no Yemenites or Bedouin in this population. This difference is present in all age groups, and it was not explained by the serum cholesterol levels.

Another piece of evidence was obtained from another sociological study in which we examined 400 people who had been consecutively autopsied. We sent the sociological investigators to the homes of the first-degree relatives, who were asked this same question. "Did the deceased have work problems in the past?" In this group of 398 consecutive autopsied people of whom we could find first-degree relatives, 30% had a myocardial infarct, proven at autopsy, when they had many work problems, and only 17% had an infarct among those who had none or few work problems. For the males, the numbers were 31 and 20; the females in this group were so few that we can't be sure of the significance.

One wonders whether the difference between the ethnic groups in Israel in their proneness to coronary heart disease could relate not only to such factors as nutrition, serum cholesterol, or exercise, but also to the fact that some ethnic groups have problems in their work, while others have less of these problems.

In comparing the prevalence of coronary heart disease among the Bedouin in the Niger desert, a group of Arab villagers, and this same group of Port of Haifa workers, there were 744, 253, and 510 male individuals between 30 and 70. Among the Haifa Port workers, almost all of them Jewish, there were 22.9%

unhappy individuals who said that they had very many or many work problems, and 77% said they had none. However among the Bedouin, only 2% said they had problems in their work; 75% never had any problems, and 21% had never worked. The Arab villagers were in between. We have, indeed, a clear differentiation of these three populations as regards work problems.

Now let us compare the prevalence of coronary heart disease. Among 510 Bedouin, there was only one case of myocardial infarction, that is 0.2%. He was in the group containing some or no work problems. Among 253 Arab villagers, three had a myocardial infarct (1.2%). Of those, two were in the no work problem group and one was in the many work problem group. Among the 744 Jews of Haifa, there were 171 with very many and many work problems. They had 5.8% with myocardial infarcts (10cases). The other group of 573 with no work problems had 1.5% infarcts. The sociologists have concluded, and I feel they had the same right as we had with our cholesterol studies, that myocardial infarct was related to having had work problems in the past.

There is insufficient time to show you the results of the complete study. It has only been touched upon as an answer to Dr. Wolf's question: "What can we do in the future?" One of the things that we could and should do is build into our epidemiological, especially the longitudinal, incidence studies, measurements of so-called psychosocial factors that have been hypothesized as playing a role in causation of the disease. It is usually said, "Yes, but I don't know how to measure these factors." The problem is not in measurement alone, although this is a very difficult problem, but whether we are willing to be taught by others how to develop the methods to measure them!

Let me finish with an anecdote. Here in America, about a year ago, a new President was elected. Every time this happens, I am filled with admiration for the accuracy with which the political/social scientists predict, although the ballot is secret, not only who is going to be elected, but even quantitatively by what percentage of the votes. It seems to me these social scientists have progressed further in determining the "risk" of being elected President of the United States than we have in determining the risk of coronary disease.

Dr. Wolf: Thank you, Dr. Groen, for pointing out the toxic factor in exercise. To further emphasize the problems of fatigue, I remind you that Wexler found spontaneous atherosclerosis predominantly in repeatedly bred male and female rats [1539].

With respect to psychological forces, of course, the nervous system becomes relevant, and we have at least two studies in which stimulation or damage to the brain is associated with acceleration of atherosclerosis, one by Gunn, Friedman and Byers, and one by Somoza [586, 1385].

To further understand the process of atherosclerosis we need to know what mechanical forces do to the metabolism of the arterial wall, and particularly what pulsatile flow may do. We have been shown that a proliferation of smooth muscle cells occurs in the normal aorta at the bifurcation. Such cellular proliferation is thought to be a very early sign of atherosclerosis. I call attention to Bjurulf's study from Lund, Sweden, in which he correlated the occurrence of cerebral arteriosclerosis with the height of individuals [185].

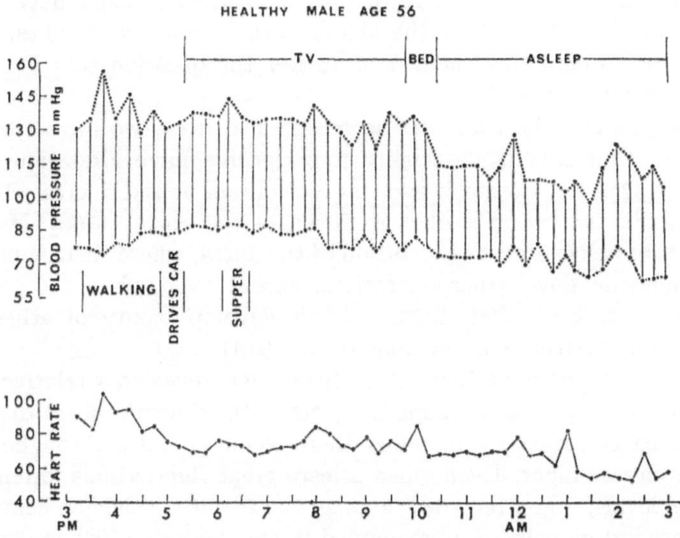

Fig. 1. Automatically recorded blood pressure in a healthy control subject over a 12-hour period

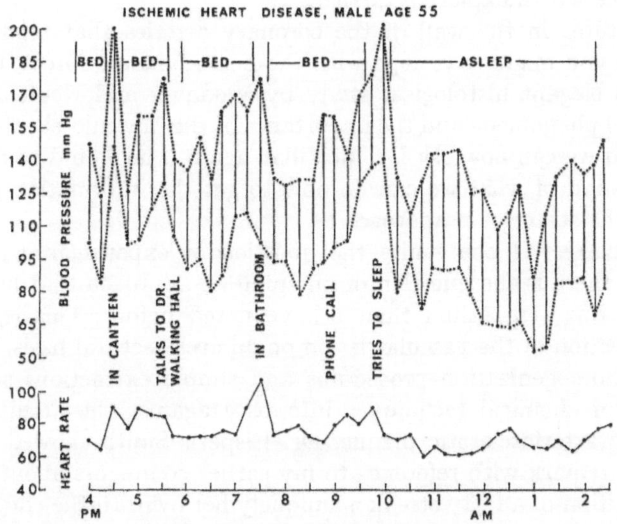

Fig. 2. Marked variability of blood pressure as automatically recorded in a subject with ischemic heart disease

It has been nearly sixty years since the first feeding experiments of Ignatowski produced atherosclerosis in rabbits [733]. Many thousands of rabbits and samples of their blood have been studied since then, and yet mechanical factors secondary to alterations in the composition of the blood have not been looked for very vigorously. Collaborative studies might have illuminated possible hemodynamic effects of altered composition of blood.

It would also have been interesting to have accompanied developing biochemical changes in the wall of the artery with histological studies. Such collaborative efforts might have helped to answer the question that Dr. McMillan has raised as to what came first.

To further pursue the leads in the mechanical area, we have the evidence of Daly et al., that rats made renally hypertensive have alterations in aortic metabolism [352]. Dr. Neufeld and his coworkers found increased coronary atherosclerosis in the presence of coarctation of the aorta [1506]. Mestel et al. have shown that below a partial occlusion of the aorta, where there is presumably a reduced pulsatile flow, atherosclerosis is absent even when the animals are fed a highly atherogenic diet. Such animals develop plenty of atherosclerosis above the partial obstruction, but none below [914].

Studies by a colleague of mine, R. A. Schneider, revealed a relatively greater variability in blood pressure among subjects with ischemic heart disease than among matched controls. He recorded their blood pressure throughout twelve hours of the day or night. Even when asleep, great fluctuations, often reaching hypertensive levels, were recorded among those with ischemic heart disease, although these individuals, when examined in the doctor's office under ordinary circumstances, were not hypertensive (Figs. 1 and 2). From all these fragments of evidence, it would appear that the variability in stress on the walls of the arteries may be worth exploring further.

The structures in the wall of the coronary arteries that tend to resist the stretching or, you might say, cope with the hemodynamic forces, have been the subject of an elegant histological study by Vlodaver and Neufeld. They stress developmental phenomena and the importance of the musculo-elastic layer [1505].

I wonder if we can now ask Dr. McMillan again if he would go a little further with the question of what we can do now to get the information that we need. What about the strategy of approach?

Dr. McMillan: If one limits the question of experimental approaches to pathogenesis, there is the question of pursuing an approach that has been better developed at this symposium than I have noted before. This is, namely, the chemical dissection of the vascular lesion on an architectural basis, moving away from simple homogenization procedures and simple extractions so as to bring the elegance of chemical techniques into play against the architectural background of the arteriosclerotic plaque. Dr. Elspeth Smith showed something of this. I should remark with reference to my earlier comments about fatty streaks that her definition of a fatty streak is uniquely her own. In the common parlance of fatty streaks they are judged by the naked eye. She requires that one look at them microscopically in order to identify those that have fat-filled cells as opposed to those that have a perifibrous deposition of lipid. Leaving this aside, there appears to be the opportunity now to match both qualitatively and quantifiably architecture and chemical properties in a detail that has not been possible before; this can be pursued.

The problems I referred to were human problems, more particularly the question of progression of adolescent lesions into those of adult life and human clinical disease. I don't believe that there is an equivalent animal model at the present time. The problem has not attracted enough attention to know whether there is an animal model that would serve to determine critically what there may be about this period of late adolescence and young adult life that allows progression of lesions, if indeed this is what happens. The question of regression can be approached in the animal model. Few of us have had the patience even to think about it.

The possibility of attempting to leap-frog detailed pathogenic information is very real. As Dr. Keys pointed out, most of us would agree that preventive interventions and evaluation trials are important issues before us. If intervention and field trial evaluations had shown that one could prevent the complications of atherosclerosis or the progression of atherosclerosis, much of the detailed knowledge of pathogenesis would have been leap-frogged.

Dr. Wolf: Dr. Kritchevsky, will you tackle the question of strategy?

Dr. Kritchesvky: To attack the question of arterial metabolism, it would be best if a suitable *in vitro* model were available. Tissue culture systems could be one answer to this. Today knowing what we do about the chemical differences between the normal and diseased artery, we could test these factors for their effect on the metabolism of this suitable model. We could attack the problem, not only from the standpoint of cholesterol metabolism, but also to assess the influence of phospholipids and fatty acids, and furthermore, to see what the effect of the amount and type of lipoproteins in the medium may be. This type of experiment could tell us something about cellular metabolism, but we must always be brought back to the entire animal model. In contrast to the current biological vogue in this field, we have to worry about mega-molecular biology, the whole animal.

The exact function of factors in the diet must also be studied more fully. As Dr. Ahrens clearly pointed out, it is much easier to quantitate what goes in than what comes out. The matter under consideration is not only quantitative but also qualitative differences. Rabbits can be fed a diet in which saturated fat has been added to laboratory chow, and they may not develop either hyperlipemia or atheromata. The same proportion of protein, fat, and carbohydrate in a semisynthetic diet will cause atherosclerosis, and the severity of the lesion can be further affected by the type of fat and carbohydrate used. Evidently, other factors in the diet play an important role. Perhaps one factor is simply dietary bulk. Maybe many of the "native populations" which are being studied are perambulating ion exchange columns. I feel that we may all be captives of our past dietary history and that it may be dangerous to construct too many theories based on drastic alterations in diets of laboratory animals.

Dr. Wolf: In addition to suggesting the possibility that alteration of the composition of blood may have mechanical effects, it is also possible that atheromata have a mediating mechanism in the liver. Another possibility is chemical receptors in the vessels themselves. There has been so much interest attached to receptors in the carotid sinus, arch of aorta, the heart and pulmonary vessels that it has used up the time of many investigators. There is the possibility that alterations in chemical composition of the blood may alter receptor mechanisms and produce reflex changes which express themselves in a trophic way. Most trophic changes in tissue, such as cell renewal, depend on innervation. Therefore, study in this direction may be profitable.

Dr. Groen, would you care to comment further on strategy?

Dr. Groen: Another gap in our knowledge is the hemodynamics of the circulation and especially of the heart during emotional interhuman conflicts. There is a discrepancy between the large amount of knowledge about how the heart and circulation behave during effort as compared with the little information about how the heart behaves during emotional conflict. Yet hyperactivity of the heart during conflict is a matter of daily experience. There are tremendous changes in the heart action during emotional conflicts. Whereas during effort the heart increases its minute volume by an increase in rate so that the stroke volume remains the same, during (especially inhibited) emotion the increase in cardiac output, which can be just as large as during effort, is to a large extent achieved by an increase in stroke volume with a much smaller rise concomitant in rate. An increase in stroke volume is a greater strain on the heart and vessels, especially the coronary vessels. If the peripheral resistance remains the same, it means an increase in systolic pressure. When the peripheral resistance is also increased during emotion, the increase in blood pressure is even greater. This great increase in systolic and often diastolic pressure must cause a great increase in stretch of the coronary and aortic vessels. I wonder if such a stretch of the vessel isn't the trauma which locally damages the intima and the elastica so that platelet aggregation begins.

Thus, I see a useful goal in the future study of the hemodynamics of the circulation during inhibited or self-controlled emotion. That is what I would like to study in animals and man.

Dr. Wolf: This is reminiscent of what we learned yesterday. Dr. Millikan placed a great deal of emphasis on vasomotor regulation with respect to cerebrovascular disease. This is not fashionable in the coronary arteries but it might be very important to restudy them with this in mind.

Finally, a general remark about strategy might be made. First, we have studied mainly why people and animals get atherosclerosis, knowing that many species and individuals are very resistant to it. It might be useful to direct intensive effort toward a study of resistance to atherosclerosis. What factors are involved. This reminds me of the difference between Sherlock Holmes and Sargeant Lastrade. Mr. Lastrade put data together in the most logical way to propose a mechanism and then, when people raised objections, to explain away the thing that didn't fit in a logical manner. This was the technique of Sargeant Lastrade with a murder, and he was always wrong. Sherlock Holmes looked for the thing that didn't fit, and pursued this. Holmes was always right.

Section XV

RECENT ADVANCES IN DRUGS AFFECTING LIPIDS, PLATELETS AND AUTONOMIC NERVE MEDIATORS

DRUGS INHIBITING CHOLESTEROL BIOSYNTHESIS, WITH SPECIAL REFERENCE TO CLOFIBRATE*

DANIEL STEINBERG

Rather than attempt an inclusive and therefore possibly superficial review of drugs affecting sterol biosynthesis, I have chosen to discuss primarily the evidence on the mode of action of clofibrate. This is by all odds the most widely used drug that inhibits cholesterol synthesis, but clearly it has additional biological effects, some as yet unexplained. Before launching into that discussion, however, it may be useful to cast a retrospective eye on the way in which this new area in pharmacology has developed and comment on the directions it may take in the future.

In 1956, when interest in the possibilities of treating hypercholesterolemia with inhibitors of sterol synthesis began to grow, there was great hope that in view of our extensive knowledge of the intimate details of the cholesterol biosynthetic pathway it would be possible to devise specific inhibitors in an intelligent and logical fashion. As a matter of fact, a great deal of work has been done and, at least at the laboratory level, done successfully exactly along these lines. On the other hand, it is a bit humbling to note that the two compounds that have received the greatest attention entered our armentarium by the back door, as it were. Thus, triparanol represented originally a compound that might retain the cholesterol-lowering effects of estrogenic hormones without having, at the same time, their feminizing properties. Its structure is related to that of diethylstilbesterol, but its mechanism of action, of course, turned out to be quite different. It is neither estrogenic nor anti-estrogenic. Its rather specific activity as an inhibitor of sterol Δ^{24}-reductase was unexpected and could not easily have been predicted on structural grounds. In retrospect, now that a number of additional inhibitors acting on the same enzyme have been discovered, a pattern can be discerned involving a diethylaminoethanol or dimethylaminoethanol substitution on a bulky aromatic or steroidal nucleus.

Clofibrate (CPIB), the ethyl ester of p-chlorophenoxyisobutyrate, was prepared by J. M. Thorp and his collaborators at Imperial Chemical Industries again on the basis of its general structural relationship to an estrogenically active allenolic acid derivative. It had no intrinsic estrogenic activity, and the original studies in species other than the rat were disappointing. The pattern of results in rats suggested that the compound might be active by potentiating endogenous hormone activity, perhaps activity of endogenous androsterone [1467]. Androsterone and CPIB combined seemed to be more reliably and reproducibly effective and the combination, Atromid, was brought through the experimental stages to the

* The work herein has been supported in part by U.S.P.H.S. NIH Grant HE-12373.

clinic. Only after clinical trials were well under way was it shown by Hellman and his coworkers [662] and by Oliver [1119] that the androsterone was quite unnecessary and that CPIB alone, Atromid-S, had just as much activity as the combination.

Thus, the basis on which these two important drugs came under study originally was serendipitous. The right drugs became objects of interest for wrong reasons. At the same time, shelves full of compounds had been prepared as structural analogues of known intermediates in sterol biosynthesis and tested for their ability to block that process. Many of them have indeed proven to be effective inhibitors in *in vitro* systems. However, only very few have proven to be effective in experimental animals and still fewer have come to clinical trial.

It would be a mistake to conclude from this that one ought to abandon all attempts at rationality in further pharmacologic research along these lines. In both of these cases, the compounds were originally chosen for study because they were in the right ball park, i.e. they did bear some structural relationship to compounds active in one way or another in relationship to cholesterol metabolism. CPIB, for example, was probably chosen for intensive study in part because of its structural relationship to a previously studied inhibitor, alpha-phenylbutyric acid, which inhibits acetate activation. As it turns out, CPIB *does* have a rather potent activity as an inhibitor of cholesterol synthesis but at a different and more useful point in that pathway. While we certainly have to admit that serendipity has been a valued handmaiden in much that has been accomplished, we need not apologize for doing our groping in the dark, at least in an area where we can reasonably expect to find something. Fleming's discovery of penicillin was a happy accident, intelligently interpreted and pursued, but it would scarcely have been possible if Fleming had not at least been working with bacteria!

Now a few words about which part of the ball park we ought to be in. A great deal of evidence points to the reduction of hydroxymethylglutaryl-CoA to mevalonic acid as the rate limiting step in cholesterol biosynthesis under most circumstances. Consequently, I think we would all be happiest if the target for any drug treatment could be this normally rate limiting reaction, However, the luck of the draw has been such that compounds designed to inhibit at that stage have not proven effective *in vivo*, perhaps because they cannot penetrate the liver cell. We have seen instead a large number of compounds developed that inhibit in the later stages of cholesterol synthesis, subsequent to cyclization of squalene. Because of the earlier disappointing experience with Δ^4-cholestenone and with triparanol, both of which led to accumulation of unwanted sterols with their own potential for atherogenesis, we are all justifiably skeptical about the possible value of inhibitors of this kind. Certainly replacement of cholesterol by dihydrocholesterol, as with Δ^4-cholestenone, or by desmosterol, as in the case of triparanol, represents only a Pyrrhic victory over hypercholesterolemia. However the pendulum may have swung too far on this score. First, it does not necessarily follow that every inhibitor in the later stages of cholesterol biosynthesis will necessarily lead to accumulation of intermediates *in the plasma*, even though the intermediates may accumulate in the liver. Secondly, the atherogenecity of other sterol intermediates has not been explicitly studied, and there may be some that do not share the atherogenic potential of cholesterol and desmosterol. And, finally, it is not certain that toxic side effects of drugs like triparanol are rightly attributable to either the inhibition of sterol synthesis *per se* or to the accumulation of sterol intermediates. In the case of triparanol, there are unacceptable side effects, but there is some reason to believe that these are due to concurrent and possibly independent metabolic effects of the drug and not due to the desmosterol accumulation resulting from inhibition. If this were to be the case, then other compounds might be found that are effective inhibitors, possibly even at the same step, and yet lack the additional metabolic effects that lead to serious side effects. Obviously, one would have to be extremely careful in evaluating and demonstrating safety, but it is not out of the question.

A good deal of research, in fact, continues on inhibitors in the latter stages of cholesterol synthesis. The biochemists have enjoyed a field day using these compounds as tools for study of cholesterol metabolism. Dempsey, Frantz and their collaborators in Minneapolis and Avigan, Goodman and myself in Bethesda have found these inhibitors valuable tools in studying the pathway of sterol modification beyond lanosterol. Recently there has also been an interesting spin-off in an ingenious clinical application resulting from the findings on triparanol and desmosterol reductase. Paoletti and coworkers have taken advantage of the fact that relatively undifferentiated brain tumors, like fetal brain, show a relatively high rate of sterol biosynthesis and have a relative deficiency of desmosterol reductase, resulting in accumulation of desmosterol. In contrast, normal adult brain contains no desmosterol and synthesizes sterol only very slowly. Triparanol accentuates the accumulation of desmosterol in brain tumors but only traces at most appear in normal brain. By pretreating patients with triparanol and then looking for desmosterol in cerebrospinal fluid they find that they can rather regularly establish a correct clinical diagnosis of brain tumor [1150]. However, we still do not have a nontoxic, clinically effective inhibitor acting on the later steps of sterol transformation.

Now I would like to turn to a discussion of clofibrate. The drug is administered as the ethyl ester, but this is rapidly hydrolyzed; it is primarily the free acid that appears in plasma. It is hardly necessary here to review its gratifying clinical effectiveness, demonstrated first by Oliver and his coworkers in Edinburgh and since confirmed and extended in many clinics around the world. Instead I would like to limit myself to a discussion of the mode of action of this widely used drug in lowering lipoprotein levels. Table 1 lists some of the mechanisms of action that have been proposed, each supported by some experimental evidence. The list is rather discouragingly long and it is probably not complete. I will try to comment on the evidence for each of these and the strength of it. I don't think we can, at the present time, single out any one mechanism as being the most important, but we may be able to rule out some as being unlikely.

Like many other anions, the free acid of CPIB binds to serum albumin and to other serum proteins. Thus it could theoretically compete with and displace other substances normally transported as protein complexes. Since the metabolic activity of, for example, thyroxine relates to the concentration of the unbound or "free" form rather than the total concentration, such competition could increase effective metabolic activity.

Thorp's original experimental studies, indeed, suggested a mechanism of this kind, specifically that CPIB was potentiating the activity of endogenous androsterone and so the combination of CPIB and androsterone was marketed. As discussed, it was soon found that the androsterone was quite unnecessary and that the CPIB ester alone, Atromid-S, was fully as active as the combination. Moreover, CPIB is effective in the absence of the adrenals or the gonads [147]. Thus, I think we can strike 1 A from our list as "case not proved".

What about displacement of thyroxine? The acid test would be to determine whether or not CPIB is effective in the complete absence of the thyroid hormone. Harrison and Harden [620] reported two such cases, i.e. patients with untreated myxedema who failed to respond to CPIB until some thyroxine was added to

Table 1. *Some mechanisms of action proposed for the hypolipidemic effect of CPIB*

1. Enhancement of endogenous hormone activity secondary to competition for binding sites on plasma proteins
   A. Androgens
   B. Thyroid hormone
2. Decrease in rate of FFA mobilization
3. Decrease in rate of hepatic cholesterol biosynthesis
   A. Block between acetate and mevalonate
   B. Block between mevalonate and cholesterol
   C. Diversion of acetoacetatyl CoA to free acetoacetate
4. Increase in rate of hepatic cholesterol oxidation
5. Decrease in rate of hepatic release of lipoproteins
6. Increase in rate of peripheral uptake of lipoproteins

their regimen. On the other hand, Danowski and Alley [360] reported a perfectly fine response to CPIB alone in a patient with complete primary myxedema. At very high molar ratios CPIB does displace thyroxine from human albumin but the therapeutic levels, which are about 200 μg/ml, correspond to a molar ratio of only 1:1.

Chang et al. [301] and Musa et al. [1059] have been unable to demonstrate any interference with binding of thyroxine (T_4) to the primary carrier, the thyroid-binding globulin and two recent studies in man, those of McKerron et al. [956] and of Barbosa and Oliner [92], fail to reveal any significant effects on free (that is, effective) thyroxine levels in man. Thorp and others [1468] have called attention to a disproportionate shunting of T_4 to the liver and suggest that the liver might be specifically "hyperthyroid". In view of the evidence just mentioned, I wonder if that "shunting" might reflect not a change in T_4 binding but rather a consequence of the profound changes in liver morphology and size. In any case, the effects of CPIB can't be attributed *exclusively* to a T_4-like effect. For example, the latter *increases* the rate of cholesterol synthesis, while CPIB treatment *inhibits* it.

Finally, I would point out some very telling differences between the responses in man to CPIB and to T_4. The former, as nicely shown by Strisower and Strisower [1429], primarily reduces S_f 20–400 lipoproteins (LP); the latter primarily reduces S_f 0–20 LP. CPIB increases HDL_3 while T_4 decreases it. Moreover, as CPIB reduces S_f 20–400 LP, it causes an *increase* in S_f 0–20 LP whereas T_4 *reduces*

S_f 0–20 LP. Finally, Strisower [1426] showed that adding T_4 to CPIB treatment does not enhance its effect on the S_f 20–400 class. The effects of the two drugs appear to be additive with respect to the S_f 0–20 class but not with respect to the S_f 20–400 class [148]. While there may be some subtle effects of CPIB on thyroid hormone metabolism I think we have to consider 1B as also not proved

Still another hypothesis that has been presented regarding the mode of action of CPIB is that it acts through an effect on free fatty acid transport. Speake has shown that CPIB *in vitro*, at concentrations comparable to those reached in the plasma during treatment with ordinary doses, inhibits the epinephrine or norepinephrine stimulated release of free fatty acids (FFA). Barrett and Thorpe have shown that the increment in FFA due to catecholamine injections in dogs is reduced but by no means completely abolished by prior treatment with CPIB. On the other hand, Duncan, Best and Robertson found only a very minimal effect of CPIB on catecholamine-induced FFA rises in man, effects that were much smaller than those produced by nicotinic acid. It should be mentioned here that some of the confusion in the early literature on this topic relates to the fact that the CPIB acid is extracted partially and titrated in the usual Dole method or the Trout modification of it. Since the concentrations of CPIB rise to as high as 1 μEq/ml and something like 30% of it is extracted, it is apparent that a significant error can be introduced and that the FFA levels must be corrected appropriately. Before discussing the acceptability of this hypothesis, the mechanism presumed to be involved should be mentioned.

How strong is the evidence that there is any cause-and-effect relationship between FFA mobilization and lipoprotein levels? This is a proposition that was first put forward some years ago as a result of studies done by Drs. Shafrir and Sussman in our laboratory. It was supported by a correlation between FFA and lipoprotein levels under the influence of hormonal stimulation. The presumption is that when FFA flux to the liver is increased, the rates of deposition of FFA, the rates of FFA oxidation, and the rates of secretion of plasma lipoproteins all increase. There has been support from perfused liver studies as well as a number of *in vivo* studies for the operation of such a mechanism. However, I would stress that it is not yet proved *under physiologic conditions* that the rate of FFA mobilization represents an important determinant of steady state lipoprotein levels. If we could raise the peripheral levels without using agents that have other physiologic effects, we might be convinced. Dr. Johan Kotzé in our laboratory is applying a new technique for direct FFA infusion to try to get a direct answer to this problem. I was pleased to see Dr. Havel's data (see p. 210) correlating FFA flux to the liver and the VLDL flux out, but there was no manipulation there within the same individual. So, the case is strong, but not proven conclusively.

If CPIB does limit FFA mobilization, how does it do so? The effect has been attributed by some to the binding of CPIB itself to albumin, something analogous to the displacement of thyroxine, making binding sites unavailable to FFA. I think this is unlikely on theoretical grounds, which I won't have time to discuss, but also on experimental grounds.

Recently Drs. William B. Greenough and Stephen R. Crespin in our laboratory have done experiments infusing FFA into animals, raising the levels up to 1 and

2 μEq/ml by infusing sodium oleate, using a new continuous-flow blood centrifuge that lets one introduce FFA into separated plasma at a high rate. In some of these experiments, we measured the concentrations of the nonoleate fatty acids to see if the adipose tissue was continuing to release in the presence of the imposed high FFA level. The results are shown in Table 2. In this experiment the total FFA was raised from 0.49 to 1.55 by infusion of oleate, the latter comprising the bulk of the fatty acid, of course. The essential point is that the nonoleate fatty acids did not go down; if anything, they increased slightly. Thus FFA themselves loaded onto the albumin did not seem to suppress FFA mobilization. Since FFA bind more tightly than CPIB, I think it is very unlikely that CPIB could work by this mechanism.

Table 2. *Failure of elevated FFA levels to limit continuing release of endogenous FFA*

	Basal μEq/ml	During oleate infusion μEq/ml	Change μEq/ml
Total FFA	0.49	1.55	+1.06
Oleate	0.15	1.00	+0.85
All other FFA	0.34	0.55	+0.21

Table 3. *Inhibition of cholesterol biosynthesis by prior CPIB treatment of rats*

Precursor	Percentage inhibition
Liver slices	
Acetate-1-^{14}C	82%
Mevalonate-2-^{14}C	(+5%)
In vivo	
Acetate-1-^{14}C	51%
$^{3}H_2O$	36%

Finally, there is something to be learned by comparing CPIB and nicotinic acid. The latter is a very powerful inhibitor of FFA mobilization as shown by Carlson. It is equally effective in reducing levels both of beta and prebeta lipoproteins, whereas CPIB, as we have discussed, has its most striking effects on the latter only. If the mechanism of action of both compounds were the same, namely limited to effects secondary to suppression of fatty acid mobilization, should not their clinical effects be more similar? If their effects on free fatty acid metabolism are relevant to their hypolipidemic effects (and that has not been *proven* in either case) then either one or the other, or both, must have at the very least some additional mechanism by which it influences plasma lipoprotein levels.

The third general mechanism of action proposed is through inhibition of cholesterol biosynthesis. That CPIB does decrease rates of cholesterol synthesis is generally agreed although there is some disagreement as to the site of action. The first thorough study was that of Avoy, Swyryd and Gould [78] although an effect had been noted earlier by Boyd [1469]. Avoy et al. showed both *in vivo* and *in vitro* that acetate incorporation into liver cholesterol was markedly inhibited whereas mevalonate incorporation was unaffected (Table 3). Dr. Richard Dexter in our laboratory at the National Heart Institute confirmed these findings *in vivo* (Dexter and Steinberg, unpublished results). As shown in Table 4, incorporation of intraperitoneally administered ^{3}H-acetate into sterol was strongly inhibited but incorporation of labeled ^{14}C-mevalonate, given simultaneously, was unimpaired. Neither in the studies of Gould's group nor in ours was acetate incorporation into fatty acids impaired; if anything, it was increased. These results strongly imply a site of action at HMG CoA reductase but do not prove it. Indeed Burch [267] has reported an *increase* in acetoacetyl-CoA deacylase activity

Table 4. *Effect of CPIB (0.25% in diet) on cholesterol biosynthesis in the rat*

Precursor	Radioactivity in liver sterols (dpm/g wet weight)		
	controls	CPIB-treated	
Tritium-labeled acetate	9,174	1,297	$p \ll 0.001$
Carbon-14 labeled mevalonic acid	4,810	4,070	
	Radioactivity in liver fatty acids (dpm/g wet weight)		
Tritium-labeled acetate	3,260	4,056	$p = 0.1$

in livers of CPIB-treated rats and suggested diversion of substrate to ketone body production as a mechanism for decreased sterol synthesis. However, there is still no evidence that this deacylase activity can ever become rate limiting. Moreover, elsewhere White (see p. 545) has presented more direct evidence that HMG CoA reductase is specifically inhibited by CPIB. Azarnoff, Tucker and Barr [80] found a decrease in mevalonate incorporation in rats fed CPIB. This result, contrasting with those of Avoy et al. and our own, may relate to the longer period of CPIB treatment prior to testing (21 days) and reflect secondary changes.

The fourth mechanism that has been considered is enhanced cholesterol oxidation. Kritchevsky and Tepper [827] found that isolated mitochondria prepared from livers of rats fed CPIB for 21 days oxidized cholesterol-26-^{14}C more rapidly on an absolute basis than did normal mitochondria, but when results were expressed per milligram of mitochondrial nitrogen the differences disappeared. Mitchell, Truswell and Bronte-Stewart [1013] found no increase in fecal bile acid excretion in CPIB-treated patients although there was some increase in fecal sterol excretion. Ahrens and coworkers at Rockefeller University have also measured fecal bile acid excretion and found no effect of CPIB (personal communication). Thus, there is on balance no basis to accept the fourth proposition.

The fifth possibility—a direct effect on release of lipoproteins from the liver—is an intriguing one, well supported experimentally and raising questions about the underlying mechanism that is affected. Duncan, Best and Despopoulos [412] showed clearly that perfused livers from CPIB-fed rats secreted newly-synthesized lipoprotein triglyceride into the perfusate at about one-half the normal rate, even though the rate of uptake of free fatty acid was normal. This effect in experimental animals has been amply confirmed and extended by several groups [80, 558, 1009, 1336].

Data in man are limited. The results of Nestel, Hirsch and Couzens [1087] are compatible with this mechanism in that the slope of the lipoprotein cholesterol-^{14}C curve decreased under the influence of CPIB, but this could simply reflect inhibition of cholesterol biosynthesis. The recent clinical results of Scott and Hurley [1324] using iodinated lipoproteins indicate a decrease in net turnover of LDL plus VLDL (although most of the label was in the LDL fraction). In contrast, Ryan and Schwartz [1271] concluded from their kinetic studies that CPIB *increased* clearance of triglycerides without affecting production and secre-

Table 5. *Observed effects of administration of CPIB*

Decrease in plasma lipoprotein levels
Decrease in plasma fibrinogen levels
Decrease in platelet adhesiveness; increase in platelet survival
Increase in body weight
Increase in liver weight

tion rate. On balance, a good case has been made for an effect on liver secretion. This effect deserves further investigation for the light it might cast on the still poorly understood mechanism of lipoprotein secretion.

Finally, evidence has been presented for enhanced rates of peripheral removal of lipoproteins. The clinical study of Ryan and Schwartz has just been mentioned. Nestel and Austin [1085] report increased *in vivo* rates of uptake of palmitate-labeled chylomicrons by epididymal fat pads from CPIB-fed rats. This was not accompanied by a measurable increase in lipoprotein lipase activity, and they suggested a primary effect on fatty acid reesterification. In contrast, a preliminary report by Tolman and Tepperman [1473] notes a doubling of lipoprotein lipase activity in fat pads of their CPIB-fed rats.

If we refer back to our menu of mechanisms (Table 1) and attempt to summarize. It seems the case for Mechanisms 1, 2, 3B, 3C and 4 is weak; the case for 6 is still preliminary and data conflicting; the case for 3A and 5 is quite strong. Thus, at least two mechanisms may be operative and possibly several others contributory.

We have limited discussion to the effects on lipid transport but, as shown in Table 5, there are a number of other striking effects of CPIB administration that require explanation. Especially striking is the impressive increase in liver weight that occurs so rapidly with increases in the number of microbodies or peroxisomes [677, 1444]. These are certainly not effects common to other inhibitors of cholesterol synthesis, nor is it easy to see why suppression of lipoprotein secretion should lead to such profound changes in cytoarchitecture. To the reviewer it seems more likely that CPIB exerts a profound effect on cell membranes or their metabolism that secondarily leads to manifold metabolic consequences, including the effects on lipoprotein transport that happen to interest us most.

The fact that these profound changes in cell structure and size are not accompanied by observable toxic effects on a macrolevel and that they seem to be readily reversible is remarkable. Certainly the final word on the mechanism of action of this drug is not in, despite the attention the problem has received. From the pragmatic point of view, the drug is acceptable by all the usual criteria applied in clinical pharmacology. However, because it is so widely used, further attempts to understand its action at the molecular level would be in order.

DRUGS AFFECTING BILE ACID AND CHOLESTEROL EXCRETION*

Tatu A. Miettinen

The formation of atheromatous plaques in the walls of coronary arteries initiates development of coronary heart disease. These lesions consist of lipid, primarily cholesterol, which is generally believed to be deposited from the circulating blood. Thus, the cholesterol of atheromata has been shown to be in equilibrium with serum cholesterol [309]. Infiltration of the latter into atheromatous lesions is assumed to take place at a rate directly correlated with the serum cholesterol concentration. This assumption is supported by a great many investigations which have clearly shown that patients with coronary heart disease have higher serum cholesterol levels than healthy subjects and that the higher the serum cholesterol level the higher the frequency of coronary heart disease or the greater the likelihood that ischemic heart disease will develop. Atheromatous arterial disease appears to occur with very high frequency in subjects with familial hypercholesterolemia, Type II hyperlipoproteinemia [489]. Thus, reduction of the elevated serum cholesterol level might logically be expected to prevent the development of atheromatous lesions or their progression. Reduction in the size of these deposits can be expected, provided there is sufficient decrease of serum cholesterol, and particularly if it is associated with increased elimination of cholesterol from the body, i.e., with enhanced fecal excretion of bile acids and/or neutral steroids derived from cholesterol. As a matter of fact, recent studies have revealed that the ileal by-pass operation, which increases cholesterol elimination by about 2 g/day [992], reduces the size of both the rapidly and the slowly miscible pools of exchangeable cholesterol to normal [1027]. The cholesterol of atheromata belongs to the latter pool. Though decrease of serum cholesterol by dietary means appears to be associated with a reduced recurrence rate of

* The study herein is supported by grants from the Sigrid Jusélius Foundation, the National Research Council for Medical Sciences, Finland, and by Grant R05 TW00218, U.S.P.H.S.

myocardial infarction [857] or initial episodes of coronary heart disease [1479], no conclusive evidence exists so far that treatment of hypercholesterolemia with drugs has a similar favorable effect. Yet the use of hypocholesterolemic agents is generally accepted.

Drugs may reduce serum cholesterol either by inhibiting synthesis or by stimulating elimination of cholesterol as fecal steroids. Redistribution of cholesterol from plasma to tissues may also occur. Elimination may be augmented

Table 1. *Effect of various nonabsorbable and absorbable hypolipidemic drugs on cholesterol metabolism in man*

Site of action	Drug	Fecal steroids			Cholesterol synthesis	Cholesterol absorption
		neutral	acidic	total		
Intestine	Cholestyramine	− +	+	+	+	−
	Neomycin	= +	+	+	+	−
	Methyl neomycin	+	+	+	+	−
	DEAE Sephadex	+ −	+	+	+	−
Liver	Clofibrate	+	−	+	− ?	=
	Nicotinic acid	+ =	=	+ =	− ?	=
	Thyroid hormones	+	= +	+	+	=

\+ increased; − decreased; = unchanged.

by (1) enhanced excretion of cholesterol and bile acids via the bile (and intestinal wall) into the gut, (2) inhibited intestinal absorption of both endogenous and dietary cholesterol, and (3) reduced reabsorption of bile acids.

Table 1 illustrates the most commonly used hypolipidemic drugs, which have been reported to increase elimination of cholesterol from the body as either acidic or neutral fecal steroids. The drugs are divided into two groups, those which are unabsorbed and exert their effect in the intestinal lumen, primarily by interfering with reabsorption of bile acids and those which are absorbed and act primarily by stimulating excretion of cholesterol into the bile, apparently also interfering with synthesis of cholesterol.

UNABSORBABLE AGENTS

Cholestyramine. Cholestyramine, an anion exchange resin with a polystyramine skeleton, was first shown to reduce serum cholesterol in man by Bergen et al. [138]. The resin is unabsorbable and binds bile acids both *in vitro* and in the intestinal contents [1458]. Thus, it interrupts the enterohepatic circulation of bile salts and can accordingly result, via bile salt deficiency, in inadequate micellar solubilization of digested fats in the intestinal lumen. Enhanced conversion of cholesterol to bile acids, however, restores the bile acid pool, so that no gross abnormality of fat absorption ensues unless large doses of resin are consumed [354, 627]. This augmented synthesis of bile acids usually exceeds the corresponding compensatory stimulation of cholesterol synthesis leading to reduction of serum cholesterol.

That cholestyramine actually increases fecal bile acid excretion in man was first shown by Carey and Williams [279], who reported an eightfold increase of fecal desoxycholic acid output in a normal man. Hashim and Van Itallie [627] observed a manyfold elevation in bile acid excretion (mono-, di- and trihydroxy bile acids) induced by the resin in two female patients and in one normal man. The neutral steroid fraction, consisting of cholesterol and plant sterols and their respective bacterial conversion products, remained unchanged. Using the isotope technique, Moore et al. [1026] observed no change in the neutral steroid output while fecal bile acid excretion was augmented about threefold. The elimination of cholesterol from the body was increased about twofold, i.e. by approximately 800 mg/day. Two subjects apparently homozygous for hyperlipoproteinemia of Type II, studied by Moutafis and Myant [1045] with the isotope technique, increased their fecal steroid excretion by 1.1 to 1.3 g/day in response to cholestyramine, the increment being primarily due to a change in bile acid output and, to a lesser extent, to an elevation of neutral steroid elimination. The increment was continuous during the study, which was continued for several months, indicating that the augmented elimination of cholesterol was compensated by increased synthesis, particularly because no change was detected in serum cholesterol or in the size of the exchangeable cholesterol pool. Plasma cholesterol turnover, determined by Goodman and Noble [546] on the basis of the disappearance of radioactive cholesterol from the circulation, also indicated that cholestyramine increased the production rate by about 1 g/day, suggesting that the rate of cholesterol excretion from the body was augmented by the same amount. The size of the rapidly miscible cholesterol pool was minimally affected. Increased bile acid excretion and cholesterol turnover have also been reported by Grundy et al. [584].

Our own studies, with direct measurement of end-products of cholesterol metabolism, have revealed that in patients with hyperlipoproteinemia of Type II, maintained on a low cholesterol diet (82–122 mg/2,400 cal), 32 g of cholestyramine daily resulted in a 25% decrease in serum cholesterol and in a 1 g increment of fecal steroid excretion [985, 986]. The latter was due solely to enhanced bile acid excretion. Since cholestyramine decreases intestinal absorption of exogenous and endogenous cholesterol [731, 1398], the finding suggests that excretion of endogenous cholesterol from the liver and/or intestinal wall might have been reduced, probably because of an enhanced requirement for bile acid synthesis. Studies carried out on normocholesterolemic subjects indicate that, in spite of the low absolute decrement of serum cholesterol by cholestyramine, the increment of cholesterol elimination is about twice that found in hypercholesterolemia. Accordingly, though hypercholesterolemic patients are able to markedly increase their bile acid excretion and synthesis, this ability appears actually to be less strong than in normal subjects. The observation supports the view that Type II hyperlipoproteinemia may be due to partial failure to convert cholesterol to bile acids [994].

A marked reduction of the $^{3}H/^{14}C$ ratio in the serum cholesterol after intravenous administration of a ^{3}H-mevalonate-^{14}C-acetate mixture indicated that synthesis before mevalonate, probably between hydroxymethyl glutarate and mevalonate, was increased threefold by the resin [990, 992]. Though the activity of the enzymes after mevalonate does not limit the rate of cholesterol synthesis [556], the accumulation of liver and serum methyl sterols during cholestyramine treatment in the rat and in man, this suggests that during grossly enhanced synthesis the later intermediary steps of the synthetic pathway may become rate-limiting [991]. The primary site of enhanced synthesis may be the liver [725, 991], though reduction of intestinal bile acid concentration, probably caused by cholestyramine, also stimulates intestinal cholesterogenesis [392].

Since cholestyramine increases elimination of cholesterol in every patient, mobilization of tissue cholesterol and particularly enhanced synthesis between acetate and mevalonate are the factors which ultimately determine the final serum cholesterol level. The isotope studies did not indicate a decrease of the tissue pools. Clinical observations that xanthelasma, and cutaneous and even tendon xanthomata disappear or are reduced in size during long-term treatment suggest, however, that some mobilization is actually taking place. The problem of hypercholesterolemia and the mobilization of accumulated tissue cholesterol could easily be solved if the compensatory enhancement of synthesis before mevalonate could be inhibited by another drug gven simultaneously with cholestyramine. Agents such as nicotinic acid and clofibrate appear to be unsatisfactory in this respect. Because cholestyramine alone is effective in a very high percentage of cases, is well tolerated by patients and, acting "outside" the organism, has very few if any harmful side effects, it is a convenient agent for the treatment of hypercholesterolemia. Furthermore, the drug is ideal for studies designed to explore the regulation of cholesterol metabolism not only in patients with hypercholesterolemia but also in normal subjects.

Neomycin. Since the report by Samuel and Steiner [1289] that neomycin significantly reduces the serum cholesterol level in man, this almost unabsorbable antibiotic has been found to decrease serum cholesterol by 10–36% [1287]. In doses of 1–2 g daily it is relatively well tolerated, larger doses (6–12 g) resulting in diarrhea and the malabsorption syndrome. The latter may be associated with partial villous atrophy of the jejunal mucosa [742] but are also found without any detectable alterations in mucosal histology [861].

The decrease of serum cholesterol by neomycin, even in doses of 2 g/day, has been related to its capacity to induce mild malabsorption, which could explain the increased elimination of cholesterol as bile acids and neutral steroids into the feces [1195]. Increased fecal loss of bile acids by neomycin may reduce sterol and fat absorption in the same way as cholestyramine, i.e., via bile acid deficiency. Another explanation for the increased fecal steroid excretion is that this antibiotic alters the intestinal flora, thus interfering with bacterial action on sterols and bile acids in the intestine and hence with their absorption [543, 1195]. This mechanism of action seems unlikely, however, because N-methylated neomycin, which is a basic neomycin derivative without antibacterial action, was equally effective in reducing serum cholesterol and markedly increased fecal excretion of neutral steroids and bile acids in man [1491]. Since neomycin and its N-methylated derivative were able to precipitate bile salts *in vitro*, it was suggested that the polybasic neomycin molecule might interfere with reabsorption of bile acids and indirectly with neutral steroids. It is noteworthy, however, that though neomycin effectively reduces serum cholesterol in man and in germ-free and conventional chicks, it is ineffective or even hypercholesterolemic in the rat. It augments fecal bile acid excretion correspondingly in the two former species, but is ineffective and even reduces bile salt output in germ-free and conventional rats, respectively [445]. Thus, the bile acid-binding capacity, though clear *in vitro*, particularly for dihydroxy bile acids, is insignificant in the rat intestine.

No information appears to be available on the relationship between the decrement of serum cholesterol and increment of fecal steroid excretion, primarily because fecal steroid determinations were carried out with nonspecific methods in the earlier sterol balance studies. The question of a compensatory increase of cholesterol synthesis would also be interesting to study in view of the possible direct or indirect action of neomycin on the metabolism of the intestinal wall and its cholesterogenesis. In contrast to experiments with cholestyramine, the size of the "intermediate" pool of cholesterol was decreased almost 40% by neomycin in man, while the half time of the serum cholesterol radioactivity decay curve did not change consistantly [1288].

Other Agents. Augmented residues of undigested fiber in stools have been considered to increase elimination of cholesterol from the body by making stools bulkier or by interfering more specifically with absorption of either bile acids or cholesterol. As a matter of fact, many large-molecular compounds, primarily polysaccharides, appear to decrease serum cholesterol and increase fecal steroid excretion [874, 1146]. A hydrophilic colloid derived from the blond psyllium seed markedly reduces serum cholesterol in man, concomitantly increasing fecal bile acid excretion threefold [479]. Lignin binds bile acids, particularly if the hydroxyl moieties on the phenyl-propane units are made less polar by methylation, and, when given to a patient with massive resection of the small intestine, controls diarrhea, apparently by binding bile salts in the colon [416]. Dextran and cellulose anion exchangers, which act in essentially the same way as cholestyramine, will probably be the most useful agents of the high-molecular polysaccharide class. These agents effectively bind bile acids, reduce serum cholesterols in cockerels and dogs, and increase fecal bile acids in hypercholesterolemic cockerels [1152]. According to our own limited experience, oral administration of DEAE-Sephadex lowers serum cholesterol and increases fecal bile acid excretion in hypercholesterolemic patients to an extent which, depending on the dose, resembles that obtained with cholestyramine.

ABSORBABLE AGENTS

Nicotinic Acid. While lowering serum cholesterol in a very high percentage of even Type II hypercholesterolemics, it is frequently effective on elevated triglycerides and powerfully inhibits lipolysis in adipose tissue [43, 282, 489]. Since the drug reduces the flow of free fatty acids to the liver, its hypolipidemic action has been related to this effect. Many animal experiments, both *in vivo* and *in vitro*, have indicated that nicotinic acid inhibits cholesterol synthesis at an early stage, probably between acetate and mevalonate; other studies showed, however, that synthesis was unchanged or even stimulated [700].

Earlier sterol balance studies in man indicated that a nicotinic acid-induced fall in serum cholesterol was not accompanied by any significant increase of fecal bile acids and neutral steroids, so that the drug obviously lowered serum cholesterol by inhibiting cholesterol synthesis [1001]. The latter assumption was supported by reduced conversion of ^{14}C-acetate to serum cholesterol during nicotinic acid treatment in man [700]. It has been reported, however, that in a group of 20 atherosclerotic patients the decrease of serum cholesterol was associated with increased fecal bile acid and cholesterol excretion [1]. Our own studies showed that nicotinic acid increased fecal neutral steroids derived from blood cholesterol, while bile acid output and absorption of dietary cholesterol did not change consistently [985]. Thus, the drug appears to stimulate cho-

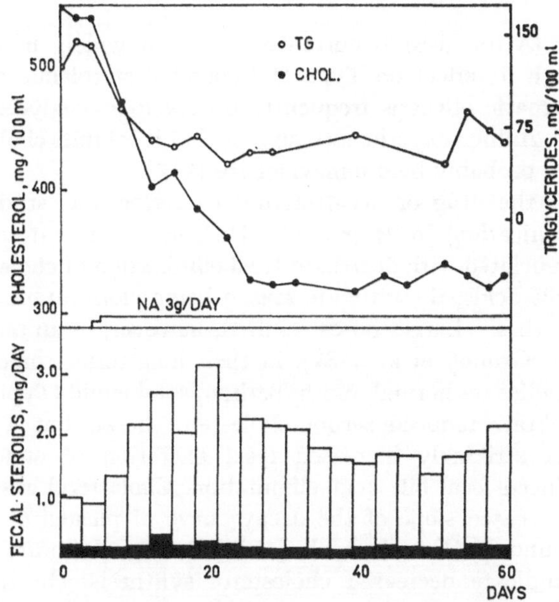

Fig. 1. Effect of nicotinic acid on serum lipids, and on excretion of fecal bile acids (black bars) and neutral steroids (white bars) in a hypercholesterolemic woman. Diet contained 95 mg of cholesterol

lesterol excretion, probably via the biliary tract. This stimulation is perhaps nonspecific, because excretion of tocopherol, an exogenous compound, also appears to be enhanced. Nicotinic acid might stimulate catabolism of serum lipoproteins and/or inhibit their formation, thus leading to augmented excretion of cholesterol into the bile. In some cases the increment of fecal cholesterol elimination exceeded the decrement of serum cholesterol, suggesting that cholesterol was mobilized from tissues or that synthesis was increased; in others the increment accounted insufficiently for the decrement in serum, probably owing to reduced synthesis. The decreased or unchanged slope of the serum cholesterol radioactivity-time curve during therapy suggested that synthesis was decreased, though a similar effect is obtained even in the presence of increased synthesis, provided that tissue cholesterol with a high specific activity is mobilized.

Our more recent studies have indicated that nicotinic acid increases cholesterol elimination in more than three-fourths of the patients with familial hypercholesterolemia. The increment of the elimination correlated significantly with the decrement of serum cholesterol level ($r = 0.76$). Serum cholesterol reduction and increased fecal neutral steroid excretion were also found during a total fast, suggesting that the effect was not due to decreased synthesis, because the latter was already suppressed [986, 987]. Fig. 1 shows that the increase of cholesterol elimination can be sustained, suggesting that it is balanced, partly at least, by increased synthesis. Studies with a ^{14}C-acetate-^{3}H-mevalonate mixture in man indicated that, in contrast to earlier findings, nicotinic acid might stimulate cholesterol synthesis between acetate and mevalonate or reduce the acetate pool [987].

Clofibrate. It (Atromid-S) is currently the most widely used hypolipidemic drug, even though its effect on Type II hypercholesterolemic patients may be negligible; a dramatic effect is frequently observed in triglyceridemic subjects [489, 1427, 1428]. Animal experiments suggest that it inhibits cholesterol synthesis at an early stage, probably before mevalonate [557].

The effect of the drug on fecal steroid excretion was studied by Mitchell (personal communication) in 21 patients. He concluded that serum cholesterol reduction was associated with decreased fecal elimination of cholesterol, primarily in the form of bile acids, the ultimate reason being clofibrate-induced inhibition of cholesterol synthesis. Larger doses resulted, however, in an increase in neutral steroid excretion. Grundy et al. [583], in their long-term (three to six months) sterol balance studies on normal and hyperlipoproteinemic (Types I–V) patients, found that clofibrate reduced serum cholesterol in all but Type I hypertriglyceridemics. It strikingly increased fecal excretion of endogenous neutral steroids and reduced fecal bile acid elimination. Cholesterol absorption was not changed. The decreased slope of the decay curve of plasma cholesterol specific activity, also found by Nestel et al. [1087] during clofibrate treatment, was interpreted to indicate decreased cholesterol synthesis. On the basis of this finding the increased fecal cholesterol elimination, which exceeded the corresponding decrement of plasma cholesterol, was considered to be balanced mainly by mobilization of tissue cholesterol. Accordingly, clofibrate seems to stimulate excretion of cholesterol as such from the circulation to the gut lumen, either via the bile or through the intestinal wall. The ultimate mode of action, the mechanism by which cholesterol transfer from lipoproteins to the intestine is stimulated by clofibrate, is still unknown. Similarly, it remains to be shown whether in long-term treatment increased cholesterol elimination is ultimately balanced by increased synthesis or returns to the pretreatment or reduced level.

Thyroid Hormones. These, including d-thyroxine, reduce the serum cholesterol level not only in hypothyroid patients but also in hypercholesterolemic subjects; they are relatively ineffective in patients with triglyceridemia [489, 1427, 1428] and their use is limited by worsening angina in patients with coronary heart disease, even when d-thyroxine is used.

Animal experiments, and studies with radioactive acetate and cholesterol in man indicate that thyroid hormones enhance elimination of cholesterol from the body, synthesis being relatively less strongly stimulated [1073]. That oxidation of cholesterol to bile acids is increased is indicated by enhanced cholic acid turnover in hypothyroid patients treated with thyroid hormones [663].

Direct measurements of fecal end-products of cholesterol metabolism have shown that thyroid hormones induce sustained enhancement of neutral steroid excretion in patients with myxedema, while acidic steroids increase less consistantly [989]. This is also seen from Table 2, which shows, in addition, that fecal steroid excretion is subnormal in hypothyroidism and tends to be increased

Table 2. *Serum cholesterol and fecal steroids in eu-, hypo- and hyperthyroid patients (mean ± SE*[a]*)*

Treatment	Serum cholest. (mg/100 ml)	Fecal steroids, mg/24 h neutral steroids	bile acids	total
		Controls (9)		
None	209 ± 10	670 ± 87	252 ± 35	921 ± 102
		Hypothyroid (8)		
None	478 ± 25[b]	393 ± 42[b]	164 ± 33	557 ± 63[b]
Thyroxine	263 ± 23	599 ± 65	170 ± 26	807 ± 48
Change	−215 ± 26[b]	+206 ± 40[b]	+6 ± 19	+212 ± 49[b]
		Hyperthyroid (5)		
None	162 ± 20[b]	780 ± 87[b]	518 ± 268	1,298 ± 229[b]

[a] Number of subjects in parentheses.
[b] $P<0.05$ for differences between hypothyroid and control or hyperthyroid patients, and between hypothyroids with and without treatment.

in hyperthyroidism. Furthermore, the serum cholesterol decrement is significantly correlated with the increment of fecal steroid output ($r=0.87$). Since absorption of dietary cholesterol remains practically unchanged, it is obvious that thyroid hormones decrease serum cholesterol by enhancing excretion of cholesterol via the bile or intestinal wall. Animal experiments have actually shown a marked augmentation of cholesterol output via bile fistula in response to thyroid hormones, the change in total bile acid excretion being less significant. As is the case during a nicotinic acid, or clofibrate-induced fall in the serum cholesterol level, the slope of the radioactivity-time curve of serum cholesterol decreases or remains unchanged in thyroxine-treated hypothyroid patients [989]. This suggests that the increased fecal excretion is not balanced fully by increased synthesis but that there is also a flux of cholesterol from the tissues to the circulation. The mode of action of thyroid hormones in reducing serum cholesterol may be the same in both hypothyroidism and Type II hypercholesterolemia.

PHARMACOLOGIC CONTROL OF FREE FATTY ACID MOBILIZATION AND PLASMA TRIGLYCERIDE TRANSPORT

L. A. Carlson

I would like to begin with the free fatty acids (FFA). I feel that it is appropriate to spend some time on indicating the possible role of FFA in the pathogenesis of atherosclerosis as this has not been previously discussed at this symposium on atherosclerosis. FFA is a rather neglected but in many ways an attractive candidate in the pathogenesis of atherosclerosis.

One major reason that FFA have been neglected in the past is the lability of this plasma lipid fraction. This means that there are considerable difficulties in getting values of FFA which are meaningful and representative for a given person. We have, for instance, very few data on this labile fraction during the 24-hour period. Studies like those presented by Dr. Schlierf (see p. 459) are thus highly desired. We certainly have no data whatsoever on FFA levels during a man's lifetime before clinical atherosclerosis appears.

On the other hand, FFA is an attractive candidate in the pathogenesis of atherosclerosis, because we know that the levels of FFA in blood plasma may increase rapidly in response to many of the environmental factors that have been discussed at this symposium and are believed to carry a high risk for development of atherosclerosis. To mention some conditions or situations recognized as risk factors where high plasma FFA levels may be the pathogenetic link between risk and disease, we can start with metabolic disorders such as diabetes, carbohydrate intolerance, and obesity. We can look at "emotional stress" or as Dr. Gröen put it (see p. 493) "work problems" as conditions which may enhance FFA mobilization and thus raise FFA levels. We can regard smoking as another factor in this context. We can look at feeding and eating habits as factors which certainly have profound influence on the variation of plasma FFA levels and last, but perhaps not least, we may consider lack of exercise and physical training as other possible major factors in this regard.

In what way may high FFA levels in plasma be a pathogenetic link between risk factors and atherosclerosis? A number of possible mechanisms have been listed in Table 1. This table contains some conditions or areas of potential interest in atherosclerosis where FFA may be of importance.

The plasma triglyceride area is one of these, as hypertriglyceridemia is common in patients with atherosclerosis. The plasma triglyceride level may well increase when the mobilization of FFA is increased and plasma FFA levels raised [283, 287]. Furthermore the concentration of triglycerides decreases when the free fatty acid mobilization is inhibited by agents such as nicotinic acid [283, 285, 288]. Tissue triglycerides behave in a way very similar to plasma triglycerides in relation to plasma FFA levels [283, 285, 287]. I think that it would be a quite fruitful and interesting area to study the lipid content of the arterial wall in relation to enhanced and inhibited FFA mobilization.

It is interesting that the work of Dr. Nikkilä [1103] and of Dr. Robinson [1559] has suggested a relationship between lipoprotein lipase activity and FFA mobilization. The work of Randle has suggested that the glucose tolerance may decrease in response to excessive FFA mobilization [1209]. Decreased glucose tolerance is very common in patients with atherosclerotic manifestations. Insulin secretion, as shown by Dr. Steinberg and coworkers [567] may well increase in response to high FFA levels. It is of clinical importance that the oxygen consumption

Table 1. *FFA and areas of potential interest in atherosclerosis*

Area	FFA mobilization	
	excessive	inhibited
Plasma TG	Increase	Decrease
Tissue TG (arterial wall ?)	Increase	Decrease
Lipoprotein lipase	Decrease	Increase
Glucose tolerance	Decrease	?
Insulin secretion	Increase	?
Oxygen consumption	Increase	Block of increase
Cardiac arrhythmias	Increase	?
Thrombosis	Increase ?	?

Table 2. *Hormonal stimulation of fat mobilizing lipolysis in adipose tissue*

Type of action	Mode of action
Fast (minutes)	
Catecholamines	Increase in cyclic AMP
ACTH and other peptide hormones	
Delayed (hours)	
Glucocorticoids	Decreased FFA-re-esterification
Growth hormone	Protein synthesis ?
Facilitates/permissive	
Glucocorticoids	Cyclic AMP system ?
Thyroid hormones	

may be raised by high FFA [287]. Thanks to the work of Dr. Oliver and coworkers, it now appears possible that certain deleterious cardiac arrhythmias may be related to high FFA levels [1124]. Finally we have the difficult question of the relation between thrombosis and FFA concentration.

The concentration of FFA is raised when the mobilization of FFA is increased. The FFA mobilization is regulated by three factors, the fat mobilizing lipolysis, fatty acid esterification and blood flow in adipose tissue. This review has to be confined to the first of these e.g. fat mobilizing lipolysis and ways in which this can be modified pharmacologically.

Table 2 shows that fat mobllizing lipolysis can be influenced by a number of hormones. The action of these hormones can be described as being either a *fast* mobilizing action, a *delayed* action or a *facilitated/permissive* action. I will only have time to discuss the fast action. The fast mobilizing lipolysis appears to be related to the levels of cyclic AMP in adipose tissue [272]. Compounds that interfere with the fast stimulation of fat mobilizing lipolysis can be grouped

Table 3. *Inhibitors of FFA mobilization metabolites*

Glucose
Lactate, pyruvate
Ketone bodies
RNA and ATP

Table 4. *Inhibitors of FFA mobilization: Hormonal*

Hormones	Pancreatic	Insulin
	Neurohypophyseal	Vasopressin Oxytocin
	Adenohypophyseal	Prolactin
Peptides	Plasma globulins	Angiotensin II (Hypertensin)
Prostaglandins		PGE_1, PGE_2, PGE_3

Table 5. *Inhibitors of FFA mobilization: Pharmacological agents with direct effect on adipose tissue (adrenergic blocking agents)*

a-Blockers	Dibenamine
	Dibenzyline
	Phentolamine (Regitine)
	Ergot alkaloids
β-Blockers	Dichloroisoproterenol (DCI)
	Pronethalol (Nethalide = Alderlin)
	Propranolol (Inderal)
	INPEA
	Kö 592
Others	Isopropyl- and
	Butyl-methoxamine

Table 6. *Inhibitors of FFA mobilization: Pharmacological agents with direct effect on adipose tissue*

Nicotinic acid [a]	Quabain
Salicylates [a]	Phenformin
Pyrazoles [a]	Sulfonylurea ?
Isoxyzoles [a]	Clofibrate ?

[a] And derivatives.

in the three main categories. Table 3 shows that there are several metabolites which are active in inhibiting FFA mobilization. Table 4 lists a variety of hormones which inhibit FFA mobilization. I would like to suggest that perhaps the most important ones in this regard are insulin and the prostaglandins.

The pharmacological agents inhibiting FFA mobilization may be divided into those acting within adipose tissue with a direct effect on the tissue and those having an indirect effect outside adipose tissue. Of course, a variety of adrenergic blocking agents, as exemplified in Table 5, can inhibit free fatty acid mobilization. I think, however, that the compounds listed in Table 6 are of greater pharmacological interest. These compounds have all been shown to have

Table 7. *Inhibitors of FFA mobilization: Pharmacological agents with indirect effect on adipose tissue*

1. Action on CNS	Meprobamate Pentobarbital Chlorpromazine
2. Sympathetic ganglionic blocking agents	Hexmethonium Azamethonium (Pendiomide) Trimethaphan (Arfonad) Agentit
3. Action on sympathetic nerve terminal	Reserpine Guanethidine (Ismelin) Bretylium
4. Local anesthetics	e.g. spinal anesthesia
5. Sulfonylureas	Tolbutamide Chlorpropamide

Table 8. *Effect of CH 13,437 on plasma TG and on the intravenous fat tolerance (fractional removal rate, K_2)*

Patient no.	Before		During	
	TG (mmol/l)	K_2 (%/min)	TG (mmol/l)	K_2 (%/min)
1	4.6	2.1	1.7	3.2
2	4.5	1.6	2.3	5.5
3	3.9	1.0	2.3	8.1
4	3.8	3.7	2.4	6.9
5	3.3	4.6	2.6	5.7
6	2.6	4.5	2.0	6.8
7	2.3	2.8	1.2	5.8
8	2.3	4.2	2.0	8.0
9	1.9	6.2	1.4	4.8
Mean	3.2	3.4	2.0	6.1

a direct effect on adipose tissue. Some of these, such as nicotinic acid and salicylates, have been used clinically in the treatment of hyperlipidemia.

Finally Table 7 shows that there are a variety of compounds which may have indirect effect on fat mobilization from adipose tissue. They may have their primary action on the central nervous system or on the endocrine glands.

To leave the free fatty acids and continue with plasma triglycerides I would like to stress the possibility that the triglycerides may be of considerable importance in the pathogenesis of atherosclerosis. Hypertriglyceridemia is, at least, in Sweden the most common form of hyperlipidemia in clinical atherosclerosis [281, 289]. Hypertriglyceridemia appears to be about twice as common as hypercholesterolemia (Type II) in this regard in Sweden.

Several lines of evidence during recent years suggest that a major cause of hypertriglyceridemia is a defect in removal of the triglycerides from the blood stream. Because of that, it is highly desirable to have a method to determine plasma triglyceride removal, and it would be especially valuable to have such a method in the evaluation of various pharmacological compounds affecting plasma triglyceride levels. We have been working recently on a method which

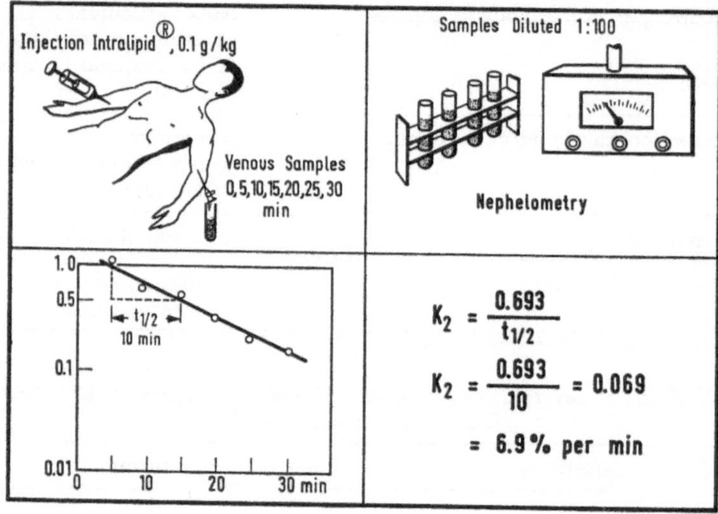

Fig. 1. The intravenous fat tolerance test is carried out as follows: Intralipid (0.1 g/kg) injected intravenously (top left) and the concentration of exogenous triglycerides in blood is determined by nephelometry (top right). The concentration of exogenous triglycerides is plotted against time and $t_{1/2}$ estimated (bottom left). The fractional removal constant, K_2, is then calculated (bottom right)

measures removal of exogenous triglycerides from the blood. I will briefly describe this method which we call the *intravenous fat tolerance test* [199, 286] and also the effect of pharmacological compounds on triglyceride removal. The intravenous fat tolerance test is in many ways very similar to the intravenous glucose tolerance test. The procedure of the test is outlined in Fig. 1. We give an intravenous injection of a fat emulsion called Intralipid. This emulsion has properties which are very similar to chylomicrons; therefore we have good reason to believe that the removal kinetics that we observe after injection of this fat emulsion traces the behavior of chylomicrons. After the intravenous injection we estimate the amount of exogenous triglycerides present in the blood at various times by nephelometry. Plotting the data in a semilogarithmic plot we can then estimate the $t_{1/2}$ for the removal in the usual way and calculate the fractional removal constant from the $t_{1/2}$ (Fig. 1). If we apply this method to subjects with triglyceridemia and look at this removal rate constant, we observe that the fractional rate constant, K_2, decreases with increasing triglyceride concentration [199]. The relationship between plasma triglyceride levels and K_2 was found to be hyperbolic [199] which suggests that the product of triglycerides times K_2 is constant. This product might be related to the turnover rate of plasma triglycerides if K_2 reflects the fractional removal not only of exogenous triglycerides but also of endogenous.

What happens when patients with hypertriglyceridemia are treated with compounds lowering plasma triglycerides? At present the two most efficient compounds that lower plasma triglycerides are clofibrate and nicotinic acid. We have used a compound called CH 13,437 which is a structural analog to clofibrate. We have given this compound to nine patients. The results are shown in Table 8. The triglyceride levels were reduced on the average from 3.2 to 2.0 mmol/l. At the same time the initially low fat tolerance, 3.4%/min, on the average increased to 6.1%/min [198]. These findings suggest that this compound lowers triglycerides by increasing peripheral removal. This assumption is strengthened by other observations such as determination of triglyceride turnover in some of these patients and of free fatty acid turnover and lipoprotein lipase levels, fast and slow acting, which all were unchanged [198].

In summary, if we believe that high levels in plasma of free fatty acids and triglycerides play a role in the pathogenesis of atherosclerosis, the situation presently looks promising. We soon should have available effective chemotherapy against high levels of free fatty acids and triglycerides.

DRUGS INTERFERING WITH PLATELET FUNCTION

G. V. R. Born

Measurement of Changes in Adhesiveness of Platelets. A central problem has been to find out why platelets, which are normally separate from each other in the circulating blood, acquire a tendency to adhere to vascular endothelium and to clump together under certain circumstances. The nature of these circumstances are also of concern. It seems that platelets acquire this tendency whenever they come into contact with a "foreign" surface, which presumably is everything except normal vascular endothelium. Platelets adhere to the endothelium when it is damaged, and when removed from the circulation they tend to adhere to glass and to other surfaces. Recent evidence [327] suggests that the foreign surface which initiates platelet thrombosis is subendothelial tissue exposed by the sudden rupture of an atheromatous plaque.

Quantitative investigations of changes in platelet adhesiveness were first made in 1941 by Dr. Helen Payling Wright. She introduced a method that measures the adhesiveness of platelets to glass. Fresh blood containing a suitable anticoagulant is rotated slowly in a glass bulb. At the beginning and after increasing intervals the platelets are counted, and their adhesiveness is indicated by the decrease in the counts, the missing platelets having stuck to the glass. With this method she demonstrated that clinical states that predispose to thrombosis are associated with increased adhesiveness. This method is still much used either as originally described or in a modified form. For example, platelets may be counted before and after passing blood or platelet-rich plasma through a column of glass beads [657].

A different method was introduced later [205]; light is made to pass through platelet-rich plasma, or through platelets suspended in artificial media, and the amount transmitted is continuously recorded. The platelets are kept uniformly suspended in the plasma by rapid stirring, which does little or no damage to them. When the platelets clump the amount of transmitted light increases and when the clumps break up the amount decreases. Thus, changes in the optical density provide measures of the rate and extent of aggregation of the platelets. This method has been and is still being used all over the world both in research departments and in clinical laboratories, and it has provided much new information about platelets [981].

Platelet Aggregation by Adenosine Diphosphate and Its Inhibition. It has been known for a long time that the "stickiness" of platelets towards each other and towards glass and other surfaces is greatly increased by thrombin. It was thought, therefore, that thrombin was responsible in some way for the development not only of the coagulation type of thrombus in veins but also of the conglutination thrombus found in arteries, and it was postulated that thrombin was formed temporarily in the plasma. More recently, other naturally occurring substances, including fatty acids and adrenaline, have been found to increase the adhesiveness of platelets. In 1960 Hellem discovered that it is markedly increased by a substance present in erythrocytes. This was subsequently identified by Hellem and his colleagues [508] as adenosine diphosphate (ADP), which is present in all the cells of the body and is increased in injured cells. Some years earlier it had been shown that platelets contain extraordinarily high concentrations of adenosine triphosphate (ATP) and that this disappears during clotting [204] or when platelets undergo the changes known as viscous metamorphosis [1600]. Since ADP is the first breakdown product of ATP, these observations suggest that the increase in adhesiveness brought about by ADP might underlie the physiological mechanism responsible for the formation of hemostatic platelet plugs and the pathological mechanism responsible for thrombosis [205]. This hypothesis is now supported by considerable evidence [207, 926].

The platelets of all species of mammals tested so far are rapidly aggregated by ADP in very low concentrations. There is evidence that the ADP mechanism underlies the aggregating action of the various other agents such as thrombin and fatty acids. Elegant experiments by Haslam [629], now at the ICI Research Laboratories, have shown that these agents fail to cause aggregation of platelets in the presence of an enzyme system that ensures the rapid removal of ATP. The aggregating mechanism appears to be specific to ADP. It requires the presence of calcium and of at least one plasma protein, almost certainly fibrinogen;

and aggregation is inhibited by lack or excess of ionic calcium, deficiency or inactivation of the plasma protein, and deficiency or inactivation of a component of the platelets.

The aggregation of platelets in plasma is reversible which suggested that the ADP is broken down [205], a suggestion since confirmed directly in the Thrombosis Research Group [1003]. The products of this breakdown (which is catalysed by at least two enzymes, see below) are adenosine monophosphate (AMP) and adenosine. Adenosine was found to inhibit aggregation [205, 212].

Specific Receptor or Binding Sites for ADP and Certain Nucleoside Inhibitors. [218]. The only nucleotides related to ADP which are so far known to cause aggregation are deoxy-ADP which is less potent, and 2-chloroadenosine diphosphate which is more potent than ADP by one order of magnitude [900]. The effect of the 2-chloro derivative was discovered some time after it had been found that aggregation by ADP was specifically inhibited by adenosine and some closely related substances of which 2-chloroadenosine was the most potent [206]. The specificity of aggregation by the nucleotides suggested that it is caused by their complexing with equally specific chemical groupings, or receptors on or within the platelet surface membrane [207], because ADP cannot penetrate through intact cell membranes. The structural similarity of the inhibitory nucleosides suggested that their inhibition is competitive [210]. This idea has received some support from the kinetic properties of the inhibition [1373, 1600].

The following affinity constants ($\times 10^7$) have been calculated for the postulated receptor-nucleotide or nucleoside complex: 2-chloroadenosine diphosphate 5.61; ADP 0.58; 2-chloroadenosine 0.26; and adenosine 0.007 [900]. Inhibition by adenosine increases in the first few minutes in a manner similar to its uptake by platelets. The kinetics of this uptake were used to calculate the number of receptor sites for ADP as about 2×10^5 per platelet [207]. This agrees remarkably well with a calculation, based on effect of ADP on the electrophoretic mobility of platelets, of about 1×10^5 [602].

Recent work has cast some doubt on the competition hypothesis [1266]. Aggregation by ADP is not inhibited by adenosine monophosphate which is more similar to ADP than is adenosine, and Holmsen's alternative hypothesis proposes that phosphorylation of adenosine depletes the platelet of ATP required for the aggregation mechanism. This still leaves intact the requirement that adenosine and its inhibitory analogues must interact with a specific site although this may now be thought of either as the enzyme adenosine kinase or as a channel or carrier by which adenosine moves through the platelet membrane. This last possibility is analogous to the hypothesis for explaining the effects of 5-hydroxytryptamine on platelet aggregation [102]. Recently we have found [217] that the uptake of adenosine by platelets can be completely prevented without effect on its inhibitory action on aggregation; this observation seems to invalidate Holmsen's hypothesis. Furthermore, a specific receptor which reacts with ADP on the platelet membrane is still required. It has been proposed [207] that the mode of action of ADP can be best accounted for by assuming that ADP forms very short-lived complexes with a component of the platelet membrane, similar to the assumption made to account for, say, the action of acetylcholine on a smooth muscle membrane [268]. In relation to this proposal, arguments that platelets do not "bind" ADP [1285] are invalid since they depend on the meaning of binding in terms of time.

Mechanism of Platelet Aggregation. One hypothesis put forward to explain ADP aggregation suggests that a complex composed of ADP, calcium and a plasma protein, perhaps the von Willebrand factor, makes bridges connecting adjacent platelets [1372]. Another hypothesis [207] is that bombardment by ADP molecules produces a configurational change in another component of the system, probably a protein on the platelet surface, and that this change enables bonds to be formed between the platelets and molecules of the protein co-factor in the plasma, presumably fibrinogen.

It seems that the platelet membrane is altered by its reaction with ADP without the involvement of calcium. Evidence for this is that ADP (and 5-HT) in the presence of high concentrations (up to 10^{-2} M) of EDTA cause a rapid morphological change in the platelets, during which they become more spherical and extrude numerous processes. Calcium and fibrinogen are then required for the binding of platelet to platelet. The fibrinogen molecule is long enough (about 700 Å) [193] to make it an attractive and likely candidate for the material which forms bridges between loosely aggregated platelets; this has, however, still to be established.

A major problem is the nature of the forces that could bind the end of a fibrinogen molecule to a constituent of the platelet surface. The actual binding could come about through the establishment either of ionic, including hydrogen, bonds or of covalent bonds. Two possibilities are ionic binding via calcium between acidic groups on the glycopeptide (gamma)-chain of fibrinogen and a glycoprotein on the platelet; or covalent disulphide binding via a reactive thiol group in the fibrinogen "knot" [193] and another thiol of a platelet protein.

To distinguish between these possibilities, I have recently determined the effect of changes in the ionic strength of plasma on platelet aggregation. The platelets in 1 ml samples of citrated human plasma were made to aggregate at 37° by the addition of ADP ($1–2 \times 10^{-6}$ M) and aggregation was followed by the photometric method [205]. At increasing times, 0.03 ml volumes of the following 5 M solutions were added rapidly into the stirred plasma: sodium chloride, potassium chloride or potassium nitrate; or 0.015 ml of 10 M choline chloride. In this way the ionic strength was suddenly doubled. The effects of doing this with the different salt solutions were very similar. During the first phase of aggregation [899, 1004] there was an immediate increase in the optical density of the plasma suggesting that the platelet aggregates were dispersing; this was confirmed microscopically. This result favors the view that the adhesive forces which bind the platelets to each other during their aggregation initially are electrovalent rather than covalent. When the salt solutions were added during the second phase of aggregation [1004], there was only an immediate small increase in optical density which thereafter did not change more than that of control samples. This suggests that the second phase of aggregation, which is associated with the release of various constituents from the platelets, brings other binding forces into play as well.

Platelet Aggregation in Thrombogenesis. It can be concluded that the adhesiveness of platelets can be greatly and rapidly increased by various naturally occurring substances acting via the ADP mechanism. However it does not inevitably follow that this process is responsible for the pathological adhesiveness of platelets that results in thrombosis. It is necessary to find out, first, whether conditions that predispose towards thrombosis cause the circulating platelets to be exposed to one or more aggregating agents. Secondly one must discover whether such exposure can start a "chain reaction" [207] by which, once a few platelets have adhered to the vessel wall, others adhere to them in rapidly increasing numbers, thereby producing the build-up of a conglutination thrombus. The hypothesis of the chain reaction proposes, therefore, that an initial exposure to one or more of the naturally occurring aggregating agents, including ADP, causes the release of more aggregating agent, presumably ADP, from the platelets themselves. This hypothesis was required because of the rapid dilution and breakdown of ADP in plasma.

Various conditions thought to predispose to thrombosis are directly associated with rises in the concentrations of aggregating agents in the plasma, for example, heavy meals increase fatty acids, and stress increases adrenaline. Other conditions could bring about the appearance of such agents indirectly through their release from damaged cells, such as the endothelial cells of the vessel wall, the circulating blood cells, and the platelets themselves.

Platelets do not adhere to completely *normal* endothelium. However, even in normal vessels, platelets tend to adhere to the basement membrane when they can come in contact with it through gaps between endothelial cells [496]. Whether such platelet adhesions can lead to their intravascular aggregation is not yet known. When endothelium is removed, layers of platelets adhere to the underlying connective tissue, the collagen of which releases ADP from platelets. Damage of such magnitude would activate Hagemann factor (which is involved in the initiation of blood coagulation on contact with foreign surfaces) and release tissue thrombokinase, so as to lead to the formation of thrombin.

Hardly anything is known about the role of leucocytes except that fresh platelet thrombi are often covered by polymorphs to which platelets are also occasionally seen adhering in the peripheral blood.

When erythrocytes are destroyed, as in hemolytic diseases, ADP is presumably released and, indeed, thrombosis is a common complication of these diseases. However, red cells also increase platelet adhesiveness in the absence of demonstrable hemolysis; this effect is antagonized by adenosine, so ADP can apparently be released from essentially intact cells. The red cells represent by far the largest pool of adenine nucleotides in the blood. The continuous release of a small proportion of this pool could explain the frequency of platelet thrombi under conditions liable to affect the red cell membrane, for example turbulent flow, lipemia [219], homocystinuria [897], and osmotic effects such as occur in renal failure and in diabetes.

As to the postulated chain reaction, recent work has indicated that it does indeed exist. When ADP is added at certain critical concentrations the aggregation of the platelets occurs in two phases [899]; the first phase is caused by the added ADP, the second by ADP that is released from the platelets. During the second phase aggregation becomes irreversible. Interestingly, the effectiveness of ADP in causing aggregation is potentiated by adrenaline [59, 1113], which greatly decreases the ADP concentration required to produce irreversible aggregation [218]. These observations clearly increase the probability that the ADP mechanism is involved in thrombogenesis.

In spite of so much circumstantial evidence that thrombogenesis involves ADP, it is unlikely because of rapid breakdown to be demonstrable in plasma *in vivo*. To establish that the ADP mechanism is at work it is presumably enough to demonstrate *in vitro* that ADP *could* be released and *in vivo* that its effect is abolished by adenosine. In this role therefore ADP may be regarded as a "local hormone", the release of which is assumed because its effects are abolished by specific antagonists.

The wider implications are interesting. Presumably the original function of this local hormone was entirely physiological, that is, to arrest bleeding; but now, through the operation of predisposing conditions that did not exist originally (such as higher levels of fatty acids and adrenaline in the blood), it seems that this local hormone has become involved in the pathological process of thrombosis.

Effects of Drugs on Platelet Function. As might be expected, drugs that prevent coagulation are more effective in venous than in arterial thrombosis since successful treatment of the latter must include dispersion of the platelet masses. Substances that are known to inhibit platelet aggregation might be expected to disperse platelet masses and efforts have been made to demonstrate this. It is necessary to test the substances in animals with experimentally induced thrombi and, so far, no method is known for reproducing in animals the sequence of events that is believed to cause thrombosis in man, However, it is possible to produce with complete consistency platelet thrombi in blood vessels that are mechanically injured [472, 705]. Such platelet thrombi grow into "white bodies" that embolize intermittently in the blood stream. The rate and duration of embolization can thus be used as a measure of the thrombus-producing activity of the injured vessel.

When *in vitro* inhibitors of platelet aggregation, such as adenosine or 2-chloroadenosine, are infused into rabbits or rats the thrombus-producing activity of an injured vessel is rapidly diminished and soon disappears [209]. Adenosine analogues that are ineffective as inhibitors of aggregation *in vitro* also fail to inhibit "white body" formation *in vivo*. These observations provide direct evidence that platelet aggregation can be prevented and reversed intravascularly as well as indirect evidence that the ADP mechanism is involved in thrombogenesis, at least in that associated with trauma. Adenosine analogues that are effective as inhibitors of platelet aggregation are also vasodilators and, in man, their relative potencies for both effects is the same [214]. Much work is now being done in attempts to discover adenosine analogues that inhibit platelet aggregation and are otherwise harmless. Very recently, it has been claimed that a newly-synthesized analogue, viz. 2-methylthioadenosine-5'-phosphate, is a potent inhibitor of platelet aggregation *in vitro* without causing significant cardiovascular effects *in vivo* [981]. If this is confirmed it provides new hope that a substance of this type may have the desired therapeutic property of inactivating the function of platelets only, under thrombogenic conditions.

Since platelet aggregation is an important factor in arresting bleeding it had always been feared that drugs such as these might prevent normal hemostasis as well as platelet aggregation in a thrombus. Fortunately, however, it has been found that adenosine and its analogues inhibit thrombus formation in the lumen of injured vessels without interfering with the formation of hemostatic plugs and without causing prolongation of the bleeding time. This finding supports the conclusion that such intravascular aggregation involves ADP alone in the first-phase mechanism; and it suggests, furthermore, that extravascular aggregation involves other agents as well, collagen and thrombin for example, which rapidly bring about other less reversible changes in the platelets.

Several other types of substance, including drugs, inhibit platelet aggregation *in vitro* and interfere with their adhesion and aggregation in the hemostatic function *in vivo*. These substances are listed in several review articles [601, 658, 981]. Some of the substances occur naturally in the body and may, therefore, influence the behavior of normal circulating platelets. These endogenous sub-

Table. *Inhibitors of platelet aggregation (A) and release (B)*

Endogenous	Exogenous	
Adenosine	Adenosine analogues	(A)
Prostaglandins	Local anaesthetics	(A)
Fibrinogen degradation products	Thiol reagents	(A)
	Metabolic inhibitors	(A)
	Guanidine derivatives	(A)
	Membrane stabilisers	(B)
	Anti inflammatories	(B)

stances (Table) inhibit only the primary aggregation process. The most effective inhibitor of aggregation known at present is prostaglandin E_1, [811] but it cannot be used therapeutically because of its hypotensive effect and its rapid disappearance from the circulation. Some of the exogenous substances also inhibit aggregation; these include several drugs used as vasodilators which accelerate the reversal of platelet aggregation [601]. Other drugs inhibit the release reaction which forms the basis of the chain reaction, *viz.* imipramine and chlorpromazine and related compounds [1006] and acetylsalicylic acid, i.e. aspirin [443]. The release of nucleotides from platelets is inhibited by these drugs in concentrations which do not affect aggregation; the drugs interfere, therefore, with the positive feedback mechanism by which ADP released from aggregating platelets can cause further aggregation.

The effect of aspirin is particularly interesting. It consists in the prevention of the release reaction in response to ADP or to adrenaline and in inhibition of aggregation by collagen. Moreover, the release of platelet factor No. 3 by all these agents is diminished. A similar defect in platelet function is produced by an acetylating agent, i.e. acetic anhydride. Moreover, when platelets are incubated with acetyl-1-^{14}C salicylic acid, the platelets become radioactive showing that acetate is taken up by them. Aspirin has these effects whether it is incubated with platelets *in vitro* or ingested in the usual therapeutic doses. After ingestion of a single dose of aspirin the circulating platelets remain abnormal for several days; this suggests that the drug affects the platelets permanently and that the reappearance of normal reactions represents the appearance of a new platelet population. If this is so, a drug exists which has a long-lasting disabling effect on platelets. Clearly, therefore, this action of aspirin is potentially useful in preventing the formation of platelet thrombi. This possibility is being investigated clinically. The effect may contribute to the well-recognized tendency of aspirin treatment to cause bleeding; that would be an undesirable side-effect.

Another antipyretic drug (sulphinpyrazone) also inhibits platelet aggregation *in vitro* [1381]. This and similar substances are still more toxic than aspirin, and unlikely to be useful clinically as anti-thrombotic agents. Sulphinpyrazone increases the mean survival of circulating platelets [1381]. It is possible that the prolongation of the life-span of platelets is due to the diminution in their reactivity caused by the drug. Recently it has been found that colchicine [1387] diminishes platelet adhesiveness in aggregation and accelerates disaggregation; and that the vinca alkaloids of the periwinkle cause a rise in the blood platelet count. Both colchicine and the vinca alkaloids interfere with contractile proteins by inhibiting the polymerization of actin and they alter the structure of microtubules. It has just been suggested [1386] that these are the actions by which colchicine and the vinca alkaloids diminish the reactivity of platelets and that the alkaloids might, therefore, be considered for investigation as possible anti-thrombotic drugs.

DRUGS AFFECTING CATECHOLAMINE METABOLISM AND STORAGE IN THE ADRENERGIC NEURONE

P. A. SHORE

The past fifteen years have witnessed great advances in the understanding of the biochemistry and physiology of the adrenergic neurotransmitter system, and, of more pragmatic importance, have seen the development of a number of drugs which interact more or less specifically with discrete steps in the catecholamine metabolic pathways or storage mechanisms. Such drugs include certain antihypertensives, sympathomimetics, antidepressants and major tranquilizers.

The following brief review presents a necessarily truncated description of the current state of knowledge of this rapidly advancing field. No attempt has been made to review the literature thoroughly. Cited references are restricted mainly to pertinent review articles. Of special interest may be the proceedings of the Second Catecholamine Symposium, 1966 [9].

CATECHOLAMINE BIOSYNTHESIS

The biosynthetic pathway of catecholamines has been known for a number of years, but only recently have all of the enzymes been demonstrated directly.

Fig. 1 shows the biosynthetic pathway leading to norepinephrine (NE) and epinephrine (E) and identifies the enzymes involved in each biotransformation. The initial step, the hydroxylation of tyrosine by the enzyme tyrosine hydroxylase to form dihydroxyphenylalanine (dopa), is in a sense the most important of the several links in the biosynthetic chain, as good evidence exists that it is the rate limiting step in the entire biosynthetic pathway. This enzyme is quite specific in its substrate requirement, and the distribution of the enzyme in tissue follows, in general, catecholamine distribution. The decarboxylation of dopa by aromatic L-amino acid decarboxylase results in the formation of 3,4-dihydroxyphenylethylamine (dopamine), itself a substance of considerable importance in extrapyramidal function. Aromatic L-amino acid decarboxylase, as its name suggests, is quite unspecific, effecting the decarboxylation of 5-hydroxytryptophan, histidine, and tyrosine as well as dopa. The conversion of dopamine to NE,

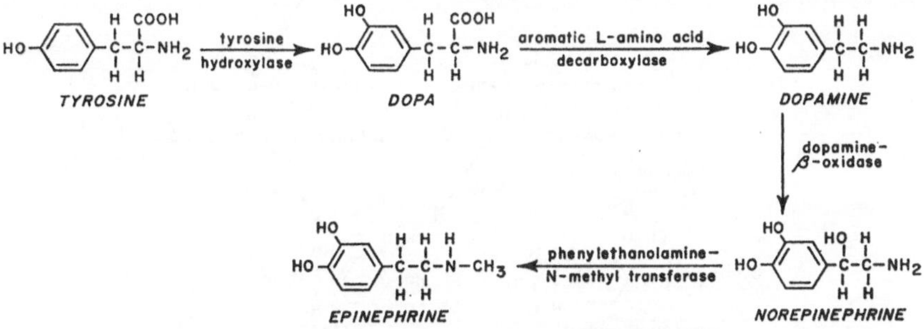

Fig. 1. Pathway of catecholamine biosynthesis

the most important catecholamine and the adrenergic neurotransmitter, occurs by the action of the copper-containing enzyme dopamine-beta-oxidase, which might better be called hydroxyphenylethylamine-beta-oxidase, as the enzyme can also effect the conversion of tyramine to octopamine, and alpha-methyl-m-tyramine to metaraminol. NE in chromaffin tissue may be converted to E by the action of phenylethanolamine-N-methyltransferase, utilizing S-adenosylmethionine as the methyl donor. Drugs interfering with the various enzymic steps are discussed hereafter. Detailed discussions may be found in recent reviews [195, 456].

CATECHOLAMINE METABOLISM

The major routes of metabolism of NE in the body are depicted in Fig. 2. Two major initial pathways of catecholamine catabolism exist in the body. NE may initially undergo oxidative deamination by the action of monoamine oxidase (MAO) to form dihydroxymandelic acid (through the intermediate dihydroxymandelaldehyde), or it may undergo ether formation by the action of catechol-O-methyl transferase (COMT). The latter involves transfer of the methyl group from S-adenosylmethionine to the 3–0-function of the benzene ring of norepinephrine to form normetanephrine. The product of either of these enzymic actions may undergo further changes by the other enzyme to form ultimately 3-methoxy, 4-hydroxymandelic acid which is commonly referred to by the misnomer vanilyl-mandelic acid (VMA). The pathway of E metabolism is essentially similar, the product of COMT action being N-methylnormetanephrine (metanephrine). Intermediate products may also undergo conjugation or reduction reactions. The final excretion products of NE thus may include a complex mixture of products along with a small portion of unchanged NE. The major excretion product of endogenous NE in the body is VMA. As described herein, much of the NE released following nerve stimulation is taken up by the adrenergic nerve terminals and stored again. Drugs interfering with each of these major pathways are also discussed.

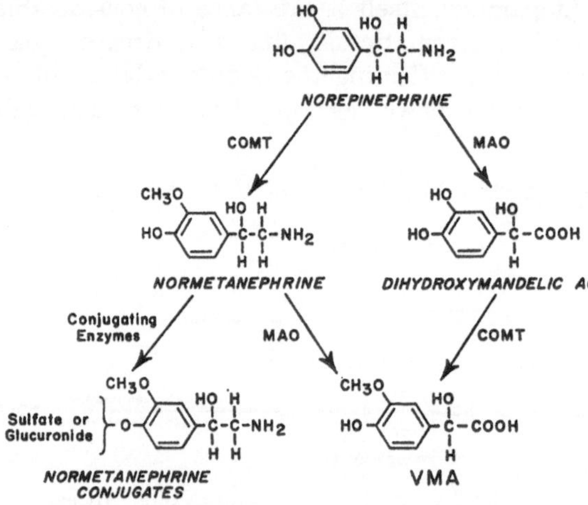

Fig. 2. Major pathways of norepinephrine metabolism

STORAGE OF NOREPINEPHRINE IN THE ADRENERGIC NEURONE

Investigations of the past decade have revealed a great deal of information regarding the mode of storage of NE in the adrenergic neurone. A schematic picture illustrating the NE concentrating and storage mechanisms is shown in Fig. 3.

NE is stored in granular vesicles of about 500 Å in diameter in the adrenergic neurone by a still poorly understood granular mechanism which is highly sensitive to the action of reserpine. This storage mechanism is often referred to as the granular concentrating mechanism or the intraneuronal concentrating mechanism. After release of NE from the nerve terminal following nerve stimulation, much of the released NE, it is currently thought by most investigators, is taken up again across the neuronal membrane by a Na^+-requiring amine carrier mechanism which is inhibited competitively by a number of drugs including cocaine and tricyclic antidepressants such as desipramine and amitriptylline. This membrane amine transport system is also inhibited by ouabain and other cardiac glycosides, apparently by virtue of diminished net Na^+ movement across the membrane. Once in the neurone, the amine is reconcentrated in the granulated vesicles by the reserpine-sensitive system. The membrane transport system appears to be quite unspecific, as a variety of catecholamine congeners may be transported into the neurone. The storage granules, on the other hand, exhibit much more stringent stereochemical requirements, and, consequently, only a very few NE congeners are stored in this intraneuronal system.

A portion of the NE synthesized in the neurone gradually leaks from the storage granules into the axoplasm where it is metabolized intraneuronally by the action of MAO. A similar fate awaits most of the NE released intraneuronally by reserpine. That portion of NE reaching the circulation following, for example, nerve stimulation, may be taken up again by the membrane transport system or may be destroyed extraneuronally by COMT. To a lesser extent, the amine may diffuse away to be metabolized by liver MAO or excreted unchanged.

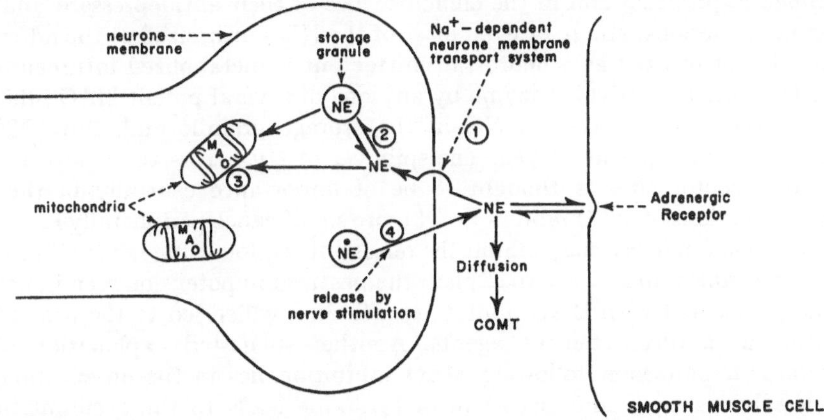

Fig. 3. Schematic model of norepinephrine uptake and storage mechanisms in the adrenergic neurone. ① Inhibited by cocaine, tricyclic antidepressants and cardiac glycosides. ② Inhibited by reserpine and guanethidine. ③ Inhibited by MAO inhibitors. ④ Inhibited by neurone blocking drugs

Pertinent discussions may be found in the following reviews: Bloom and Giarman [195], Ferry [456], Muscholl [1060] and Kopin [817].

DRUGS AFFECTING NE METABOLISM

Drugs Affecting Biosynthetic Pathways

Tyrosine hydroxylase activity is inhibited by alpha-methyl-tyrosine. Treatment with this agent lowers NE levels in the body without affecting the NE uptake and storage mechanisms. Thus the rate of decline of NE after treatment with alpha-methyl-tyrosine gives an estimate of the turnover of norepinephrine.

Dopa decarboxylase (aromatic L-amino acid decarboxylase) may be inhibited by a number of drugs, but it has proven difficult to cause sufficient inhibition of this enzyme to alter NE stores. At one time it was thought that the antihypertensive and NE depleting drug, alpha-methyldopa, was acting by virtue of its decarboxylase inhibitory action. Current evidence has shown that this is not the case, but rather, that alpha-methyldopa is itself transformed by the decarboxylase and dopamine-beta-oxidase to nordefrin (alpha-methyl-norepinephrine), a compound which depletes NE from its storage granules (see false transmitters below).

Dopamine-beta-oxidase may be inhibited by treatment with disulfiram which is reduced in the body to diethyldithiocarbamate, an agent which acts by chelation of the copper moiety of the enzyme. Although this enzyme is present in low activity compared to dopa decarboxylase, it remains difficult to alter NE levels by inhibiting this enzyme, as it is not the rate limiting step of the biosynthetic sequence.

Drugs Affecting NE Catabolism

MAO inhibitors have been studied extensively both in the laboratory for experimental purposes and in the clinic because of their antidepressant and antihypertensive actions. Much, or even most of the NE synthesized at the adrenergic neurone is not utilized as a neurotransmitter but is metabolized intraneuronally by MAO. Inhibition of this enzyme by any one of several potent MAO inhibitors increases the concentration of NE in the storage granule and, since MAO is blocked, in the axoplasm as well. The spillover of NE across the neuronal membrane to receptor sites is thought to be of importance centrally in the antidepressant actions of MAO inhibitors. Of more significance peripherally is evidence that free axoplasmic NE may inhibit the release of NE following nerve stimulation. Such a mechanism may serve to explain the postural hypotension seen in patients chronically treated with MAO inhibitors, a finding which led to the use of MAO inhibitors as antihypertensive agents. Another suggested explanation of the orthostatic hypotension following MAO inhibition lies in the observation that after MAO blockade, administration of tyramine leads to the accumulation in adrenergic neurones of the beta-hydroxylated derivative, octopamine, a substance which may act as a "false transmitter" to blunt the efficiency of the sympathetic nervous system (see the following for discussion of false transmitters).

COMT may be inhibited competitively by other catechols such as pyrogallol. While COMT inhibition has proven useful in the laboratory to help elucidate the importance of metabolic pathways, no clinical usefulness of these compounds exists. Detailed reviews of these subjects may be found in previously cited reviews.

DRUGS AFFECTING NE UPTAKE AND STORAGE MECHANISMS

Agents Acting on Granule Storage Function

Depleting Agents. Reserpine and other active Rauwolfia alkaloids, guanethidine, and tetrabenazine act mainly on the intracellular storage mechanism (see reviews by Muscholl [1060], Carlsson [290], and Shore [1357]). The exact mechanisms by which these drugs act on the storage granules to block their ability to store NE is not known. Reserpine has been the most studied of these agents as it initially appeared that the pharmacological effect of the drug (amine depletion) persisted far longer than the presence of the drug. Evidence has been presented, however, that small amounts of reserpine persist during the time of NE depletion, and recently it has been demonstrated [41] that minute quantities of reserpine are irreversibly bound in tissues with adrenergic innervation, and that a linear relationship exists between the degree of NE depletion and the concentration of persistently bound reserpine. It has been demonstrated in rat heart that one molecule of persistently bound reserpine is associated with the depletion of about 500 NE molecules. Assuming that the persistently bound reserpine is attached only to amine storage granules, it can be calculated that about 20 molecules of reserpine interact with each affected granule.

A clue to the biochemical mechanism of action of reserpine lies in the demonstration that low concentrations of this drug inhibit the Mg^{++}-ATP-stimulated binding of catecholamines by isolated adrenal medullary granules [290]. More recently, it has been proposed that reserpine may interfere with a specific Na^+-dependent amine carrier system operating intraneuronally [1440].

The mechanism of the NE depleting action of guanethidine is even less clear, although it has been demonstrated that the uptake of small quantities of guanethidine are associated with NE depletion.

False Transmitters. As mentioned, it is now known that the active depleter of NE after administration of the antihypertensive drug alpha-methyldopa, is its metabolic product nordefrin (alpha-methyl-NE). The latter compound, and its close congener metaraminol, are active NE depletors whose mechanism of action is better understood (see Muscholl [1060]). These agents, which are not substrates of MAO, are readily transported by the adrenergic neuronal membrane amine carrier into the axoplasm where they compete with NE for granular storage sites. As NE is a substrate for MAO the net result is stoichiometric displacement of NE from the storage sites by the false transmitter. This name is awarded such compounds because they occupy NE storage sites and are, like NE, released following sympathetic nerve stimulation. As their effect on the adrenergic receptor is markedly less than NE, the net result is decreased efficiency of the sympathetic nervous system. Thus, even though metaraminol displaces NE and is a sympathomimetic amine widely used as a pressor agent in the treatment of shock, small daily doses of metaraminol have been shown to be antihypertensive in man (Crout et al. [348]).

Agents Acting on Adrenergic Neurone Membrane Transport System

As described previously, cocaine and the various tricyclic antidepressants such as desipramine, inhibit amine transport into the neurone by competing with the amine for the Na^+-dependent amine carrier. It is currently held that the antidepressant effect of the tricyclic antidepressants is related to this action as they are the most potent antagonists of the amine carrier function. These compounds are looked upon as potentiating the effect of released NE by virtue of inhibition of NE uptake, a major mode of termination of the action of released NE. Cardiac glycosides also inhibit by virtue of their actions on Na^+ movement, and have proven useful in laboratory investigations into the biochemical nature of the amine transport system. It should be stressed that this effect of the glycosides occurs in drug concentrations higher than those which produce an inotropic effect on the heart. Effects on NE storage mechanisms may, however, play some role in cardiac arrhythmias produced by cardiac glycosides.

Drugs Inhibiting Release of NE by Nerve Stimulation

A relatively new class of drug known as adrenergic neurone blocking drugs has the characteristic of preventing the release of NE following nerve stimulation, possibly by stabilization of the NE storage granules (Boura and Green [231]). Included in this category of compounds are bretylium, debrisoquin and guanethidine, the latter having this effect as well as that of causing NE depletion. It is not yet clear as to how these agents prevent NE release, but it has been shown recently that a number of these agents are MAO inhibitors and are also accumulated in tissues with adrenergic innervation to the extent that they may act in part at least by blockade of MAO (Medina et al. [968]).

Sympathomimetic Amines Acting by Release of NE

Certain drugs transiently release NE in an active form from storage sites, but unlike metaraminol and nordefrin, are not themselves stored. These drugs have been termed "indirectly acting" sympathomometic amines, as all or part of their pressor or stimulatory activity is derived from the released NE (see Burn and Rand [269]). The prototype of the indirectly acting sympathomimetic amine is tyramine, which has no effect of its own on the adrenergic receptor, but transiently displaces NE from adrenergic neurons. A serious hazard in the clinical use of MAO inhibitors is the paroxysmal hypertension occurring after ingestion of certain foodstuffs such as cheeses containing tyramine and other indirectly acting sympathomimetic amines which would normally be destroyed after ingestion by MAO, but after MAO blockade survive to exert a pharmacologic effect. Other drugs acting indirectly on peripheral sites include amphetamine

Table. *Clinically useful drugs interacting with NE storage mechanisms*

Clinical use	Drug	Site of action
Antihypertensive	*NE depletors* Reserpine Guanethidine	Intraneuronal storage granules by blockade of storage mechanism
Antihypertensive	*False transmitters* α-Methyldopa	Intraneuronal storage granules by substitution of NE by amine product of drug
Antihypertensive	*MAO inhibitors* Pargylline	Block MAO; may produce false transmitter, or free NE may inhibit NE release
Antihypertensive	*Neurone blockers* Bretylium Debrisoquin	Prevent NE release by nerve stimulation. May act in part by MAO inhibition
Sympathomimetic	Amphetamine Ephedrine	Act entirely or in part by NE release from granules onto receptors
Antidepressant	*Tricyclic antidepressants* Imipramine, Amitriptyline and others	Competitive inhibition of central adrenergic neuronal membrane amine carrier system
Tranquilizer	Reserpine	Deplete NE and serotonin centrally from storage granules. Questionable if this is entirely pertinent to central action

and epinephrine, the latter being a "mixed action" sympathomimetic drug in that it acts in part through released NE and in part *per se* on the adrenergic receptor.

A list of various clinically useful drugs and their modes of interaction with NE storage mechanisms may be found in the table.

Discussion Following Dr. Shore's Paper

Dr. Moutafis: The treatment of homozygous Type II hyperbetalipoproteinemia continues to present a very difficult therapeutic problem. We have studied the effect of several drugs on several parameters of hyperlipoproteinemia Type II. We studied the effect of cholestyramine on cholesterol metabolism in such a female patient 16 years old. We followed the serum ^{14}C cholesterol specific activity for seven weeks, then gave 20 g of cholestyramine per day. This caused an increased excretion of fecal steroids; but, in spite of that, the serum cholesterol concentration remained unchanged, and the size of the xanthomata remained the same. We have reason to believe that this treatment failure is due to the fact that increased endogenous synthesis compensates for the increased sterol losses.

In contrast to cholestyramine, nicotinic acid lowered the serum cholesterol concentration substantially with a 50% reduction within three weeks time. Nicotinic acid inhibits the synthesis of cholesterol in the liver. Since nicotinic acid may upset liver function, we are trying to determine the dose of nicotinic acid which will lower the cholesterol level of the serum without disturbing the liver function tests.

Dr. Walton: We carried out studies with the protein moiety labeled with ^{131}I and in cases of hyperlipidemia. Clofibrate was given to a patient with Type III hyperlipoproteinemia. The absolute catabolic rate was greatly elevated before treatment. After a month's treatment, in addition to the total serum lipoproteins coming down, the absolute catabolic rate was restored to normal.

Another case, which corresponded to Frederickson's Type II, was more or less completely resistant to treatment with clofibrate. In this case, after a month's treatment, the serum concentration remained high and the absolute catabolic rate showed no change.

In view of the fact that the protein moiety is the same for the S_f 0–20 and the S_f 20–400, it would seem that the effect of clofibrate is probably not on the synthesis or catabolism of the protein portion of this molecule, but the effect may be through secondary mechanisms whereby this protein is loaded with triglyceride or its other lipid components.

Dr. Kritchevsky: I would like to clarify our findings on the effect of Atromid on the oxidation of cholesterol by rat liver mitochondria to which Dr. Steinberg alluded. In the complete system there really is no difference between the mitochondria prepared from Atromid-fed and normal rats; i.e. the oxidation per milligram of mitochondrial nitrogen is equal. These data are really in accord with all the others. When the supernatant factor is omitted, then there is an increase in the oxidation by the mitochondria prepared from Atromid-treated rats, but this observation will help us to understand better the nature of the supernatant rather than the action of clofibrate.

Dr. McDONALD: Dr. Keen of London, England, discussed the clinical use of tolbutamide in relation to atherosclerosis in patients with hyperglycemia. In our laboratory, we have, over a period of years, investigated, *in vitro* and *in vivo*, the effect of several oral hypoglycemic compounds, including tolbutamide, chlorpropamide and phenethylbiguanide, on the biosynthesis of both cholesterol [Dalidowicz and McDonald, Biochemistry 4, 1138 (1965)] and proteins [DeChatelet and McDonald, Biochem. Pharmac. 18, 595 (1969)]. These studies utilized, principally, ^{14}C-labeled precursors in the case of cholesterol and leucine-^{14}C in the case of proteins.

To summarize the results, all the oral hypoglycemic compounds were found to inhibit the biosynthesis of cholesterol in animal experiments. This effect would, by itself, be advantageous to users of the substances. Unfortunately, they all also inhibit protein biosynthesis, the effect being exerted at the microsomal level. I should like to ask Dr. Steinberg whether chlorpropamide or phenethylbiguanide have been found to inhibit cholesterol biosynthesis in man.

Dr. STEINBERG: I am not aware of any studies that establish whether or not oral hypoglycemic agents affect cholesterol biosynthesis in man. The studies that have been done on the effects of oral agents on blood lipid levels are to some extent conflicting. However, it is my impression that the best controlled studies failed to show any effect of, at least, tolbutamide on blood lipid levels. For example, the studies done in Bierman's laboratory, which included a double blind design with the use of placebo, failed to show any significant effect even in patients who had initially elevated cholesterol levels. Consequently, it seems unlikely that the effects *in vivo* are of a sufficient magnitude to influence plasma levels.

Dr. CUCUIAM: I wish to mention the results we have obtained in Hamilton with some pyramidine compounds. RA 233 and RA 433 inhibit release of nucleotides in the ambient fluid of rabbits and pigs. These were most potent inhibitors of nucleotide release and also lowered the concentration of ADP. The dipyridamole inhibited nucleotide release in the pig but did not affect platelet aggregation. Another compound that is released by thrombin is serotonin. RA 233 and RA 433 inhibit its release in both species, while persantine does not. This is explained by the fact that persantine or dipyridamole inhibits the uptake of serotonin from the ambient fluid.

Dr. BORN: These are very interesting results. I was aware of the results with RA 233 and RA 433, and these compounds are well worth investigating.

Dr. SAILER: The very simple intravenous fat tolerance test seems to be of great clinical value. In order to evaluate the significance of the lowered K_2 after CH 13, 437 treatment, I would like to ask Dr. Carlson if he measured the fractional removal rate of K_2 in other examples, whereby the pool size was different before and after dietetic or other therapeutic measures.

Dr. CARLSON: No.

Section XVI

SELECTED PAPERS ON DRUG EFFECTS

A CONCEPT OF ANTI-THROMBOTIC THERAPY BASED ON THE PHARMACOLOGICAL EFFECTS OF DRUGS PREVENTING PLATELET AND RED CELL AGGREGATION

H. I. BICHER

ANTI-ADHESIVE DRUGS

In previous reports [153, 155, 156, 158] we described the properties of a group of chemically nonrelated substances, such as Phenylbutazone, Chloropromazine, local anesthetics, etc. to prevent blood cell aggregation of the type that may lead to thrombosis, namely red cell and platelet aggregation. These properties were present both *in vivo* and *in vitro* and seemed to be mediated by some type of membrane action [158]. They were termed "Anti-Adhesive Drugs".

Several ketolactone derivatives [1451] exhibit these properties. Based on low toxicity and potency of action we selected 2-methyl-2-tert-butyl-beta-ketolactone (2–4 BMK) for further experimentation. This drug prevents *in vitro* platelet to glass adhesiveness and ADP-induced platelet aggregation at a concentration of 1 mg/cc (as tested using modifications of the methods of Wright [1579], Swank [1446]) and red cell aggregation at 100 γ/cc (tested with a modified Thorsen method).

The effective dose_{50} *in vivo* to prevent both platelet and red cell aggregation is 200 mg/kg. At this dose, the compound markedly improved the peripheral circulatory disturbances induced by intravascular red cell aggregation (sludge), as shown by vital microscopy in the cat's omentum.

PREVENTION BY ANTI-ADHESIVE DRUGS OF THROMBOSIS AND ANOXIC TISSUE DAMAGE

In the present experiments attempts have been made to prevent *in vivo* thrombus formation or tissue damage induced by the blood cell aggregation processes. Microthrombi in lungs and respiratory death were produced in the rat according to the technique of Nordoy (1964). Adenosine diphosphate (ADP) was injected at a dose of 17 mg/kg into the femoral vein of 24 animals, twelve of which were pretreated with 2–4 BMK. The mortality rate of the ADP control animals was 9/12, that of the drug pretreated group was 3/12. Histological sections of the lungs showed platelets and red cell aggregates plugging the small vessels in almost all animals of the first group, and only occasionally in rats pretreated with 2–4 BMK.

Sludge-induced vein thrombosis was provoked in cats using the method of Borgstrom [202]. This technique is a combination of ligation of both femoral veins (to produce venous stasis) with trauma-induced intravascular red cell aggregation. Venous thrombi developed in the ligated veins after 24 hours. The experiments were performed on three groups of ten animals each. In the first group vein ligation only was performed, and two thrombi were found. In the second group vein ligation was combined with trauma, and 18 thrombi were found. The animals of the last group were given 2–4 BMK before and 12 hours after being exposed to the two previous procedures: only nine thrombi were found. Observations of the peripheral circulation confirmed the presence of intravascular red cell aggregation in animals of the second group only.

The induction of intravascular red cell aggregation causes anoxic myocardial damage in the atherosclerotic rabbit [157] demonstrable in the ECG and histological sections. Pretreatment of the atherosclerotic rabbits with 2–4 BMK before the sludge induction prevented this effect.

A new ultramicro-oxygen electrode (2 μ tip) has been developed. The external surface of a glass micropipette is coated with a thin layer of platinum that acts as an oxygen cathode when covered, but for the tip, by a second layer of an oxygen impervious material [154]. A reference Ag-AgCl electrode can be placed either externally in the animal tissue or in the KCl filled glass micropipette.

Using this electrode, it can be shown that the compensatory response of the circulation to brain cortex anoxia has two phases, a quick phase that returns cortex PO_2 to pre-anoxic levels (reoxygenation time), and a second slow "overshoot" phase wherein the PO_2 exceeds the pre-anoxic base line. Induction of intravascular red cell aggregation by the intravenous administration of high molecular weight dextran dampens the second phase of the response, holding it under the baseline PO_2 levels, and considerably prolonging the "reoxygenation time". The intravenous injection of 2–4 BMK, 200 mg/kg, counteracts the effects of intravascular red cell aggregation and restores the "reoxygenation time" to normal values.

THROMBOTIC PROCESS

The classic concept of thrombosis—the intravascular formation of fibrin, leading to blood cell entrapment, vessel occlusion and tissue death—should be interpreted in view of the increased amount of evidence describing the behavior of the blood cells flowing in the small peripheral vessels. These vessels are ultimately responsible for the delivery of amounts of oxygen adequate to keep the tissue alive. A likely sequence of events for the thrombotic process based on the current literature and the preceding facts follows (see Fig. 1).

Phase a: Intravascular Red Cell Aggregation (Combined With Atherosclerosis or Transient Hypoxia). The absence of intravascular red cell aggregation during health has been confirmed in man [813]. Based on microscopic observations of microthrombotic occlusions in capillary vessels showing marked sludging of blood cells, a relation between sludge and thrombosis has been suggested. Experimental studies [202] and clinical observations [191, 606] have confirmed this relationship. Since sludge is present in thrombotic disease, the obvious question is: Is it a consequence or the beginning of the thrombotic process?

Gelin [521] summarized the possible pathogenetic mechanisms by which sludge could induce tissue injury. Our present experiments show that when sludge is combined with atherosclerosis or a period of transient hypoxia, anoxic tissue damage is the consequence, both in brain and heart.

Phase b: Anoxic Damage to Vascular Endothelium. In the postcapillary venules and the venous limb of the capillary the delivery of oxygen is normally very precarious. It is in this region that hypoxic damage to vessel walls by the restricted blood flow of vasoconstriction or intravascular agglutination, or by both of these plus atherosclerosis is more easily evidenced. Knisely [712] has described this damage that leads to an endothelial lesion and protein leak. Recently, Reneau [1221] developed a mathematical model in which the factors influencing oxygen diffusion to tissue were analyzed and predicted the formation of minute hypoxic areas at the venous ends of brain capillaries under pathological conditions.

Phase c: Platelet to Vessel Wall Reaction (Platelet Adhesiveness Phase). Contact is established through a "leaky" endothelium between platelet and tissue factors (collagen, etc.) that enhance platelet adhesiveness, thus initiating a more active chain of events in the thrombotic process. Platelet adhesiveness has been correlated with collagen-induced platelet aggregation. Native collagen fibrils aggregate platelets in citrated plasma. The fibrils release considerable amounts of ADP from the platelets, and the aggregation is inhibited by AMP [712]. Evidence has also been obtained that collagen releases serotonin from platelets and renders platelet factor 3 available [1389]. The electron microscopic studies of Hovig [712] indicated that the platelet membrane remains intact during interaction with collagen, while the intracellular granules disappear. The release is therefore probably due either to an increased membrane permeability to ADP and serotonin or to an extrusion of platelet granular material without membrane rupture. Recent work by Johnson [751] has provided further details of this complicated process. The release of these factors leads into the next steps of thrombus formation.

Phase d: Platelet Aggregation. The importance of platelet aggregation for hemostasis and for the pathogenesis of thrombotic processes is well established. It is associated with release of more endogenous platelet aggregation factors (EPAF), platelet factor III, minor red cell trapping, and enhanced local anoxia. Changes in platelet reactivity to ADP, the chemical agent most frequently considered to be the natural platelet aggregation-inducer, has been determined in a number of hemorrhagic and thrombotic conditions [1070]. with the aid of methods that lend themselves to a quantitative determination of platelet function. Platelet clump embolism is also considered to be part of the mechanism leading to atherosclerosis, according to Duguid's theory [411].

Once the process is initiated, more endogenous ADP and other aggregation factors are liberated, and the process tends to perpetuate itself. Our experiments demonstrated that red cells are trapped in the platelet aggregates, becoming a major factor to increase the mass of the microemboli and probably the local hypoxia.

At this point, coagulation factors liberated from tissue (thromboplastin), platelets (factors III, V) and red cells probably initiate changes in plasma proteins which lead to:

Phase e: "Cascade" or "Thrombin Activation" Process of Fibrin Formation. These well known theories [898, 1335], not discussed herein, demonstrate the manner in which the needed coagulation factors are made available by the hypoxia aggregation process, which can, being reversible in nature, regulate the amounts and availability of these factors.

Phase f: Formation of "Red Thrombus". French [496] has described how the actual length of a thrombus is determined by the mass of red cells trapped in it. This is similar to the trapping of phase c, but the cells are incorporated in a more major way into the fibrin mesh.

SITE OF ACTIVITY OF ANTI-ADHESIVE DRUGS

According to this scheme of thrombus formation, we propose that the anti-adhesive drugs exert their anti-thrombotic action on phases a, b, c, d and f of the thrombotic sequence (marked with X in Fig. 1).

X *Phase a*	*Intravascular red cell aggregation* combined with atherosclerosis and/or transient hypoxia
	↓
X *Phase b*	*Anoxic damage to vascular endothelium*
	↓
X *Phase c*	*Platelet to vessel wall reaction-ADP* and serotonin release (epaf)
	↓
X *Phase d*	*Platelet aggregation*—further epaf, platelet factor III liberation, minor *blood cell trapping*
↓	↓
Phase e	*Fibrin formation*
	↓
X *Phase f*	*Major blood cell trapping*

X-Phases prevented by the action of antiadhesive drugs

Fig. 1. The thrombotic process

HYPOCHOLESTEROLEMIC AND OTHER EFFECTS OF METHYL CLOFENAPATE, A NOVEL DERIVATIVE OF CLOFIBRATE

J. M. Thorp

It is increasingly apparent that differing types of *gross* lipoprotein abnormality do not respond similarly to any particular treatment, and that adequate characterization of the disorder is a prerequisite to the application of the appropriate therapy [489, 1427]. This may have tended to obscure the fact that useful hypolipemic responses can be achieved in the far more commonly encountered minor lipoprotein abnormalities. Nevertheless, more selective and effective methods of treatment seem to be needed, particularly in the case of hyper-beta-lipoprotein-

Table 1. *Mean results for groups of eight male rats each treated for one month with methyl clofenapate administered by oral dosage once daily*

Dose (mg/kg/day)	Initial body (g)	Final body (g)	Liver weight / body weight (g/100 g)	Plasma cholesterol (mg/100 ml)	Plasma TEFA (mEq/l)	Plasma fibrinogen (mg/100 ml)	Serum clofenapic acid (μg/100 ml)
0	138.5	300	4.3	75.5	8.4	292	0
0.25	146.0	280	4.65	60.0	8.3	276	16.0
0.50	140.0	263	4.85	54.5	6.9	268	28.5
1.0	143.5	280	5.35	52.5	6.95	237	53.5
2.0	150.0	276	6.1	44.5	6.95	212	83.0

emia, classified as Type II [489], groups 1 and 2 [1427], or S-type (Stone, unpublished data). This type of abnormality has features in common with those seen in hypothyroidism, and is to a certain extent responsive to treatment with thyroid-active substances. Our studies over the last decade of the structure-activity relationships of aryloxyisobutyrate derivatives has led us to postulate a key mechanism involving the binding of thyroxine to albumin [1468]. We have therefore sought for compounds in this series showing both intense and selective (in relation to competition with thyroxine) binding to albumin. This report deals with the compound ICI. 55,695 (methyl clofenapate, I), chosen for clinical evaluation on the basis of these and related studies. Chemically, it is methyl-2-[4-(p-chlorophenyl)phenoxy]-2-methylpropionate, and is a closely related analogue of "Atromid-S" (clofibrate). As with clofibrate, it is metabolized *in vivo* to the corresponding acid, ICI. 54,856 (clofenapic acid, II) which is the active moiety.

The selection of the methyl ester (I) for oral administration was based on the finding that it was more uniformly absorbed than the free acid (II). Doses are therefore expressed in terms of I, while serum concentrations refer to II, which was also the form (generally as a solution of its sodium salt) used for *in vitro* studies. Screening tests had indicated that persistence *in vivo* was inversely related to the solubility in water of the acids in a given series. The exceptionally low solubility of II ($<0.001\%$) was associated with marked persistence in the rat (half-life 15–20 days). At effective concentrations II was found to be extensively ($>99\%$) bound to albumin; it has a highly specific effect in reducing by 50% the primary association constant of the binding of L-thyroxine to human albumin. In accordance with this, it was found to have a volume of distribution in the rat, dog, and man corresponding to the albumin space (8–12% of the body weight). Moreover, it caused a significant redistribution of labelled thyroxine from serum into liver of the rat. While in the rat and dog the compound is excreted mainly in bile, in man it is excreted in urine, partly as the glucuronide conjugate which is its major metabolite.

The response of rats on a normal diet to treatment with I is shown in Table 1. The increase of liver weight with increasing dosage was found to be associated with the typical histological, enzymatic, and biochemical changes previously observed with other oxyisobutyrate derivatives, including clofibrate. Detailed analysis of liver lipids revealed no accumulation of desmosterol or other precursors of cholesterol. Increase of dosage beyond 2 mg/kg daily produced no further increase in hypolipemic activity. A noteworthy feature is the reduction of plasma fibrinogen achieved at serum levels of **II** taken to represent the "therapeutic" range (50–80 μg/ml).

Curiously, no hypocholesterolemic activity was observed at any dosage of **I** in our strain of mice, in which species the half-life was 2–3 days. In the dog, oral doses of 1.5–3 mg/kg daily gave a maximum hypocholesterolemic response (to about 60% of control levels) at serum levels of **II** (50–80 μg/ml) similar to those required in the rat. The half-life was 9–10 days.

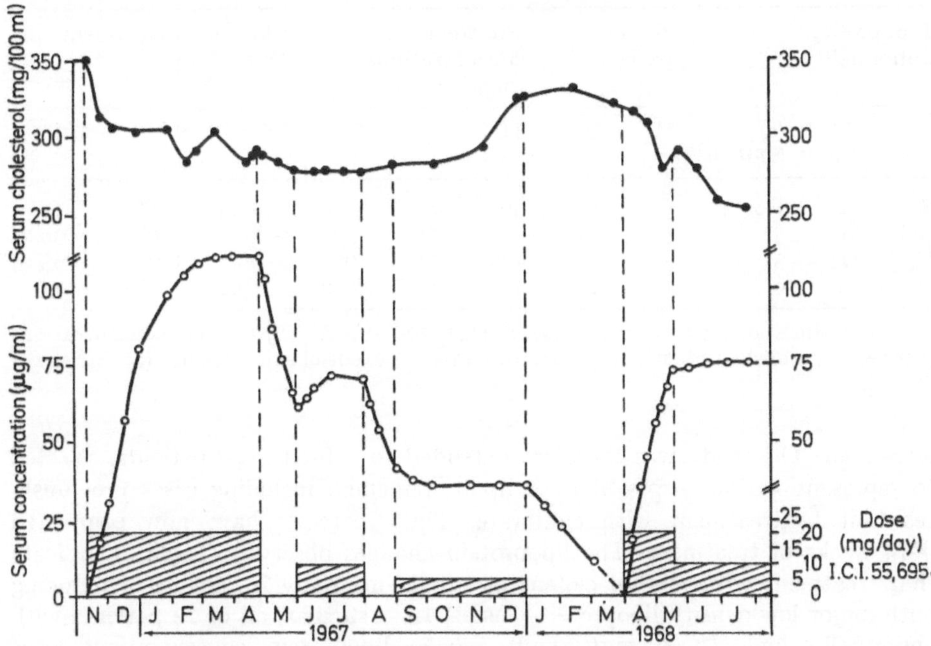

Fig. 1. Serial studies in one subject (body wt. 76.5 kg) of serum cholesterol with clofenapic acid concentrations during and between treatments with various dosages (cross-hatched areas) of methyl clofenapate

In man serum levels of **II**, following a single oral dose of **I**, decay with a half-life of 30–40 days. It was thus calculated that doses of 10–20 mg daily should give an equilibrium concentration in the "effective" range, based on the findings in the rat and dog. Fig. 1 shows the results of serial studies in a subject with a mild Type II hypercholesterolemia, previously resistant to other treatments. These suggest that an effective response can be maintained at a dosage of 10 mg (0.13 mg/kg) daily, giving a serum concentration of **II** of about 70 μg/ml (similar to that found in the rat and dog). In the later part of the study this serum level was achieved by an initial period of treatment at 20 mg daily for six weeks, followed thereafter by the maintenance dose of 10 mg. As the hypocholesterolemic effect appeared to be persistent, this pattern of dosage was adopted for subsequent clinical investigations.

Detailed examinations, made twice weekly, were completed in three of four male subjects (one subject being withdrawn due to intercurrent illness, unrelated to administration of the compound) during a two-week pretreatment and 13-week treatment period. At a mean concentration of II in serum of 67.5 μg/ml there was a reduction of 21% in total cholesterol and 51% in triglyceride. No significant side-effects or adverse alterations in serum enzymes or hematology were noted. Apart from the lipid changes, small but consistent reduction of plasma fibrinogen, euglobulin lysis time, alkaline phosphatase, bilirubin, and hematocrit

Table 2. *Observed lipoprotein changes*

Lipoprotein abnormality[a]			No. of patients		Pre-treatment concentrations (mg/100 ml)			Change on treatment (%)		
(a) SM	(b) FR	(c) STR	M	F	TC	S	M	TC	S	M
S	II	I or 2	6	9	393	785	150	−24.5	−25	−11
SM	II	5	5	3	426	822	338	−20.4	−19.5	−36.2
M_3	III	3	2	2	406	331	998	−30.4	+19.7	−65.4
M	IV	4	1	1	335	312	1,440	−19.2	+56.5	−75

[a] Classifications on basis of: (a) S (S_f 0-20) and M (S_f 20–400) concentrations (Stone, unpublished data), (b) electrophoresis (Fredrickson [489]); (c) Strisower [1425]).

were seen. The study was therefore extended to a further 29 patients, selected to represent various types of hyperlipoproteinemia, including cases previously resistant to treatment with clofibrate. These patients have now completed 6–14 weeks of treatment. The lipoprotein changes observed (Table 2) indicate that treatment with methyl clofenapate at 10 mg daily is capable of reducing both major low-density lipoprotein classes. In particular, all of 22 patients with abnormally high (>500 mg/100 ml) S_f0–20 lipoprotein concentrations have shown a reduction in this fraction, including those previously resistant to treatment with clofibrate. Further studies are required to define dose-response relationship, and to exclude the possibility of delayed or unforeseen side-effects, toxicity, or "escape".

MECHANISM OF CLOFIBRATE INHIBITION OF HEPATIC CHOLESTEROL BIOSYNTHESIS*

Lawrence W. White

Hypercholesterolemia is considered a major risk factor in the development of atherosclerosis. Consequently, prevention of atherosclerosis and its complications has included attempts to influence the concentration of plasma cholesterol. Recently, several pharmacological agents have been introduced which appear to decrease plasma cholesterol concentration by inhibiting hepatic cholesterol biosynthesis; however, too little consideration has been given to the potential consequences of interference with this process. Interference with certain steps (e.g. acetate activation) may be ineffective, interference beyond MVA[1] may lead to accumulation of intermediates with limited alternate pathways, and interference beyond the stage of cyclization of squalene may result in accumulation of precursors with atherogenic potential. Furthermore, partial inhibition of sites that are not rate-limiting may be associated with no net decrease in cholesterol synthesis. Consequently, knowledge of the biochemical sites of action of pharmacological agents used to inhibit cholesterol synthesis is essential; when correlated with information regarding physiological and pathological regulation of cholesterol synthesis, rational therapeutic approaches to the problem of atherosclerosis will be feasible.

Recently, several workers have suggested that cholesterol synthesis is regulated chiefly by the enzyme system catalyzing formation of MVA from HMG-CoA (HMG-CoA reductase); a regulatory role has also been demonstrated for the preceding reaction involving condensation of Ac-CoA and AcAc-CoA to form HMG-CoA, HMG-CoA condensing enzyme [White, L. W., Rudney, H.: Biochem. (1970A), in press].

Clofibrate (ethyl ester of p-chlorophenoxyisobutyrate), an agent that decreases cholesterol concentration in rat plasma and liver [1469] and decreases plasma cholesterol and triglyceride concentration in patients with hyperlipidemia [1118], appears to act at least in part by inhibiting hepatic cholesterol synthesis at a relatively early stage [78]. Decreased incorporation of Ac-^{14}C, but not MVA-^{14}C into hepatic cholesterol indicates an effect prior to MVA formation, but definitive assays of the various possible sites of action between Ac and MVA have not been performed. In this investigation, the effect of clofibrate feeding on reactions involved in MVA formation has been evaluated.

* The work herein was done during the tenure of an Established Investigatorship of the American Heart Association, and was supported by grants from the National Institute of Arthritis and Metabolic Diseases (AM 11574) and the Heart Association of Northeastern Ohio, Inc.

1 The following abbreviations are used throughout the text: HMG and HMG-CoA for 3-hydroxy-3-methyl glutaric acid and its CoA ester; MVA for mevalonic acid; Pyr for pyruvate; Ac and Ac-CoA for acetate and its CoA ester; AcAc and AcAc-CoA for acetoacetate and its CoA ester.

METHODS

Liver slices and cell-free fractions were prepared from male Sprague-Dawley rats. Treated animals were fed clofibrate at a level of 0.3% of the diet for one to 18 days. To study the overall pathway of cholesterol synthesis as well as selected segments, liver slices were incubated in 5 ml Krebs-Ringer bicarbonate buffer containing 0.02 M glucose and either 0.004 M Ac-1-^{14}C, 0.005 M Pyr-2-^{14}C, or 0.01 M MVA-2-^{14}C. Formation of AcAc and incorporation of labelled substrate into cholesterol, CO_2, and fatty acids were measured, In some experiments, 0.02 M MVA (unlabelled) was present to trap MVA ^{14}C formed from other substrates.

To determine the biochemical sites of action more precisely, cell-free preparations were used. Individual reactions between Ac and MVA were studied by using Ac-^{14}C, Ac-CoA^{14}C, or HMG-CoA ^{14}C as substrate and by separating the microsomal fraction (which contains HMG-CoA reductase) from the soluble fraction (which contains other enzymes including HMG-CoA condensing enzyme). Preparation and incubation of homogenate fractions, and isolation, purification, and assay of HMG and MVA were performed by methods detailed elsewhere [White, L. W., Rudney, H.: Biochem. (1970B), in press].

Altered rates of incorporation of isotopically labelled precursors may not necessarily indicate altered rates of synthesis, since dilution of intermediate pools (e.g. Ac-CoA) by endogenous unlabelled substrate will also contribute to altered incorporation. Accordingly, specific activities of HMG and MVA were determined indirectly by measuring specific activity of AcAc as previously described (White, unpublished data).

RESULTS

Clofibrate feeding was associated with lowered plasma cholesterol concentration in all treated animals, with an average decrease of 33%. The effect of clofibrate administration on incorporation of labelled substrate into products by liver slices is shown in Table 1. Incorporation of Pyr-2-^{14}C but not MVA-2-^{14}C into cholesterol was depressed, indicating an effect on the segment of the pathway prior to MVA formation. This is confirmed by decreased incorporation of both Ac-1-^{14}C and Pyr-2-^{14}C into MVA. Depressed incorporation of both substrates into MVA suggests that the site of inhibition is beyond Ac-CoA, and increased formation of AcAc indicates an inhibitory action beyond AcAc-CoA synthesis.

In fractionated liver homogenates, clofibrate was associated with decreased incorporation of Ac-^{14}C into cholesterol in a preparation containing soluble and microsomal fractions (10,000 $\times$ g supernatant). Changes in activity of HMG-CoA condensing enzyme are summarized in Table 2. With soluble fraction (105,000 $\times$ g supernatant) and Ac-1-^{14}C as substrate, incorporation into HMG was decreased by clofibrate feeding. However, incorporation of Ac-CoA-^{14}C into HMG was not significantly influenced, indicating that effects with Ac-1-^{14}C were related to decreased Ac activation.

Effects of clofibrate administration on activity of HMG-CoA reductase are shown in Table 3. In the presence of microsomes and a TPNH generating system, clofibrate feeding resulted in depressed incorporation of several substrates into

MVA, including Ac-1-^{14}C, Ac-CoA-^{14}C, and HMG-CoA^{14}C, indicating inhibition of HMG-CoA reductase. These changes occurred within 24 hours.

Clofibrate administration was associated with increased AcAc formation by soluble fraction, soluble + microsomes, or soluble + microsomes + mitochondria,

Table 1. *Effect of clofibrate administration on incorporation of substrate by rat liver slices* [a]

Duration of feeding	Substrate	Product	Control	Clofibrate	Percentage change
3 days	Pyr-2-^{14}C	Chol.	10,742 (4)	4,663 (4)	↓57
	MVA-2-^{14}C	Chol.	48,950 (4)	46,050 (4)	↓ 5.9
	Pyr-2-^{14}C	MVA	125 (4)	78.4 (4)	↓36.5
	Ac-1-^{14}C	MVA	118 (4)	68.2 (4)	↓42.3
	Pyr	AcAc	1,840 (8)	2,462 (8)	↑33.7
	Ac	AcAc	1,829 (4)	2,453 (4)	↑34
7 days	Pyr-2-^{14}C	MVA	95 (3)	61.7 (3)	↓35
	Pyr-2-^{14}C	CO_2	15,000 (3)	13,400 (3)	↓10.7
	Pyr	AcAc	303 (3)	531 (3)	↑75

[a] Values for cholesterol are expressed as cpm/mg cholesterol; for CO_2 or MVA as mμmoles substrate incorporated per gram tissue; and for AcAc as mμmoles formed per gram tissue. Figures given are average values for number of rats indicated in parenthesis.

Table 2. *Effect of clofibrate administration on HMG-CoA condensing enzyme activity in rat liver homogenate fractions* [a]

Substrate	Duration of feeding	Substrate incorporation into HMG mμmoles		
		Control	Clofibrate	Percentage change
Ac-^{14}C	7 days	32.0	18.4	↓42
	10 days	66.8	27.5	↓59
	18 days	31.8	13.6	↓57
AcCoA-^{14}C	3 days	16.1	14.0	↓13
	7 days	13.3	14.9	↑12
	9 days	28.1	33.5	↑19
	18 days	65.2	54.5	↓17

[a] Each value given represents average obtained with 4 rats. Soluble fraction (105,000 × g supernatant) was used in all experiments.

when Ac was substrate. However, when AcAc-CoA was substrate, no significant increase in AcAc formation occurred. By combining microsomes from treated rats with soluble fraction from control or treated rats, changes were localized to specific tissue fractions (Table 4). Effects of clofibrate on HMG-CoA reductase were associated with the microsomal fraction; however, depression of Ac activation and increased AcAc formation were dependent on addition of soluble fraction from clofibrate-treated animals.

In both slice and homogenate experiments, specific activity of AcAc was not influenced by prior clofibrate administration. Consequently, changes in incorporation of ^{14}C into HMG or MVA reflected altered synthesis of these intermediates, rather than changes in specific activity of precursor pools associated with altered

Table 3. *Effect of clofibrate administration on HMG-CoA reductase in rat liver homogenate fractions*

Tissue fraction	Substrate	Duration of feeding	Substrate incorporation into MVA mμmoles		
			Control	Clofibrate	Percentage Decrease
Soluble fraction (105,000 × g supernatant) + microsomes	Ac-^{14}C	1 day	14.4 (4)	1.9 (4)	87
		1 day	59.6 (4)	11.4 (4)	81
		3 days	84.9 (4)	5.4 (4)	94
		7 days	26.1 (4)	6.31 (4)	76
		9 days	108.4 (4)	54.1 (4)	50
		10 days	77.2 (4)	15.6 (4)	80
Soluble + Microsomes	AcCoA-^{14}C	1 day	4.42 (4)	2.52 (4)	43
		1 day	2.17 (4)	1.63 (4)	25
		7 days	11.7 (4)	7.58 (4)	35
		9 days	67.1 (4)	36.4 (4)	46
Microsomes	HMGCoA-^{14}C	1 day	6.92 (4)	1.90 (4)	72
		1 day	75.1 (4)	21.9 (4)	71
		3 days	41.2 (3)	4.0 (3)	90
		3 days	90.0 (4)	31.1 (4)	65
		9 days	47.3 (4)	19.9 (4)	58

Table 4. *Effect of clofibrate administration on rat liver slices: comparison of microsomal and soluble fractions*

Soluble fraction	Microsomal fraction	Ac-^{14}C incorporated into HMG mμmoles	Ac-^{14}C incorporated into MVA mμmoles	AcAc formed mμmoles
Normal (8)	Normal (8)	25.6	24.7	233
Clofibrate (4)	Clofibrate (4)	6.7	6.3	399
Normal (4)	Clofibrate (4)	23.9	15.8	242

endogenous substrate metabolism. When rates of synthesis were calculated in slice experiments, clofibrate feeding was associated with 31.2% and 29.4% reduction in MVA formation, with Ac-1-^{14}C or Pyr-2-^{14}C respectively as substrate.

Some workers have suggested that effects of clofibrate feeding on lipid metabolism may be indirectly mediated via other metabolic alterations. In preliminary experiments in which the soluble sodium salt of clofibrate was added to liver slices *in vitro*, incorporation of Pyr-2-^{14}C and Ac-1-^{14}C into cholesterol or MVA was decreased. These effects, similar to those associated with clofibrate administration *in vivo*, indicate a direct mechanism of action.

DISCUSSION

Because of the potential therapeutic importance of clofibrate, considerable effort has been devoted to studying its mechanism of action. Effects of clofibrate on cholesterol synthesis in man have been suggested by studies that show a decreased rate of decline of cholesterol-^{14}C specific activity [1087], and decreased incorporation of Ac-1-^{14}C into cholesterol [694]. To account for inhibition of cholesterol synthesis, several biochemical sites of action have been proposed, including interference with conversion of Ac to MVA [78], MVA to isopentenyl pyrophosphate [80], and increased removal of AcAcCoA by enhanced formation of AcAc [267]. We have shown an effect on hepatic microsomal HMG-CoA reductase by definitive examination of reactions involved in MVA formation. In addition, increased ketone formation in both slice and cell-free systems follows clofibrate-feeding and is dependent on soluble factors. Since this is demonstrable with Ac, but not AcAc-CoA as substrate, it would appear that the effect is not secondary to enhanced activity of AcAc-CoA deacylase.

While decreased cholesterol synthesis occurs following clofibrate-feeding, its importance with respect to prevention of atherosclerosis and its complications remains to be determined. In this regard, other demonstrated actions of clofibrate may also be important, including effects on mobilization of free fatty acids from adipose tissue, on the vascular wall, and on platelet adhesiveness and coagulation mechanisms.

STUDIES OF THE MECHANISM OF ACTION OF p-CHLOROPHENOXYISOBUTYRATE (CPIB)

Joseph N. Pereira and Gerald F. Holland

CPIB was described by Thorp and Waring [1469] as a potent hypocholesteremic agent in rats. Studies since that first report have established hypolipemic activity in other species, including man. However, numerous investigations have failed to elucidate the mechanism of action of this interesting agent. Several of these have provided clues indicating that hepatic triglyceride synthesis and/or release are affected by the administration of CPIB (Azarnoff et al. [80]). The results of Duncan and Best [412] coupled with those of Spritz and Lieber [1400] suggest that the administration of CPIB to rats depresses hepatic triglyceride synthesis.

To date, all studies of the mechanism of action of CPIB have involved long-term dosage schedules which produce hepatomegaly and increases in hepatic triglyceride concentrations. These effects occur late in relation to the plasma lipid changes and are, therefore, likely to be secondary and irrelevant to the mechanism of action of CPIB. In order to investigate the primary, short-term effects of this interesting agent, the single dose studies reported here were undertaken.

METHODS AND MATERIALS

Sprague-Dawley rats (180–220 g) obtained from Charles River Breeding Laboratories were used throughout the study. Blood for lipid analyses was drawn from the abdominal aorta. Plasma and liver triglycerides were determined by the methods of Van Handel and Zilversmit [1492] and Butler et al. [274], respectively. The method of Carr and Drekter [293] was used to determine plasma cholesterol concentrations. Isolated livers were perfused by the method of Miller [1000]. Blood for perfusion was drawn from the abdominal aorta of nonfasted rats. Two parts of whole heparinized blood were diluted with one part of Krebs-Ringer bicarbonate buffer pH 7.4 containing 1% albumin. Liver donors (250–275g) were heparinized just prior to liver excision. Perfusions were of one hour duration. The viability of the livers was assessed by bile production and appearance. Perfusate triglycerides were isolated by thin-layer chromatography. Radioactivity in perfusate triglycerides and fatty acids derived from those triglycerides was counted by standard liquid scintillation techniques. Glyceride glycerol was determined by difference. Hepatic alpha-glycerophosphate concentrations were determined by the method of Nikkilä [1101]. The Lee and Lardy [852] technique was used to measure mitochondrial alpha-glycerophosphate dehydrogenase activity. Protein was measured by the biuret method.

RESULTS AND DISCUSSION

Earlier studies with CPIB in rats have revealed that administration for seven or more days caused liver enlargement and depressed plasma lipid concentrations. Since the complete time course of the onset of these changes has not been reported, rats were fed CPIB, 0.25% in ground Purina chow for periods up to 10 days. Groups of rats were sacrificed after 1, 2, 3, 4, 5, 8 and 10 days. The results of these studies are presented in Table 1. Plasma triglyceride and cholesterol concentrations are depressed by CPIB after one overnight feeding period and remain depressed throughout the entire 10-day period. No significant changes in liver triglyceride levels were observed. The liver weight of control animals was maintained throughout the observation period at 4.2–4.4% of body weight. On the other hand, the livers of CPIB-treated rats increased in size after three days and progressed to sizes 30–35% larger than control animals.

Since the effects of CPIB on plasma lipid concentrations could be observed after one overnight feeding period, the effects of single intraperitoneal doses were investigated (Table 2). Plasma triglyceride levels were depressed as early as three hours after an intraperitoneal dose of 250 mg/kg. Plasma cholesterol concentrations were also reduced but the response was delayed so that significant reductions were observed after six hours. These lipid depressions were maintained for more than 24 hours. Due to the fact that these lipid changes could be produced by single doses of CPIB, all of the studies reported here utilized single intraperitoneal administration.

The work of Duncan and Best and Spritz and Lieber suggested that the rate of triglyceride synthesis was decreased by long-term administration of CPIB. In addition, Westerfeld et al. [1538] has clearly demonstrated the effect of long-term (seven or more days) administration of CPIB on the mitochondrial

Table 1. *Effects of CPIB, 0.25% in ground food, on liver size, plasma and liver triglyceride and plasma cholesterol levels of adult, male rats; n = 5*

Days	Treatment	Body weight (g)	Liver size (percentage body wt.)	Plasma triglycerides (mg-%)	Liver triglycerides (mg/g)	Plasma cholesterol (mg-%)
1	Control	223	4.4	61	5.8	65
	CPIB	221	4.3	21	6.2	42
2	Control	229	4.3	100	6.1	58
	CPIB	231	4.4	52	5.7	39
3	Control	234	4.2	35	4.6	61
	CPIB	236	4.7	9	5.5	35
4	Control	239	4.4	53	5.3	59
	CPIB	242	5.2	6	5.2	33
5	Control	243	4.2	26	4.2	66
	CPIB	249	5.5	5	3.7	41
8	Control	262	4.4	40	5.9	65
	CPIB	259	5.9	19	7.3	32
10	Control	281	4.4	76	6.4	63
	CPIB	276	5.8	32	5.9	33

Table 2. *Effects of CPIB, 250 mg/kg, i.p. on plasma triglyceride and cholesterol concentrations in rats given free access to food*

	Plasma lipid (mg%)	Time (hours) 0	3	6	9	12	18	24
CPIB, i.p.,	C[a]	—	55± 7	43±10	37± 4	43± 5	49± 8	45± 9
250 mg/kg	T[b]	—	32±11	40±17	33±12	37±16	22± 7	32±11
Control	C	61± 6[c]	58± 6	58± 5	62± 7	65± 6	57±10	66± 3
	T	63±16	63±12	76±26	51±17	46±12	49±13	55±22

[a] Total cholesterol.
[b] Triglycerides.
[c] Mean ± S.D.; $n = 5$.

enzyme, alpha-glycerophosphate dehydrogenase (MGPD), and postulated a role for thyroid hormone in that response. Due to the obvious importance of hepatic alpha-glycerophosphate levels (GP) in triglyceride synthesis, the effects of single doses of CPIB on the activity of this enzyme were studied. Fig. 1 demonstrates that increases in enzyme activity could be observed as early as four hours after drug administration and increased to a maximum after 24 hours. This increase represents a twofold increase over baseline activity. During exactly the same time period, hepatic GP concentrations were depressed, reaching a maximum reduction of approximately 50% after six hours (Fig. 2) and persisting for more than 15 hours. Because such a reduction in hepatic GP levels would be expected to decrease the rate of triglyceride synthesis, the effects of CPIB pretreatment on palmitate incorporation into triglycerides by the isolated, perfused rat

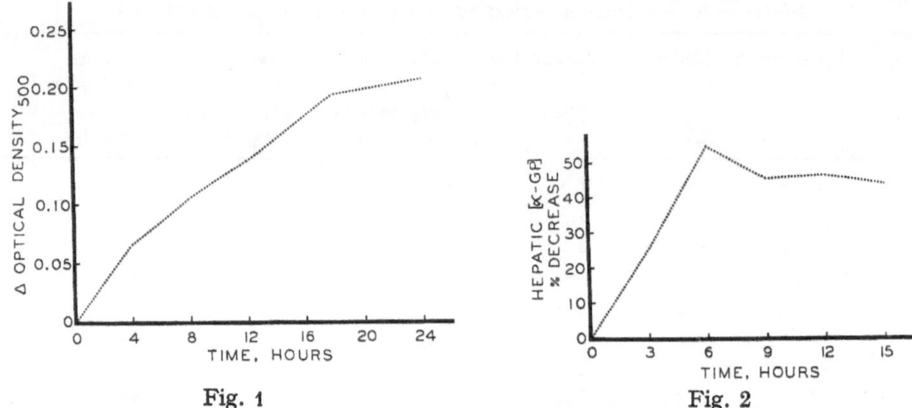

Fig. 1 Fig. 2

Fig. 1. Time course of the effect of CPIB, 250 mg/kg, i.p., on the activity of mitochondrial α-glycerophosphate dehydrogenase. Activity measured as optical density changes at 500 mμ wavelength. Changes in O.D. related to formazan production

Fig. 2. Time course of the effects of a single dose of CPIB, 250 mg/kg, i.p., on hepatic α-glycerophosphate concentrations

Table 3. *Effect of CPIB, 250 mg/kg, i.p. eight hours before perfusion on the incorporation of labeled palmitate and glucose into triglyceride fatty acids (TGFA) and triglyceride-glycerol (TG-G), respectively. N = 6, mean ± S.D.*

Precursor	Product	Percentage incorporation		Percentage of decrease
		control	CPIB	
Palmitate-1-^{14}C	TGFA	8.5 ±1.7	3.6 ±1.1	58
Glucose-U-^{14}C	TG-G	0.042 ±0.012	0.019 ±0.007	55

liver were examined. Liver donor rats were given CPIB, 250 mg/kg, i.p., and the livers excised and perfused with palmitate for one hour. The livers of CPIB-treated rats exhibited a markedly reduced (58%) capacity to incorporate palmitate (Table 3) into perfusate triglycerides at that time when hepatic levels of GP were also reduced.

If the activity of MGPD were important in controlling the rate of triglyceride synthesis, the incorporation of GP precursors into the glycerol moiety of triglycerides would be expected to be reduced. Therefore, livers were perfused with glucose, an important GP precursor. CPIB pretreatment (eight hours) reduced by more than 50% the incorporation of glucose into glyceride glycerol.

The results described here provide strong evidence that CPIB reduces plasma triglyceride concentration by increasing the activity of MGPD thereby reducing the availability of GP for triglyceride synthesis. The reduced rate of triglyceride synthesis limits the formation and secretion of plasma lipoproteins, the main lipid transport forms. The means by which CPIB influences plasma cholesterol concentrations are somewhat more indirect than the effects on plasma triglycerides but appear to be explicable in terms of the findings described.

Cholesterol in the parenchymal cell is at a branch point and can be incorporated into lipoproteins and secreted into the plasma or excreted into the bile as bile acids or neutral steroids. Factors influencing the direction in which cholesterol is metabolized have not been carefully defined, but it appears obvious that deficiencies in the supply of lipoprotein components (protein, phospholipid, triglycerides) will tend to favor the accumulation of cholesterol. When such conditions prevail, two possible results may be expected to follow. First, the excess

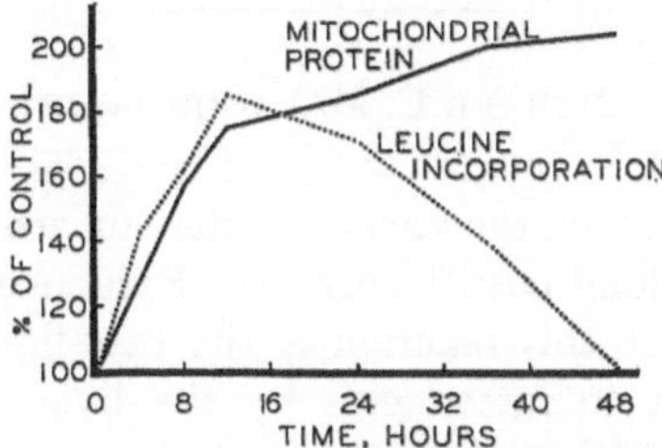

Fig. 3. Time course of the effects of a single dose of CPIB, 250 mg/kg, i.p., on leucine incorporation into mitochondrial protein and the increase in mitochondrial protein content

cholesterol might exert a negative feedback effect and thereby blunt the accumulation of cholesterol. However, a diversion of the excess cholesterol into the biliary flow represents a second mechanism. In fact, the recent findings of Grundy et al. [583] indicate that, in man, increased biliary output of neutral steroids may be the major, if not the sole, mechanism of the hypocholesteremic effects of CPIB. Studies of factors influencing the direction of hepatic cholesterol metabolism are in progress.

The results of Westerfeld et al. suggest that the increased activity of MGPD observed after repeated administrations of CPIB is due to the synthesis of new enzyme protein. In order to investigate this effect further, uniformly labeled leucine was administered intravenously at various times following the intraperitoneal administration of CPIB. An examination of the incorporation of leucine into the protein of the nuclear, mitochondrial, microsomal and cytoplasmic fractions indicates a specific stimulation of the synthesis of the mitochondrial protein (Fig. 3). The stimulation reaches a peak at 12 hours and declines so that no enhancement of leucine incorporation can be observed 48 hours after CPIB administration. The rate of decline may be a measure of the decay rate of messenger RNA since recent studies indicate that RNA synthesis precedes the observed stimulation of protein synthesis. We are continuing our studies of the molecular mechanism of CPIB in an attempt to elucidate the means by which CPIB facilitates the expression of genes controlling the synthesis of mitochondrial proteins.

In summary, studies of the primary, short-term effects of CPIB indicate that this agent produces its hypolipemic actions by a mechanism involving the induction of synthesis of mitochondrial proteins, one of which is MGPD. As a consequence of this de-repression mechanism, triglyceride synthesis is decreased and, indirectly, plasma cholesterol concentrations are reduced.

ON THE MODE OF ACTION OF LIPID LOWERING AGENTS*

MICHAEL E. MARAGOUDAKIS

The critical importance of the carboxylation of acetyl-CoA to malonyl-CoA in lipid biosynthesis has long been recognized. Evidence from many laboratories [1488, 1515] suggests that this reaction is the rate-limiting step in the overall conversion of acetyl-CoA to fatty acids by the liver. Acetyl-CoA carboxylase (ACC), the enzyme catalyzing this carboxylation reaction, is regulated by a feed-back mechanism involving the end-products, palmitoyl- and stearyl-CoA [1112], and is activated by certain TCA-cycle intermediates such as citrate and isocitrate [935]. Furthermore, it has been pointed out that in metabolic conditions in which fatty acid synthesis is depressed [221, 1547]. ACC has been found to be the locus of this effect.

Recently, we have reported on the inhibitory effect of the lipid-lowering agents, TPIA (potassium-2-methyl-2-[*p*-(1,2,3,4-tetrahydro-1-naphthyl)-phenoxy] propionate), CPIB (potassium-2-[*p*-chlorophenoxy]-2-methyl-propionate) and CDIB (potassium-2-methyl-2-[*p*-(*p*-chlorophenyl)-phenoxy]-propionate) on ACC purified from avian or rat liver [918, 920]. The inhibition of ACC by these compounds has provided a possible explanation at the molecular level for the hypolipidemic activity of these drugs *in vivo*.

RESULTS AND DISCUSSION

In vitro Experiments. The plasma lipid-lowering activities of TPIA, CPIB and CDIB have been well documented in experimental animals and in the clinic [152, 557, 675, 855, 1469]; their mechanism of action, however, is not understood, although many hypotheses have been advanced.

* The abbreviations used herein are: DIB for potassium 2-methyl-2-(*p*-phenylphenoxy)-propionate; CDIB for potassium 2-methyl-2-[*p*-(*p*-chlorophenyl)-phenoxy]-propionate; and CPIB for potassium-2-(*p*-chlorophenoxy)-2-methyl-propionate. This compound is also known as clofibrate. TPIA is for potassium 2-methyl-2-[*p*-(1,2,3,4-tetrahydro-1-naphthyl)-phenoxy]-propionate. This compound is also known under the code number Su-13437; and ACC for acetyl-CoA carboxylase.

We have assessed ACC as a possible enzymatic locus of action of these drugs. This enzyme is strongly inhibited by TPIA, CPIB and CDIB and their inhibitory potency is TPIA > CDIB > CPIB, as shown in Table 1. The inhibition is evident at all stages of purification of the enzyme and over the whole range of pH where the activity is measurable. Prolonged contact of drug with the enzyme does not result in irreversible inactivation of ACC. There are structural requirements

Table 1. *Inhibition of rat liver acetyl-CoA carboxylase by hypolipidemic drugs*

Compound	Abbreviation	Concentration for 50 % inhibition (I_{50})
CH_3 —O—C—COOH CH_3	(TPIA)	8.5×10^{-5}M
Cl —O—C—COOH CH_3 CH_3	(CDIB)	2.5×10^{-4}M
CH_3 —O—C—COOH CH_3	(DIB)	4.2×10^{-4}M
Cl —O—C—COOH CH_3 CH_3	(CPIB)	7.5×10^{-4}M

Activity is expressed as CPM incorporated into malonyl-CoA per 5 min. Incubation mixture contained 40 μmoles of Tris-HCl (pH 7.5), 12 μmoles of $MgCl_2$, 14 μmoles of potassium citrate, 0.8 μmoles of 4 mercaptoethanol, 0.6 mg of bovine serum albumin, and rat enzyme, purified 600 fold, in a volume of 0.52 ml. After preincubation at 37° C for 30 min, 1.4 μmoles of ATP, 0.1 μmole of acetyl-CoA and 12 μmoles of [^{14}C]-HCO_3 (4.2×10^5 CPM/μmole) were added, yielding a total volume of 0.66 ml. After incubation for 5 min at 37° C, 0.1 ml of 6 N HCl were added and the radioactivity was determined after drying.

for the inhibition of ACC and hypolipidemic activity as exemplified by a drop in inhibitory potency and hypolipidemic activity for DIB, when DIB is compared to CDIB, which differs from the former only by the presence of chlorine. It is also of interest that both TPIA and CDIB exert their hypolipidemic properties *in vivo* at doses lower than CPIB.

A detailed kinetic analysis of the inhibition of avian liver ACC [919] reveals that the inhibition is competitive for acetyl-CoA and citrate or isocitrate and noncompetitive for ATP and HCO_3^-. Competitive inhibition with respect to acetyl-CoA and isocitrate or citrate suggests that the drugs interfere with the ACC activity either by competing with the substrate acetyl-CoA or the activator citrate or isocitrate for the same active site on the enzyme protein. Kinetic constants are low and in the range of the apparent Michaelis constants for acetyl-CoA and citrate or isocitrate, indicating that at physiologically possible concentrations of the drugs *in vivo* the inhibition on ACC could be quite pronounced. Because both acetyl-CoA and citrate compete with the drugs, even small decreases of the *in vivo* levels of either substance would accentuate the drug-inhibition of ACC. It is not clear from our data whether interference of the drugs with the activation process of ACC or competition with acetyl-CoA at the substrate level brings about the inhibitory effect on ACC *in vivo*. In fact, both may be functioning at certain acetyl-CoA and citrate or isocitrate levels.

The question of whether the same or different sites on the ACC protein are involved in the interaction with the different compounds is of importance. Different binding sites could forecast a possible synergistic effect. Mixed inhibition studies, however, with CPIB and TPIA show that the sites of interaction with ACC are the same for both drugs. These sites are different from the site of interaction with CoA esters of long chain fatty acids, which inhibit ACC but by a different mechanism.

The activation of ACC by citrate or isocitrate is accompanied by a marked increase in sedimentation rate of the enzyme, due to the aggregation of inactive protomers to an active polymer. The effect of TPIA and CPIB on the sedimentation patterns of ACC shows that the drugs prevent the aggregation of the subunits. Arrhenius plots, and other thermodynamic parameters studied, make it seem plausible that small conformational changes, caused by binding of drug to the enzyme protein, result in disaggregation of the active form of ACC by the drugs [919].

In vivo Data. The inhibition of ACC by TPIA and CPIB is also demonstrable *in vivo*. As shown in Table 2, levels of ACC in drug-treated animals are significantly lower than the controls. The differences are significant at $p < 0.001$, whether activity is expressed per aliquot of the preparation or per liver. It is important to note that ACC activity was measured in preparations of the enzyme at the second ammonium sulfate stage. When a two-hour dialysis against citrate-containing buffer is performed, the ACC activity in the preparations from treated animals rises almost to the levels of similarly treated preparations from control animals. This indicates that the drug causes inhibition of ACC by means of a reversible association with the enzyme. Undoubtedly, some drug is lost during the purification of ACC prior to assay, and the difference in enzyme activity between the control and the treated animals may be even greater than the one recorded in Table 2. Unfortunately, we cannot obtain reliable measurements of ACC activity in the crude liver extract.

TPIA and CPIB have no inhibitory effect on the fatty acid synthetase multienzyme complex and several other enzymes tested [919]. If none of the other enzymes involved in lipid biosynthesis and degradation is affected by these drugs, both lipogenesis from acetate and total lipids should be depressed in drug-treated animals. Lowered total lipids will result from the inhibition of a critical biosynthetic step (ACC) while degradation of the lipids proceeds at an unaltered rate. Both biosynthesis and degradation of fatty acids are unidirectional processes, each involving its own specific enzymes and intermediates. These expecta-

Table 2. *Hepatic ACC activity in TPIA and CPIB-treated rats vs. controls*

Drug treatment	ACC activity[a] before dialysis		ACC activity after dialysis	
	CPM/25 λ	CPM/liver	CPM/25 λ	CPM/liver
TPIA-treated	1,523 ± 261	$5.02 \times 10^5 \pm 7.92 \times 10^4$	5,262 ± 534	$1.89 \times 10^6 \pm 2.10 \times 10^5$
Controls	4,299 ± 463	$1.08 \times 10^6 \pm 1.04 \times 10^5$	6,820 ± 407	$1.77 \times 10^6 \pm 1.25 \times 10^5$
p for test of significance[b]	< 0.001	< 0.001	0.03	N.S.
CPIB-treated	2,233 ± 259	$3.76 \times 10^5 \pm 4.82 \times 10^4$	6,495 ± 786	$2.12 \times 10^6 \pm 2.91 \times 10^5$
Controls	4,906 ± 499	$7.41 \times 10^5 \pm 7.38 \times 10^4$	11,223 ± 731	$3.21 \times 10^6 \pm 2.45 \times 10^5$
p for test of significance	< 0.001	< 0.001	< 0.001	< 0.01

[a] Ten adult male rats approx. 150 g were included in each group. Treated animals received 25 mg/kg/day of TPIA or 75 mg/kg/day of CPIB by intubation for 18 days and were maintained on regular diet. Control groups were intubated with the same solution but no drug. Animals were deprived of food for 48 hours, while on medication, and were fed for 48 hours before sacrifice. The livers were removed and ACC was extracted from the individual animals under identical conditions. The enzyme activity was measured at the first ammonium sulfate purification stage because in the crude extract the enzyme assay gives erratic results.

[b] Results were analyzed on square root transformation and expressed as means plus or minus standard error.

Table 3. *Carcass lipids and lipogenesis from acetate-1-^{14}C in TPIA-treated vs. control mice*[a]

	Body weight		Carcass		
	initial (g)	final (g)	weight (g)	lipids mg total lipids/g tissue	lipogenesis CPM/g carcass tissue
TPIA-treated	23.3 ± 0.3	25.5 ± 0.4	16.4 ± 0.4	125.3 ± 8.1	4,486 ± 294
Controls	23.5 ± 0.2	27.4 ± 0.4	18.1 ± 0.3	157.6 ± 9.5	6.388 ± 318
p for test of/significance	N.S.	0.01	0.01	0.02	< 0.001

[a] Fourteen mice were treated for 14 days with 25 mg/kg/day of TPIA which was mixed with "fat free diet" (Nutritional Biochemical Corp., Cleveland, Ohio). Control group (14) was maintained on the same diet without drug. Lipogenesis was measured as radioactivity incorporated into total extractable lipids ($HCCl_3$:CH_3OH, 2:1) [475] under the following conditions. The food was removed from the animals for 10 hours and then TPIA-treated animals were intubated with 25 mg/kg TPIA in 50% sucrose (250 mg sucrose per mouse). Control animals received only sucrose solution. Two hours later each animal received 2 μC of Acetate-1-^{14}C (specific activity 0.25 mC/10.3 mg) and after two hours the animals were sacrificed, their intestines removed and carcasses frozen at −20° C for lipid analysis. Data were analyzed on square root transformation and expressed as means ± standard error.

tions, which are based on theoretical considerations, were fully born out experimentally. Table 3 shows that mice treated with TPIA have lower capacity in synthesizing lipids from acetate. Total carcass lipids are also lower in TPIA-treated animals than the controls, and this is reflected in the carcass and body weights.

In summary, our results support the contention that reduction not only of circulating but also of total body lipids in TPIA- or CPIB-treated animals is associated with inhibition of ACC. This inhibition has been proposed as a possible mechanism of action of these agents.

EFFECT OF CHOLESTYRAMINE ON FECAL STEROID EXCRETION AND CHOLESTEROL SYNTHESIS IN PATIENTS WITH HYPERCHOLESTEROLEMIA*

Tatu A. Miettinen

Administration of cholestyramine, an anion exchange resin, to normo- and hypercholesterolemic patients results in a significant reduction of the serum cholesterol level [138, 354]. No effect is seen in the severe form of hypercholesterolemia, particularly in homozygous subjects with hyperlipoproteinemia of Type II [798]. The resin binds bile acids in the intestinal content, interfering with their reabsorption. Thus, fecal excretion of bile acids has been shown to rise [279, 581, 627] and elimination of radioactive cholesterol from the blood into the feces, primarily as bile acids, to increase, the excretion of radioactivity in neutral steroid fraction remaining practically unchanged or increasing only slightly [546, 581, 1026, 1045]. Since the resin treatment results in continuous augmentation of cholesterol elimination from the body [1045], this loss must be balanced by enhanced mobilization of tissue cholesterol (from the tissues themselves, or from xanthomata or atheromata) and/or by increased synthesis of cholesterol. Accordingly, cholestyramine appears to be a convenient tool not only for treatment of hypercholesterolemia but also for studies designed to reveal possible abnormalities in the capacity of hypercholesterolemic patients to enhance their cholesterol elimination and subsequently increase their cholesterol synthesis. In the present investigation sterol balance studies have been carried out before and during cholestyramine therapy, using serum methyl sterols and conversion of a ^{14}C-acetate-^{3}H-mevalonate mixture to serum cholesterol as additional indicators of enhanced cholesterol synthesis and liver cholesterol concentration as an index of changes in the size of the readily exchangeable tissue cholesterol pool.

* The work herein is supported by grants from the Sigrid Jusélius Foundation, and the National Research Council for Medical Sciences, Finland.

MATERIAL AND METHODS

Six control subjects and thirteen patients with Type II hyperlipoproteinemia [489] were investigated in this sterol balance study and five additional subjects in other experiments. Their ages ranged from 4 to 60 years, all but a 4 year old girl having clinical and/or ECG signs of coronary heart disease. The girl appeared to be homozygous; the other subjects were probably heterozygous.

The patients were hospitalized and put on a low-cholesterol (82–122 mg/ 2,400 cal), solid food diet. After administration of Cr_2O_3 and beta-sitosterol as internal markers for correction of fecal flow, continuous three-day stool collections were made. Cholestyramine (Cuemid) was administered in four doses daily, of 8 g each; the little girl received 6 g four times daily. The treatment was well tolerated by most patients, though some constipation occurred and one subject had mild diarrhea. Percutaneous liver biopsy was performed in eleven subjects with the Menghini technique [972] before and after 10–14 days on the treatment.

Dietary sterols, and fecal neutral and acidic steroids were quantitated with the gas chromatographic method [581, 993]. Serum methyl sterols were determined as presented earlier [984]. The possibility that cholesterol synthesis was activated before mevalonate was studied in four subjects, using the double label technique [988]. Thus a dose of ^{14}C-acetate-^{3}H-mevalonate mixture was injected intravenously before and during the treatment and the ratio $^{3}H/^{14}C$ was determined serially in serum free and esterified cholesterol. A decrease in the ratio indicates activation of cholesterol synthesis between acetate and mevalonate. Liver lipids (triglycerides, and esterified and free cholesterol) were quantitated from the biopsy specimens according to Reunanen et al. [1224].

RESULTS

Serum cholesterol decreased in all subjects, except in the homozygous 4-year-old girl the average reduction being 62 mg% in controls and 104 mg% in patients (Table 1). Serum triglycerides and fecal neutral steroid excretion remained unchanged. In the hypercholesterolemic subjects, fecal bile acid output tended to be subnormal, particularly when related to body weight (3.7 ± 0.5 mg/kg/day for controls and 2.3 ± 0.3 mg/kg/day for hypercholesterolemics), and tended to show a negative correlation with the corresponding serum cholesterol level ($r = -0.51$). However, it was markedly stimulated by cholestyramine in every subject, including the girl who showed no decrease in serum cholesterol. The average increment of 1,913 mg/day in the controls was almost twice that (1,010 mg/day) in the hypercholesterolemics (Table 1). Since neutral steroid excretion remained unchanged, the results indicate that hypercholesterolemic patients are able to increase elimination of cholesterol from the body but to a lesser extent than normocholesterolemic controls. The increment of bile acid excretion did not appear to depend on the decrement of serum cholesterol but was correlated with initial bile acid output values ($r = 0.56$).

The marked increase in cholesterol catabolism coupled with the lack of any association between the decrement of serum cholesterol and the increment of cholesterol elimination suggest that the latter was balanced by mobilization of tissue cholesterol and/or increased synthesis. The results of the liver biopsy

Table 1. *Effect of cholestyramine on serum cholesterol and fecal steroid excretion in normo- and hypercholesterolemic subjects (mean ± SE)* [a]

Treatment	Serum chol. (mg/100 ml)	Fecal steroids, mg/24 h		
		bile acids	neutral steroids	total
		Control subjects (6)		
None	209 ± 11	238 ± 50	638 ± 106	876 ± 118
Resin	146 ± 7	2,151 ± 231	730 ± 100	2,881 ± 234
Difference	−62 ± 6	+1,913 ± 200	+93 ± 46	+2,006 ± 230
		Hypercholesterolemic patients (13)		
None	482 ± 61*	156 ± 26	693 ± 72	849 ± 80
Resin	378 ± 70*	1,166 ± 292*	659 ± 44	1,825 ± 319*
Difference	−104 ± 16*	+1,010 ± 280*	−34 ± 65	+976 ± 306*

[a] Significant differences ($P < 0.05$) from controls are indicated by *. Number of subjects in each group is presented in parentheses.

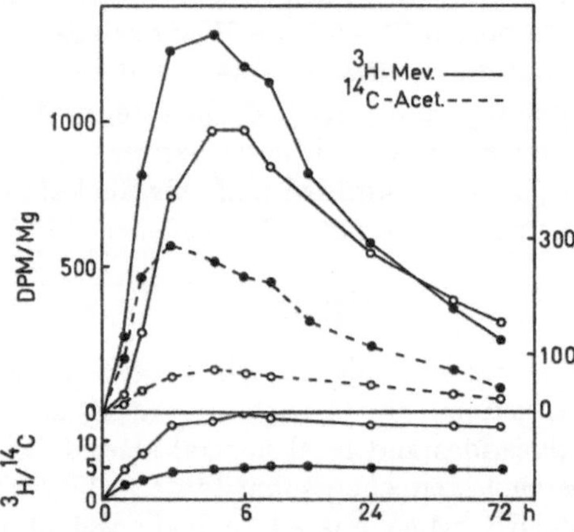

Fig. 1. Effect of cholestyramine on the incorporation of a ^{14}C-acetate-^{3}H-mevalonate mixture into serum free cholesterol in a hypercholesterolemic patient. The values before treatment are indicated by circles and those during treatment by dots. The residue of the radioactivity (DPM/mg) of the first experiment was subtracted from the values of the second experiment by evaluating the rate of disappearance of radioactivity from the slope of the specific activity-time curve before the second labeling

Table 2. *Effect of cholestyramine treatment on liver lipids in subjects with hypercholesterolemia (mean ± SE)*

Group	Triglycerides, as a percentage	Cholesterol, mg/100 g		
		free	ester	total
Before	2.39 ± 0.52	258 ± 11	104 ± 12	362 ± 19
During	2.35 ± 0.38	226 ± 18	82 ± 8	308 ± 21
Difference	−0.04 ± 0.49	−32 ± 23	−22 ± 10	−54 ± 27

Table 3. *Serum cholesterol and methyl sterols before and during cholestyramine treatment in five hypercholesterolemic patients (Mean ± SE)*

Treatment[a]	Serum chol.	Serum methyl sterols[b] (μg/100 ml) I	II	III	IV	V	Total
None	399 ± 24	31 ± 6	31 ± 4	24 ± 2	33 ± 4	14 ± 2	134 ± 10
Resin	285 ± 24	84 ± 20	94 ± 15	32 ± 6	54 ± 4	47 ± 11	310 ± 35
Difference	−114 ± 21	+53 ± 18	+63 ± 13	+8 ± 5	+21 ± 3	+33 ± 9	+176 ± 29

[a] Duration of cholestyramine treatment ranged from 10—57 days.

[b] According to mass spectrometric analysis, composition of subfractions was as follows: I dihydrolanosterol and two methostenols, II monounsaturated dimethylsterol, III diunsaturated dimethylsterol, and traces of monounsaturated trimethylsterol and monounsaturated monomethylsterol, IV lanosterol and V diunsaturated dimethylsterol.

analysis (Table 2) showed that the reduction of hepatic cholesterol concentration during cholestyramine treatment by 54 mg% (15%) was not statistically significant, though the total cholesterol level was decreased in 8 of 11 subjects studied. Conversion of ^{14}C-acetate to serum cholesterol in relation to that of ^{3}H-mevalonate increased on an average threefold (an experiment is illustrated in Fig. 1), indicating threefold stimulation of synthesis between acetate and mevalonate by the resin. Fecal steroid excretion, measured in three of the subjects, was increased from 1.3 to 1.9 times only. The few *in vitro* studies as yet carried out suggest that hepatic cholesterol synthesis is increased by about tenfold. Table 3 shows that increased synthesis is also seen in serum methyl sterol concentration. The total amount is elevated approximately twofold, subfraction V, containing a diunsaturated dimethyl sterol, being increased threefold.

DISCUSSION

The cholestyramine-induced increment of cholesterol elimination determined by direct analysis of fecal steroids in the hypercholesterolemic subjects of the present study is of the same magnitude as that reported by others with less direct methods [627, 1026, 1045]. In accordance with the earlier observations [991, 994] the basal bile acid excretion tended to be subnormal in subjects with familial hypercholesterolemia, a finding which did not appear to be attributable to possible differences in body weight but was suggested to indicate a defect in bile acid production [994]. Cholestyramine, however, induced a marked increase in bile acid production in hypercholesterolemic patients. That this augmentation was less than in normocholesterolemic subjects may have been due to the relative defect in hepatic bile acid synthesis, though effective intestinal reabsorption of bile salts could also have reduced their fecal loss during the resin treatment.

One of the chief goals of the treatment of hypercholesterolemia is to prevent the development of arterial atheromata or even to reduce their size. Studies with radioactive cholesterol have indicated, however, that the pool of exchangeable cholesterol, in which arterial atheromata can be included, may not be changed consistently by cholestyramine treatment [546, 1045]. On the other hand, the ileal bypass operation, which stimulates cholesterol elimination from the body by essentially the same mechanism as cholestyramine but more effectively [992], has been reported to reduce both the rapidly miscible and the slowly miscible cholesterol pools to normal size in subjects with hypercholesterolemia [1027]. The liver biopsy analyses of the present study suggest that the pool of rapidly miscible tissue cholesterol may actually have been reduced slightly, even by such relatively short-term cholestyramine treatment.

The serum methyl sterol concentration, and particularly the conversion of the labeled acetate-mevalonate mixture to serum and liver cholesterol, indicated that cholesterol synthesis was stimulated by cholestyramine more than was indicated by the sterol balance studies. This could indicate, as already suggested [992], that synthesis is enhanced, primarily in the liver, which may normally contribute relatively little to the fecal sereoids in man.

Discussion Following Dr. Maragoudakis' Paper

Dr. Steinberg: I think the biochemical studies presented by Dr. Maragoudakis are very elegant, and they show a very nice competitive effect with regard to the citrate influence on the acetyl-CoA carboxylase (ACC) aggregation. I would quarrel with the extrapolation to the whole animal, and reiterate, that in CPIB-treated rats the rate of acetate incorporation into fatty acids is not only not depressed but is actually *increased*, as shown by Gould, Dexter in our lab and by Duncan and Best. The perfused liver takes up palmitate and converts it to glycerides at a normal rate, and yet the glyceride concentration in the liver is increased.

I would suggest that Dr. Maragoudakis got this result for one of the following reasons. The activity of ACC is very much influenced by food intake, and I wonder, first, if the animals were controlled with regard to this at the time they were sacrificed. Another possible explanation may lie in the profound changes in liver morphology occurring in CPIB-treated rats that may lead to a different subfractionation of the ACC.

My third specific question is whether he measured the rate of Acetyl-CoA incorporation into fatty acids in the crude homogenates where there would be no chance of losses of enzyme.

Dr. Maragoudakis: In our hands the incorporation of acetate into total lipids is always depressed in drug-treated animals. This depression in carcass-lipids is true not only for free fatty acids, but also for all the other major classes of lipids. The enzyme activity was measured under identical and very carefully controlled dietary conditions of the animals, and the differences in enzyme activity can not be accounted for by differences in food intake.

I doubt that changes in the morphology of the liver, because of the drug-treatment, can cause any profound changes in the fractionation of the enzyme. The drug is actually bound to the enzyme protein, as shown by TPIA-^{14}C-treated animals and following enzyme activity and TPIA-^{14}C in the fractionation of the liver homogenate.

Dr. Steinberg: Did you measure the rate of acetate conversion to fatty acid in either slices or whole homogenates?

Dr. Maragoudakis: No, this was done in whole animals, under conditions of optimal lipogenesis.

Dr. SCHWEPPE: We have heard a great deal about different drugs, such as CPIB, nicotinamide, nicotinic acid, but nothing about D-thyroxine. Granting that experimental atherosclerosis in a rabbit is not comparable to humans, would anyone discuss the therapeutic application or the prophylaxis of the development of atherosclerosis by CPIB, D-thyroxine, nicotinamide or any other agent of this sort?

Dr. STEINBERG: No, the national coronary drug project is under way, and I think that they may have an answer in a few years.

Dr. GETZ: Dr. Pereira, in your statement that CPIB has an effect on RNA metabolism, were you referring to the RNA in the mitochondria?

Dr. PEREIRA: No, I am referring to a messenger RNA which is apart from mitochondrial RNA. The protein synthesis which we see, takes place on the cytoplasmic ribosome. The mitochondrial proteins are then incorporated into the mitochondrial structure. There is no effect on mitochondrial protein synthesis.

Dr. STEINBERG: I would like to ask Dr. Thorp, since we have presented two different assessments of the importance of the thyroxine-binding, whether it is his feeling that this effect, which is only clearly demonstrated on thyroxine binding to albumin, is acceptable to him as an explanation of all of the actions of CPIB. Could the effect on albumin binding be enough, in fact, to explain changes in thyroxine effects when the binding to thyroxine-binding globulin (TBG) seems not to be affected? We have to explain the decrease in cholesterol synthesis, we have to explain liver hypertrophy, and we have to explain the fact that patients gain weight, whereas thyroid makes them lose weight.

Dr. THORP: I think we have a very valid system for selecting compounds on the basis of *in vitro* activity, and this is borne out in practice by the results we have seen with this later series of compounds. On the other hand, I don't think thyroxine binding by itself accounts for all of the drug's activity. I am certain that there are other substances transported by albumin to which these compounds are selectively bound, and this would possibly include effects of fatty acid transport. The very big difference between thyroxine effects and the effects of compounds like CPIB is that, in contrast to the thyroxine-treated animal where there is a marked increase in lipolysis, the animals treated with CPIB show a fall in free fatty acid level and a decrease in turnover of free fatty acid. Thus, the liver in these animals is essentially a fasting liver and this can be further recognized in the low glycogen content of the liver.

When one considers effects on thyroxine distribution by CPIB, one finds a situation which is not in fact comparable and which might lead to the observed effects of an increase in body weight and a relative hypothyroid effect outside of the liver and an increase in TBG capacity. Since some of these compounds do not interfere with thyroxine binding to TBG, it is hardly surprising that no real effect is seen in plasma.

Dr. REISEL: I would like to ask Dr. Thorp whether this new agent is working in animals rendered hypothyroid, as in the case of clofibrate.

Dr. THORP: It is known that in hypothyroid animals CPIB does not have an effect, as is also true, to a large extent, in man. We haven't specifically tested the effect of this new compound in such animals.

Discussion Following Dr. Miettinen's Paper

Dr. KHACHADURIAN: How do you reconcile your findings with the clinical observation that cholestyramine causes a decrease in the size of the xanthomata in these patients?

Another question I would like to ask is whether these methylated steroids are arising from tissues during cholestyramine therapy.

Dr. MIETTINEN: Most of these studies are not long-term studies, so that as far as xanthomata are concerned, we have no data. In other studies, we have observed that xanthomata decrease in size over a period of one year or more. As far as removal of tissue cholesterol during treatment is concerned, it is very difficult to determine the extent of its mobilization during cholestyramine treatment, and I just don't know whether it can be done.

Dr. AHRENS: I would like to comment on the sensible approach that Dr. Miettinen has taken in his estimates of changes in cholesterol synthesis. Many experiments in the past have been based upon measurement of the conversion of radioactive acetate to radio-cholesterol. The numbers obtained are deceptive; they should not be taken very seriously because the sizes of the immediate precursor pools are never known. He has attempted to improve these crude estimates by two means: by measuring the ratio of ^{3}H to ^{14}C in cholesterol after pulse labeling with radioactive ^{3}H-acetate and ^{14}C-mevalonate; and by measuring the amounts of the methyl sterols that are precursors in cholesterol biosynthesis. This combination of methods represents very real improvement in precision, and through their use Dr. Miettinen has shown that after cholestyramine (and presumably after ileal bypass) there is a large increase in cholesterol synthesis. Nevertheless, it is still impossible to know how much of the increase in fecal steroid excretion is due to increased *de novo* cholesterol synthesis, and how much is due to the flux of cholesterol out of tissue stores. This is, to my mind, a major unsolved problem—how to measure the amount of cholesterol stored in the tissues and how to measure the effects of various interventions on these stores. This is a major difficulty in evaluating the usefulness of drugs or diets: do these interventions reduce the amount of cholesterol stored in various tissues, or are they merely stimulating cholesterol synthesis? I am afraid that the means of differentiating these two causes of increased fecal steroid excretion are not yet at hand.

Dr. LINDSTEDT: Do you have any data on the specific radioactivity of bile acids in these experiments? Isn't it quite possible that you are measuring an estimation of bile acid flux, because there is no increase in cholesterol synthesis in the liver which is producing this increase in fecal bile acids? There is a change in the equilibrium between liver and blood cholesterol in this situation.

Do you find a very high specific activity for hepatic bile acids in relation to specific activity of fecal bile acids and serum cholesterol such as we usually find?

Dr. MIETTINEN: Unfortunately, we did not determine specific activity of bile acids and sterols in studies with ^{14}C-acetate-^{3}H-mevalonate. Most of the sterol balance studies were carried out without isotopes.

Section XVII

PROGRESS IN THE CONTROL OF ATHEROSCLEROSIS

DESIGN OF PRIMARY AND SECONDARY PREVENTION TRIALS*

Jerome Cornfield

Experimental design has been a familiar concept in many branches of science and technology for several decades. We have it on the authority of no less a person than the President of the Royal College of Surgeons of England that its adaptation to the clinical trial "was as important and valuable as the discovery of penicillin" [73]. The body of ideas and experience associated with this concept points to numerous design characteristics that appear necessary to assure repeatability and interpretability of results, although sufficiency is of course another matter. A review of some of the design characteristics of special importance for prevention trials in cardiovascular disease follows.

Random Allocation. Control and experimental patients must be alike in all relevant factors if differences in their subsequent experience are to be attributed to the intervention under study. The only safe way now known to achieve this comparability is by random allocation, with or without prior stratification on relevant variables. Substitutes, such as matching without randomization, assume either that all important determinants are accounted for by the matching variables, or that the important remaining ones will somehow average themselves out. However, the extreme selection effects that are possible in human populations makes dependence on matching without randomization hazardous.

An indication of the possible magnitude of selection effects is provided by a recent randomized trial of linseed versus sunflower oil reported by Natvig and colleagues [1080]. Mortality from all causes during the study year in the industrially employed men aged 50–59 enrolled in this trial was, as shown in Table 1, well below that expected on the basis of overall mortality statistics among all males of this age group, but those employed men who refused participation had a mortality experience above expectation. A hypothetical trial comparing the effects of a treatment on those willing to be enrolled with a "control" group consisting of those who refused participation could thus have "demonstrated" a difference of 55% for a totally ineffective intervention. It remains to be shown that matching on known risk factors could eliminate selection effects of this size.

Because such of selection effects study populations will rarely be representative of any desired target group in the general population. Randomization assures that any differences found can be attributed to the experimental intervention (or, as discussed below, to other variables confounded with it) in the study population. One cannot generalize from study to target population with equal rigor as pointed out by the Diet-Heart group [1079]. Such generalization must necessarily rest on a less compelling argument, i.e. the lack of plausible scientific

* The work herein has been supported by NIH Grant GM-15004.

Table 1. *Deaths from all causes during observation year and deaths expected on the basis of mortality in Oslo and in Norway, 1961—65*

	Observed	Expected	
		Oslo	Norway
A. Randomized. Sunflower seed	40	79.3	65.3
B. Randomized. Linseed	43	79.7	65.5
C. Not randomized. Sunflower seed	1	1.6	1.4
D. Willing, but no allotment	12	16.2	13.3
E. Refused participation	25	20.7	16.9
	121	197.5	162.4
Ratio: observed to expected			
A+B+D	—	0.54	0.66
E	—	1.21	1.47
Ratio of ratios	—	0.45	0.45

reasons for expecting an intervention to be successful in study, but not target, populations.

The comparability of randomly allocated control and experimental patients can be seriously compromised by subsequent drop-outs and nonadherence to the experimental regimens, unless all persons originally randomized are retained in the final analysis. For this to be possible follow-up procedures which ascertain the outcome for each member of the originally randomized study group are necessary. When drop-out and nonadherence rates are high, such retention will dilute whatever real experimental effects are present. Eliminating them from the analysis to avoid dilution will introduce biases arising from differences between drop-outs and nonadherence on the one hand and continuing adherers on the other. That these differences may be considerable is suggested by the experience in the National Diet-Heart Study in which 6.8% of the noncigarette smokers, but 11.4% of the smokers dropped out (First and Second Study combined).

An often employed device to reduce the drop-out and nonadherence rate is to have a prerandomization dry run in which the irresolute and faint of heart are shaken out.

The use of institutional rather than free-living populations has the apparent attraction of providing greater control over adherence to the experimental regimen. Thus in the National Diet-Heart Study adherence among participants in the Fairbault State School and Hospital appeared more satisfactory than among free-living participants—as judged by falls in serum cholesterol. But these participants were mental defectives and other groups, e.g. schizophrenics, might be less cooperative. In the study by Dayton et al. of the semi-institutional population of domiciled veterans [384] only about one-fourth of the participants ate 80% or more of their meals in the study dining room and mean adherence was 56% for the control group and 49% for the experimental. This reflected both discharge from the institution and nonadherence even though present. Even aside from questions of generalizability, therefore, the use of institutional populations is not without special problems.

Adequate Numbers. It has been by no means unusual for prevention trials to find at the end of a long and difficult investigation that the sample size used was too small to supply clear-cut answers to the questions asked. To the extent that it is possible, it is clearly advantageous to estimate the numbers required before the trial starts. The following framework for such estimation is finding increasing acceptance [597, 1079, 1315].

It starts with the obvious remark that once data are in, it is desirable to test the observed difference in event rate between treated and control groups for statistical significance, i.e. to compute the probability of finding by chance alone a difference as large as or larger than that observed when there is no true difference. Conventionally the observed difference is accepted as significant if this probability is less than some small quantity, say one in one hundred, the significance level adopted for the Coronary Drug Project (later an alternative approach to presented). Call this probability α.

Specifying a small value for α, is only part of the story, however. One would also like to assure that if a true difference does exist, the probability of finding a significant difference is high. Call this second probability $1-\beta$. Thus, α is the probability of judging an observed difference significant when none in fact exists, while β is the probability of failing to judge an observed difference significant when a true difference does exist. Unless the sample size is sufficient to make both probabilities small, a nonsignificant observed difference may mean either that no true difference exists or that a difference as large as or perhaps larger than the observed difference does exist, but that the sample size was too small to permit it to be judged significant.

Methods are available [597] for computing required sample size once both probabilities have been specified. But an essential ingredient has yet to be mentioned. The second probability β, obviously depends on the magnitude of the true difference and cannot be specified without specification of this magnitude. At first sight one seems to be involved in a circular argument. The trial cannot begin until β and hence the magnitude of the true difference is specified but this magnitude cannot be known (at best) until the trial is completed. However there is, in fact, nothing circular in the joint statement: (a) the magnitude of the true difference is unknown, but (b) if it is as large as Δ the probability of not finding a significant difference, β, should be some suitably small quantity.

The specification of Δ is in reality a judgment, affected in part by consideration of what size reductions would be of public health importance, if achieveable, and in part by consideration of the epidemiologic evidence relating event rate and the level of the risk factor or factors to be affected by the intervention. Thus in Framingham the incidence of new coronary events is proportional to about the $2^1/_2{}^{\text{th}}$ power of the serum cholesterol level [330] so that an intervention that lowered serum cholesterol by 10% might, if the Framingham relation is in fact causal, lead to a lowering in the incidence of new coronary events of $(1-0.9^{2.5}) \times 100\%$, or about 23%. Of course, even to the extent that this relation is causal, it presumably reflects a life-time relationship, and a lowering of serum cholesterol by 10% for five years after attaining middle age might be less effective and some provision for this possible reduction in effectiveness needs to be made. Although there are conjectural elements in this calculation, it does force a realistic appraisal of what may be achieved by lipid-lowering interventions. The increasing size of newly initiated or proposed trials appears to be at least in part a consequence of the spread of this kind of thinking.

For a specified true percentage difference to be detected at significance level α with probability $1-\beta$ the required sample size is nearly inversely proportional to the ratio of the event rate in the controls to the complement of that rate. Table 2 shows for $\alpha=0.01$, the sample sizes required to detect with probability 0.95 ($\beta=0.05$) an effective reduction of 20% (i.e. after allowance for dropouts and the number of years required to achieve the full Framingham effect) for various event rates in the controls.

Important economies can clearly be achieved by selecting study populations with high control event rates. This is, in fact, a major reason for studying secondary rather than primary prevention, since a reduction of at least five-fold in required sample sizes is achievable. Even in primary prevention a selection of men with serum cholesterols above 250 mg/100 cc leads to not inconsiderable differences in incidence (Table 3). The higher risk group so defined constitutes somewhat more than one-fourth of all men in each age group.

Table 2. *Dependence of sample size on control rate*

Rate in control group	Total number required
0.05	27,100
0.10	12,900
0.20	5,800
0.40	2,300

Table 3. *Twelve-year incidence of new coronary events in Framingham men by initial cholesterol level*

Serum cholesterol	Age	
	40–49	50–62
>250	17.5%	25.8%
<250	9.9	17.0
All	11.9	19.8

Of course the problem of generalizing from results in high risk groups to target populations of more general interest remains. Few for example would interpret a negative result in secondary prevention as necessarily meaning that no effect was achievable in primary prevention. But such an answer would be of value in its own right, and a positive answer, while of equal intrinsic value, would almost certainly be judged relevant to primary prevention as well.

Standardization of Procedures. The number of patients required for clear-cut answers will often be beyond the capacity of a single investigator or institution and multi-institution studies will accordingly be called for. But unless comparability of procedures among the participating institutions can be assured, the decrease in data quality consequent upon the increase in numbers will prove self-defeating. The wide-spread recognition of the necessity for planning for such standardization from the very start stems in part from the experience of the Cooperative Study of Lipoproteins and Atherosclerosis in the 1950's [541] in which embarrassingly large variations in lipid determinations from laboratory to laboratory emerged during the course of study and greatly complicated the final analysis.

Common protocols, central laboratory determinations, coordinating centers which review results for comparability, performance-monitoring visits to participants and a small decision-making executive group are becoming increasingly common features of multi-institutional trials. A recent authorative review of this aspect of cooperative studies is given in the report to the National Advisory Heart Council by the Heart Special Project Committee [1395].

Double-Blinding. In a double-blind study neither the patient nor the treating physician knows the therapy to which the patient has been assigned. Such

Table 4. *Effect of diet on different end points in Leren's study of secondary prevention*

	Diet group	Control group
	Number of events	
Death from all causes	42	55
Sudden death	27	27
Myocardial reinfarctions	43	64
Acquired angina pectoris	10	29

blinding is designed to avoid two possible errors, bias in evaluation of outcome and confounding of treatment effects with the effect of other variables.

"Cold stone dead hath no fellow" and an intervention that significantly reduces mortality from all causes can hardly be explained by bias in evaluation. However, in primary prevention noncardiovascular causes of death are numerous, and can become a source of noise which seriously reduces the sensitivity of the trial. But if the end point is to be mortality from cardiovascular disease, an evaluation of cause of death is required, and the possibility of bias can no longer be overlooked. In secondary prevention noncardiovascular causes of death are less frequent and mortality from all causes is a reasonably sensitive end-point. Even here problems can arise, as illustrated by Paul Leren's admirable but nondouble-blind study of diet in secondary prevention. As shown in Table 4 a nonsignificant lowering in mortality from all causes and none in sudden death is accompanied by a marked and significant lowering in myocardial infarction and new cases of angina pectoris. The softer the end-point, the larger the apparent effect. In the absence of double-blinding these results are difficult to interpret particularly since the epidemiologic evidence shows that, if anything, the risk of developing angina is less dependent on serum cholesterol levels than it is for the other end-points [332].

The other possible source of error in nondouble blind studies, the confounding of treatment effects, arises because an experimental intervention can be accompanied by changes in other risk factors. As shown in Table 5 the participants in the National Diet Heart Study experienced decreases in weight and blood pressure and almost one-fourth of the cigarette smokers stopped entirely. In a blind study these concomitant changes would occur in both treated and control group and any differences in event rate that were found could not reasonably be attributed to them. In a nonblind study this need not be the case and the possibility that the effects found are not specific to the experimental intervention under study is at least in principle an open one.

It need hardly be added that double-blinding can present operational and/or ethical difficulties and that the final decision in any particular study must be based on balancing pros and cons.

Statistical Analysis of Results. Most analyses of clinical trials utilize the classical theory of hypothesis testing, i.e. *P*-values. But it has become increasingly apparent that the structure of such trials is more complex than has been assumed

Table 5. *Effect of diet intervention on weight, blood pressure and smoking (National Diet-Heart Study)*

Change in	All open centers	Faribault
Wt. (lb)	−4.7	+1.0
Blood pressure, systolic (as a percentage)	−1.8	−9.0
Blood pressure, diastolic (as a percentage)	−4.7[a]	−11.9
Cigarette smoking (as a percentage discontinued)	−23	NA

[a] Not corrected for equipment failure in Twin Cities.

in that theory. In actual clinical trials unforeseen but essential compliactions can arise; the detailed analysis of results discloses interesting, but unanticipated relationships, etc. There is nothing sinful about having data suggest new hypotheses. But the *P*-value assigned by the traditional calculation to hypotheses so suggested does not have the usual interpretation of the relative frequency with which a true hypothesis would be erroneously rejected. The relative frequency can be much greater than the nominal *P*-value. Small *P*-values, therefore, do not make the inferences as safe as they seem.

Many of the new statistical techniques of the last 25 years (sequential analysis, multiple comparison procedures, multivariate methods) can be considered as attempts to deal with special aspects of this general problem. A more general solution is needed however, and as part of the continuing data monitoring and analysis task of the Coronary Drug Project, an attempt has been made to develop one. Some details are given in a recent Biometrics article [331].

CONCLUSION

It should be emphasized, in conclusion that even with randomization, adequate numbers, standardization of procedures, double-blinding and sophisticated statistical analysis, prevention trials are not push-button affairs, but call for the highest exercise of scientific judgment, since the possibilities of independent repetition are often severely limited by the costs and time involved.

CONTROL OF ATHEROSCLEROSIS: PROGRESS IN PRIMARY DIET TRIALS

Osmo Turpeinen

The prevention of atherosclerotic disease is usually regarded as having two aspects: the primary prevention, i.e., prevention among a presumably healthy population, at least with respect to previously experienced clinical manifestations of atherosclerotic disease, and the secondary prevention, i.e., prevention among survivors of one or more attacks of this disease. From a theoretical point of view, such a division may not be entirely justified. We know that the atherosclerotic disease has a long latent period and thus our "healthy" population may not be truly healthy. The line of demarcation between the two phases of the disease, the latent and the manifest one, is not always clear, and the differentiation depends to a large extent on the criteria chosen. In practice, however, it may be useful to make such a distinction, as these two phases of the disease carry rather different prognoses and, accordingly, the chances for prevention may also be quite different. *A priori*, it seems that the chances of prevention should be better among presumably healthy persons, and it could even be argued that a clinical manifestation of atherosclerosis as such indicates a pathologic process too far advanced to be appreciably influenced by preventive measures.

Although the title of this paper refers to atherosclerotic manifestations generally, the main body of this presentation will be devoted to the most prevalent manifestation, namely, ischemic heart disease, because it has been studied much more extensively than the other clinical manifestations of atherosclerosis.

The studies which provide the now available evidence on the possibilities of primary prevention of ischemic heart disease through diet were started about ten years ago. At that time there already was much epidemiological and other indirect evidence to favor the hypothesis that the incidence of ischemic heart disease could be decreased by a suitable change in the fat composition of the diet. It had been found that in populations experiencing high incidence of ischemic heart disease, serum cholesterol values tended to be high, and the dietary intake of fats of the saturated type was usually also high. Furthermore, it had been definitely demonstrated that serum cholesterol level could be influenced by dietary means, particularly by the quality and quantity of dietary fats. However, the hypothesis had not been put to test by means of direct experiments in which the diet of a population group had been changed to satisfy the requirements of the hypothesis and the development of manifestations of ischemic heart disease had been observed over a sufficiently long period.

Three dietary trials aiming at primary prevention of ischemic heart disease which I am going to review are: the Anti-Coronary Club Project of New York, the clinical trial at Los Angeles Veterans Administration Center, and the mental hospital study in Helsinki.

The latest report on the Diet and Coronary Heart Disease Study Project (usually known as the Anti-Coronary Club) has been published by Rinzler [1227].

The study was started in February, 1957 in New York City. The subjects of the study were free-living men in the age group 40 to 59 years. They were recruited among volunteers who responded initially to a radio and press call for participants. For this experimental group a diet was constructed ("prudent diet") in which foods with predominantly saturated fatty acids were reduced in quantity or eliminated, and replaced by those with predominantly unsaturated types of fatty acids. In the experimental diet the percentage of fat was reduced from the initial 40% to 33% of the total energy, and the distribution of the fatty acids was changed into: saturated acids 33%, monoethenoid acids 33%, and polyethenoid acids 34%. The overweight subjects were placed on a diet that averaged 1,600 calories and contained only 19% of the total energy as fat. When weight reduction was completed, this was changed to the standard diet.

The control group, which was started in 1959, was recruited from men who had voluntarily appeared for examination at the Cancer Detection Clinics of the New York City Department of Health. These subjects were considered similar to the experimental subjects in that they showed health consciousness and were willing to participate in a health program.

The latest report available gives the accumulated evidence as of November 30, 1967. Up to that time 1,242 volunteers had enlisted for the study. On entry to the study 301 subjects had been excluded because of a history of clinical or electrocardiographic evidence of coronary heart disease. The remaining 941 subjects who were free of evidence of clinical coronary heart disease constituted the experimental group. Up to the previously mentioned date these men had accumulated 3,954 person-years of experience while in an active status, i.e. regular attendance for examinations and consultations. By the end of the period of observation 532 of the 941 subjects had lapsed into an inactive status, in which they had accumulated 3,207 person-years of experience. Subjects in an inactive status were appraised annually as to health and nutritional status but did not return regularly for the examinations. The control group included in the study consisted of 457 subjects who showed no initial evidence of coronary heart disease by the same criteria applied to the experimental group.

Serum cholesterol values in the experimental group showed a highly significant drop of about 30 mg/dl from an average initial level of 260 mg after one year in the study. Thereafter the concentration leveled off at about 225 mg. In the control group the cholesterol level fell about 7 mg during the first two years but rose thereafter, so that by the end of the fourth year the average level had returned to the initial concentration. The difference between the cholesterol levels of the two groups appears to have been approximately 25 mg on the average.

The pattern of fatty acids in the adipose tissue lipids were determined in 78 subjects who had followed the experimental diet for one to four years. The major change associated with prolonged adherence to the study diet was in the polyethenoid fatty acid components of the depot fat and particularly in the proportion of linoleic acid, which was increased about twofold, from a mean of 9.7% initially to 18.9% in the group of subjects who had been on the diet more than three years. The increase in the linoleic acid and the more highly unsaturated fatty acids was achieved at the expense of myristic, palmitic and oleic acids. The analyses of depot fat, since it is related to the linoleic content of the diet, has served as a useful method in distinguishing between adherence and nonadherence to the experimental diet.

Incidence of new coronary events was assessed in both groups. The 941 experimental subjects had accumulated 3,954 person-years of active experience and shown 17 new coronary events. This represents an overall incidence rate of 430 per 100,000 person-years. Similarly the 457 men of the control group had accumulated 3,122 person-years of experience and 32 new coronary events, resulting in an overall incidence of 1,025 per 100,000 person-years. The incidence in the inactive group, 748 per 100,000 person-years, was intermediate between that of the active experimental and control subjects.

To validate the comparison of coronary heart disease incidence in the experimental group on the diet used in the study and the control group that maintained its normal diet, a study on a number of factors, such as demographic and risk factors associated with coronary heart disease as they exist in the two groups on entry, was carried out. Such a study indicated that the significantly lower incidence observed in the experimental group compared with the total control group could not be ascribed to demographic differences. The groups were also compared regarding entry levels of three risk factors identified by the Framingham Study and other studies, i.e., hypercholesterolemia, hypertension and obesity. The two groups were quite comparable regarding the proportion with initial hypercholesterolemia. However, the experimental group had higher proportions with initial obesity and hypertension than did the control group. In view of these findings, it would be expected that the experimental group might experience a higher frequency of coronary heart disease than the control group.

The data presented indicate that the incidence of new coronary events among initially coronary-free full participants in the Anti-Coronary Club's program was significantly lower than that among its control group. The authors think it reasonable to attribute this difference primarily to the effects of the Anti-Coronary Club's program, the major feature of which was supervised adherence to the study diet.

The results of the Los Angeles clinical trial have recently been published in detail by Dayton et al. [384].

The subjects of this study were elderly (mean age 65.5 years) domiciled male veterans. Volunteers were allocated randomly to control and experimental groups. Participants numbered 422 in the control group and 424 in the experimental group. The two groups were indistinguishable at the outset of the study in almost all observations.

The control diet was similar to the regular institutional diet. It provided 40.1% of calories as fat, having a mean iodine value of 53.5; cholesterol intake was 653 mg/day. The experimental diet provided 38.9% of calories as fat, with an iodine value of 102.4, and had a cholesterol content of 365 mg/day. Linoleic acid contents of the two diets were 10% and 39% of total fatty acid, respectively.

The experimental diet induced a prompt drop in serum cholesterol level and sustained a difference between the experimental and control groups amounting to 12.7% (29.5 mg/dl) of the starting level.

Mean linoleic acid concentration of adipose tissue was initially 10.9%. During the latter part of the trial, which lasted eight years for some subjects, linoleic acid concentration in adipose tissue approached an asymptomatic level of 33.7% among good adherers.

Clinical follow-up was carried out on a double-blind basis.

The number of men sustaining events in major categories, in the control and experimental groups, respectively, was: definite silent myocardial infarction, 4 and 9; definite overt myocardial infarction, 40 and 27; sudden death due to coronary heart disease, 27 and 18; definite cerebral infarction, 22 and 13. The difference in primary end-point of the study, sudden death or myocardial infarction, was not statistically significant. However, when these data were pooled with those for cerebral infarction and other secondary end points, the totals were 96 in the control group and 66 in the experimental group; $P = 0.01$. Fatal atherosclerotic events numbered 70 in the control group and 48 in the experimental group; $P < 0.05$. Life-table analysis in general confirmed these conclusions.

The results of the Finnish mental hospital study have been published by Turpeinen et al. [1479]. The study was started in 1958 in two hospitals. In one, designated as Hospital N, the diet was changed so that a large part of milk fat was replaced by soybean oil; the other hospital, Hospital K, was kept as the control without any intentional dietary change. In 1965, when the experimental diet had been in use in hospital N a little over six years, this hospital was returned to the normal diet, and Hospital K was placed on the experimental diet. The roles of the hospitals in the experimental design were thus reversed.

The subjects of the study were male patients aged 34 to 64 years at the outset. Their total number during the first phase of the trial was 327 in the experimental hospital and 254 in the control hospital.

Before the start of the experiment the diets in both hospitals were fairly similar and contained relatively large quantities of fat of the saturated type derived mainly from whole milk and butter. The total fat content was 31 to 36% and milk fat contributed about 17% of the total food energy. The dietary change in hospital N increased the quantity of polyethenoid fatty acids about threefold and decreased that of saturated fatty acids by one half. Thus the dietary fatty acid compositions of the hospital diets were rendered greatly different.

Samples of subcutaneous adipose tissue were taken at intervals from patients in each hospital. The fatty acids which showed the greatest difference between the two populations were myristic acid (derived mainly from milk fat) and linoleic acid (derived mainly from soybean oil). At the end of the first period of the study the linoleic acid content in the experimental hospital had risen to 27%, whereas this value at the control hospital was 10%. The relative quantities of myristic acid were just opposite (1.5% vs. 3.8%). The reversal of the diets was followed by the reversal of the fatty acid compositions as well, with a rise of linoleic acid and a fall of myristic acid in the experimental hospital and the opposite changes in the new control hospital. The changes, however, were slow and at the latest sampling nearly four years after the reversal of the diets, a final equilibrium did not seem to have been fully reached yet.

Of the blood lipids the most consistent studies were devoted to serum cholesterol, the blood lipid admittedly best correlated with the incidence of coronary heart disease. The cholesterol values were at all times lower in the subjects on the experimental diet. This was the case during the first period of the experiment; the reversal of the diets brought about a reversal of the cholesterol values as well, and during the second period the new experimental hospital showed consistently lower values. The mean difference in serum cholesterol levels was 51 mg/dl during the first period and 35 mg/dl during the second period.

Serum triglyceride values, on the contrary, behaved differently. During the first period they were lower in the experimental hospital, but the reversal of the diets caused no definite change. This lipid fraction seemed to be rather insensitive to the changes in fatty acid composition of the diet. At all times the triglyceride levels were higher in hospital K.

In the assessment of the incidence of coronary heart disease in the two subject groups ingesting different diets the chief reliance was placed on electrocardiography. Electrocardiographic studies were regularly carried out among the patients of both hospitals. In the classification of records the system known as the Minnesota Code was used. This system, even if not free from observer variability, provides a method for a relatively objective classification of electrocardiographic findings.

The incidence of new electrocardiographic patterns, presumably due to coronary heart disease, were judged by the use of several criteria of different levels of discrimination. It was found that the incidence of new electrocardiographic patterns presumably due to coronary heart disease was by all the criteria used markedly and significantly lower in hospital N, where the diet had been changed. The difference in incidence between the hospitals was greatest when the more rigorous criteria were applied, but even the use of milder criteria revealed significant differences in incidence.

In addition to electrocardiographic signs, another criterion of coronary disease was used, namely, the coronary death. The number of coronary deaths was, however, too small to reveal a statistically significant difference between the hospitals. But if the incidences of electrocardiographic signs and of coronary deaths were pooled, a definitely lower total incidence for the experimental hospital was found, and the difference was statistically highly significant. (Annual incidence rates per 1,000 were 14.4 in the experimental group and 33.0 in the control group.)

What has been said about the incidence of coronary heart disease refers to the first phase of the study. The evidence from the second phase, i.e., the period after the reversal of the diets, is not yet sufficient for significant conclusions. This evidence, however, seems to indicate that the new experimental hospital is experiencing a lower incidence of electrocardiographic signs and also a lower coronary mortality than the new control hospital.

All the three studies just reviewed have produced evidence which is favorable to the hypothesis that the incidence of atherosclerotic manifestations could be decreased by appropriate changes in the fatty acid composition of the diet. All these studies were started more than ten years ago, and they have been called "the first generation studies". Their experimental design admittedly shows various shortcomings, and the evidence obtained may not yet be conclusive. Even so, they have perhaps fulfilled their purpose and also pointed the way for new, larger and better studies.

DIET AND ISCHEMIC HEART DISEASE: PROGRESS IN SECONDARY PREVENTION DIETARY TRIALS

SEYMOUR DAYTON

It is possible to trace several major phases in work on dietary prevention of ischemic heart disease (IHD). In the early 1950's there were two important developments. First of all, epidemiologic studies provided mounting evidence for an important correlation between plasma cholesterol level and the risk of developing overt IHD. Secondly, and more or less simultaneously, experiments in clinical nutrition demonstrated which dietary variables were important in regulating the plasma cholesterol level in man. As this information unfolded, several dietary attempts at secondary prevention were undertaken, using either diets low in total fat content or diets containing predominantly unsaturated fat. Results of some of these studies were available even before 1960. Although these early clinical trials in this difficult field were not fully controlled, they were encouraging in that their results suggested that the course of IHD might be influenced, even after clinically overt, by diets of modified fat composition. The combined impact of information from all these sources led a number of workers, shortly before 1960, to consider the formidable task of undertaking more rigorous clinical trials. Several such trials were in time begun and the harvest has been reaped in the last four years.

This discussion will be devoted largely to a review of several secondary prevention trials, reported since mid-1965, having in common the most important characteristic of a clinical trial: control and treatment groups were established by random allocation of individuals in the study population. Furthermore, these more recent trials have employed techniques designed to minimize the influence of observer bias. In addition to reviewing these four trials which were aimed specifically at study of secondary prevention, I shall present some results of our own trial which bear on the secondary prevention question.

The first of these experiments to be reported was the small but carefully executed study of Rose et al. [1256]. Their subjects were free-living persons who manifested either electrocardiographic evidence of myocardial infarction or a clear history of angina of effort. They were allocated at random to three groups: a control group receiving a conventional diet, and two groups receiving a basic low-fat diet which was supplemented in the one instance by olive oil and in the other instance by corn oil. Serum cholesterol levels fell about 26 mg/dl in the corn oil group but there was no significant serum cholesterol change in the other two groups.

This trial was partially blindfold in that the observers knew whether a subject was receiving oil, but they did not know which oil he was receiving. The duration of the trial was two years. Clinical results are summarized in Table 1. The olive oil group fared slightly worse than did the control subjects, and the corn oil group worse still. These results are discordant from those of the several larger trials which will be described shortly. It is not possible to identify major operational defects on which to blame this relatively unique outcome. However, the trial was, after all, a small and brief one. In view of the better experience of treated groups in other trials, one may suppose that the results shown in Table 1 are at variance with the others to be described because of the operation of chance in a small study population.

The second of these trials was a cooperative test of a low-fat diet in a group of London hospitals [1222]. Here, too, the subjects were free-living individuals,

Table 1. *Clinical results in the trial of Rose, Thomson, and Williams* [1256]

	Diet		
	control	olive oil	corn oil
Number of subjects at start	26	26	28
Number of subjects developing:			
Sudden death	1	2	3
Fatal myocardial infarction	0	1	2
Definite nonfatal myocardial infarction	3	4	3
Probable nonfatal myocardial infarction	2	2	4
"Other significant cardiac pain"	5	2	3

Table 2. *Clinical results in the cooperative London trial of a low-fat diet* [1222]

	Diet	
	control	low-fat
Number of subjects at start	129	123
Number of subjects developing:		
Definite myocardial infarction	27	27
Probable myocardial infarction	7	4
Possible myocardial infarction	10	12
Deaths (all causes)	24	20

in this instance, middle-aged survivors of myocardial infarction. The effect of the dietary modification on serum cholesterol concentration was a modest one: there was a mean drop of 23 mg/dl in the control group and 40 mg/dl in the low-fat group. During the follow-up period of three years, evaluation of end-points was carried out in a semi-blindfold fashion, in that the evaluating physician was unaware of the dietary assignment.

The outcome of this study of low-fat diet is summarized in Table 2. There was no appreciable difference in the clinical experience of the two groups. Although this too was a carefully controlled trial, the net effect[1] of the experimental diet in lowering serum cholesterol was sufficiently small so that one must be quite cautious about generalizing from the negative outcome of this study.

1 Presumably the net effect is the decrement in the experimental group minus the decrement in the control group, a net decrement of 17 mg/dl.

Major contributions to the literature on secondary prevention dietary trials are provided by two rather similar studies, one carried out by Leren [857] in Oslo and the other by a research committee of the Medical Research Council in London [967]. In the Oslo trial, the participants were 412 free-living male survivors of myocardial infarction. The subjects had higher serum cholesterol levels than those commonly observed among typical myocardial infarction patients in England and the United States. the levels averaging 296 mg/dl in both groups. The experimental subjects were instructed in preparation of a diet involving major substitution of unsaturated vegetable oils for much of the saturated fat of the conventional diet, whereas the control group received no dietary instruction. There was a small serum cholesterol drop amounting to 3.7% in the control group as compared with 17.6% in the treated group.

Table 3. *Clinical results in the trial by Leren* [857]

	Diet	
	conventional	unsaturated fat
Number of subjects at start	206	206
Number of subjects[a] developing:		
Sudden death	27	27
Myocardial infarction	54	34
New angina pectoris	29	10
Number of subjects with relapse:		
Total	90	64
Excluding angina pectoris	81	61

[a] Some subjects had relapses in more than one category, and are included more than once in the tabulation.

Diagnoses of myocardial infarction were evaluated by a blindfold diagnostic committee but this was not true of angina pectoris. The results of this trial are summarized in Table 3. There is a statistically significant difference in total relapse, due entirely to myocardial infarction and acquired angina pectoris, there being no difference whatsoever in numbers of sudden deaths. If attention is confined to relapse manifested either by sudden death or by myocardial infarction (in order to eliminate the uncertainties and possible biases in the angina pectoris results), one finds 81 such instances in the control group as compared with 61 in the experimental group—a significant difference ($p < 0.05$) by the chi-square test.

The cognate trial in London [967] involved a design very similar to that employed by Leren. The subjects were male survivors of myocardial infarction who were allocated at random to control and experimental groups. The latter group received instruction concerning rigorous restriction of saturated dietary fat and inclusion of 85 g of soybean oil daily in the diet, while control subjects were kept on conventional diets. In the control group the mean starting serum cholesterol level was 273 mg/dl and the mean level during the trial 258; the experimental group started with a mean level of 272 mg/dl and displayed a mean level of 221 during the test period. The trial period lasted between 2 years and $6^3/_4$ years. Questions of coronary heart disease relapse were evaluated by a blindfold committee.

The major results of this trial are presented in Table 4. The experimental diet had no measurable effect upon the incidence of myocardial reinfarction nor upon the number of deaths from cardiovascular disease. There was, however, a moderate reduction in "other non-fatal relapses".

Efforts to reconcile these results with the somewhat more encouraging outcome of Leren's trial have generally emphasized the differences in the study populations. In the London trial, starting serum cholesterol levels were lower, the time from the initial infarct to the start of the trial was shorter, the subjects were younger, and hypertensive patients were excluded. These differences, individually or together, appear to be a poor explanation for the more favorable results in Oslo, but the difference in outcome of the two trials could readily have been a result of chance.

Table 4. *Clinical results in the cooperative London trial of a diet containing soybean oil as the major fat* [967]

	Diet	
	control	experimental
Number of subjects at start	194	199
Number of first relapses:		
Fatal	14	15
Nonfatal definite reinfarctions	25	25
Other nonfatal relapses	35	22
All deaths from cardiovascular disease	25	27

Our own contribution in the field of secondary prevention has been limited. Our group has carried out a controlled, double-blind dietary trial in an institutionalized population, employing an experimental diet low in saturated fat and high in unsaturated fat. The primary objective of the trial was to test the primary prevention question. However, 30% of the participants were found at the outset to have either definite evidence or some suspicion of overt atherosclerosis at some site, and these may be viewed as a secondary prevention group of a sort. The total length of time in the trial was variable, up to a maximum of $8^1/_3$ years. Mean serum cholesterol level was similar for the two groups at the start (241 mg/dl in those subjects with definite or possible preexisting complications of atherosclerosis). During the period of dietary modification, the experimental group maintained mean levels 13% lower than those of the control group.

The results of interest in the present context are given in summary form in Fig. 1. This figure presents the combined incidence of definite myocardial infarction, definite cerebral infarction, and sudden death due to IHD as cumulative incidence figures, computed by the life table method after stratification of the study population by presence or absence of pre-existing complications.

The group designated "with pre-existing complications" includes all subjects with definite or possible complications at any site. In the stratum without pre-existing complications, a statistically significant difference between the two incidence curves was observed, in favor of the experimental diet. This was not true of the stratum with pre-existing complications. However, during most of the follow-up period, the incidence in this stratum was lower in the experimental group even though not at a statistically significant level. The high *P*-value for

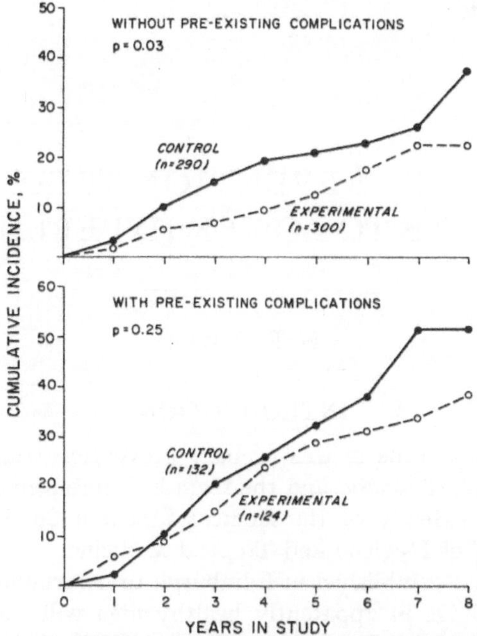

Fig. 1. Combined cumulative incidence of sudden death due to coronary heart disease, definite myocardial infarction, and definite cerebral infarction, after stratification based on evidence of pre-existing complications of atherosclerosis at the initial examination (Los Angeles Veterans Administration trial). Subjects were allocated to the group with pre-existing complications if the initial examination revealed evidence of any definite or possible manifestations of atherosclerosis at any site. *P*-values were computed by a permutation technique and applied to comparison of the entire curves. Reprinted from the American Journal of Medicine by permission [383]

subjects "with pre-existing complications" may have been due as much to the relatively small size of this stratum as to any other factor. It is impossible to state from inspection of these incidence curves that the group with pre-existing complications derived less benefit from the experimental diet than did the group without pre-existing complications. Examination of fatal acute atherosclerotic events stratified in the same fashion leads to the same conclusion. This trial is documented in greater detail in another publication [384].

The state of affairs may thus be summarized in the following terms. The last several years have given us results of five dietary trials involving secondary prevention, having as common characteristics randomization of subjects into control and experimental groups and measures for minimizing observer bias. Three of these trials yielded evidence suggesting that the experimental diet did indeed lower the incidence of relapse, albeit to only a modest degree. The other two trials yielded discordant results. However, one of these involved small groups of patients, and the other was a trial of a low-fat diet in which only a small net reduction in serum cholesterol level was achieved. It thus appears that diets low in saturated fat and high in unsaturated fat probably do yield small benefits. It is not clear that these benefits are great enough to justify a major change in a patient's way of life.

A PRIMARY PREVENTION TRIAL USING CLOFIBRATE TO LOWER HYPERLIPIDEMIA

M. F. OLIVER

INTRODUCTION

In presenting the outline of this primary prevention trial, I am acting as a spokesman for Dr. W. G. Macfie and the team in Edinburgh and Professor J. N. Morris and Dr. J. A. Heady of the Medical Research Council Social Medicine Unit, London School of Hygiene and Tropical Medicine.

In 1965 a trial was established in Edinburgh to determine whether reduction of elevated serum lipids in apparently healthy men will lead to a decrease in the expected incidence of ischemic heart disease (IHD). This trial was extended in 1967 to Prague[1] and Budapest[2]. It is now coordinated by the World Health Organization.

The study is designed to control only one risk factor, hyperlipidemia. Advice is not given to the participants about altering their way of living in order to modify other risk factors, such as excess cigarette smoking, obesity, or physical inactivity.

The method chosen for the control of hyperlipidemia is the use of a drug and no change is advised in the usual diet. Clofibrate [1118, 1120, 1449, 1466] (Atromid-S) was selected at the inception of the study and is still regarded as the drug of choice. Should a better one be developed, the design of the study permits its introduction. We are not testing Clofibrate as such but using it as an acceptable method of lowering elevated lipid levels in the free-living population.

Design. Male volunteers, 30–59 years, are admissible to the Trial. They must conform to certain criteria of health (listed in the Working Manual)[3] and are

1 Institute for Cardiovascular Research, Prague (Drs. Z. Hejl and H. Geizerova).

2 Hungarian Institute for Cardiology, Budapest (Drs. G. Gábor, G. Lamm and I. Gyárfás).

3 Copies of the Working Manual can be obtained on request.

excluded if, on clinical or electrocardiographic examination, they have features of ischemic or other heart disease (aortic valve disease, for example); if they have a disease requiring treatment (severe diastolic hypertension, for example) or if they have a disease which has a poor prognosis for life.

Men are selected for entry according to their serum cholesterol levels, measured at a screening visit, according to the design outlined in Fig. 1. All whose serum cholesterol is in the top one-third of the distribution of the population under study are acceptable and they are randomized into treatment (Clofibrate) and placebo groups. A random half of the lowest one-third are also admitted to the trial and receive the placebo, olive oil. The remaining half of this third and all of those with serum cholesterol levels in the middle third of the population, i.e. half

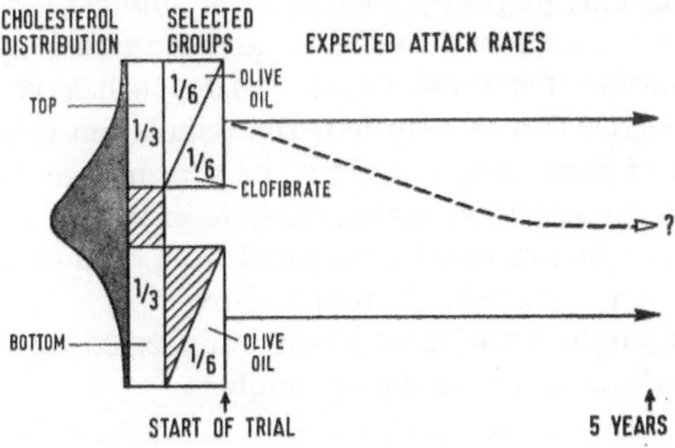

Fig. 1. Design of the Edinburgh-Prague-Budapest primary prevention Trial. Men with serum cholesterol levels in the middle third of the normal distribution and a random half of those in the lower third are not included in the Trial. Three groups of equal size, two with high and one with low serum cholesterol levels, comprise the Trial

the total population originally screened, are not accepted. Nonacceptance might raise doubts and anxiety in the mind of a volunteer and so the decision about selection is made before interview. The inclusion of a low cholesterol group serves two purposes. It provides a second control group against which changes in the high cholesterol treated group can be contrasted. It also avoids the problem of inducing a cholesterol neurosis. Participants are told, if they inquire, that men with high and with low-serum cholesterol levels are recruited into the trial and that the examining doctor does not know the level of any individual.

To allow for seasonal variation in serum cholesterol, the cutting-points for the top and bottom one-third groups are assessed every month from groups of about 500. The system used takes into consideration levels obtained from the immediately adjacent months. This also helps to reduce variation due to small numbers.

The trial is "blind" with respect to treatment group, and in the high cholesterol groups is, thus, a conventional "double blind" randomized trial. The capsules are prepared to look identical and contain either Clofibrate, 400 mg or the placebo, olive oil. Two are taken in the morning and evening.

Specifications. Any trial of this kind should be designed to meet certain specifications and these are set out in Table 1.

Table 1. *Specifications of the Trial*

1. Numbers must permit detection of a fall of 33% or more in incidence of IHD in Clofibrate-treated group at the 1% significance level (alpha value) with 95% confidence (beta value).
2. The incidence of IHD is 1% per annum in untreated hypercholesterolemic controls.
3. Each man agrees to collaborate for a period of five years.
4. The "drop-out" rate from the trial will be 30% over five years, 10% during the first year, and 5% during each subsequent year.

Sample Size. In order to meet these specifications it will be necessary for 15,000 men to enter the five-year trial. Of those approached in Edinburgh about 25% cannot be admitted; of these, 20% show no interest, 2% are regarded by their family doctors as unfit or unsuitable, and a further 2–3% are found to be unfit on examination. On these figures, 20,000 will have to be approached in order to admit 15,000. Since only half the population originally screened is approached, a total of about 40,000 need to be screened to identify the appropriate numbers with high and low serum cholesterol levels.

It is planned that 5,000 should be recruited from each of the three centers—Edinburgh, Prague and Budapest. Currently (November, 1969), 4,000 have been recruited from Edinburgh, 3,500 from Prague and 2,500 from Budapest—some 10,000 in all or two-thirds of the requisite numbers.

PROGRESS IN EDINBURGH

Plainly, this Trial has presented a considerable organizational problem, and the main report at present is that it has proved feasible and is working satisfactorily. No results concerning the effect of Clofibrate on IHD are yet available. Such results shall not be divulged until the Trial's statistician Dr. J. A. Heady at the M.R.C. Social Medicine Unit considers either that a significant trend or that anything untoward is emerging, or that an agreed period of study has been completed. He makes regular assessments of the progress.

There are, however, other features which can be reported and these are listed in Table 2.

Side effects have been few and equal in all groups. Indigestion and bowel looseness are the main symptoms but have occurred in less than 2% of the men. Impotence has been reported on several occasions but is as common in the control as in the Clofibrate-treated group.

One case of severe alopecia and one of partial hair loss have been seen; both men were receiving olive oil. No example of cardiac arrhythmia has been seen.

Muscle pain has been reported as a possible toxic effect. The clinical follow-up procedure includes the London School of Hygiene questionnaire [1255] on intermittent claudication and leg pain. From the answers to this it can be stated that there has been no excess of muscular pain (at least in the legs) in the Clofibrate-treated group and so far no man has specifically complained of muscle pain.

Elevation of serum creatine kinase and of serum aspartate aminotransferase has been reported in other studies [839, 1118]. These enzymes, together with serum alkaline phosphatase, were estimated "blind" in 296 men and no signi-

Table 2. *Progress in Edinburgh*

Index	High cholesterol groups		Low cholesterol group
	Clofibrate (I)	olive oil (II)	olive oil (III)
Total nos. (September, 1969)	1,218	1,141	1,204
Side effects sufficient to remove	19	15	23
Opted out	71	54	52
Left district	17	24	19
Se. cholesterol (mean fall in $1^1/_2$ years)	−18 %	−5 %	−4 %
280 mg-%	−27 %	—	—
260–279 mg-%	−21 %	—	—
230–259 mg-%	−17 %	—	—
230 mg-%	− 8 %	—	—
Se. triglycerides[a] (mean fall in 1 year)	−28 %	−4 %	−5 %
Weight (3-year figs.)	+1.2 kg	+0.3 kg	+0.2 kg
Positive blood test for CPIB	95 %	—	—

[a] Based on a 10 % sample.

Table 3. *Serum enzyme levels in healthy male blood donors after six months participation in Trial*

Groups	No. of patients	Serum creatine kinase (IU/l)			Serum alkaline phosphatase (K.A. units/100 ml)			Serum aspartate aminotransferase (R.F. units/ml)		
		mean	S.D.	range	mean	S.D.	range	mean	S.D.	range
1. Clofibrate-treated high cholesterol group	101	57.2	32.5	8–196	7.0	2.3	3–15	27.4	10.4	11–86
2. Control high cholesterol group	110	58.9[a] (53.8)	47.7[a] (29.0)	18–360 (18–176)	9.8	2.7	3–20	26.8	11.2	16–70
3. Control low cholesterol group	85	49.7	27.8	4–164	9.5	2.9	3–20	24.8	13.0	13–55

[a] This group includes 2 results of 320 IU/l and 360 IU/l. The figures in parenthesis are those obtained if these two results are ignored.

ficant elevation of the former two was seen (Table 3)[4]. Serum alkaline phosphatase was reduced in men taking Clofibrate, as has been reported previously [662].

4 This study has now been published—Smith, A. F., Macfie, W. G., Oliver, M. F.: Clofibrate, serum enzymes and muscle pain. Brit. med. J. **1970 II**, 86.

SUMMARY

An account is given of progress in a trial of the effect on the incidence of ischemic heart disease by reducing elevated serum lipids in healthy men; Clofibrate is used for this purpose. 10,000 men, aged 30–59, have now been admitted to the study which is based in Edinburgh, Prague, and Budapest.

In Edinburgh, 85–90% of men are still participating after three years. The degree of reduction of elevated serum lipids is regarded as satisfactory; and no side effects of any consequence have occurred.

CONTROL OF HYPERLIPIDEMIA

4. PROGRESS IN DRUG TRIALS OF SECONDARY PREVENTION WITH PARTICULAR REFERENCE TO THE CORONARY DRUG PROJECT

Authors: The Coronary Drug Project Research Group* **

The purpose of this report is to review the current status of mass field trials aimed at assessing safety and efficacy of therapy for coronary patients with antihyperlipidemic drugs.

* Presented for the Coronary Drug Project Research Group by Jeremiah Stamler Chairman, Steering Committee, Coronary Drug Project.

** The Coronary Drug Project Research Group is under the leadership of the following professional personnel: E. Cowles Andrus, M.D., Samuel Baer, M.D., Allan H. Barker, M.D., Jacob E. Bearman, Ph.D., Kenneth G. Berge, M.D., David M. Berkson, M.D., Donald Berkowitz, M.D., Reuben Berman, M.D., William H. Bernstein, M.D., Henry Blackburn, M.D. (Director, ECG Center), Edwin P. Boyle, M.D., Paul L. Canner, Ph.D., Thomas Chalmers, M.D., Ralph E. Cole, M.D., Elmer E. Cooper, M.D., Gerald Cooper, M.D. (Director, Central Laboratory), Theodore Cooper, M.D. (Director, National Heart and Lung Institute), Mr. Jerome Cornfield, Mr. Fred Ederer, Leo Elson, M.D., Dean A. Emanuel, M.D., Irving Ershler, M.D., Eloise Evanson, M.D., Charles K. Friedberg, M.D., Nicholas J. Galluzzi, M.D., Mario Garcia Palmieri, M.D., Mr. Salvatore D. Gasdia, Peter C. Gazes, M.D., Fred I. Gilbert, Jr., M.D., James Gillette, M.D., Arthur J. Gosselin, M.D., Lawrence Gould, M.D., Ernst Greif, M.D., Robert J. Grissom, M.D., Jacob I. Haft, M.D., Adrian Hainline, Ph.D., Max Halperin, Ph.D., Olga M. Haring, M.D., Richard J. Havlik, M.D., Stephen J. Herbert, M.D., Richard J. Jones, M.D., Gerald Klatskin, M.D., Christian R. Klimt, M.D. (Director, Coordinating Center), Gennel Knatterud, M.D., Robert M. Kohn, M.D., William F. Krol, Ph.D., Thomas A. Landau, M.D., Ward Laramore, M.D., Louis Lasagna, M.D., Charles A. Laubach, Jr., M.D., Sidney A. Levine, M.D., Robert Levy, M.D., Bernard I. Lewis, M.D., Irving M. Liebow, M.D., Donald McCaughan, M.D., Jessie Marmorston, M.D., Alan Mather, M.D., Louis B. Matthews, Jr., M.D., Gordon L. Maurice, M.D., Curtis L. Meinert, Ph.D. (Co-Chairman, Safety Monitoring Committee), Charles B. Moore, M.D., David Z. Morgan, M.D., Frank W. Mowry, M.D., Elliot Newman, M.D., Milton Z. Nichaman, M.D., William B. Parsons, Jr., M.D., Thaddeus E. Prout, M.D., Bernard A. Sachs, M.D., Paul Samuel, M.D., Robert C. Schlant, M.D., Henry K. Schoch, M.D., Ralph C. Scott, M.D., Charles W. Silver-

GENERAL REVIEW OF STUDIES

As is well known, many pharmacologic agents lower serum levels. Several have been extensively investigated in man and animals, and have been made available for prescription use. These include clofibrate, estrogens, heparin, nicotinic acid, plant sterols, thyroid hormones and dextrothyroxine [1406]. While a vast literature exists on these and other substances, definitive knowledge is not available concerning long-term safety and efficacy of any preparation. Until recently, few field trials had been undertaken to obtain the critically needed information. The earlier studies on efficacy dealt exclusively with estrogens [930, 1122, 1406, 1411, 1413]. Carried out in the 1950s, they produced contradictory and inconclusive results, almost certainly because of their small sample sizes.

In recent years, more extensive studies have been launched. For the most part, these are still in progress, or at least their findings have not yet been reported. One is a double-blind controlled trial of clofibrate for secondary prevention of CHD (H. A. Dewar, personal communication). After six years of investigative work, this trial in the north of England was brought to completion in July, 1969 and results should be available shortly.

A similar trial has been in progress under the aegis of the Scottish Society of Physicians. Again, information is not yet available from the study concerning efficacy of clofibrate for secondary prevention in patients with myocardial infarction (M. F. Oliver, personal communication).

A multidrug CHD secondary prevention trial was undertaken several years ago as a national cooperative effort by the Veterans Administration research programs in the United States. This double-blind investigation is still in progress. It involves 570 men randomly assigned to six treatment regimens—low dosage estrogen, aluminum nicotinate, dextrothyroxine, estrogens plus nicotinate, and estrogens plus dextrothyroxine (H. Schnaper, personal communication). Data are not yet available concerning its long-term findings.

The national cooperative Coronary Drug Project in the United States is the most extensive trial ever undertaken of secondary prevention of atherosclerotic coronary disease with pharmaceutical agents [54]. The remainder of this report deals with this endeavor.

THE CORONARY DRUG PROJECT (CDP)

Background, Development and Organization. Planning of this study was undertaken in 1960 at the initiative of the National Advisory Heart Council of the National Heart Institute (NHI). During the next years, extensive deliberations proceeded concerning design, organization, implementation and operations, resulting in the development of a formal Protocol and Manual of Operations. Initial

---

blatt, M.D., William M. Smith, M.D., Jeremiah Stamler, M.D. (Chairman, Steering Committee), Reuben Straus, M.D., Bernard Tabatznik, M.D., Suketomi Tominaga, M.D., Joseph A. Wagner, M.D., James R. Warbasse, M.D., Donald L. Warkentin, M.D., Robert W. Wilkins, M.D. (Chairman, Policy Board), C. Basil Williams, M.D. and William J. Zukel, M.D.

The project is proceeding as a collaborative study with the support of the National Heart Institute.

field work was begun in March, 1965. Thereafter, the study was progressively expanded to encompass 53 investigative centers. The CDP is proceeding under the operational scientific leadership of a Steering Committee, and under the supervision of a Policy Board. It is financed by the National Heart Institute as a collaborative study, with the NHI an active participant through assignees from its professional staff. A Coordinating Center is located at the Institute of International Medicine, University of Maryland School of Medicine. The study is also serviced by an ECG Center at the Laboratory of Physiological Hygiene, University of Minnesota, by a Central Laboratory for biochemical determinations at the Communicable Disease Center of the U.S. Public Health Service in Atlanta, Georgia, and by a Central Drug Procurement and Distribution Facility at the U.S.P.H.S. Supply Service Center, Perry Point, Maryland. Effective liaison and coordination are accomplished through the Steering Committee, with representatives from all key groups of the Project, including the Principal Investigators responsible for the 53 field research centers. All the latter, as well as leaders of other operational units of the study, are members of the Technical Group, meeting semiannually. Another key body is the Safety Monitoring Committee, with responsibility for bi-monthly review of confidential interim data on the end-points of the study.

Aims and Objectives. The primary objective of the CDP is to test the efficacy and safety of several drugs in the long-term therapy of coronary heart disease (CHD) in men age 30–64 with proved previous myocardial infarction. The pharmacologic agents under investigation (with their abbreviated designations) are: mixed conjugated equine estrogens—2.5 mg/day (ESG1); mixed conjugated equine estrogens—5.0 mg/day (ESG2); clofibrate—1.8 gm/day (CPIB); dextrothyroxine—6.0 mg/day (DT4); nicotinic acid—3.0 gm/day (NICA); placebo (PLBO). The primary end-point for assessment of therapeutic value is five-year total mortality rate. In addition, many other end-points are being monitored in relation to drug efficacy and toxicity, e.g. incidence and mortality rates of myocardial infarction, congestive heart failure, stroke, ECG changes; biochemical data relating to possible toxicity of drugs (see below).

Assessment of the efficacy of drugs in this controlled study requires the simultaneous long-term observation of a group randomly assigned to placebo treatment, in fact the largest study population of postmyocardial infarction patients ever assembled. A key objective, therefore, is to take fullest possible advantage of this opportunity for accruing new information on the natural history of coronary heart disease.

The large sample of patients required for a definitive assessment of drug efficacy could be assembled only through a national cooperative undertaking involving many research groups. A third basic aim of this investigation, therefore, is to acquire additional experience and knowledge concerning the total methodology of such large-scale, long-term collaborative clinical trials for assessing therapy of chronic noninfectious cardiovascular diseases.

General Plan. Patients randomized into the CDP are men age 30–64 with evidence of one or more myocardial infarctions (MI), categorized as Class I or II of the functional classification of the New York Heart Association, and free from a specified list of excluding diseases and conditions. All patients were classified as to long-term risk. Risk 1: Men with a single infarction free of serious complications during the acute episode. Risk 2: Men with a single infarction who during the acute episode did have one or more complications, as well as men with two or more myocardial infarctions.

Patients still eligible at the end of a two-month control period were randomly allocated to one of the six medication schedules. A separate random allocation schedule was utilized by the Coordinating Center for each of the two risk groups within each participating clinic. Each schedule was designed to assure approximately equal numbers of patients in the five drug groups and approximately five patients in the placebo group for every two patients in any of the other groups.

The study is conducted as double blind in the sense that neither the patient nor the clinic staff is informed of patient drug allocation, except as required in a verified medical emergency. Initial prescription of assigned medication is three capsules per day, supplying one-third of ultimate full dosage (see preceding), and is increased at monthly intervals to six and then to the maximum of nine capsules per day, unless the managing physician alters the regimen for specified reasons.

Each patient is to be followed for a period of five years. He reports to the clinic every four months for a follow-up visit. Complete routine examination, including ECG, is done annually. Complaints and findings suggestive of illness or toxicity are thoroughly evaluated by the research clinic. In all circumstances, the Protocol and Manual allow full leeway for optimal medical care for patients with myocardial infarction.

Data sent to the Coordinating Center from the clinics are monitored for events such as death, recurrent myocardial infarction, angina pectoris, ECG changes, etc., as well as toxic and side effects, e.g. flushing, feminization, nausea, and jaundice (see below).

Available Findings to Date. The first major task of the CDP was *recruitment* of the required number of eligible patients. In accordance with the sample size estimates originally made by CDP statisticians, the investigators in the clinical centers had pledged to enroll 8,210 patients. Intake of new patients ceased on June 30, 1969. At the time of this Symposium, the last of these patients were being randomly assigned to their treatment groups with enrollment of 8,341 men.

One of the key concerns is to verify *comparability* of study groups, i.e. whether the process of stratified randomization has indeed resulted in six groups of patients essentially similar in regard to cardinal characteristics known or suspected to influence long-term prognosis of middle-aged men with a previous history of myocardial infarction. To evaluate this matter, detailed tabulations by treatment group have been done for baseline findings, considered singly and in various combinations. Data available as of August 1, 1969, with 7,536 patients enrolled in the CDP, show that randomization of this large number of men has resulted in marked similarity of the six treatment groups with respect to baseline demographic, medical, biochemical and electrocardiographic findings.

As indicated, one fundamental objective of the study is to collect information concerning *natural history* of coronary disease. The baseline measurements in the CDP yield vast quantities of information for this purpose, and multiple analyses are in progress. For example, data available cast light on one matter of current interest, i.e. patterns of serum lipids and their relationship to CHD (Table 1). With the cutting points specified for gross hypercholesterolemia and hypertriglyceridemia[1], approximately one half the CDP men are frankly hyperlipidemic, with these 50% about evenly divided into men with hypercholesterolemia and no hypertriglyceridemia, and men with hypercholesterolemia plus hypertriglyceridemia. These two groups may be regarded respectively, as roughly equivalent to Type II and Types III–IV (predominantly IV in all likelihood) in the classification of hyperlipoproteinemia based on paper electrophoresis [489]. It is of course recognized that these estimates are crude, both because the cutting points are arbitrary, and because approximation of type is of limited validity based only on serum cholesterol and triglyceride measurement. For example, moderate hypertriglyceridemia may be present in Type II.

It is further evident from Table 1 that about 40% of the CDP men did not manifest gross hyperlipidemia, as defined, and about 11% had hypertriglyceridemia without hypercholesterolemia. Of course, as prospective epidemiologic studies unequivocally indicate, use of arbitrary cutting points to define hyperlipidemia is a gross oversimplification, since risk of disease is a curvilinear function of serum lipid levels practically throughout their range [1406]. The main point of interest in these data, therefore, is the indication as to relative rates of different types of frank hyperlipidemia-hyperlipoproteinemia in middle-aged men with coronary disease. Specifically the data suggest that myocardial infarction among middle-aged men is associated about equally often with nonhypertriglyceridemic and hypertriglyceridemic hypercholesterolemia, i.e. hyperlipoproteinemia Types II and Types III–IV.

Table 1. *Baseline patterns of serum lipids coronary drug project*

Serum cholesterol (mg/dl)	Serum triglycerides (meq/l)	No. of men	Rate per 100
<250	<6.0	1,917	39.5
<250	$\geqq 6.0$	560	11.5
$\geqq 250$	<6.0	1,252	25.8
$\geqq 250$	$\geqq 6.0$	1,125	23.2

The data at entry also shed light on another matter of current interest, i.e. the relationship between relative weight and pattern of hyperlipidemia. Prevalence of hypertriglyceridemia, but not hypercholesterolemia, in CDP patients increased with relative body weight. This relationship between relative weight and risk of hypertriglyceridemia was found both for men under age 55, and patients age 55 and over. Prevalence of hypertriglyceridemia, with or without hypercholesterolemia, was approximately double for men with relative weight of 1.25 or greater, compared with men at desirable weight. The simple correlation coefficient between relative weight and serum triglycerides was 0.20, and the partial correlation was 0.12 (after factoring out the confounding effect of age, blood pressure, serum cholesterol, uric acid and glucose). Relative weight was

1 The cutting point of 6.0 meq/l for serum triglycerides is equal to approximately 175 mg/dl.

also significantly associated with plasma glucose, serum uric acid and blood pressure.

As indicated earlier, one of the key aims in the CDP is to enhance knowledge concerning factors influencing *prognosis* after myocardial infarction. Since average duration of observation of CDP patients was only about one year as of August 1, 1969, the data currently available permit only the most preliminary evaluation of these matters. This report then must be viewed as merely an indicator of the types of analyses being developed, and of completely preliminary and tentative findings.

These initial data indicate that both risk and age influence mortality, as anticipated (Table 2). They further show a marked relationship between New York Heart Association classification category and mortality. Thus, of 1,165 and 1,340 men in the placebo group classified N.Y.H.A. 1 and 2 respectively, the

Table 2. *Age, risk and early mortality, placebo group, coronary drug project, August 1, 1969*

Age	Risk	No. of men	No. of deaths	Percentage deceased
<55	1	905	33	3.6
<55	2	460	27	5.9
$\geqq 55$	1	734	42	5.7
$\geqq 55$	2	406	31	7.6
<55	Both	1,365	60	4.4
$\geqq 55$	Both	1,140	73	6.4
All	1	1,639	75	4.6
All	2	866	58	6.7
All	Both	2,505	133	5.3

proportions deceased as of August 1, 1969, were 3.3 and 7.0% respectively. Similarly, status with respect to angina pectoris (AP) at entry appears to be related to subsequent mortality. Thus, for placebo patients with no angina pectoris, 3.9% were deceased as of August 1, 1969, whereas for men with definite AP, 7.0% had died.

In contrast, one other medical finding, duration since last myocardial infarction, has thus far not been found to relate to mortality. When the placebo group was stratified into four groups based on duration since last MI (3–12, 13–36, 37–60 and $\geqq 61$ months) the proportions deceased as of August 1, 1969 were 5.6, 4.6, 5.3 and 5.3% respectively.

There is a paucity of data as to the predictive significance of hyperlipidemia *after* recovery from myocardial infarction, in contrast to the demonstrated relationship with risk of first MI [1406]. A similar lack of data prevails with respect to other cardinal coronary risk factors, e.g. hypertension, cigarette smoking, hyperglycemia, hyperuricemia, overweight, singly and in combination and their impact on long-term risk of dying for patients recovered from previous myocardial infarction. The question is of the utmost significance both theoretically and practically, in terms of pathogenetic mechanisms and secondary preventive approaches to the disease once it has become manifest in the major form of clinical myocardial infarction. Unquestionably the CDP will eventually make a major contribution to clarifying this most important matter.

Initial findings on relationship between serum lipids and early mortality in the placebo group are presented in Table 3. They suggest that hypercholesterolemia considered as a single factor may be associated with increased risk of dying during the first year after a myocardial infarction, i.e. as of August 1, 1969, men with levels of ≧250 mg/dl had experienced an approximately 30% greater mortality than men with levels <250. No consistent association seems apparent between hypertriglyceridemia, considered as a single variable, and early mortality.

Table 3. *Serum lipids and early mortality, placebo group, coronary drug project, August 1, 1969*

Serum lipid	No. of men	No. of deaths	Percentage deceased
Cholesterol mg/dl			
< 200	298	15	5.0
200–249	924	46	5.0
250–299	763	51	6.7
≧ 300	343	21	6.1
Triglycerides meq/l			
< 3.0	277	14	5.1
3.0–4.9	898	52	5.8
5.0–6.9	556	26	4.7
≧ 7.0	599	41	6.8
Cholesterol < 250 mg/dl			
Triglycerides < 6.0 meq/l	902	40	4.4
≧ 6.0	320	21	6.6
Cholesterol ≧ 250			
Triglyceride < 6.0	595	40	6.7
≧ 6.0	511	32	6.3

However, when the placebo group was stratified by these two serum lipid measurements simultaneously, all three hyperlipidemic subgroups (hypertriglyceridemia without hypercholesterolemia, hypercholesterolemia without hypertriglyceridemia, and hypercholesterolemia plus hypertriglyceridemia) seem to have an approximately 50% greater risk of dying, compared to the subgroup with neither hypertriglyceridemia nor hypercholesterolemia. These initial findings seem to be in agreement with those reported from Oslo, and in disagreement with those reported from Toronto and New York [857, 884]. Obviously, additional experience of the CDP placebo group over the years ahead will greatly clarify this situation.

Initial data on other risk factors are also intriguing. Thus, the data to date indicate that both hyperglycemia and hyperuricemia are predictive of increased risk of dying during the first year for middle-aged men recovered from myocardial infarction (Table 4). For relative weight, no association is apparent, at least with regard to overweight; the data suggest that leanness may be associated with increased risk. The present data with respect to diastolic blood pressure appear equivocal. Thus there is a suggestion that mortality may indeed be greater in patients with diastolic blood pressure in the range 100 and greater, and further that men with diastolic readings under 80 may be at greater risk, i.e. these initial findings suggest a possible U-shaped curve. Perhaps diastolic pressure under 80 reflects impairment of myocardial function. Obviously further analyses, together with accumulation of additional data over time, are needed to evaluate these matters more definitively. Finally, the current data indicate

Table 4. *Risk factors for first MI events and early mortality, placebo group, coronary drug project, August 1, 1969*

Risk factor	No. of men	No. of deaths	Percentage deceased
Plasma glucose, 1 hour mg/dl			
< 140	569	25	4.4
140–169	527	31	5.9
170–199	487	34	7.0
≧200	565	41	7.3
Serum uric acid mg/dl			
< 6.0	601	23	3.8
6.0–6.9	626	43	6.9
7.0–7.9	517	37	7.2
≧8.0	410	28	6.8
Relative weight			
< 1.00	301	23	7.6
1.00–1.14	1,039	47	4.5
1.15–1.29	807	44	5.5
≧1.30	350	19	5.4
Diastolic B.P. mm Hg			
< 80	856	53	6.2
80–89	937	40	4.3
90–99	501	26	5.2
≧100	211	14	6.6
Cigarettes/day			
None	1,561	80	5.1
1–20	665	40	6.0
≧21	278	14	5.0

no association between cigarette smoking and prognosis during the first year for men recovered from a myocardial infarction.

It has been amply shown by the large scale prospective studies that susceptibility to first episodes of myocardial infarction in middle-aged men is related particularly to combinations of the foregoing risk factors [1406]. Therefore, a few initial tabulations have been done with respect to this matter for men recovered from previous myocardial infarction. The data on serum cholesterol and plasma glucose suggest that the combination of hyperglycemia plus hypercholesterolemia is associated with marked increase in mortality.

It is appropriate to re-emphasize that these data are very preliminary. No conclusions can be drawn at this juncture, both because the period of follow-up is as yet too brief, and because detailed evaluations have not been made of comparability of the subgroups identified in the stratifications of Tables 3 and 4. Obviously, analyses of these types are meaningful and valid only if these groups are reasonably comparable with respect to other factors influencing prognosis for patients with previous myocardial infarction, e.g. age, risk, New York Heart Association classification, status with respect to angina pectoris. At this juncture, the number of deaths does not permit a meaningful report based on additional stratifications along such lines. They will be presented at later stages of the study. In addition, detailed comparability studies will be completed, and multifactor analytical methods applied to the data [1477].

One of the key tasks of the CDP is to study and assess data possibly indicative of toxicity induced by drugs. For this purpose, extensive laboratory measurements

Table 5. *Percentage of patients in placebo group with laboratory findings in "alert" or "toxic" range—coronary drug project, all follow-up visits combined—August 1, 1969*

Test	"Alert" limit	Rate, as a percentage	"Toxic" limit	Rate, as a percentage
Total bilirubin	>0.8	19.5	>1.7	0.8
Direct bilirubin	>0.4	14.1	>0.7	1.3
SGOT	>40	17.2	>70	3.1
Alkaline phosphatase	<4	2.4	<3	0.4
Alkaline phosphatase	>10	13.1	>16	0.8
Uric acid	>8	24.5	>10	4.5
Urea nitrogen	>20	19.5	>30	0.7
Plasma glucose, fasting	>110	21.3	>120	10.5
Plasma glucose, one hour	>220	17.1	>240	9.5
Hematocrit	<38	1.6	<36	1.0
WBC	<5,000	11.3	<3,000	0.1
ANC	<3,500	29.8	<1,800	1.1
ANC/WBC	<0.5	14.2	<0.4	2.4
Urine glucose	+	5.2	+	5.2
Urine protein	>Trace	7.5	>1+	3.0

are made, both centrally and locally, from specimens collected at interval visits. In addition, of course, clinical symptomatology and signs, including ECG findings, are utilized for this purpose. Table 5 details some of the biochemical and hematologic measurements, and the "alert" and "toxic" levels used in assessing the data. When values are in the "toxic" range for measurements made at the Central Laboratory, physicians in the clinics are informed of the findings by special communications. As is evident from Table 5, a sizeable proportion of placebo group patients have values above the "alert" and "toxic" limits. These findings clearly indicate the crucial importance of a random control group in a clinical trial of drug safety and efficacy.

In addition to its key role in monitoring aspects of possible toxicity, the Central Laboratory is also responsible for biochemical measurements to assess trends of serum lipids and adherence to treatment regimens. Thus, it has a crucial role in the study. Quality of its work and the regular assessment of this is obviously of great importance. Two general approaches are used for *quality control,* i.e. internal and external monitoring. The former involves procedures carried out systematically and routinely by the Central Laboratory itself to evaluate proficiency of staff and methods. The latter entails submission of control samples as unknowns from the clinics to the Central Laboratory, for the dual purposes of evaluating reproducibility and long-term trends of measurement. Periodic reports show that the Laboratory is functioning in a highly satisfactory fashion. This laboratory experience is making a fundamental contribution to the third main objective, i.e. the contribution of the study to the basic methodology of long-term national cooperative mass field trials of therapy for chronic non-infectious diseases.

Finally of course, the CDP, particularly through its Safety Monitoring Committee and its Policy Board, is regularly reviewing the extensive data accruing on critical end-points, i.e. rates of toxicity, disease and mortality by treatment group. In accordance with the design of the Coronary Drug Project, these are confidential. However, the study is continuing according to its original Protocol, and this approach was reaffirmed based on data review at the meetings of the Safety Monitoring Committee and the Policy Board in the Fall of 1969. The conclusion implicit in this fact can be stated explicitly, i.e. no trends to date are of a nature or significance to warrant discontinuance of any treatment groups because of either positive therapeutic effects or negative toxicity findings.

CONTROL OF MILD HYPERTENSION

EDWARD D. FREIS

About 15 years ago antihypertensive drug therapy reached a stage of development where effective control of blood pressure could be obtained in the majority of hypertensive patients. It was soon demonstrated that it was possible to change the course of malignant hypertension by drug treatment. A significant percentage of such patients could be salvaged from what was formerly an almost uniformly rapidly fatal outcome [415, 616, 1166, 1383].

In hypertension of lesser severity, however, some physicians still adopt a wait-and-see attitude. Evidence of prevention of morbid events is much more difficult to obtain in essential hypertension because of the long life history and the great variability amongst patients in the rate at which these complications develop. Such skepticism has been well expressed in a volume devoted to controversies in internal medicine in which the editor [1219] concludes that evidence for the effectiveness of drug treatment in prolonging life or preventing complications still is lacking in essential hypertension. Recently, however, several long-term prospective control studies have brought forth evidence demonstrating the value of antihypertensive drugs in the treatment of patients with essential hypertension who have higher than average levels of diastolic blood pressure. Similar evidence still is lacking in mild hypertension although several control studies are currently in progress. At present, we can only extrapolate from the results of clinical trials obtained in the more severe forms of the disease and to utilize additional pertinent experimental and clinical observations as a basis for evaluating the possible benefits of antihypertensive drug treatment in patients with mild hypertension.

As a general rule, the type of complication causing death in hypertension bears some relation to the height of the blood pressure. In untreated accelerated hypertension with severely elevated diastolic blood pressure, death is often the result of renal or cardiac failure or of a vascular catastrophe such as dissecting aneurysm of the aorta or cerebrovascular hemorrhage. When the hypertension is mild, however, the course is prolonged and such patients tend to develop complications associated with atherosclerosis, the most frequent being the manifestations of coronary artery disease.

Studies carried out on the natural history of hypertension prior to the era of antihypertensive drug treatment do not provide a consistent picture of expected morbidity and mortality in hypertensive patients. Palmer and his associates [1147], found over an eight-year period of follow-up that 22% of patients with "mild" hypertension had died and that the rate of mortality increased with more severe grades of hypertension. On the other hand, Perera [1164] observed a mortality of only 17% in patients with all grades of severity after an average of 12 years of follow-up (from documented inception of hypertension). Sokolow [1384] indicated a mortality of 36% over a five-year period in an unselected series of hypertensive patients. Some of the variability of the results may be due to differences in the duration of hypertension prior to enrollment in the follow-up study. Also, the actual year of onset of hypertension often is unknown.

The wide variations in mortality reported by different investigators makes it impossible to utilize data gathered in the pretreatment era as a basis for assessing the value of antihypertensive drug therapy. Even if the data were more uniform it is not certain that patients studied in one decade in time as compared to another or in different regions will exhibit the same rates of morbidity and mortality.

These various considerations lead to the establishment of the Veterans Administration Cooperative Study on Antihypertensive Agents [1498]. The purpose was to compare prospectively the incidence of morbid events in a series of patients treated with antihypertensive drugs as compared to another group receiving only symptomatic treatment. Because of the importance of its conclusions this study will be described in some detail.

Long-term therapeutic trials in out-patients present a number of difficult problems. There is no continuous control over the patient as there is in in-patient trials. Obviously, the results of a study will be invalid if a considerable proportion of the patients neglect to take their pills or take them only sporadically or irregularly. Certain precautions can be taken to minimize this difficulty, the most effective being careful selection of patients. Of great value in making such a selection is the utilization of a prerandomization trial period.

In the Veterans Administration study obviously unreliable patients such as vagrants, alcoholics and antagonistic personalities were excluded immediately. The remaining patients, all of whom were males, entered a two to four month out-patient trial period in which they received placebos of the antihypertensive agents. Pill counts were carried out at monthly clinic visits. The placebos contained riboflavin which produces fluorescence of the urine when viewed under ultraviolet light. Acceptability for randomization into the therapeutic trial required two successive clinic visits in which pill counts were satisfactory and the urine exhibited fluorescence.

The prerandomization trial period served an additional useful function in the elimination of many potential dropouts. The highest percentage of dropouts generally occurs in the first few months of follow-up. Furthermore, the procedures described for selecting cooperative patients permits randomization of the more reliable and conscientious individuals who are less liable to default. The success of these techniques in minimizing the dropout problem in the VA study is indicated by the fact that only 8% of the patients defaulted during the trial.

The study was designed to encompass all patients with pretreatment diastolic blood pressures averaging 90 through 129 mm Hg. Results are available at present only in the subgroup of patients with diastolic blood pressure averaging 115 and above. In this latter group the study was terminated because of the great difference in morbid events developing in the untreated as compared to the treated group. The evaluation of antihypertensive therapy still is proceeding in the larger group of patients with diastolic blood pressures averaging less than 115 mm Hg.

There were 143 patients who fulfilled the criteria for randomization and who also exhibited diastolic blood pressures averaging between 115 and 129 mm Hg during the prerandomization period when all of the patients received only placebos. Of this number 73 were randomized on active drugs. The therapeutic regimen consisted of hydrochlorothiazide 50 mg plus reserpine 0.1 mg combined in a single tablet given twice daily. In addition, these patients received hydralazine 25 to 50 mg given three times daily. The 70 other patients received placebos of these medications. The method of administration was double-blind. The reduction of blood pressure achieved in the actively treated patients averaged 43/30 mm Hg as opposed to no significant change in the placebo treated patients.

During a follow-up period averaging approximately 18 months the following morbid events developed in the 70 patients making up the placebo treated group: four patients died; one of "sudden death," two of dissecting aortic aneurysm and one of a ruptured abdominal atherosclerotic aneurysm. Nonfatal events occurred in the following: eight patients developed hypertensive neuroretinopathy, two other patients exhibited increasing azotemia, another sustained a cerebrovascular hemorrhage and one patient had a disabling cerebrovascular thrombosis. Three additional patients exhibited progression of blood pressure to dangerously high levels although no clinically apparent morbid events developed. In all, 21 patients developed "terminating" events in the placebo treated group, the majority of these events being manifestations associated specifically with hypertension.

Morbid events associated with atherosclerosis were considerably less frequent consisting of myocardial infarction in two patients, cerebrovascular thrombosis in two, and transient ischemic attacks in one. The total number of patients developing either hypertensive or atherosclerotic events in the placebo treated group was 27. By contrast, only 2 of the 73 patients receiving antihypertensive drugs developed complications. One of these was related to side effects of the antihypertensive agents consisting of hyperglycemia presumably associated with hydrochlorothiazide and depression apparently related to reserpine. The other patient developed hypotensive syncopal attacks immediately following the institution of active drug treatment. He persisted in the treatment without informing his physician and after two weeks developed a hemiparesis which slowly cleared following dosage adjustment of the antihypertensive drugs.

The results of this trial provided convincing evidence of the value of antihypertensive therapy in the prevention of morbid events in male patients with essential hypertension and higher levels of diastolic blood pressure. The proportion of such events developing in these patients randomly assigned to one regimen or the other was 27 in the untreated group as compared to two in the treated.

Essentially similar results have been reported by Hamilton and his associates [599] who followed 61 patients, 22 males and 39 females with essential hypertension and diastolic blood pressures averaging 120 mm Hg or higher on several clinic visits. Alternate cases received antihypertensive agents with ganglion blocking agents or guanethidine supplemented with thiazide diuretics when needed while the remainder received only symptomatic treatment without antihypertensive drugs.

Over a two to six-year period of follow-up none of the 10 treated male patients developed morbid events. Of the 12 untreated males, four developed strokes, one suffered a myocardial infarction and one exhibited increasing left ventricular enlargement. Eight of 19 untreated female patients suffered morbid events similar in type to those observed in the males. However, in contrast to the male patients five of the 20 treated females developed complications of which three were strokes. However, the blood pressure was not adequately controlled in four of these five patients since their diastolic levels never were recorded below 110 mm Hg. Pill counts or marker substances were not used in this study so that it is not possible to estimate whether the failure of blood pressure reduction was due to poor cooperation or drug resistance. In all of the other treated patients the blood pressure was well controlled. If reduction of diastolic blood pressure to levels below 110 mm Hg is used as the basis of comparison, then one of 26 patients maintaining such a reduction developed a morbid event as compared to 19 of the 35 patients whose diastolic levels were not reduced.

It should be emphasized that myocardial infarction was a relatively uncommon morbid event in both the VA study and in Hamilton's series. The untreated patients with higher levels of diastolic blood pressure tend to develop complications more specifically associated with hypertension such as accelerated hypertension, left ventricular enlargement and congestive heart failure, cerebrovascular accidents, dissecting aneurysm and renal failure.

On the other hand, it is well known that hypertension predisposes to coronary artery disease [435, 773]. There is a large body of evidence both experimental and clinical that hypertension accelerates the rate of development of atherosclerosis [491].

It would appear, however, that atherosclerosis being a slowly developing process does not have time to manifest itself in untreated patients with moderate to severe elevations of diastolic blood pressure. Hypertensive complications develop at a more rapid rate than do atherosclerotic events in these patients with considerably elevated diastolic blood pressures. Coronary artery disease is a more frequent complication in the patients with lesser degrees of hypertension which has been present for many years without producing hypertensive complications.

Hodge and Smirk have compared the causes of death occurring in their hypertensive patients before and after the advent of effective antihypertensive therapy. Prior to the antihypertensive drug era the most common causes of death were congestive heart failure, cerebrovascular hemorrhage and uremia. Since the advent of drug therapy, coronary artery disease including "sudden death" has become the leading cause of mortality accounting for approximately half of the total deaths. Such observations suggest that antihypertensive treatment is not as effective in combatting atherosclerotic events, particularly coronary artery disease, as it is in preventing hypertensive complications.

The stage of the disease at which antihypertensive drug treatment is initiated may be important in the prevention of atherosclerotic complications. Pathological studies have demonstrated that when hypertension has been present for some time changes occur in the walls of the large arteries similar to those found with aging. These changes include fragmentation and loss of elastic fibers with replacement by connective tissue, dilatation of the arteries, and loss of compliance of the vessel wall. It is possible that these changes render the arterial wall more susceptible to the development of atherosclerosis. If such is the case it would provide an argument for the early treatment of hypertension.

The final evaluation of the effectiveness of antihypertensive drug treatment in the prevention of coronary artery disease must in the last analysis depend on well controlled prospective trials in the milder forms of hypertension and in a relatively early stage of the hypertensive process. This will require large numbers of patients followed for a considerable period of time. Studies of this type are urgently needed. Those currently in progress, such as the VA study in patients with mild hypertension, may not provide adequate information with regard to prevention of atherosclerosis since no effort was made to select patients in the early stages of the disease.

Early reduction of elevated blood pressure with presently available antihypertensive agents appears to be a rational but unproven approach toward reducing the increased risk of atherosclerotic complications. In view of the lack of definitive evidence that antihypertensive treatment reduces the incidence of coronary artery disease, a large scale therapeutic attack on mild hypertension does not appear justified at present. However, in the presence of additional risk factors favoring the development of atherosclerosis, such as diabetes mellitus, family history of coronary artery disease or an elevated serum cholesterol, the treatment of mild, early hypertension may well be justified on the basis of the available, admittedly circumstantial, evidence.

Discussion Following Dr. Freis' Paper

Chairman Oliver: This session is entitled "Progress in the Control of Atherosclerosis". In fact, this is not precisely what we have considered. We discussed control of the complications of atherosclerosis, in particular of ischemic heart disease. These act as the end-points for the atherosclerotic process, so far as any primary or secondary prevention trials are concerned.

It is important to make a clear distinction between primary and secondary intervention trials. One can define a primary intervention trial as one established to control one or more risk factors in apparently healthy people, thereby reducing their likelihood of developing disease. The secondary prevention trial could be defined as an attempt to control one or more risk factors in those who have already developed the features of the disease in the hope of slowing its progress.

Both of these present discrete and different problems. The main problem of the primary prevention trial is its burden of imposing some alteration in the normal way of living, some disciplinary regimen, on apparently healthy people in order to prevent them from getting a disease which they may not, in fact, ever get.

The principal problem of the secondary prevention trial is that there is population self-selection. We have evidence from a survey of acute heart attacks in Edinburgh that only 59% of those that presented an acute heart attack would be available later to enter a prevention trial. By six months, 49% of those who had a heart attack had died. This means that a secondary prevention trial instituted nine months or one year after the heart attack would include less than 50% of those available to a primary prevention trial. Further, we cannot assume that the risk factors that were operating before the heart attack developed are the same after it has occurred.

The second problem of secondary intervention trials is that the control of risk factors which have been shown to be important in the development of the disease may be irrelevant once it has developed. For example, there is some suggestion, that the prognosis of patients who have had a myocardial infarction is independent of cholesterol levels. There may be a whole new set of different factors operating which are of less or no importance before a heart attack occurs, such as impaired myocardial contractility or a major thrombogenic tendency. I would like you to bear in mind, therefore, that the results and the potential yield of primary and secondary intervention trials have to be regarded differently.

Dr. Oglesby Paul: I would just like to make three points which may be pertinent here. First, I don't believe we must wait for ultimate proof before applying those presumably preventive measures which are clearly safe, for which there is reasonable evidence of their effectiveness and which are available and inexpensive. This can include the omission of tobacco, exercise under supervision, and weight control. Next, there is tremendous need for better documentation of the benefits of nearly all measures designed to alter morbidity and mortality; not only the diets which we have discussed, and all drugs, but also the role of exercise. Finally. I would point to the concept of the critical age for entrance into a primary prevention program. In rheumatic fever, the critical age is in childhood. In chronic bronchitis it is probably the same, and in the disease process which we are discussing today, it is really not clear whether we are aiming at the prevention of plaque formation, or complications thereof, or both.

Dr. Kohn: I would like to offer an alternative hypothesis to the diet studies. Those persons put on experimental diets may become so depressed over taking this diet that they have an increased incidence of taking antidepressant medication, or they develop so many headaches that they take more aspirin. As you heard, both antidepressant medication and aspirin have an effect on clotting factors and platelets.

Consequently, a group taking these medications might be expected to exhibit fewer thromboembolic events than a group not exposed to these agents. It is such considerations that add to the difficulty of evaluating controlled intervention studies.

Dr. WISSLER: I would just like to point out that the diets that are quite effective in lowering serum cholesterol don't have to be "depressing". They can be delectable. It takes skill on the part of the physician and the nutritionist to make them that way.

Dr. MACMILLAN: Earlier in the symposium, Dr. Frank was unable to show an association between serum cholesterol and second heart attacks. I wonder if this experience supplies a reason why secondary trials to date have been inconclusive.

Dr. STAMLER: The Coronary Drug Project is looking at this question very carefully. Based on very short follow-up, I think that our data about cholesterol are equivocal. At this point we are not sure we are getting a clear differentiation, but there is about a 20% or 30% higher mortality rate for the higher cholesterol man (>250 mg%) with control of other factors, but I think it is a little too early for us to come to any firm conclusion.

Dr. GOTTLIEB: Could I ask whether or not the eating habits are being controlled as carefully as the diet is being controlled? Do we know when the people are going to eat these diets and what this relationship is to their living habits?

Dr. DAYTON: In the studies involving free-living persons, the best evidence that they did, indeed, eat the diets is given partly in the changes in adipose tissue, linoleic acid and by the changes of serum cholesterol concentrations. In our studies, having the advantages that go along with institutional situation, we had the additional information derived from attendance records at the dining room, indeed, the adherence based on this measure was about 50% of total possible adherence for experimental subjects. So, in summary, there is evidence of group adherence, although hardly anybody knows exactly what adherence is for any individual even in an institutional study.

Dr. KATZ: Dr. Stamler, how do you make your study with estrogens really blind when there is so much breast enlargement and loss of libido in your treated patients?

Dr. STAMLER: Yes, of course, such studies only start out double blind in terms of random allocation. As certain side effects occur, particularly in the estrogen groups and in the nicotinic acid group, a degree of blindness is lost. However, the placebo group always does show the "typical side effects" of drugs at a low rate. It is precisely because of this problem that we have made the key end point in this study total mortality.

Chairman OLIVER: The Chairman has the prerogative of trying to reach a conclusion. I would suggest that we at the present moment have no clear lead with regard to the control of hyperlipidemia.

It seems to me that there are two acceptable lines of action. One is that we agree that the design of the existing studies is good enough, and we wait for their results. The other is that obviously the design is not good enough, and therefore, there is a *prima facie* case emerging for another new and very large study.

In my view there is no place for the other two possible courses which would be to ignore the presence of hyperlipidemia or to conclude that the case for prevention and control of hyperlipidemia has been proved. I also would like to stress that we mustn't confuse judgment with subjective impressions, and that if a negative result comes out of these trials, it might be just as scientifically valuable as a positive result, although, of course, more disappointing.

Section XVIII

PROGRAM PLANNING FOR CONTROL OF ATHEROSCLEROSIS

PERSPECTIVES IN INTERNATIONAL PROGRAM PLANNING

Zdenek Fejfar

Atherosclerosis and resulting diseases of the vital organs and tissues are particular problems, the solution of which should be speeded up by international cooperation. The motivation, possibilities, organizational framework and obstacles to international planning of research in atherosclerosis and its complications are discussed from the viewpoint of ten years' experience in an international organization.

MOTIVATION

Diseases associated with atherosclerosis are an increasing problem in most parts of the world and, as with many other problems of today, are becoming more and more urgent for the younger generation. Although the most serious complications in the heart and brain usually become manifest in adults, atherosclerosis develops gradually from childhood and, from the point of view of research today and prevention tomorrow, it is becoming a pediatric problem [1431, 1578].

Mortality from ischemic heart disease shows a positive correlation with the level of national income. Statistics further indicate that there has been an increase in deaths from ischemic heart disease in countries where 10–15 years ago the mortality rates were low, the relative increase being greater in the younger than in the older age groups (WHO Programme Review: "Cardiovascular Diseases", 1969). In developing countries atherosclerosis and ischemic heart disease occur in the upper socioeconomic strata of the population, the trend being similar to that in highly industrialized countries where the disease has already reached the common man. The frequency in the latter areas can be seen from a WHO autopsy study in Malmö (Sweden), Prague (Czechoslovakia), and Ryazan (USSR), in which ischemic heart disease was found in 39% of males in the age group 40–59 years and in 22% of females in the same age group.

In subjects who died suddenly, ischemic heart disease has been found far more often, in 78% of males and 49% of females, and the high frequency did not change with age.

Available information indicates that atherosclerosis occurs in all ethnic groups. Its development and complicating conditions are positively correlated with rising standards of life and ways of living in affluent societies. The rapid trend towards industrial development throughout the world indicates that atherosclerosis and its complications may soon result in the greatest epidemic mankind has ever faced unless we are able to reverse the trend by concentrated research into their causes and prevention.

POSSIBILITIES

Although atherosclerotic lesions, ischemic heart and ischemic brain disease occur universally, marked differences in their incidence and severity have been recognized in epidemiological, clinical and pathological investigations. In high incidence areas, environmental and other factors known to influence the development, intensity, and manifestation of these conditions are usually grouped together. It is therefore difficult, if not impossible, to separate the essential from the contributing factors, those involved in the underlying processes from those which trigger clinical disease in the target organs.

In low incidence areas, on the other hand, the extent of known etiological factors can be distinguished. In most places with a low frequency, ischemic heart disease, arterial (though not necessarily essential) hypertension, is common, and its most frequent consequence is cerebrovascular lesions at ages usually lower than those at which brain infarction occurs in areas with frequent atherosclerosis [454]. At the same time, the average blood cholesterol is usually lower than in areas with a high frequency of ischemic heart disease.

Good possibilities for investigations in such areas have been already confirmed in several studies promoted by WHO. Studies of the population groups in Jamaica pointed to a number of subjects with an enlarged heart, with clinical and laboratory signs of ischemic heart disease but not myocardial infarction. Studies among the Polynesians showed the differences in blood pressure levels and other circulatory characteristics, related to the nutritional habits, and to the way of living in the groups of the same origin, subjected to faster or slower processes of what we call "civilization". Variations in the blood pressure levels with age, the prevalence and etiology of hypertension in different African population groups, and mechanism of thrombosis and vascular diseases were investigated by the WHO Cardiovascular Research and Training Centre in Kampala, Uganda. Population studies in Peru confirmed that arterial hypertension and ischemic heart disease are uncommon among people living at high altitude.

The high frequency of ischemic heart disease in Indians as compared with that in the local populations from Singapore and Fiji, shows another opportunity for investigating the pathogenic mechanisms in different ethnic groups living in the same environment.

Rapid industrial development in many low incidence areas is associated with a tremendous change in the life of large groups of people, who are transformed from village hunters and farmers into modern city dwellers. The opportunity to observe the effect of such changes in health and particularly in cardiovascular diseases, has not been adequately utilized, even though only a couple of years of observation in the WHO Research and Training Centre in Kampala had shown a rise in blood pressure levels among young warriors, a few years after leaving their traditional life and becoming soldiers in the capital [1343]. Perhaps ischemic heart disease may be observed even in this generation in the near future.

The various recognized predisposing causes of atherosclerosis and its consequences need further investigation in relation to their pathogenesis. Cooperative studies on the role of trace elements are an example of what has been done [937]. Without such investigations the recent statement that "Epidemiological investigations suggest a multifactorial etiology which amounts to little more than the evils of civilization added to diseases common in middle age" [130] would be fully justified.

The necessity for a differential diagnosis of the causes of fever was accepted a long time ago, that of hypertension much later, but differentiation of the various causes leading to atherosclerosis is still a matter of research. An international cooperative study may well uncover several new etiologies and provide a hierarchy of causative factors, those of basic importance and those which further the disease and trigger the complications.

Cooperation is particularly needed in studies aiming to prevent the occurrence of ischemic heart disease or to delay arrest or reverse the progress of the established disease. There are several reasons for this. Preventive trials require large numbers of subjects to be studied for a long period of time, and it is difficult to find them in one place only. For example, 15,000 subjects have to be enrolled in the WHO sponsored trial on the primary prevention of ischemic heart disease with Clofibrate in Edinburgh, Prague and Budapest, in order to enable statistically significant differences to be brought out. Multicenter trials at the same time provide important information on the attitude towards treatment of the population studied, as well as on local differences in living habits, dietary customs etc. Furthermore, it is becoming obvious that population group prevention trials can be done more easily and cheaply in areas where the health services are organized by the community as opposed to countries where the treatment is more or less in the hands of private physicians. The example of polio vaccine invented in the United States, but first applied on a nation-wide scale in several countries in Europe, clearly showed the advantages of international cooperation in medical research. However, until now such cooperation has been insufficiently, and perhaps reluctantly, obtained in the field of atherosclerosis and ischemic heart and ischemic brain disease.

Multifactorial, multicenter studies aiming at preventing ischemic heart disease by controlling several established and etiological factors, trials on the control of arterial hypertension, and investigations on the effect of a prolonged or periodic stay at high altitudes, of increased physical activity, or of altered dietary habits in various ethnic groups living together in different etiological set-ups indicate the kind of cooperative studies that should be of immediate importance and confirm or invalidate current hypotheses.

The WHO autopsy study of populations mentioned is another example demonstrating the feasibility and utility of international cooperation. It covers demographically defined groups of people, and thus provides information on the extent of atherosclerosis and its organic complications that cannot be achieved in areas where, for cultural and other reasons, autopsies can be performed only in a small number of subjects who die in hospitals.

The community program on acute myocardial infarction, promoted by WHO primarily in the European Region, shows other advantages and aspects of international cooperation [1577]. It includes registration of every case suspected of having acute myocardial infarction in a given community during a one-year period: it also includes the diagnosis, treatment, and rehabilitation of survivors, and the autopsy diagnosis and retrospective analysis of the dead, with particular attention to the investigation of sudden death. The data will be analyzed centrally by WHO. Information is expected on the extent of the problem, on the need for community control programs at the hospital level and at the patients' homes, on the attitude of health workers and the behavior of the general public, and on the early diagnosis of acute myocardial infarction, etc. Comparison of the progress and problems in community programs will help to improve the diagnosis and treatment facilities. It should further promote cooperation and also a better understanding of the different problems of life in communities of varying cultural and socioeconomic structures.

The examples quoted should suffice to show that cooperative studies in properly selected environmental and ecological situations have many advantages. Among the possibilities created are: (a) a demonstration of the relative weight of established etiological factors and of the role of pathogenic mechanisms; (b) the utilization of such special situations and of the structure and organization of health services for prevention trials and for the establishment and evaluation of community control programs; and (c) a greater understanding of communities rapidly being transformed from rural, agricultural into urban industrialized, thereby undergoing an evolution similar to that for which affluent societies are paying such a toll in increasing atherosclerosis, ischemic heart disease, and ischemic brain disease.

ORGANIZATION

Good motivation and excellent possibilities may remain unused if an organizational framework does not exist for communication and cooperation between interested institutes. This applies equally to the coordinating center at a country level as well as internationally, the latter having the additional problems of how to overcome national, cultural, and political boundaries.

The traditional channels of scientific communication such as publication in scientific journals or reporting at international congresses, have become too slow in relation to the enormous expansion and accelerated output of new scientific work. Close personal contacts between people working in similar fields with prior circulation of material for publication, "invisible colleges", or bilateral and multilateral exchanges between scientific institutes also no longer suffice to cope with the accumulation of new results or adequately cover interdisciplinary contacts. Thematic conferences or symposia, such as this one are, however, a very useful break in the daily routine of work, giving time for creative thinking and reflection and for critical review and revision of one's own ideas and work through contact with other researchers working on parallel lines.

The need for the energetic promotion of concentrated research on burning local problems that have been studied only in isolation by independent scientists and institutions, leads to the establishment of national medical research councils. The logical next step was the creation of an international agency for coordination of the work being carried out all over the world. The Twelfth World Health Assembly in 1958 recommended further expansion of WHO research, and this resulted in the establishment of the WHO Unit, whose task it has been to promote the prevention and control of cardiovascular diseases through international cooperation.

For obvious reasons atherosclerosis and ischemic heart and ischemic brain disease are given top priority. Cooperation is being promoted in several respects in improving communication between scientists, in training, in research itself, and in the rapid application of new knowledge in the community (WHOProgramme Review: "Cardiovascular Diseases", 1969).

As for research itself, the World Health Organization assists governments and national institutes in planning national research programs. It also promotes and conducts cooperative studies carried out on an international scale. Duplication of national effort is avoided as far as possible.

Collaboration in research is provided through investigators in national institutes and laboratories. In one example, each investigator carries out the same investigation using an agreed operating procedure; in another, each institute carries out a particular piece of research, contributing an item of knowledge to the whole. In both kinds of investigation, the central collection, storage, analysis, and reporting are done when required in WHO headquarters.

A network of collaborating centers and laboratories selected according to their suitability to tackle specific problems has been gradually built up in all regions of the world. There are at the moment 18 institutes designated as such, and there are many more with which WHO has direct contact. If trained personnel are lacking in a suitable area for research, WHO has the possibility of sending one or more members of a research team and can assume the training of local personnel who in time will take over responsibility for the research. An example of this is the WHO Research and Training Centre in Kampala, Uganda, to which the WHO Cardiovascular Research Team has been attached.

As a matter of principle, WHO's function is catalytic; studies are initially supported by the Organization in varying proportions, but later on the responsibility is taken over by the local institution. A balance is maintained between studies of obvious immediate applicability at the community level and those where more basic knowledge on etiology and pathogenesis is needed prior to attempts at prevention at the community level.

WHO, with a total of 131 Member States, has an unrivalled opportunity for receiving cooperation in all aspects of its program throughout the world. Apart from cooperation at the governmental level, the Organization enjoys excellent working cooperation with international scientific organizations such as the International Society of Cardiology, the Councils of this Society, and national societies of cardiology, and it also has direct contact with scientists of all cultures. Ten years of experience with WHO's activities in the field of cardiovascular diseases has proven that a central agency, concerned with a world-wide program aiming to prevent major cardiovascular diseases, has been accepted and plays an increasingly important role. Further expansion of its activities is both needed and requested.

It has not yet been settled whether and when it will be necessary to create regional or international institutes for research on atherosclerosis, and ischemic heart disease on the lines of and with similar justification and structure as the International Agency against Cancer. The advantage of the Agency is that it is a part of WHO but administratively and economically independent. Its budget is provided by countries who are members of the Agency.

OBSTACLES

Fear that scientific freedom and individual initiative will be lost has persisted from the time of free scientific enterprise. It would be justified if coordination were to be replaced by direction of scientists from an administrative office, thereby limiting their individuality and creativity. Proper coordination assumes a role similar to that of the central nervous system in recording, storing, and evaluating seemingly independent events with an appropriate feed-back mechanism and in keeping highly specialized experts abreast of new achievements, trends and developments in their subject. It is meant to aid and facilitate research, to make new independent studies more productive by avoiding repetition of work and mistakes made by others, and by showing narrow specialists the way through the jungle of detailed analytical studies, thus avoiding incomprehension and misunderstandings. Not infrequently the defense of "scientific freedom" conceals personal incompetence and fear of its detection in studies compared and directly evaluated when done in cooperation with others.

Bureaucratic management, which might become a purposeless self-perpetuating "establishment" instead of a tool, is a real danger that must constantly be kept in mind. There are many examples of this happening in other fields of man's activity. So far the best form of prevention appears to be a clear-cut open agreement on mutual responsibilities in cooperative projects, control of professional managers by groups of scientists and layman advisers selected by rotation, and periodic public checking of work achieved.

The concept of one world and of a cooperative effort for the solution of common medical problems is recent. Its realization is hampered by lack of experience on how to cope with the diversity of economic, cultural, social, and political differences, and by the very fact that new ideas generally need long periods of incubation.

The contrast between the agreed support for medical research within a country, and the reluctance to contribute to the same purpose outside the national boundaries is striking. It is striking even if one knows that better opportunities for an investigation are to be found elsewhere than at home. The work promoted by WHO in the field of atherosclerosis, ischemic heart and ischemic brain disease, indicates that much faster progress could be attained if the best existing opportunities for international cooperation were utilized. The resources required would only be a negligible fraction of those spent annually in individual countries.

CONCLUSIONS

1. The motivation, possibilities, organizational framework, and difficulties of international planning of research in atherosclerosis and related diseases have been discussed in the light of 10 years of experience while working within WHO.

2. The increasing problem of cardiovascular diseases associated with atherosclerosis represents an imminent danger in most parts of the world, affecting more and more of the younger population. Environmental factors governing the development, intensity and manifestation of atherosclerosis and ischemic heart and ischemic brain disease have been demonstrated in many studies. The positive correlation of these conditions with an increase in the national income forecasts the rise of the conditions in less developed areas now possessing a low incidence.

3. Examples have been given to demonstrate that properly planned cooperative studies in selected environmental set-ups can clarify the relative weight of the known etiological factors and the pathogenesis. This applies particularly in communities which are in the process of transformation from rural to industrialized urban life.

4. Experience has shown that preventive trials and community control program can be achieved through international cooperation. Such studies are easier and cheaper in countries with certain health service structures.

5. International cooperation requires adequate organizational framework. WHO is a unique overall health agency with 131 Member States and access to all parts of the world. Atherosclerosis, ischemic heart disease and vascular lesions of the central nervous system, have been among the top priorities in the WHO cardiovascular research program since 1959. International cooperation is promoted in communication, training, research and the rapid application of new knowledge at the community level.

6. Some of the obstacles to achieving more intensive international cooperation are fear of the loss of scientific individuality, fear of bureaucratic administration, and the gulf between support for cardiovascular research within the country and reluctance to contribute towards research outside. Traditional thinking and the lack of experience in professional management of research are being gradually overcome.

7. Experience has also shown that the allocation of only a small fraction of the resources available for national research on atherosclerosis and allied conditions for internationally coordinated studies could rapidly provide the information needed on the etiology, pathogenesis, and prevention of cardiovascular diseases.

CRITERIA FOR PROGRAM EVALUATION

D. D. REID

Enthusiasm is growing for the control of atherosclerotic heart disease, e.g. by dietary change or drugs. Some even press for immediate wide-scale adoption of their favorite prescription for the public's cardiovascular health. This is, therefore, the time for a cold appraising look at the pros and cons of the methods proposed from the viewpoint both of the individual and the community. My task is to review some of the criteria of profit and loss that have been or could be used in such an appraisal.

Estimating Likely Benefits. Observational studies usually give the first estimate of the potential scope for a preventive program. Cornfield and Mitchell (unpublished data), for example, used the fact that death rates in Scandinavian countries among men under the age of 55 are less than half those in the United States to suggest that a change in the American way of life towards the Scandinavian mode might halve the death rate from coronary heart disease. More specifically, they calculated that, on the basis of Framingham experience, lowering blood cholesterol levels from 250 to 220 might reduce the risk of coronary heart disease of a man in his thirties by 50%.

The use of computer simulation studies applying available observational data to mathematical models are simply an extension of such calculations. The arithmetic may be eased and realism increased by the introduction of some random element when estimating the likely outcome of a series of changes in either the specific factor or the nature of the population concerned. The essential problem of an observational as opposed to an experimental basis remains because the observed association between risk factors such as diet or blood cholesterol and cardiovascular morbidity has, as yet, not been conclusively proven to be one of cause and effect. To take an extreme example, although red hair and pulmonary tuberculosis are traditionally associated because of the susceptibility of the Celts to the disease, no one has proposed that cutting off red hair would prevent it.

Observational studies cannot give more than a reasoned estimate of the likely limit of the benefits that might be achieved by specified changes in either external risk factors such as high fat diet or smoking or innate physical characteristics like blood pressure or cholesterol. Public health practice must be more firmly based on the trial by ordeal that is the controlled field experiment.

Field Trials in Program Assessment. In such field trials of methods of coronary heart disease prevention, the criteria of benefit used are, of course, crucial. Their choice will depend on the immediate objectives of the trial. These objectives can be, in Schwartz and Lallouch's [1321] terms, either "explanatory" or "pragmatic". If the prime interest is in the effect of drugs on pathogenetic mechanisms, one is especially interested in the relative frequency of some specific clinical phenomenon in treated and untreated groups. Thus one looks for changes in blood pressure in a trial of hypotensive agents or of thrombotic episodes in trials of long-term anticoagulant administration in the aftercare of patients who have survived infarction. If, on the other hand, the aim of the trial is the pragmatic one of balancing the saving of life against the investment in medical manpower needed to achieve it, the death rate from all causes would be the overriding criterion. In practice, however, the dichotomy is not so clear-cut, and it is usual to employ a range of measures depending on the degree of interest in pathogenesis, in occupational recovery, or death from specific or all causes as well as on the stage of development of the preventive program.

The first practical question that a field trial seeks to answer concerns feasibility; and this may depend on the particular population to which the program is applied. In the United States National Diet-Heart Study [1079], for example, the adherence to the special diets was markedly better in institutionalized hospital groups than in the free-living population. Thus, both the degree of adherence to a prophylactic regime and the limited ability to generalize from specific populations are important.

Next, effectiveness must be assessed usually by the result of the regime on a predisposing or risk factor itself. The effect of diet changes on fat metabolism has been measured by methods ranging in sophistication from changes in body weight through serum lipid assay to gas-liquid chromatography of fatty acids in subcutaneous fat aspirated from the buttock. The choice of method will depend on the scale of the trial for large field trials usually necessitate simple methods that are readily and widely applicable.

Clinical Criteria in Prophylactic Trials. In pragmatic terms, however, the term "effectiveness" must apply to the results of prophylaxis on the incidence or severity of coronary heart disease. Here again, a wide range of measures have been used. In general, the precision with which a clinical end-point can be determined is proportional to its severity. The presence of angina is an evanescent phenomenon in the same individual over a period of time and subject to observer variation even when standard clinical questionnaires are used [1253]. Even electrocardiographic interpretation by experts, particularly in detecting reinfarction, is a precarious business, although it provides material for independent review by unbiased observers [966]. At the extreme end of the clinical scale lies death. Most studies concentrate on cardiovascular modes of dying, presumably because these are the most relevant and because their clinical nature may indicate a specific effect of the regime on, for example, pulmonary embolism or ventricular fibrillation. Always one looks for consistency in the direction of the difference between experimental and control groups in the presence of symptoms and signs of cardiovascular disease in survivors at follow-up or in fatal cardiovascular complications in those who died. Post-mortem evidence is usually obtained for only a small proportion of deaths, and it is a better index of changes in pathogenesis that the trial regimen may have produced than of that regimen's overall value in disease prevention.

On the other hand, although a clinical and pathological review may help to explain results, the pragmatic aims of a field trial make the death rate decisive. In prophylactic trials in cardiovascular disease, deaths from this cause are likely to form more than half of the total number of deaths from all causes so that it is worth considering both specific and total mortality. In the diet-heart study by Dayton and his colleagues [384], for example, there was a significant reduction in the special diet group in the frequency of cardiovascular signs and sudden death. But there was none in deaths from all causes. Unforeseen effects on non-cardiovascular deaths of chance differences e.g. in cigarette smoking, may occur even with a random allocation procedure; and these may obscure a real effect of changes in diet. Both deaths from other causes and presumed cardiovascular deaths have thus to be looked at with special care. In the study by Dayton et al., the authors emphasized the difficulty of defining "sudden death" and expressed the fear that observers might have been biased in their allocation of deaths to that category. As they plaintively asked, "... if sudden death is susceptible to bias, what clinical end-point [other than death *per se*] is not?" We have taken this argument to its logical conclusion in our international collation of data from trials of anticoagulants in the long-term prophylaxis after infarction by concentrating on death from all causes as the most decisive end-point when comparing the experience of treated and control series. (International Anticoagulant Review Group.[1])

1 Collaborative analysis of long-term anticoagulant administration after acute myocardial infarction. Lancet **1970** I, 203.

Economic Criteria in Program Assessment. In relating the benefits and costs of methods of cardiovascular disease prevention to community resources, economic as well as humanitarian considerations arise. Premature death or permanent disability before the usual age of retiring represents the loss of the productive capacity of men often at the height of their career. Although several American and European studies [168, 572, 678] have shown how the speed of a man's return to work depends in part on the color of his collar, much less is known about the economic savings that effective prevention would provide. Against such savings must be put the cost of diverting medical and other professional personnel from routine medical care to screening, health education, and similar aspects of preventive medicine. Moreover, specific methods of preventing cardiovascular disease may have their own risks. The possible long term side effects of cholesterol-lowering drugs cannot be ignored. Giving up smoking may increase obesity and neurosis. But it is also likely to reduce the risk of chronic bronchitis and lung cancer. In such circumstances, only the death rate from all causes will strike a true balance. Thus in the global assessment of new ways to combat heart disease the consequences both for national economy and national health must be taken into account. The crucial criterion is the saving of life and since we cannot measure its worth in human terms the community is forced to count its gain from preventive medicine by setting the reduction in absences from work and the extension of useful working life against the cost of achieving them.

THE GORGONZOLA DIET AND THE PREVENTION OF MYOCARDIAL INFARCTS

Osler L. Peterson

There is no doubt about the importance of atherosclerotic heart disease as a cause of death. There is similarly no doubt about the value that could accrue to individuals and to society if a substantial proportion of these deaths could be prevented, because many of them occur at younger, productive ages. The important questions are whether their preventibility is established and, if established, whether it is feasible.

If we are to properly assess the potential for prevention of atherosclerotic disease and its fatal manifestations, we must understand under what circumstances preventive medicine has been effective. It has been dramatically successful and its application to atherosclerosis is, therefore, an attractive goal. Santyana defined certain strictures pertaining to people who ignore history, so I will therefore examine the major historical mechanisms of disease change.

In a classical study, MacKeown examined the changes in death rates in England and Wales between 1851 and 1900, a period when longevity and population were increasing because of declining death rates [955]. During this period, improvement was due entirely to reduction in deaths from infectious diseases (Table). The percentages in this table totalled somewhat more than 100%, because certain infectious disease deaths (pertussis, measles and diphtheria) increased concurrently with these declines. MacKeown, after study of housing, sanitorium care and the like, concluded that the 47% improvement in tuberculosis mortality could best be attributed to improved nutrition. Typhoid and dysenteries were water and food borne, and since pure, piped water was preferred over impure water carried in pails and good food over spoiled food the solution was an attractive and popular one. John Snow had worked out the mechanism of cholera transmission in 1848–49, and this knowledge no doubt speeded sanitation. There was no effective treatment of scarlet fever in the 19th century and variation of streptococcal virulence is the most likely explanation for the observed decline. The decline in smallpox death rates was attributed to immunization.

Table. *Percentage decline in death rates 1851–1900 England and Wales*

Tuberculosis	47%
Typhus, enteric fever, typhoid	23%
Scarlet fever	20%
Diarrhea, dysentery, cholera	9%
Smallpox	6%
All other	2%

Between 1900 to 1953, the U.S. age-adjusted death rates for all cases declined by 30% (from 1,178 to 811/100,000 population). In this period, food and water borne infections have declined twentyfivefold and, tuberculosis, sixteenfold [1502].

The 20th century has produced one other important death rate change by a different mechanism. The U.S. pneumonia death rates which have declined eightfold are not an example of prevention but are, nevertheless, pertinent to our problem as an example of effective action. This death rate dropped quite definitely in the early 1930's (antipneumoccal serum) and again between 1937–1938 (sulfapyridine) and further in the mid-40's when penicillin became generally available. This is one of the few instances where an effective treatment is reflected in a major death rate change. To these we might add immunizations for a number of infectious diseases such as diphtheria, pertussis, and measles. The death rates from these diseases were for the most part declining before immunization became available and the effect of the immunizations has been to hasten the disappearance of these deaths.

In summary, there are several mechanisms that have been effective: (1) general social changes, (2) sanitary measures, (3) immunizations, and (4) effective, safe drugs. These mechanisms share several common characteristics. They were all very simple to carry out. Problems stemming from population cooperation were minimal or absent. Medical care can postpone other deaths. However, its effect has been modest when compared with these measures.

Most studies of ischemic heart disease prevention have been concerned with persons over age 40 when the incidence of myocardial infarctions (MI) and death rates are increasing sharply. Among U.S. males in 1966, there were nearly 350,000 deaths from a disease No. 420 (arteriosclerosis), most of which are MI or coronary disease [1501]. About 35% of these occurred at ages under 65. For the two-thirds that occurred at ages 65 and over, prevention is less promising for reasons unrelated to the effectiveness of any action. All death rates are high at this age. If Disease A is eliminated, individuals are still exposed to risks of death from Diseases B, C, etc. which are high and rise rapidly with age.

The diet trial of Dayton and his colleagues is particularly interesting in this respect [384]. The administered diet lowered cholesterol and was associated with significantly fewer myocardial infarctions, sudden deaths, and cerebral infarctions. There were also consistently, though not significantly, fewer deaths from atherosclerotic events. Despite this apparent effect on one group of diseases, the total deaths in the treated and control groups were very similar, reflecting the possible effects of highly competing mortality rates mentioned.

The interesting and remarkable pathophysiological studies of Enos and of McGill et al. emphasize the early onset of atherosclerosis [434, 952]. Preoccupation with atherosclerosis beginning at age 40 is too late. From the pathological studies just cited and, on the general theory that primary prevention is more effective than secondary, it would seem that the value of case finding and preventive action would be greater at younger ages.

I will now consider the implication of prevention in relation to several of the indicators that put persons in the high risk groups.

THE GORGONZOLA DIET

The relationship between the level of serum cholesterol or other lipids and the risk of MI has received more attention than any other indicator. I will, therefore, use it as an example of the issues raised by preventive programs.

We have already emphasized the simplicity of the mechanisms, curative or preventive, that have affected major death rates. For example, the patient with lobar pneumonia is sick, often has pain, and therefore seeks his doctor's help. A single injection or a handful of pills are all that are needed to convert a high risk to a very low risk. The child who is immunized against a possible fatal infectious disease is normally brought to the doctor by its mother who is fulfilling her parenteral obligation. It is not very important if some mothers neglect it, since herd immunity will assure the child of a low risk. I have chosen these examples of prevention and treatment because they involve personal services which more nearly resemble the problems posed by MI than the acceptance of safe food and water.

We can predict that the finding of patients with high serum cholesterol will be more difficult. Chest x-rays, for example, were widely available when TB was an important problem, but the response from the population was disinterested and sluggish. We could depend upon the practitioners to screen patients for high cholesterols. After all, about 70% of the population sees a physician every year. We have the example of cytology screening which in some areas has been extended to nearly 80% of the female population at risk after years of intense effort [25].

The doctor who finds a number of persons with elevated cholesterol must then prescribe a diet and arrange for follow-up of the patient to ascertain that the diet is followed, and the expected change of cholesterol is obtained. The British MRC Report commented tersely that a polyunsaturated fat diet was not easy to follow [967]. In societies where the population can afford large quantities of food and rich foods, Gruyere and Gorgonzola cheese, bacon and eggs, and the like, inducing an asymptomatic person identified as being at high risk of an MI to change his habits will not be easy.

There is evidence that doctors can influence patients to take actions which other people, such as nurses, can not; therefore planned delegation of responsibility may sacrifice effectiveness. Any diet would require constant patient support. This is especially true if young asymptomatic persons are to be the object of prevention as was suggested previously. In some countries, such as England, the medical care system has assured continuity of physician-patient care and this would help in follow-up. In other countries, such as the United States, medical care is highly fragmented and the continuity needed to change risk is often lacking. All in all, the prevention of atherosclerosis through diet would be far more complicated and difficult than any programs of preventive medicine that have succeeded so far.

I have chosen to first discuss the feasibility of preventing MI using an altered diet because feasibility is a necessary consideration. Even more important is the question of whether prescriptive screening can be ethically justified by present knowledge [1111]. Offering a screening procedure by implication also offers some benefit to the individual identified as a high risk, and this question must be faced.

Is there evidence that lowering of serum cholesterol, the most studied correlate of myocardial infarcts, will change the risk? Several rigorous clinical trials of secondary prevention have left the effect of cholesterol lowering diets unsettled. The British MRC clinical trial failed to demonstrate an effect of treatment, whereas, in Leren's trial there were significant differences in morbidity but not in the deaths [857, 967]. An effect of diet on morbidity as judged by new ECG abnormalities but not on deaths was found in the Turpeinen study [1479]. Different outcomes of different studies and lack of agreement between harder and softer end points leave the question hanging in midair. In my opinion, the evidence does not justify preventive programs of prescriptive screening.

SMOKING

The evidence that cigarette smoking increases the frequency of myocardial infarcts and that stopping diminishes their frequency is good [24]. Our position is like John Snow's in some respects; we know what to do though not how our prescription works. It differs from Snow's in that he had identified an effective preventive measure; he removed the pump handle and stopped the use of the well from which cholera was spread. We have no evidence that any action to reduce smoking is useful.

Holland has found that smoking begins at a shockingly early age in England, varies greatly by school and produces early symptoms [692]. This kind of information provides, at least, a logical basis for attacking smoking habituation. Primary prevention of smoking is the logical approach, especially since reforming the smoker is less useful as a preventive measure and also frequently unsuccessful.

THE GOOD LIFE AND OBESITY

Wealthy nations with high death rates from myocardial infarcts also have purchasing power and services which favor inactivity and obesity. This state of affairs is called, "The Good Life". Every physician knows that inducing a single obese patient to reduce is not easy and often unsuccessful. Attempts to wean a well but high risk population segment away from its energy-saving machines and from ample or excessive eating will have to contend with attitudes that physicians may deplore but which are, nevertheless, real and important. Prevention based upon widespread weight reduction or increased exercise must be put in the class of dubious feasibility.

Proposal to change national diets through educational programs or through regulations is logical and is backed by good evidence [917, 945]. Personal and unverified observations suggest that the fat content of knockwurst eaten in the United States increases regularly as the meat content disappears. If we need cheap sausages there are certainly better substitutes than animal fat. In my opinion, regulation is likely to be more effective than nutritional education. Presumably, knockwurst could be made with less atherogenic substances but even widespread substitution is unlikely to affect the excessive consumption of food. Regulation involves political processes which are occasionally dramatically successful but are almost always subject to chance. Environmental pollution and automobile safety, both political problems, are examples from the United States. Automobile safety was sparked largely by one concerned man, Mr. Ralph Nader. Pollution, on the other hand, is becoming worse.

HYPERTENSION

Drug treatment of hypertension in a well controlled clinical trial has reduced both morbidity and mortality, although the extent of its effect on MI is not established [1498]. The drugs which are used for treatment of hypertension are not as benign as penicillin which is almost a model drug because of its low toxicity and rapid effectiveness. The development of drugs of low toxicity and determination of the value of drug treatment of mild hypertensive disease are important research problems.

TWO POTENTIALLY FEASIBLE MEASURES

There are two possible preventive measures that are of interest because they are feasible ones.

The first is the discovery and confirmation in several parts of the world that hard water is associated with lower death rates from atherosclerosis [49]. More evidence on this interesting association is needed. The simplicity of the preventing MI by treating water is in the tradition of effective public health measures.

Lowering of body cholesterol stores by Atromid-S is the second [1121]. It appears to be effective. If it proves suitable for long term administration, its simplicity would make it a feasible preventive.

In passing, we should mention one other means of reducing the MI death rates, good medical care. Fig. 1, taken from a study done by A. M. Burgess and myself, shows the case fatality rates for males under age 60 in the hospitals of one area. Among the severest MI the rates were dramatically reduced in hospitals with either an intensive care unit or a coronary care unit. The unit itself is only part of a complicated explanation which, for the moment, is best characterized as good medical care.

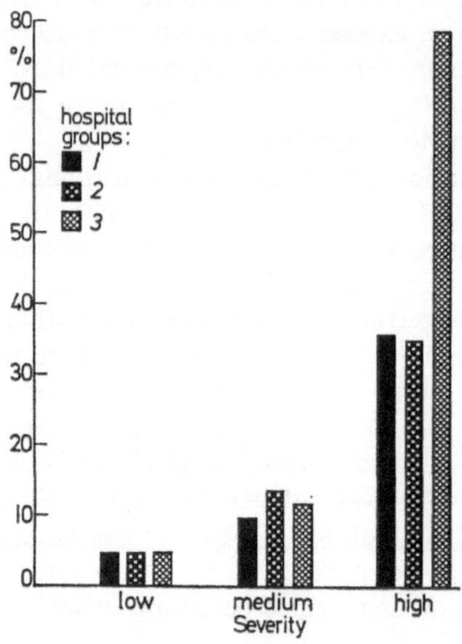

Fig. 1. Case fatality of patients with MI by severity class and by hospital group

DISCUSSION

The problems of preventing atherosclerotic diseases are different from most of the preventive programs that have been successful. Dieting to reduce cholesterol or weight, changing activity levels, stopping smoking are not easy where many characteristics of a society favor these risks. The intense desire of physicians and investigators to prevent myocardial infarcts or deaths at young ages will have to cope with the disinterest of the well population they would like to reach.

The possibilities of future prevention of myocardial infarcts and other complications of atherosclerosis need to be as pessimistic as prospects based on present studies. Pessimism is supportable only if we take the short view. We must stop and remind ourselves that our knowledge of atherosclerosis is quite recent. It is only a rather short time ago that atherosclerosis and its consequences were classed as a "degenerative disease" and therefore as an inevitable consequence of aging. This view has only recently been replaced by an attitude of inquiry. The pioneering Framingham Study, for example, is still in its "teens". Recent research on atherosclerosis has been of a remarkably high quality. Studies of pathophysiology, for example, suggest that understanding of the disease mechanism will be achieved.

The clinical trials directed at preventing myocardial infarcts have set a high standard. For good reasons these trials have dealt with very high risk individuals. Study populations that have already had myocardial infarcts or are in high age groups present a most formidable challenge to trials of prevention. The alternative of conducting trials on younger subjects who have not had myocardial infarcts but who have the characteristics which indicate their proneness to myocardial infarction will necessarily involve large numbers, more time, and effort. Such experiments which start with less of a handicap may well demonstrate that prevention is possible.

Prevention of myocardial infarcts will require a type of physician responsibility that many medical care systems are too ill equipped and poorly organized to furnish. The medical care systems of societies in which atherosclerosis is most severe were developed in response to acute diseases. As these systems are adapted to populations in which major disease problems are chronic and occur at higher ages, preventive measures which are necessarily directed at individual patients over a long period of time will become more feasible.

PROGRAM PRIORITIES IN SOCIETY

IRVING J. LEWIS

I have some difficulty in understanding exactly what my credentials for participation may be. I am not a doctor of medicine, nor have I developed a competence with respect to atherosclerosis. In fact, as I reviewed the abstracts I found myself increasingly uncomfortable about my lack of scientific credentials, until I was struck with the realization that those interested in atherosclerosis cannot function alone. If it has been true, as I suspect it has been, that professionals tend to flee the harsh world of conflicting priorities and demands upon society resources, then it is wise for this group to confront this discomfort and relate its specific interest to broader social factors that influence program priorities.

There is obviously no simple answer to so general and broad a question as the setting of social priorities. In any society, priorities are in constant flux. Their selection under the totalitarian form of government will proceed on bases far different from those found appropriate to a democratic society. In America it is certainly true that we are prepared to tolerate substantial waste in human and material resources, because we give so much weight to consumer desires. Such desires lead to consumer extravagances which could hardly be comprehended by the Soviet-controlled society, which tolerated the starvation of millions of its citizens as a byproduct of its single-minded national interest focused on capital formation.

Not only are our social priorities shaped by our desires, but they are also shaped by the availability and advances of technology, the forces of international relations, and partisan politics. In the 1950's and the early 1960's, our expanding technological capability, married to our traditional reliance upon the expectation and demands of the consumer, contributed to and was reinforced by a continually growing economy. This unparalleled economic growth provided over a long period an embarrassment of riches for the American consumer, especially the middle class consumer.

As the benefits of economic growth became more widespread, so did our understanding with respect to those elements in our society who were not being rewarded by this growth. In time the role of government has become, as a consequence of this realization, increasingly significant in helping to shape the program priorities of our society. Many interests steadily pressed upon Government for help to support particular activities to a point where many activities can no longer be conducted without this support. As a consequence of Government support across the breadth of our human endeavors, we thus tend to look for appropriate government action as a touchstone of our concern about priorities.

The vast governmental role, expressed numerically as a $ 200 billion budget against a trillion dollar Gross National Product, can neither be taken for granted nor ignored by groups such as this. Like it or not, with dependence on governmental support for biomedical research, manpower training, education, prevention and control, and the delivery of health services, this group is now part of the political process and must come to understand and live with its elements and its imperfections. The nature of this process varies with time, and this time factor is marked in our society by electoral procedures. Referring only to the national scene, this procedure has now brought forth a new administration, the essential features of which, at least in respect to domestic programs, are beginning to emerge. It would be presumptuous to assess the extent to which these features were planned or merely fortuitous, but in any case, they are reasonably clear and should be of keen interest.

Of course, the most important priority set by the Nixon Administration is the battle against inflation. The battle is waged in the money markets, in the tax hearing rooms, and in controls over Government expenditures. Expenditure controls are set because the Government budget of $ 200 billion is of such magnitude that, regardless of the purposes which individual expenditures may support, Government spending is an economic tool of major significance. While controls must be applied selectively, the primary concern with respect to the overriding priority of inflationary control is the total level of Government spending and not its particulars.

Against this background of limited Federal budgetary resources several significant features of policy can be seen. The first of these goes under the phrase of "New Federalism". This in its simplest form is the attempt to divide the labor between the levels of Government. Under this division there is assigned to the national level the problem of income support, for example, the new welfare program, and State and local governments (and I think it tends to stress government as opposed to voluntary groups) would be helped by revenue sharing and block grants whereby the Federal Government provides the wherewithal to carry out services.

The second major feature is called income strategy under which the new family assistance program would place 21 million people under Federal support as compared to 9 million on welfare. This strategy alone will mean an added

$ 4 billion annually to the Federal budget in the next few years. In addition, increased Social Security benefits are being proposed.

Finally, there is a substantial effort underway which we might call rationalization of the system of Government. Probably only the Executive Branch can produce this (and there are many who doubt the capacity of Government to govern today). This involves attempting to harmonize and integrate a recognized patchwork of programs which have developed over the years without reference to priorities. I foresee a very strong effort in this field to eliminate competing programs and to discontinue many categorically oriented programs, whether in health, education, welfare or manpower. In fact, a possible harbinger of the future is the Administration's comprehensive manpower program, which assigns major functions to States formerly reserved for the Federal Government.

I have set forth these features of the new Administration because they will be quite relevant as Administration initiatives begin to take clear shape in respect to health. There is a strong emphasis in the Government to shape program priorities on programs targeted to mothers and children, to the poor and near poor, and to activities which have a very strong preventive aspect, for example, the current emphasis in the field of nutrition. In the face of the daily statements of the crisis in the American health care system, one might well wonder why there has been no initiative in health so direct as that thus far taken with respect to family assistance or manpower. I think that this perhaps derives from efforts to understand what the crisis in health care really is.

As a social priority, health assumes a very high rating. Clearly it is a matter of value judgement as to how that rating should compare with education, conservation, recreation, and other areas of social interest. It is sufficient at this time merely to point out that the total national investment in health is $ 60 billion compared to $ 17 billion in 1955, and $ 30 billion in 1965. There are those who forecast with some confidence that this will be $ 100 billion in 1975. Of the $ 60 billion currently devoted out of the Gross National Product, $ 18 billion is a Federal expenditure. A first and most fundamental ingredient of the health care crisis is that the American consumer is asking with increasing stridency what he is obtaining for this investment. If this question is asked, he is told that the United States of America is fifteenth in the world in infant mortality and twenty second in life expectancy for males. He finds that one-half of the babies born in public hospitals are born to mothers who have had no prenatal care, and that a poor child has four times the risk of the nonpoor of dying before he reaches 30 years of age.

Facts such as these have led to a changing perception of priorities within the health field. In the 1950's and 1960's there was a predominant emphasis, which I need hardly elaborate to this audience, on generating new knowledge through biomedical research. This activity shaped the medical schools of today for good or ill, and in large measure determined the nature of today's medical practice.

As the white middle class American came to recognize "the Other America" of 40 or 50 million poor whites, blacks, Mexican American, and Indians, there began to emerge, as a social priority requiring governmental intervention, the provision and financing of medical care. In the medical community, as well as the lay sectors, the view has strongly developed that priority must be assigned to getting what we now know to the people who need it. The first response was found in the investment in financing of individual health care bills, illustrated by Medicare and Medicaid. These programs have accounted for the major Federal increase in expenditures since 1965 and coupled with the indices of health status give some sense of the nature of the crisis with respect to health care. In essence, we must concede that we do not have the capacity to match our willingness to finance health care. By capacity I include biomedical research, because manpower, facilities, and systems of health care without knowledge will not yield us quality health care systems.

Stated another way, 76% of the total Federal expenditures of health are for financing the entry into a health care system that is not capable of responding. We have been following a strategy based upon a mythology that all that prevents those who need health care from obtaining it is a lack of financial resources. We have learned to our bitter regret that in many places entrance into the system does not exist, and that added purchasing power has led to the dilution in quality of care, increase in cost, and the movement of more people into the hospital element of the system. What is first, therefore, on the agenda in dealing with the crisis in health care is the need to control methods of financing and a major effort by society (Government at all levels and voluntary at all levels) to build and shape a medical care system that matches our willingness to spend $ 60 billion or maybe $ 100 billion a year. The issue is not how much we should spend for health, for who is to say how much this should be, and what the value of health is in relation to other social values. Rather, the issue is qualitative, as to the system itself, not quantitative as to dollars.

As we move to rationalize the health care system for the 1970's and 1980's, when hard choices have to be made by a decisionmaker, he will place greater reliance upon analytical techniques that modern economics and the computer technology have developed. These techniques, parading under various names such as systems analysis, cost benefit analysis, and planning and programming will not help society choose among the broad areas of social endeavor; only our imperfect sense of values can guide us. Within any one field, and I predict these techniques have particular applicability to health, the health program most likely to compete successfully is that which can formulate its goals and objectives with clarity, specify its activities with sharp definition, permit the decisionmaker to see his alternatives and options, and furnish him with a predictable outcome of effectiveness with respect to cost. It is unlikely that the proverb "an ounce of prevention is worth a pound of cure", will win any dollars without meeting these tests for the decisionmaker in Government.

PANEL DISCUSSION ON PROGRAM PLANNING FOR CONTROL OF ATHEROSCLEROSIS

Discussion Following Mr. Lewis' Paper

Chairman McGILL: Many people are asking, "What do we need to do next?" A fairly impatient public that has been supporting basic research in atherosclerosis is demanding action, and many scientists and physicians are also recommending action. Unfortunately, the scientists and physicians are not unanimous about what action to take, and we are beginning to learn that everything that is good and desirable can not be done in this country alone. So, the focus of this panel has been on the criteria for selecting and using scientific knowledge for the control of atherosclerosis in the everyday world. Knowledge remains useless until it is used.

Mr. Lewis, it is obvious from the papers presented, and from the cautions and precautions described by Dr. Reid and Dr. Peterson regarding prevention and evaluation of these programs, that using this knowledge is going to take a great deal of work and time, and will be very expensive. It is difficult to establish priorities for what to do even among the scientific community. I would like to ask Mr. Lewis, regarding presentation of this case to the public and to the government, how we should go about it. Must we be unanimous, or can we continue to be pluralistic? Other than stating our goals would you have any additional advice for us both in the United States and in other countries? It is obvious that we have some ideas. We cannot guarantee results. The consensus seems to be that we need a demonstration to generate that degree of certainty. This is quite expensive and is of such magnitude that it will have to be considered among other national priorities.

Mr. LEWIS: I find a little difficulty in answering because I don't know about the particular disease and how the particular program could best be presented. There obviously has been a very substantial amount of work done with respect to individual diseases, the demonstrated value of which remains very much in doubt. I think merchandising on a particular categorical basis in the United States today is very, very difficult to do. The merchandising of a particular disease or a particular problem is best done within the framework of the problem of the health care system.

What we have done in this country is to begin to develop some new programs. For example with respect to the heart field, we developed a whole new program of regional medical programs for heart, cancer, and stroke, which is aimed at trying by a different mechanism to get to the people through the medical care system, presuming to dispense that which we know.

If you have a program which is a specific project aimed at a particular disease, my feeling at this point in time is that, within the United States, it runs best within the framework of the National Institutes of Health. As to the resources available to carry out the study, I do not foresee a substantial increase in resources available to carry out the work.

Dr. FEJFAR: Mr. Chairman, when we are discussing general policies, and I can speak only from the health point of view, I might mention here what the European countries have decided.

Several years ago the governments in Europe recognized that cardiovascular diseases are the No. 1 problem in Europe, and they requested WHO to work out the first longitudinal four-year program in cardiovascular diseases. They even backed it financially, so that about one-fifth of the total regular budget in the European region is devoted to cardiovascular problems. Obviously the first priority there is ischemic heart disease, and the community program which I mentioned is just one little bit of this budget.

The interesting thing is that in every government one has to judge the resources, possibilities, and desires. For example, last year in the Manila Seminar on preventable heart disease, which covered mainly those associated with infections (rheumatic fever, rheumatic heart disease, preventable hypertension), we found that this could be worked out fairly cheaply.

If we look at the problem as though we were now in a war, we know the casualty rate is such-and-such, and we have to plan against it. If we look at the major health problems we will have to face before the end of the century, I would say we will be looking at air pollution, accidents, cancer and cardiovascular diseases, and perhaps the problem of overcrowding. I have to find out which of them has a solution that can be met by existing resources. Where we do not have enough knowledge for the solution of a problem, i.e. atherosclerosis, the only program is research.

Mr. LEWIS: Putting it in terms of priorities, there is no question as to what major health problems must be dealt with in this country. The major health problems relate to mothers and children, and to the problems of infant mortality.

I think Dr. Peterson is quite right in pointing out that actually the capability of our society to deal with these may not necessarily be through what we would call classic health measures. The improvement in infant mortality in this country may come about by a much broader attack on the whole area of poverty. This doesn't necessarily allow for a program targeted on atherosclerosis.

Section XIX

SUMMARY OF SYMPOSIUM

SUMMARY

Hugh Sinclair

Some of us (but not you, Mr. Chairman) when we were students would sit up all night before an examination, looking through our notes (if any) and turning over the pages of elementary textbooks; we would then enter the examination next morning with our thoughts in glorious disarray. The task of summarizing a congress such as this puts one in the same position. He is the only person who has to attend all of the papers, in case (the cynic might say) someone inadvertently says something new; and when he hastens from the session to lunch and tries to nibble his tomato juice as he has been advised to do to avoid atherosclerosis, he only ingests a drop or two before more information is thrust down his throat. Back he comes from the lunch-time lecture to hear someone—it might be Dr. Ho from Chicago—blitz him around some field that might be slightly unfamiliar to him. This bombardment at high pressure is very dangerous to vessel walls, and I am pleased to see here one of the wisest men, my old friend Professor Groen, Professor of Psychobiology, sitting in the front row in head phones, tuned no doubt to dance music.

I asked what the task of a summarizer should be, and I was given two rather different pieces of advice. First, I was told that he might summarize the papers. There have been 109 papers, and as I have started a little late and have every intention of finishing on time, that would give me rather under three-and-a-half minutes for each paper. Most of the speakers were unable to summarize their own papers in that amount of time. The second piece of advice given was that I might compare what we know now with what we knew at the time of the Athens Conference. This, alas, is impossible for me because I was not at the Athens Conference, and I will not mention whether or not I have read the proceedings.

However I want to mention something rather interesting that the very beautiful picture by Cezanne of the fruit (which we saw last night) recalled to me. When our ancestors took their forepaws off the ground in order to eat that fruit more easily, that was their diet (with, of course, the occasional caterpillar) as, indeed, it is of the monkeys today. Then our ancestors had no problem of metabolizing saturated fat as is the case with the monkeys today, except the children of Morris' Monkey 263, one of whom (named I 699) was very properly rejected by its mother just after birth, and the other (I 569) drowned in its own cholesterol pool. When conditions got a little cooler, man ate himself; there was little else to eat. He could not eat a woolly rhinoceros (so beautifully depicted here in the Field Museum) unless he had tools with which to kill it. When he had tools he was a hunter, eating animals with little stored fat and much of it unsaturated. Domestication of animals has been quite recent; the cow, for better or worse, came from the Middle East, and most of us (except the French) are not wise enough to eat the horse which is rich in linolenic acid.

We have in this Congress been taken back twice into the Old Testament, by Fejfar to Noah and by Buchwald who quoted Leviticus I: 22–23: "The Lord spake unto Moses saying: Speak unto the children of Israel. You shall eat no manner of fat. Neither of ox, nor of sheep, nor of goat." Buchwald took that rather out of context. Fat is not being forbidden because it is harmful but because it is the choicest part of the animal, and, therefore, had to be reserved for sacrifice to God. Not being a theologian, I cannot comment on the subsequent metabolic fate of the saturated fat. In recent years, there has been a very important change in the fat, even of these domesticated animals. This was briefly referred to by Shaper who mentioned results of Michael Crawford on the difference both in the quantity and in the quality of the fat of domesticated and nondomesticated animals. There is much more fat, even hidden fat, in the type of animals we eat, and it is increasing; also, the fat is much more saturated and the polyunsaturated fats are quite rare.

In considering the subject of this Symposium we should remember that atherosclerosis and coronary heart disease are not the same; the distinction between the two has occasionally become a little blurred. Professor Schettler in his introduction made the important point that in many European countries during the war there was a fall in deaths attributed to ischemic heart disease. This was true of Britain (though there are difficulties in my country because of two alterations the Registrar-General made in 1940, both of which would tend to cause a fall). It was true in Scandinavian countries, and Professor Schettler showed that it was true for Germany. If there can be a sudden change in mortality when an episode such as a war occurs, this must be a change in the thrombotic tendency of blood rather than in so chronic a process as atherosclerosis.

Let us consider first atherosclerosis. You, Mr. Chairman, told us in your introductory remarks that "not enough attention is paid to the basic cause." We must remember that normal endothelial cells need free cholesterol and certain polyunsaturated fatty acids for growth and repair; John Poole showed many years ago, in some beautiful work with French and the late Lord Florey, that endothelial cells do divide, and this division, as Born mentioned in discussion, is particularly at sites of stress. Helen Payling Wright showed that in the aorta mitosis was twice as common in endothelial cells at junctions with collaterals. There is no difficulty in intimal cells getting cholesterol; free cholesterol readily enters and probably the cells can synthesize it (although in the rabbit fed cholesterol, synthesis is of squalene and cholestanol). There could, on occasion, be difficulty in their getting the right proportion of fatty acids, and Collins described a man who failed completely for eight months to get linoleic acid. In such pure deficiency of essential fatty acids in man, the plasma cholesterol is low; in Collins' patient it remained at 135 mg/100 ml throughout. This is also true of the lower animals, and yet there is deposition of cholesterol in certain tissues.

The mechanism of the early lesion is a matter of great interest. Another point of great importance mentioned frequently has been that the lipid in fatty streaks is intracellular and has a composition very different from that of the cholesteryl esters of plasma. A television broadcast three days ago by Drs. Wissler and Stamler and Jones seemed to take for granted that the lipids of fatty streaks come completely from the bloodstream (Kritchevsky has echoed Wissler on that), and secondly that the smooth-muscle cells migrate from the media. I would support the suggestion of Scott that the smooth-muscle cells may come from endothelial cells, though another possible source is replication of the occasional cell seen beneath the endothelial cells in the normal intima. We should decide the origin of these smooth-muscle cells. It is difficult to believe the lipid within them arises from LDL that has also passed through endothelial cells because of the composition of the lipid. Edward Lear a century and a quarter ago published his *Book of Nonsense*, and though perhaps not the most appropriate source for this Conference we might borrow a dogmatic Limerick or two:

Bob Wissler, Dick Jones et al. say
The cells from the media stray
To the intima where
Plasma lipids they snare:
But this is proved wrong by assay.

Elspeth Smith, Geer, Insull and others have shown that the intracellular lipid of fatty streaks (unlike that of the normal intima or the extracellular lipid of fibrous plaques) is rich in oleic and eicosatrienoic acids and low in linoleic; Elspeth Smith also found low levels of immuno-beta-lipoprotein within the cells of fatty streaks. The same lipid pattern is found in xanthomas. It is very difficult to believe that LDL from plasma enter the smooth-muscle cells and then lose most of their protein and cholesteryl linoleate while gaining cholesteryl eicosatrienoate. Wissler, however, stated that his immuno-fluorescent method demonstrated protein of LDL intracellularly near the lipid droplet. Zilversmit showed that whereas much of the phospholipid was locally synthesized, free cholesterol passed from the plasma at first slowly and then increasingly fast so that the accumulation was exponential. How the free cholesterol traverses the plasma membranes of endothelial cells and then smooth-muscle cells has not been elucidated.

Once inside, this free cholesterol is presumably esterified by the Glomset enzyme, lecithin cholesterol acyl transferase (LCAT), which occurs in the arterial wall and is increased in fatty streaks. The partially deacylated phospholipids must either be abnormally low in linoleic acid or retain this exceptionally, or the fatty acids transferred are locally synthesized. Geer mentioned that this synthesis is increased in lesions, and Björkerud and Chobanian respectively showed greater incorporation of both glucose and acetate. The usual method of removal of excess cholesterol from tissues is in HDL by formation mainly of cholesteryl linoleate. If this essential fatty acid is relatively deficient, cholesteryl oleate and eicosatrienoate are formed; this would occur particularly in areas where increased cell division (and therefore formation of new cell membranes) was occurring, as in stressed parts of the aorta. Perhaps we should have heard more about Glomset enzymes, especially as six cases of inborn absence of them are now known, and in these, as in Tangier disease, there is lipid deposition in the cornea. It may be that

The enzymes of Glomset, LCATs,
Are concerned with deposits of fats
Unless we eat oils,
As is shown by the toils
Of our eminent Chairman, L. Katz.

The fatty streak passes, as we now do, to the fibrous plaque in which the lipid is extracellular and undoubtedly has mainly come from plasma owing to the increased permeability. Such increased permeability is very prominent in deficiency of essential fatty acids which causes uncoupling of oxidative phosphorylation as found in the lesion, but it could arise from various causes. There is no doubt that into the later lesions lipoproteins pass from plasma: carotenoids are found which could not be locally synthesized. Therefore the extracellular lipid is characteristic of that of beta lipoproteins, the cholesteryl esters being rich in linoleate and low in oleate and eicosatrienoate. Adams, like Wissler and Zilversmit, stressed the increased permeability; and he also showed the sclerogenic effect of cholesterol and certain of its esters (monounsaturated and trans-di-unsaturated being very marked, but essential fatty acids slight). In this later lesion lipoproteins can also be demonstrated by the beautiful immuno-fluorescent technique Wissler used, and also by Walton and by Elspeth Smith. The perifibrous lipid is relatively rich in sphingomyelin, the synthesis of which is however slower than that of phosphoryl choline or inositol. Geer showed sphingomyelin increases with free cholesterol; in diseased as compared with normal aortas there is a fourfold incorporation of radioactive phosphorus into sphingomyelin (Bowyer), and also more incorporation into it of glucose (Björkerud). Why sphingomyelin accumulates remains obscure: Y. Stein thought it was through decreased hydrolysis (but why then does not atheroma occur in Niemann-Pick's disease?), whereas Portman has shown increased synthesis.

Since LDL are passing into the advanced lesion, the factors controlling them are crucial. We have had brilliant discussions of the latest work on these. Experimental animals included monkeys with an inborn error (Morris), a puppy with deficient lipoprotein lipase (Bierman), and Trappist monks so patiently ingesting different formula diets and carefully studied by Vergroesen and Thomasson.

Some believe platelets are irrelevant to atherosclerosis; others that they are fundamental. Wissler and Studer were among the latter, and Wissler showed us a platelet in the intima. However, Elspeth Smith told us how dissimilar are the lipids of platelets and of fatty streaks:

Researches, by Elspeth B. Smith
On lipids in intimas with
  Atheromas, must get
  Completely upset
Rokitansky's and Duguid's old myth.

Thrombosis, however, is fundamental in coronary heart disease as mentioned earlier in connection with Schettler's excellent address. Diet can affect thrombosis in various ways: saturated free fatty acids greatly increase it whereas unsaturated do not affect it; deficiency of essential fatty acids causes uncoupling of oxidation and phosphorylation with consequent increase in ADP; and deficiency of EFA will also decrease PGE_1 which is the most powerful known substance for decreasing aggregation of platelets. Gottenbos, for instance, showed that the more linoleic acid he fed (as sunflower seed oil), the less the aggregation. Many years ago Ramalingaswami and I found sludging of erythrocytes in deficiency of EFA. As Marquis stated, PGE_1 increases adenyl cyclase, and cyclic AMP formed by this inhibits aggregation of platelets by ADP:

The platelets of Mustard and Born
Show stickiness in vessels torn.
To ensure they have none
Give PGE_1
Obtained from fresh semen or spawn.

Epinephrine, however, like collagen and thrombin, behaves like ADP in increasing aggregation; it inhibits adenyl cyclase. Professor Groen said that the more risk factors are known, the more they are insufficient for prediction. Wanstrup showed smoking caused anoxia, and Kjeldsen produced increased stickiness of platelets by giving medical students CO, a technique most of us have wanted to use. Various risk factors were illustrated by Schettler in his opening address. It would appear from Groen's observations that to avoid coronary thrombosis we should avoid working and wearing white collars. However everyone seems to agree that diet is the primary risk factor. Whether or not this fits the available data has also been discussed. Longitudinal epidemiological data (such as prospective trials) were discussed less than cross-sectional ones, and we had some interesting comparisons from Prior who studied persons living on different atolls: the Pukapuka and the Fakaofa both eat fish, but the latter eat much more coconut oil with its lauric and myristic acids and, therefore, have higher levels of plasma cholesterol. Ancel Keys' last slide showed the palace he had built on a very different atoll:

Aloft on a lofty atoll
Ancel Keys built his high capitol
To control all the work,
And to silence each quirk
With a generalized protocoll.

Preventive trials, both primary and secondary, have been presented, and it is quite obvious that we need not several small preventive trials but the one definitive trial that we all wish to see done. Mr. Lewis remarked on the government budget of two hundred billion dollars and the part which might be available for such absolutely essential work. This was very illuminating to the outsider, who has no right to express any view, but one reflects that the cost would be a fraction of that of a rocket. This definitive preventive trial is absolutely essential if we are to have a final answer to one of the most important problems facing the more privileged countries today. Evidence is accumulating that the primary factor is a decrease in the ratio in the body of fatty acids of the linoleic and linolenic groups (essential fatty acids) to other fatty acids which the body can make, for instance from sugar. Most would agree that the nature of dietary fat is the most important single factor in atherosclerosis and in ischemic heart disease, but we need proof.

As Dr. Paul White said: "It becomes clear that we have much to do", and that is the theme, Dr. Katz, with which we leave. However we leave with immense gratitude to you as General Chairman; to Dr. Wissler as Organizing Chairman and to Mrs. Wissler who took the trouble to meet all of us from abroad at our respective points of arrival; to Mrs. Cora Gillette who always greeted us with a smile and immense help although at the bottom of her heart she must have thought, "Oh, it's that person again;" to Dr. Richard Jones, the Editor of the Proceedings; to the members of the Ladies' Committee because it is so important to keep the wives quiet and happy; to those who so generously entertained us in their private homes; to your financial donors, to the projectionist, the microphonist and to the stenographers who have managed to deliver the typed scripts of what the participants hoped to say while the saliva was still wet on their lips.

We leave with new information, culture, admiration for this City of Chicago and gratitude for a superbly organized Congress. Thank you very much indeed.

BIBLIOGRAPHY

1. Abdurakhmanov, F. A.: Influence of nicotinic acid on the metabolism of cholesterol and bile acids in atherosclerotic patients. Med. Zh. Uzbek. **12**, 32 (1965).
2. Abdulla, Y. H.: Beta-adrenergic receptors in human platelets. J. Atheroscler. Res. **9**, 171 (1969).
3. — Adams, C. W. M., Morgan, R. S.: The reaction of connective tissues to implantation of purified sterol, sterol esters, phosphoglycerides, glycerides and free fatty acids. J. Path. Bact. **94**, 63 (1967).
4. — Adams, C. W. M., Morgan, R. S.: Differential resorption rates of subcutaneous implants of (^{3}H) cholesterol, various (^{3}H) cholesteryl esters and (^{3}H) cholesterol-(1-^{14}C) linolenate. J. Atheroscler. Res. **9**, 81 (1969).
5. — Orton, C. C., Adams, C. W. M.: Cholesterol esterification by transacylation in human and experimental atheromatous lesions. J. Atheroscler. Res. **8**, 967 (1968).
6. Abell, L. L., Levy, B. B., Brodie, B. B., Kendall, F. E.: A simplified method for the estimation of total cholesterol in serum and demonstration of its specificity. J. biol. Chem. **195**, 357 (1952).
7. Abrams, M. E., Jarrett, R. J., Keen, H., Boyns, D. R., Crossley, J. N.: Oral glucose tolerance and related factors in a normal population sample. II. Interrelationship of glycerides, cholesterol and other factors with the glucose and insulin response. Brit. med. J. **1969 I**, 599.
8. Abramson, D. I.: Blood vessels and lymphatics. New York: Academic Press 1962.
9. Acheson, G. H. (ed.): Second Catecholamine Symposium. Pharmacol. Rev. **18**, 1 (1966).
10. Acheson, R. M., Florey, C. du V.: Body weight, AB0 blood groups, and altitude of domicile as determinants of serum uric acid in military recruits in four countries. Lancet **1969 II**, 391.
11. Adam, D. J. D., Hansen, A. E., Wiese, H. F.: Essential fatty acids in infant nutrition. J. Nutr. **66**, 555 (1958).
12. Adams, C. W. M.: Atheroma lipids. J. Atheroscler. Res. **7**, 117 (1967).
13. — Vascular histochemistry. London: Lloyd-Luke 1967.
14. — Abdulla, Y. H., Morgan, R. S.: Modification of aortic atheroma and fatty liver in cholesterol-fed rabbits by intravenous injection of saturated and polunsaturated lecithins. J. Path. Bact. **94**, 77 (1967).
15. — Bayliss, O. B.: The relationship between diffuse intimal thickening, medial enzyme failure and intima lipid deposition in various human arteries. J. Atheroscler. Res., **10**, 327 (1969).
16. — — Abdulla, Y. H., Mahler, R. F., Root, M. A.: Lipase, esterase and triglyceride in the ageing human aorta. J. Atheroscler. Res. **9**, 87 (1969).
17. — — Davison, A. N., Ibrahim, M. Z. M.: Autoradiographic evidence for the outward transport of ^{3}H-cholesterol through rat and rabbit aortic wall. J. Path. Bact. **87**, 297 (1964).
18. — — Ibrahim, M. Z. M.: A hypothesis to explain the accumulation of cholesterol in atherosclerosis. Lancet **1962 I**, 890.
19. — — — Webster, M. W. (1963): Phospholipids in atherosclerosis: the modification of the cholesterol granuloma by phospholipid. J. Path. Bact. **86**, 431 (1963).
20. — Morgan, R. S.: The effect of saturated and polyunsaturated lecithins on the resorption of 4-^{14}C-cholesterol from subcutaneous implants. J. Path. Bact. **94**, 73 (1967).
21. — Tuqan, N. A.: Elastin degeneration as source of lipids in the early lesion of atherosclerosis. J. Path. Bact. **82**, 131 (1961).
22. — Virág, S., Morgan, R. S., Orton, C. C.: Dissociation of (^{3}H) cholesterol and ^{125}I labelled plasma protein influx in normal and atheromatous rabbit aorta. J. Atheroscler. Res. **8**, 679 (1968).

23. Adler, E., Adler, C., Magora, A., Shanan, J., Tal, E.: Stroke in Israel 1947–1961. Jerusalem: Polypress Ltd. 1969.
24. Advisory Committee to the Surgeon General of the Public Health Service, Report of the. *Smoking and Health*: U. S. Department of Health, Education and Welfare. Public Health Service Publication No. 1103. Washington, D. C., USA: Superintendent of Documents, Government Printing Office.
25. Ahluwalia, H. S., Doll, R.: Mortality from cancer of the cervix uteri in British Columbia and other parts. Brit. J. prev. Soc. Med. **22**, 161 (1968).
26. Ahrens, E. H., Jr.: Nutritional factors and serum lipid levels. Amer. J. Med. **23**, 928 (1957).
27. — Hirsch, J., Insull, W., Jr., Tsaltas, T. T., Blomstrand, R., Peterson, M. L.: The influence of dietary fats on serum-lipid levels in man. Lancet **1957 I**, 943.
28. — — Oetta, A., Farquhar, J. W., Stein, Y. (1961): Carbohydrate-induced and fat-induced lipemia. Trans. Ass. Amer. Phycns. **74**, 134 (1961).
29. Aladjem, F.: Immunoelectrophoretic properties of low-density human serum lipoproteins. Nature (Lond.) **209**, 1003 (1966).
30. Alaupovic, P.: Recent advances in metabolism of plasma lipoproteins: chemical aspects. Progr. Biochem. Pharmacol. **4**, 91 (1968).
31. — Furman, R. H., Falor, W. H., Sullivan, M. L., Walraven, S. L., Olson, A. C.: Isolation and characterization of human chyle chylomicrons and lipoproteins. Ann. N. Y. Acad. Sci. **149**, 791 (1968).
32. — Olson, A., Tsang, J.: Studies on the characterization of very high-density lipoproteins of human serum. Biochem. **5**, 4044 (1966).
33. — Seidel, D., McConathy, W. J., Furman, R. H.: Identification of the protein moiety of an abnormal human plasma low-density lipoprotein in obstructive jaundice. Fed. Europ. Biochem. Soc. **4**, 113 (1969).
34. Albrink, M. J., Davidson, P. C.: Impaired glucose tolerance in patients with hypertriglyceridemia. J. Lab. clin. Med. **67**, 573 (1966).
35. — Man, E. B.: Serum triglycerides in coronary artery disease. Arch. intern. Med. **103**, 4 (1959).
36. — Meigs, J. W.: Interrelationship between skinfold thickness, serum lipids and blood sugar in normal men. Amer. J. clin. Nutr. **15**, 255 (1964).
37. — — The relationship between serum triglycerides and skinfold thickness in obese subjects. Ann. N. Y. Acad. Sci. **131**, 673 (1965).
38. Allan, T. M., Dawson, A. A.: ABO blood groups and ischaemic heart diesase in men. Brit. Heart J. **30**, 377 (1968).
39. Allen, R. J. L.: Estimation of phosphorus. Biochem. J. **34**, 858 (1940).
40. Allinson, A. C., Blumberg, B. S.: Serum lipoprotein allotypes in man. Progr. med. Genet. **4**, 176 (1965).
41. Alpers, H. S., Shore, P. A.: Specific binding of reserpine: association with norepinephrine depletion. Biochem. Pharmacol. **18**, 1363 (1969)
42. Altschul, R.: Endothelium, its development, morphology, function and pathology, p. 157. New York: MacMillan Co. 1954.
43. — Niacin in vascular disorders and hyperlipemia. Springfield: C. C. Thomas 1964.
44. — Herman, I. H.: Influence of oxygen inhalation on cholesterol metabolism. Arch. Biochem. Biophys. **51**, 1 (1954).
45. American Public Health Association, Joint Session of the Epidemiology, Food and Nutrition and Statistic sections. Measuring the risk of coronary heart disease in adult population groups a symposium. Amer. J. publ. Hlth. **47**, 1 (1957).
46. Anderson, J. T.: Dietary carbohydrate and serum triglycerides. Amer. J. clin. Nutr. **20**, 168 (1967).
47. — Battachargya, A. K., Grande, F., Keys, A.: A cholesterol lowering diet. Fed. Proc. **27**, 221 (1968).
48. — Grande, F., Keys, A.: Hydrogenated fats in the diet and lipids in the serum of man. J. Nutr. **75**, 388 (1961).

49. Anderson, T. W., LeRiche, H. W., MacKay, J. S.: Sudden death: correlation with hardness of water supply. New Engl. J. Med. **280**, 15 (1969).
50. — — — Sudden death and ischemic heart disease. New Engl. J. Med. **280**, 805 (1969).
51. Andrus, E. C. (ed.): Atherosclerosis. In: *The heart and circulation*, p. 341. Second Nat. Conf. Cardiovascular Dis. I, Washington, D. C. 1964.
52. Anitschkov, N. N., Chalatov, S.: Über experimentelle cholesterinsteatose und ihre Bedeutung für die Entstehung einiger pathologischer Prozesse. Zbl. allg. Path. path. Anat. **24**, 1 (1913).
53. Anonymous: Build and blood pressure study, vol. 1. Chicago: Society of Actuaries 1959.
54. — Coronary drug project enters enrollment phase. J. Amer. med. Ass. **200**, 37 (adv.) (1967).
55. — New weight standards for men and women. Stat. Bull., Metropolitan Life Ins. Co. **40**, 1. 1959
56. — Statistical Abstract of Israel, No 19. Central Bureau of Statistics. Jerusalem: Government Press 1968.
57. Antonis, A., Bersohn, I.: The influence of diet on serum triglycerides. Lancet **1961** I, 3.
58. Aramaki, Y., Kobayashi, T., Imai, Y., Kikuchi, S., Matsukawa, T., Kanazawa, K.: Biological studies of cholestane-3β, 5α, 6β-triol and its derivatives. Part 1. Hypocholesterolemic effects in rabbits, chickens, and rats on atherogenic diets. J. Atheroscler. Res. **7**, 653 (1967).
59. Ardlie, N. G., Glew, G., Schwartz, C. J.: Influence of catecholamines on nucleotide induced platelet aggregation. Nature (Lond.) **212**, 415 (1966).
60. — Schwartz, C. J.: A comparison of the organization and fate of autologous pulmonary emboli and of artificial plasma thrombi in the anterior chamber of the eye, in normocholesterolemic rabbits. J. Path. Bact. **95**, 1 (1968).
61. Arfors, K. E., Hint, H. C., Dhall, D. P., Matheson, N. A.: Counteraction of platelet activity at sites of laser-induced endothelial trauma. Brit. med. J. **1968 IV**, 430.
62. Armstrong, M. C., Connor, W. E., Warner, E. D.: Tissue cholesterol concentration in the hypercholesterolemic rhesus monkey. Arch. Path. **87**, 87 (1969).
63. Aschroft, M. T., Beadnell, H. M. S. G., Bell, R., Miller, G. J.: Characteristics relevant to cardiovascular disease among adults of African and East Indian origin in Guyana. Bull. Wld. Hlth. Org., in press (1969).
64. Ashford, T. P., Freiman, D. G.: The role of endothelium in the initial phases of thrombosis. An electron microscopic study. Amer. J. Path. **50**, 257 (1967).
65. — — Platelet aggregation at sites of minimal endothelial injury. Amer. J. Path. **53**, 599 (1968).
66. Ashworth, L. A. E., Green, C.: The transfer of lipids between human alpha-lipoprotein and erythrocytes. Biochim. biophys. Acta (Amst.) **84**, 182 (1964).
67. Asmussen, E., Knudsen, E. O. E.: Studies in acute but moderate CO-poisoning. Acta physiol. scand. **6**, 67 (1943).
68. Astrup, P.: An abnormality in the oxygen-dissociation curve of blood from patients with Burger's disease and patients with nonspecific myocarditis. Lancet **1964 II**, 1152.
69. — Hellung-Larsen, P., Kjeldsen, K., Mellemgaard, K.: The effect of tobacco smoking on the dissociation curve of oxyhemoglobin. Scand. J. clin. lab. Invest. **18**, 450 (1966).
70. — Kjeldsen, K., Wanstrup, J.: Enhancing influence of carbon monoxide on the development of atheromatosis in cholesterol-fed rabbits. J. Atheroscler. Res. **7**, 343 (1967).
71. — Role of blood coagulation and fibrinolysis in the pathogenesis of arteriosclerosis. In: I. H. Page (ed.), *Connective tissue, thrombosis, and atherosclerosis*, p. 223. New York: Academic Press 1959.
72. — Role of blood coagulation and fibrinolysis in the pathogenesis of arteriosclerosis. In: E. C. Andrus and C. H. Maxwell (eds.), *The heart and circulation. Second*

National Conference on Cardiovascular Diseases, vol. 1. Washington, D. C.: Federation of American Societies for Experimental Biology 1965.

73. Atkins, H.: Conduct of a controlled clinical trial. Brit. med. J. **1966 II**, 377.
74. Aubert, L., Arroyo, A., Detolle, P., Cavelier, C., Picard, D., Cotte, G.: Etude clinique et cytologique d'un deuxieme cas d'IgA myelome xanthomateux avec anticorps circulant anti-lipoproteine. Sem. Hop. Paris **43**, 3014 (1967).
75. Auerbach, O., Hammond, E. C., Garfinkel, L.: Smoking in relation to atherosclerosis of the coronary arteries. New Engl. J. Med. **273**, 775 (1965).
76. Austin, W., Nestel, P. J.: The effect of glucose and insulin *in vitro* on the uptake of triglyceride and on lipoprotein lipase activity in fat pads from normally fed rats. Biochim. biophys. Acta (Amst.) **164**, 50 (1968).
77. Avigan, J., Steinberg, D.: Sterol and bile acid excretion in man and the effects of dietary fat. J. clin. Invest. **44**, 1845 (1965).
78. Avoy, D. R., Swyryd, E. A., Gould, R. G.: Effects of CPIB with and without androsterone on cholesterol biosynthesis in rat liver. J. Lipid Res. **6**, 369 (1965).
79. Azarnoff, D. L.: Species differences in cholesterol biosynthesis in arterial tissue. Proc. Soc. exp. Biol. Med. (N. Y.) **98**, 680 (1958).
80. — Tucker, D. R., Barr, G. A.: Studies with ethyl chlorophenoxyisobutyrate (Clofbrate). Metabolism **14**, 959 (1965).
81. Bagdade, J. D.: Basal insulin and obesity. Lancet **1968 II**, 630.
82. — Bierman, E. L., Porte, D., Jr.: The significance of basal insulin levels in the evaluation of the insulin response to glucose in diabetic and nondiabetic subjects. J. clin. Invest. **46**, 1549 (1967).
83. — Porte, D., Jr., Bierman, E. L.: Diabetic lipemia: A form of acquired fat-induced lipemia. New Engl. J. Med. **276**, 427 (1967).
84. — — — Acute insulin withdrawal and the regulation of plasma triglyceride removal in diabetic subjects. Diabetes **17**, 127 (1968).
85. — — — Hypertryglyceridemia: A metabolic consequence of chronic renal failure. New Engl. J. Med. **279**, 181 (1968).
86. Baglio, C. M., Farber, E.: Reversal by adenine of the ethionine-induced lipid accumulation in the endoplasmic reticulum of the rat liver. J. Cell Biol. **27**, 591 (1965).
87. Nailey, J. J.: Cellular lipid nutrition and lipid transport. In: G. H. Rothblat and D. Kritchevsky (eds.), *Lipid metabolism in tissue culture cells*. Symposium Monograph, **6**, 85. Philadelphia: Wistar Institute Press 1967.
88. Bailey, J. M.: Influence of some immunological procedures on experimental atherosclerosis in rabbits. Arch. Mal. Coeur Rev. Atheroscler. **1**, 205 (1967).
89. Baker, N., Schotz, M. C.: Quantitative aspects of free fatty acid metabolism in the fasted rat. J. Lipid Res. **8**, 646 (1967).
90. Baltaxe, H., Amplatz, K., Varco, R. L., Buchwald, H.: Coronary arteriography in hypercholesterolemic patients. Amer. J. Roentgenol. **105**, 784 (1969).
91. Bandopadhyay, A., Banerjee, S.: Plasma lipids in some cardiovascular disorders. Amer. J. med. Sci. **248**, 203 (1964).
92. Barbosa, J., Oliner, L.: Effect of clofibrate on serum thyroxine transport and free thyroxine levels. Metabolism **18**, 141 (1969).
93. Barkham, P., Silver, M. J., O'Keefe, L. M.: The lipids of human erythrocytes and platelets and their effect on thromboplastin formation. In: S. A. Johnson, R. W. Monto, J. W. Rebuck and R. C. Horn (eds.), *Blood platelets*. Henry Ford Hospital International Symposium, p. 303. Boston: Little, Brown and Co. 1961.
94. Barnard, P. J.: Pulmonary arteriosclerosis and cor pulmonale due to recurrent thromboembolism. Circulation **10**, 343 (1954).
95. — Thompson, D. H.: Focal lipid lesions in blood vessels due to erythrocytes and platelets. Experimental observations on goats and rabbits. Circulation **33**, 744 (1966)
96. Barnes, M. J., Partridge, S. M.: The isolation and characterization of a glycoprotein from human thoracic aorta. Biochem. J. **109**, 883 (1968).

97. Bassett, D. R.: Epidemiological studies of cardiovascular disease in the Pacific. Proc. 4th Asian-Pacific Cong. Cardiol., Tel Aviv 1968.

98. — Moellering, R. C., Rosenblatt, G., Greenberg, D., Stokes, J.: Coronary heart disease in Hawaii. J. chron. Dis. **21**, 565 (1969).

99. — Rosenblatt, G., Moellering, R. C., Hartwell, A. S.: Cardiovascular disease, diabetes mellitus and anthropometric evaluation in Polynesian males on the Island of Niihau—1963. Circulation **34**, 1088 (1966).

100. Basso, L. V., Havel, R. J.: Hepatic metabolism of plasma free fatty acids in normal and diabetic dogs. Clin. Res. **15**, 137 (1967).

101. Baumgartner, H. R., Born, G. V. R.: Effects of 5-hydroxytryptamine on platelet aggregation. Nature (Lond.) **218**, 137 (1968).

102. — — The relation between the 5-hydroxytryptamine content and aggregation of rabbit platelets. J. Physiol. (Lond.) **201**, 397 (1969).

103. — Tranzer, J. P., Studer, A.: An electron microscopic study of platelet thrombus formation in the rabbit with particular regard to 5-hydroxytryptamine release. Thrombos. Diathes. haemorrh. (Stuttg.) **18**, 592 (1967).

104. Baxter, J. H.: Origin and characteristics of endogenous lipid in thoracic duct lymph in rat. J. Lipid Res. **7**, 158 (1966).

105. Bazin, S., Delaunay, A.: Charactères de cathepsines collagénolytiques présentes dans les tissus enflammés du rat. Ann. Inst. Pasteur **110**, 192, 347; **112**, 419 (1966).

106. Beaumont, J. L.: L'hyperlipidémie par auto-anticorps anti-beta-lipoprotéine. Une nouvelle entité pathologique. C. R. Acad. Sci. Paris **261**, 4563 (1965).

107. — Une γ_A-globuline de myelome douée d'une activité spécifique anti-lipoprotéine. L'auto-anticorps anti-Pg. C. R. Acad. Sci. (Paris) **263**, 2046 (1966).

108. — L' activité spécifique des protéines M. Vers un nouveau critère de classification des myélomes et des macroglobulinémies. Rev. franc. Étud. clin. Biol. **12**, 319 (1967).

109. — Une speécificité commune aux alpha et beta-lipoprotéines du sérum, révélée par un auto-anticorps de myélome. L'antigène Pg. C. R. Acad. Sci. (Paris) **264**, 185 (1967).

110. — Hyperlipidemia with circulating anti-beta-lipoprotein auto-antibody in man. Auto-immune hyperlipidemia, its possible role in atherosclerosis. In: C. J. Miras, A. N. Howard, R. Paoletti (eds.), *Progress in biochemical pharmacology*, vol. 4, p. 110. Basel-New York: Karger 1968.

111. — Un deuxième type d'auto-anticorps anti-lipoprotéine de myélome: l'IgG anti-Lp Al. Sa. C. R. Acad. Sci. (Paris) **269**, 107 (1969).

112. — Aubert, L., Arroyo, H., Detolle, P., Jacotot, B., Beaumont, V.: Un deuxième cas d'hyperlipidémie par auto-anticorps antilipoprotiéine, chez un sujet atteint de myélome IgA avec xanthomatose. Presse méd. **75**, 1266 (1967).

113. — Baudet, M. F.: Présence d'un phospholipide dans le site Pg, que révèle l'IgA myélomateuse anti-lipoprotéine (anti-Pg). C. R. Acad. Sci. (Paris) **266**, 969 (1968).

114. — — Delplanque, B., Peron, F.: L'hémagglutination passive au chlorure de chrome; son emploi sans diluant macromoléculaire. Path. et Biol. **17**, 429 (1969).

115. — Beaumont, V.: Vitamin A tolerance test, fat metabolism disturbances and antilipemic drugs. In: S. Garattini, R. Paoletti (eds.), *Drugs affecting lipid metabolism*, p. 361. Amsterdam: Elsevier Publishing Co. 1961.

116. — — Antonucci, M.: Présence d'un auto-anticorps anti-beta-lipoprotéine dans le sérum d'un lapin ayant une hyperlipidémie par immunisation (l'hyperlipidémie par auto-anticorps expérimentale). C. R. Acad. Sci. (Paris) **268**, 183 (1969).

117. — — Jacotot, B.: Un nouveau cas d'hyperlipidémie par auto-anticorps. Son traitement par la D-pénicillamine. Bull. Soc. med. Hôp. Paris **118**, 709 (1967).

118, — Delplanque, B.: Methode de purification d'anticorps de lapin anti-lipoproteine humaine a partir de precipites specifiques. Immunochemistry **6**, 489 (1969).

119. — Lacotot, B., Beaumont, V.: L'hyperlipidemie par auto-anticorps: une cause d' atherosclerose. Presse méd. **75**, 2315 (1967).

120. — — — Warnet, J., Vilain, C.: Myelome, hyperlipidemie et xanthomatose. Nouv. Rev. franc. Hémat. **5**, 507 (1965).

121. Beaumont, J. L., Lacotot, B.: Vilain, C., Beaumont, V.: Presence d'un auto-anticorps anti-beta-lipoproteine dans un serum de myelome. C. R. Acad. Sci. (Paris) **260**, 5960 (1965).
122. — Lemont, N.: Purification de l' alpha-lipoproteine du serum. Ann. Biol. clin. **27**, 237 (1969).
123. — Lorenzelli, L.: L'auto-anticorps anti-lipoproteine (anti-Pg) du γ_A-myelome avec hyperlipidemie. Methode d'isolement et de purification a partir des complexes circulants. Ann. Biol. clin. **25**, 655 (1967).
124. — — Delplanque, B.: Emploi d'un detergent pour la purification d'anticorps anti-lipoproteines. Immunochemistry, in press (1969).
125. — Poullin, M. F., Jacotot, B., Beaumont, V.: Myelome et hyperlipidemie. IV. Nature de l'activite specifique anti-lipoproteine. Nouv. Rev. franc. Hémat. **7**, 481 (1967).
126. — Swynghedauw, B., Beaumont, V.: Composition chimique des lipoproteines de S_f0–12 dans l'hypercholesterolemie familiale xanthomateuse. Rev. franc. Ètud. clin. biol. **10**, 221 (1965).
127. Beaumont, V., Beaumont, J. L.: L'hyperlipidemie experimentale par immunisation chez le lapin. Path. Biol. **16**, 869 (1968).
128. Becker, C. G., Murphy, G. E.: Demonstration of contractile protein in endothelium and cells of the heart valves, endocardium, intima, arteriosclerotic plaques, and Aschoff bodies of rheumatic heart disease. Amer. J. Path. **55**, 1 (1969).
129. — Nachman, R. L.: Contractile protein of platelets and endothelial cells. J. clin. Invest. **48**, 7a (1969).
130. Bedford, E.: Harvey's third circulation. De circulo sanguinis in corde. Brit. med. J. **1968 IV**, 273.
131. Begg, T. B.: Dietary factors in ischemic heart disease. Abstracts of Wld. Med. **36**, 225 (1964).
132. Beher, W. T., Baker, G. D.: Effect of dietary bile acids on *in vivo* cholesterol metabolism in the rat. Proc. Soc. exp. Biol. Med. (N.Y.) **98**, 892 (1958).
133. Behnke, O.: Electron microscopic observations on the surface coating of human blood platelets. J. Ultrastruct. Res. **24**, 51 (1968).
134. Belknap, B. H., Amaral, J. A. P., Bierman, E.: Plasma lipids and mild glucose intolerance. I. The response of plasma triglycerides to high carbohydrate feeding and the effect of tolbutamide therapy. In: W. J. H. Butterfield and W. van Westering (eds.), *Tolbutamide after ten years*, p. 159. Amsterdam: Excerpta Medica Foundation 1967.
135. Belt, J. H.: Late sequelae of pulmonary embolism. Lancet **1939 II**, 730.
136. Bennett, C. G., Yokuyama, G. H., McBride, T. C.: Cardiovascular-renal mortality in Hawaii. Amer. J. publ. Hlth. **52**, 1418 (1962).
137. Berenson, G. S., Fishkin, A. F.: Glycoprotein from bovine aorta. Arch. Biochem. **97**, 18 (1962).
138. Bergen, S. S., Van Itallie, T. B., Tennent, D. M., Sebrell, W. H.: Effect of an anion exchange resin on serum cholesterol in man. Proc. Soc. exp. Biol. Med. (N.Y.) **102**, 676 (1961).
139. Bergström, S., Danielsson, H.: On the regulation of bile acid formation in the liver. Acta physiol. scand. **43**, 1 (1958).
140. — — Samuelson, B.: Formation and metabolism of bile acids. In: K. Bloch (ed.), *Lipid metabolism*, p. 291. New York: John Wiley & Sons Inc. 1960.
141. — Lindstedt, S., Samuelsson, B., Corey, E. J., Gregoriou, G. A.: The stereochemistry of 7α-hydroxylation in the biosynthesis of cholic acid from cholesterol. J. Amer. Chem. Soc. **80**, 2337 (1958).
142. Berkson, D. M., Stamler, J.: Atherosclerosis. In: P. J. Talso and A. P. Remenchik (eds.), *Basic mechanisms of disease*, p. 59. St. Louis: C. V. Mosby 1968.
143. — — Jackson, W. E.: The precordial electrocardiogram during and after strenuous exercise. Amer. J. Cardiol. **18**, 43 (1966).
144. — — Lindberg, H. A., Miller, W., Hall, Y.: Socioeconomic correlates of atherosclerotic and hypertensive diseases. Proc. N. Y. Acad. Sci. **84**, 835 (1960).

145. Berséus, O.: Conversion of cholesterol to bile acids in rat: Purification and properties of a Δ^4-3-ketosteroid 5β-reductase and a 3α-hydroxy steroid dehydrogenase. Europ. J. Biochem. **2**, 493 (1967).
146. — Studies on the conversion of cholesterol into bile acids. Opusc. med. Suppl. VI (1967).
147. Best, M. M., Duncan, C. H.: Hypolipemia and hepatomegaly from ethyl chlorophenoxyisobutyrate (CPIB) in the rat. J. Lab. clin. Med. **64**, 634 (1964).
148. — — Effects of clofibrate and dextrothyroxine singly and in combination on serum lipids. Arch. intern. Med. **118**, 97 (1966).
149. Bettex-Galland, M., Luscher, E. F.: Thrombosthenin—a contractile protein from thrombocytes. Its extraction from human platelets and some of its properties. Biochim. biophys. Acta (Amst.) **49**, 536 (1961).
150. Bezman, A., Felts, J. M., Havel, R. J.: Relation between incorporation of triglyceride fatty acids and heparin-released lipoprotein lipase from adipose tissue slices. J. Lipid. Res. **3**, 427 (1962).
151. Bhargwa, R. K., Husain, S. A., Dave, A. S., Natang, N. K., Banerjee, A., Gupta, U.: Incidence of heart disease in Rajasthan. J. Ass. Phycns India **14**, 14 (1965).
152. Bianchine, J. R., Weiss, P., Hersey, R. M., Peaston, M. J. T.: Metabolism of 2-methyl-2-[p-(1,2,3,4-tetrahydro-1 naphthyl-phenoxy]-propionic acid (Su-13437) in man. Clin. Res. **17**, 378 (1969).
153. Bicher, H. I.: Prevention of sludge induced myocardial damage by an anti-adhesive drug. (Abs.) Proc. V Int. Conference on Microcirculation, Gothenberg 1968.
154. — Brain tissue re-oxygenation time, demonstrated with a new-ultra-micro oxygen electrode. J. appl. Physiol. in press (1970).
155. — Prevention of sludge induced mycardial damage by an anti-adhesive drug. Bibl. anat. (Basel), **10**, 202 (1969).
156. — 2–4 butyl methyl ketolactone, a prototype anti-thrombotic drug preventing platelet and red cell aggregation. Circulation, in press (1969).
157. — Beemer, A. M.: Induction of ischemic myocardial damage by red cell aggregation (sludge) in the rabbit. J. Atheroscler. Res. **7**, 409 (1967).
158. — Licht, A.: K^+ and the platelet membrane. Relationship to platelet aggregation and its prevention by anti-adhesive drugs. Proc. of the Intern. Union of Physiol. Sci. **7**, 44 (1968).
159. Bierman, E. L., Amaral, J. A. P., Belknap, B. H.: Hyperlipemia and diabetes mellitus. Diabetes **15**, 675 (1966).
160. — Porte, D., Jr.: Carbohydrate intolerance and lipaemia. Ann. intern. Med. **68**, 926 (1968).
161. Biersleker, K.: Correlation between water hardness and cardiovascular death in Holland. T. soc. Geneesk. **45**, 658 (1967).
162. Biggs, M. W., Kritchevsky, D.: Observations with radioactive hydrogen (H^3) in experimental atherosclerosis. Circulation **4**, 34 (1951).
163. Bihari-Varga, M., Simon, J., Gerő, S.: Identification of glycosaminoglycan-beta-lipoprotein complexes in the atherosclerotic aorta intima by thermoanalytical methods. Acta biochim. biophys. Acad. Sci. hung. **3**, 365 (1968).
164. — Végh, M.: Quantitative studies on the complexes formed between aortic mucopolysaccharides and serum lipoproteins. Biochim. biophys. Acta (Amst.) **144**, 202 (1967).
165. — — Levai, J., Gerő, S.: The effect of polyunsaturated phosphatidyl choline on the correlation of serum lipid and seromucoid levels and on the thermal decomposition of atherosclerotic aortas. Clin. chim. Acta **22**, 355 (1968).
166. Billiau, A., Evrard, E., Van den Bosch, J., Joossens, J. V., DeSomer, P.: The fatty acid distribution in plasma, liver and aorta of cholesterol-fed and triton-treated rabbits. J. Atheroscler. Res. **3**, 222 (1963).
167. Biörck, G., Bostrom, H., Widstrom, A.: On relationship between water hardness and death rate in cardiovascular disease. Acta med. scand. **178**, 239 (1965).

168. Biörck, G., Wedelin, E. M.: The return to work of patients with myocardial infarction. Acta med. scand. **175**, 215 (1964).
169. Björkerud, S.: Atherosclerosis initiated by mechanical trauma in normo-lipidemic rabbits. J. Atheroscler. Res. **9**, 209 (1969).
170. — Reaction of the aortic wall of the rabbit after superficial, longitudinal, mechanical trauma. Virchows Arch. Abt. Path. Anat. **347**, 197 (1969).
171. —, Huth, F.: The incorporation of glucose and palmitic acid into lipids in human arterial intima and media *in vitro*. J. Atheroscler. Res., **10**, 179 (1969).
172. Björkhem, I.: On the mechanism of cholest-5-ene-3β, 7α-diol into 7α-hydroxycholest-4-en-3-one. Europ. J. Biochem. **8**, 345 (1969).
173. — Reaction mechanisms in bile acid biosynthesis. Opusc. med., Suppl. (Stockh.) **13** (1969).
174. — Stereochemistry of the enzymatic conversion of a Δ^4-3-oxosteroid into a 3-oxo-5beta-steroid. Europ. J. Biochem. **7**, 413 (1969).
175. — Danielsson, H.: Formation and metabolism of some Δ^4-cholestenols in the rat. Europ. J. Biochem. **2**, 403 (1967).
176. — — Einarsson, K., Johansson, G.: Formation of bile acids in man: conversion of cholesterol into 5β-cholestane-3α, 7α, 12α-triol in liver homogenates. J. clin. Invest. **47**,1573 (1968).
177. — — Issidorides, C., Kallner, A.: On the synthesis and metabolism of cholest-4-en-7α-ol-3one. Acta chem. scand. **19**, 2151 (1965).
178. — Einarsson, K., Johansson, G.: Formation andmetabolism of 3β-hydroxycholest-5-en-7-one and cholest-5-ene-3β, 7β-diol. Acta chem. scand. **22**, 1595 (1968).
179. Bjorklund, R., Katz, S.: The molecular weights and dimensions of some human serum lipoproteins. J. Amer. chem. Soc. **78**, 2122 (1956).
180. Bjorntorp, P., Bergman, H., Varnauskas, E., Lindholm, N.: Lipid mobilization in relation to body composition in man. Metabolism, **18**, 840 (1969).
181. — Hansson, L. O., Hood, B.: Polyunsaturated fatty acids in the lipids of the atherosclerotic femoral artery. Changes after corn oil supplementation of the diet. Amer. J. clin. Nutr. **10**, 217 (1962).
182. — Hood, B.: Studies on adipose tissue from obese patients with and without diabetes mellitus. I. Release of glycerol and free fatty acids. Acta med. scand. **179**, 221 (1966).
183. — Liljemark, A., Angervall, L.: Fatty acid composition of lipids of serum and aorta in the chicken on different diets. J. Atheroscler. Res. **3**, 72 (1963).
184. Bjurulf, P.: Atherosclerosis in different parts of the arterial system. Amer. Heart J. **68**, 41 (1964).
185. — Atherosclerosis and body-build with special reference to size and number of subcutaneous fat cells. Acta med. scand. Suppl. **166** (1959).
186. Blaton, V., Howard, A., Gresham, G., Vandamme, D., Peeters, H.: Lipid changes in the plasma lipoproteins of baboons given an atherogenic diet. J. Atheroscler. Res., in press (1970).
187. — Peeters, H.: Lipid and fatty acid modifications in plasma lipoproteins of baboons under atherogenic diet. Acta Zool. Path. Antverpiensia **48**, 233 (1969).
188. — — The subunits of low and high density lipoproteins. In: *Protides of the biological fluids*, vol. **16**, 707. New York, Oxford: Pergamon Press 1969.
189. — — Gresham, G. A., Howard, A. N.: Differential fatty acid composition of alpha and beta lipoproteins in baboons. Progr. biochem. Pharmacol. **4**, 122 (1968).
190. Bleyl, U.: Arteriosklerose und fibrininkorporation. Berlin-Heidelberg-New York: Springer 1969.
191. Bloch, E. H.: Microscopic observations of the circulating blood in the bulbar conjectiva in man in health and disease. Ergebn. Anat. Entwickl. Gesch. **35**, 1(1956).
192. Bloch, K., Berg, B., Rittenberg, D.: The biological conversion of cholesterol to cholic acid. J. biol. Chem. **149**, 511 (1943).
193. Blomback, B., Blomback, M., Henschen, A., Hessel, B., Iwanaga, W., Woods, K. R.: N-Terminal disulphide knot of human fibrinogen. Nature (Lond.) **218**, 130 (1968).

194. Blomstrand, R., Christensen, S.: Fatty acid composition of plasma, aorta and liver lipids in cockerels with stilbesterol-or cholesterol-induced hyperlipemia J. Atheroscler. Res. **3**, 142 (1963).
195. Bloom, F. E., Giarman, N. J.: Physiologic and pharmacologic considerations of biogenic amines in the nervious system. Ann. Rev. Pharmacol. **8**, 229 (1968).
196. Bloor, W. R.: The determination of cholesterol in blood. J. Biol. Chem. **24**, 227 (1916).
197. Boberg, J., Carlson, L. A., Freyschuss, U.: Studies on the total and splanchnic turnover of plasma triglycerides in man by means of isotopic and chemical methods. Course on synthesis and use of labelled lipids and sterols, Milan, September, 1968. Progr. Biochem. Pharmacol. **5**, in press (1969).
198. — — Fröberg, S. O., Orō, L.: Effect of a hypolipidemic drug, CH 13 437, on plasma and tissue lipids on the intravenous fat tolerance in man. J. Atheroscler. Res., in press (1970).
199. — — Hallberg, D.: Application of a new intravenous fat tolerance test in the study of hypertriglyceridaemia in man. J. Atheroscler. Res. **9**, 159 (1969).
200. — — Normell, L.: Production of lipolytic activity by the isolated perfused dog liver in response to heparin. Life Sci. **3**, 1011 (1964).
201. Borgström, B.: Quantification of cholesterol absorption in man by fecal analysis after the feeding of a single isotope-labeled meal. J. Lipid Res. **10**, 331 (1969).
202. Borgstrom, S., Gelin, L. E., Zederfelt, B.: The formation of vein thrombi following tissue injury. Acta chir. scand., Suppl. **247** (1959).
203. Born, G. V. R.: Adenosine triphosphate (ATP) in platelets. Biochem. J. **62**, 33 (1956).
204. — Changes in the distribution of phosphorus in platelet rich plasma during clotting. Biochem. J. **68**, 695 (1958).
205. — Aggregation of blood platelets by adenosine diphosphate and its reversal. Nature (Lond.) **194**, 927 (1962).
206. — Strong inhibition by 2-chloroadenosine of the aggregation of blood platelets by adenosine diphosphate. Nature (Lond.) **202**, 95 (1964).
207. — Platelets in thrombogenesis: mechanism and inhibition of platelet aggregation. Ann. roy. Coll. Surg. Eng. **36**, 200 (1965).
208. — Uptake of adenosine and of adenosine diphosphate by human platelets. Nature (Lond.) **206**, 1121 (1965).
209. — Inhibition of thrombogenesis by inhibition of platelet aggregation. In: F. Koller, F. Duckert and F. Streuli (eds.), *Pathogenesis and treatment of thromboembolic diseases*, p. 159. Stuttgart: Schattauer 1966.
210. — Mechanism of platelet aggregation and of its inhibition by adenosine derivatives. Fed. Proc. **26**, 115 (1966).
211. — Cross, M. J.: Effect of adenosine diphosphate on the concentration of platelets in circulating blood. Nature (Lond.) **197**, 974 (1963).
212. — — The aggregation of blood platelets. J. Physiol. (Lond.) **168**, 178 (1963).
213. — — Effects of inorganic ions and of plasma proteins on the aggregation of blood platelets by adenosine diphosphate. J. Physiol. (Lond.) **170**, 397 (1964).
214. — Haslam, R. J., Goldman, M., Lowe, R. D.: Comparative effectiveness of adenosine analogues as inhibitors of blood platelet aggregation and as vasodilators in man. Nature (Lond.) **205**, 678 (1965).
215. — Honour, A. J., Mitchell, J. R.: Inhibition by adenosine and by 2-chloroadenosine of the formation and embolisation of platelet thrombi. Nature (Lond.) **202**, 761 (1964).
216. — Hume, M.: Effects of the numbers and sizes of platelet aggregates in the optical density of plasma. Nature (Lond.) **215**, 1027 (1968).
217. — Mills, D. C. B.: Potentiation of the inhibiting effect of adenosine on platelet aggregation by drugs that prevent its uptake. J. Physiol. (Lond.) **202**, 41 P (1969).
218. — — Roberts, G. C. K.: Potentiation of platelet aggregation by adrenaline. J. Physiol. (Lond.) **191**, 43P (1967).

219. Born, G. V. R., Philp, R. B.: Effects of adenosine analogues and of heparin on platelet thrombi in non-lipaemic and lipaemic rats. Brit. J. exp. Path. **46**, 569 (1965).
220. Bornstein, P.: The cross-linking of collagen and elastin. In J. E. Dunphy (ed.), *Connective tissue repair*, p. 137. New York: McGraw-Hill, Inc. 1969.
221. Bortz, W., Abraham, S., Chaikoff, I. L.: Localization of the block in lipogenesis resulting from feeding fat. J. biol. Chem. **238**, 1266 (1963).
222. Boshoff, W. H.: Ergonomic aspects of traditional and modern cultivation tasks in Uganda. Proc. IV Int. Congress on Rural Medicine. Japan: Usuda (in press) 1969.
223. Böttcher, C. J. F.: Phospholipids of atherosclerotic lesions in the human aorta. In: R. J. Jones (ed.), *Evolution of the atherosclerotic plaque*, p. 109. Chicago: University Press 1963.
224. — Chemical constituents of human atherosclerotic lesions. Proc. roy. Soc. Med. **57**, 34 (1964).
225. — Boelsma-van Houte, E., Ter Haar Romeny-Wachter, C. C., Woodford, F. P., Van Gent, C. M.: Lipid and fatty-acid composition of coronary and cerebral arteries at different stages of atherosclerosis. **1960 II**, 1162.
226. — Van Gent, C. M.: Changes in the composition of phospholipids and of phospholipid fatty acids associated with atherosclerosis in the human aortic wall. J. Atheroscler. Res. **1**, 36 (1961).
227. — Woodford, F. P.: Chemical changes in the arterial wall associated with atherosclerosis. Fed. Proc. **21** (**4**), 15 (1962).
228. — — Romeny-Wachter, C. T. H., Boelsma-van-Houte, E., Van Gent, C. M.: Composition of lipids isolated from the aorta, coronary arteries and circulus willisii of atherosclerotic individuals. Nature (Lond.) **183**, 47 (1959).
229. — — — Boelsma-van Houte, E., Van Gent, C. M.: Fatty acid distribution in lipids of the aortic wall. Lancet **1960 I**, 1378.
230. Bounameaux, Y.: L' accolement des plaquettes aux fibres sousendothéliales. C. R. Soc. Biol. (Paris) **153**, 865 (1959).
231. Boura, A. L. A., Green, A. F.: Adrenergic neurone blocking drugs. Ann. Rev. Pharmacol. **5**, 183 (1965).
232. Bowyer, D. E.: Biochemical aspects of occlusive vascular disease. Dissertation for a Ph. D. degree, University of Cambridge 1967.
233. — Leat, W. M. F., Howard, A. N., Gresham, G. A.: The determination of the fatty acid composition of serum lipids separated by thin-layer chromatography and a comparison with column chromatography. Biochim. biophys. Acta (Amst.) **70**, 423 (1963).
234. Boyd, G. S., Scholan, N. A., Mitton, J. R.: Factors influencing cholesterol 7α-hydroxylase in rat liver. In: W. L. Holmes and L. Carlson (eds.), *Drugs affecting lipid metabolism*. New York: Plenum Press 1969.
235. Boyns, D. R., Crossley, J. N., Abrams, M. E., Jarrett, R. J., Keen, H.: Oral glucose tolerance and related factors in a normal population sample. I. Blood sugar, plasma insulin, glyceride, and cholesterol measurements and the effects of age and sex. Brit. med. J. **1969 I**, 595.
236. Bradley, R. F., Partamian, J. O.: Coronary heart disease in the diabetic patients. Med. Clin. N. Amer. **49**, 1093 (1965).
237. Brehmer, W., Lubbers, P.: Über eine generalisierte xanthomatose mit knochenbefall and diffuser plasmazellwucherung im knochenmark bei essentieller hyperlipämie. Virchows Arch. Abt. Path. Anat. **318**, 394 (1950).
238. Brice, J. G., Dowsett, D. J., Lowe, R. D.: The effect of constriction on carotid blood-flow and pressure gradient. Lancet **1964 I**, 84.
239. Brink, A. J.: An investigation of factors influencing repolarization of the human heart. S. Afr. J. clin. Sci. **2**, 288 (1951).
240. Brochs, H.: Experimentelle undersogelsen over lipoidaflezringen i coronarterierne hos kaniner. Copenhagen These 1945.
241. Bronte-Stewart, B., Keys, A., Brock, J. F.: Serum cholesterol, the diet and the relationship to incidence of cornary disease. Lancet **1955 II**, 1103.

242. Brown, D. J.: Blood lipids and lipoproteins in atherogenesis. Amer. J. Med. **46**, 691 (1969).
243. Brown, H. B.: The national diet-heart study—implications for dietitians and nutritionists. J. Amer. diet. Ass. **52**, 279 (1968).
244. — Farrand, M. E.: Pitfalls in constructing a fat-controlled diet. J. Amer. diet. Ass. **49**, 303 (1966).
245. — — Page, I. H.: The interaction of dietary cholesterol and polyunsaturates in practical diets for serum cholesterol reduction. Circulation, Suppl. II, **32**, 4 (1965).
246. — — — Design of practical fat-controlled diets. Foods, fat composition and serum cholesterol content. J. Amer. med. Ass. **196**, 205 (1966).
247. — Lewis, L. A., Page, I. H.: Mixed hyperlipemia, an important type of hyperlipoproteinemia. (Abs.) Circulation, Suppl. VI. **38**, 128 (1968).
248. — Page, I. H.: Variable responses of hyperlipemic patients to altered food patterns. J. Amer. med. Ass. **173**, 248 (1960).
249. — — Practical diets for serum cholesterol reduction. Proc. VIIth Int. Congr. Nutrition, Hamburg **5**, 429 (1966).
250. Brown, J. B.: Changes in nutritive value of food fats during processing and cooking. Nutr. Rev. **17**, 321 (1959).
251. Brown, W. V., Levy, R. I., Fredrickson, D. S.: Studies on the proteins of the very low-density lipoproteins. Biophys. J. **9**, A-147 (1969).
252. Brownlee, K. A.: Statistical theory and methodology in science and engineering, 2nd edition, p. 366. New York: John Wiley & Sons 1965.
253. Brunner, D.: Effect of western diet on serum cholesterol in Yeminite Jews in Israel. In: C. J. Miras, A. N. Howard and R. Paoletti (eds.), *Progress in biochemical pharmacology*, vol. 4, p. 52. Basel: S. Karger 1968.
254. — Altman, S.: Vascular disease in diabetes. Proc. 9th Int. Congr. Life Assoc. Med., Tel Aviv 1968.
255. Bucher, N. L. R., Overath, P., Lynen, F.: β-hydroxy-β-methyl-glutaryl coenzymes reductase, cleavage and condensing enzymes in relation to cholesterol formation in rat liver. Biochim. biophys. Acta (Amst.) **40**, 491 (1960).
256. Buchwald, H.: Vitamin B_{12} absorption deficiency following bypass of the ileum. Amer. J. dig. Dis. **9**, 755 (1964).
257. — Surgical treatment of the hyperlipidemic states by partial ileal bypass. In: H. R. Casdorph (ed.), *Treatment of the hyperlipidemic states* (in press). Springfield: C. C. Thomas 1970.
258. — Moore, R. B., Lee, G. D., Frantz, I. D., Jr., Varco, R. L.: Combined dietary, surgical, and bile salt binding resin therapy in the treatment of hypercholesterolemia. Arch. Surg. **97**, 275 (1968).
259. — Varco, R. L.: Ileal bypass in patients with hypercholesterolemia and atherosclerosis. Preliminary report on therapeutic potential. J. Amer. med. Ass. **196**, 627 (1966).
260. — — Partial ileal bypass operation for hypercholesterolemia. Cine Clinics Film, presented October, 1969. Available from the American College of Surgeons.
261. Buckingham, S., Maynert, E. W.: The release of 5-hydroxytryptamine, potassium and amino acids from platelets. J. Pharmacol. exp. Ther. **143**, 332 (1964).
262. Buckley, J. T., Delahunty, T. J., Rubinstein, D.: The relationship of protein synthesis to the secretion of the lipid moiety of low density lipoprotein by the liver. Canad. J. Biochem. **46**, 341 (1968).
263. Buddecke, E.: Chemistry and metabolism of aortal glycosaminoglycans. In 7th Int. Congr. Clin. Chem., Genève. Basel: S. Karger 1969 (in press).
264. — Kresse, H.: Glykosamino-Glykanohydrolasen des Arteriengewebes und ihre Aktivitätsänderungen im Alter und bei Arteriosklerose. In Centre National de la Recherche Scientifique (ed.), Colloque international sur le rôle de la paroi artérielle dans l'athérogénèse. p. 691. Paris 1967.
265. Buisson, J.: Contribution à individualisation du syndrome β_2-*A* myélome xanthomateux. These, Marseille 1960.

266. Bungenberg de Jong, J. J., Marsh, J. B.: Biosynthesis of plasma lipoproteins by rat liver ribosomes. J. biol. Chem. **243**, 192 (1968).
267. Burch, R. E.: Acetoacetyl-CoA deacylase: an enzymatic site of action of the hypercholesterolemic agent ethyl chlorophenoxyisobutyrate. J. clin. Invest. **47**, 13A (1968).
268. Burgen, A. S. V.: The drug-receptor complex. J. Pharm. Pharmacol. **18**, 137 (1966).
269. Burn, J. H., Rand, M. J.: A new interpretation of the adrenergic nerve fiber. Advanc. Pharmacol. **1**, 1 (1962).
270. Burnet, M.: The clonal selection theory of antibody production. London, New York: Oxford University Press 1959.
271. Burstein, M., Caroli, J.: Lipoprotéines sériques anormales au cours de certains ictères par rétention. Rev. franc. Étud. clin. biol. **12**, 898 (1967).
272. Butcher, R. W., Baird, C. E., Sutherland, E. W.: Effect of lipolytic and antilipolytic substances on adenosine 3′, 5′-monophosphate levels in isolated fat cells. J. biol. Chem. **243**, 1705 (1968).
273. — Scott, R. E., Sutherland, E. W.: The effects of prostaglandins on cyclic AMP levels in tissues. Pharmacologist **9**, 172 (1967).
274. Butler, W. M., Maling, H. M., Horning, M. G., Brodie, B. B.: The direct determination of liver triglycerides. J. Lipid Res. **2**, 95 (1961).
275. Butler, W. T.: Partial hydroxylation of certain lysines in collagen. Science **161**, 796 (1968).
276. Campbell, M.: Death rate from diseases of the heart: 1876 to 1959. Brit. med. J. **2**, 528 (1968).
277. Carey, J. B., Jr.: Conversion of cholesterol to trihydroxycoprostanic acid and cholic acid in man. J. clin. Invest. **43**, 1443 (1964).
278. — Haslewood, G. A. D.: Crystallization of trihydroxycoprostanic acid from human bile. J. biol. Chem. **238**, 855 (1963).
279. — Williams, G.: Relief of the pruritus of jaundice with a bile-acid sequestering resin. J. Amer. med. Ass. **176**, 432 (1961).
280. Carlson, L. A.: Determination of serum glycerides. Acta Soc. Med. upsalien **64**, 208 (1959).
281. — Serum lipids in men with myocardial infarction. Acta med. scand. **167**, 399 (1960).
282. — Consequences of inhibition of normal and excessive lipid mobilization. Progr. Biochem. Pharmacol. **3**, 151 (1967).
283. — Boberg, J., Högstedt, B.: Some physiological and clinical implications of lipid mobilization from adipose tissue. In: A. E. Renold and G. F. Cahill (eds.), *Handbook of physiology. Adipose tissue*, p. 625, sec. 5, vol. I, ch. 63. Washington, D. C.: American Physiol. Soc. 1965.
284. — Eklund, L. G.: Splanchnic production and uptake of endogeneous triglycerides in the fasting state in man. J. clin Invest. **42**, 714 (1963).
285. — Fröberg, S. O., Nye, E. R.: Acute effects of nicotinic acid on plasma, liver, heart and muscle lipids. Nicotinic acid in the rat. II. Acta med. scand. **180**, 571 (1966).
286. — Hallberg, D.: Studies on the elimination of exogenous lipids from the blood stream. The kinetics of the elimination of a fat emulsion and of chylomicrones in the dog after single injection. Acta physiol. scand. **59**, 52 (1963).
287. — Liljedahl, S. O., Wirsen, C.: Blood and tissue changes in the dog during and after excessive FFA mobilization. Acta med. scand. **178**, 81 (1965).
288. — Nye, E. R.: Acute effects of nicotinic acid in the rat. I. Plasma and liver lipids and blood glucose. Acta med. scand. **179**, 453 (1966).
289. — Wahlberg, F.: Serum lipids, intravenous glucose tolerance and their interrelation studied in ischaemic cardiovascular disease. Acta med. scand. **180**, 307 (1966).
290. Carlsson, A.: Drugs which block the storage of 5-hydroxytryptamine and related amines. In: O. Eichler and A. Farah (eds.), *Handbook of experimental pharmacology*, vol. XIX, p. 34. Berlin-Heidelberg-New York: Springer 1965.

291. Carmon, A., Lavy, S., Schwartz, A.: Correlation of clinical and angiographic findings in one hundred patients with "completed stroke". J. neurol. Sci. **4**, 111 (1967).
292. Carnes, W. H.: Copper and connective tissue metabolism. In: A. D. HALL (ed.), Int. Rev. Connect. Tiss. Res. **4**, 197 (1968).
293. Carr, J. J., Drekter, I. J.: Simplified rapid technique for the extraction and determination of serum cholesterol without saponification. Clin. Chem. **2**, 353 (1956).
294. Casley-Smith, J. R., Ardlie, N. G., Schwartz, C. J.: Electron microscopical observations on the organization of artificial thrombi in the rabbit pulmonary artery. Brit. J. exp. Path. **48**, 501 (1967).
295. Castleman, B., Bland, E. F.: Organized emboli of the tertiary pulmonary arteries. Arch. Path. **42**, 581 (1946).
296. Cederlöf, R., Friberg, L., Jonsson, E.: Hereditary factors and "angina pectoris". Arch. environm. Hlth. **14**, 397 (1967).
297. Ceriotti, G.: A microchemical determination of desoxyribonucleic acid. J. biol. Chem. **198**, 297 (1952).
298. Chaikoff, I. L., Siperstein, M. D., Dauben, W. G., Bradlow, H. L., Eastham, J. F., Tomkins, G. M., Meier, J. R., Chen, R. W., Hotta, S., Srere, P. A.: C^{14}-cholesterol. II. Oxidation of carbons 4 and 26 to carbon dioxide by the intact rat. J. biol. Chem. **194**, 413 (1952).
299. Chandler, A. B.: Thrombosis in the pathogenesis of artherosclerosis. J. med. Ass. Ga. **56**, 319 (1967).
300. — Hand, R. A.: Phagocytized platelets; a source of lipids in human thrombi and atherosclerotic plaques. Science **134**, 946 (1961).
301. Chang, Y. H., Pinson, R., Jr., Malone, M. H.: Displacement of L-thyroxine from its binding proteins in human, dog and rat plasma by α-(p-chlorophenoxy) isobutyric acid. Biochem. Pharmacol. **16**, 2053 (1967).
302. Chapman, I.: Morphogenesis of occluding coronary artery thrombosis. Arch. Path. **80**, 256 (1965).
303. Chesterton, C. J.: Distribution of cholesterol precursors and other lipids among rat liver intracellular structures. J. biol. Chem. **243**, 1147 (1968).
304. Chiang, B. N., Alexander, E. R., Bruce, R. A., Thompson, D. J., Ting, N.: Factors related to post-exericse ST segment depression in middle-aged Chinese males. Circulation, **39**, 403 (1969).
305. Chlouverakis, C., Jarrett, R. J., Keen, H.: Glucose tolerance, age and circulating insulin. Lancet **1967 I**, 806.
306. Chobanian, A. V.: Effects of serum hormones on phospholipid, RNA, and protein synthesis in the arterial intima. J. Atheroscler. Res. **8**, 763 (1968).
307. — Sterol synthesis in the human arterial intima. J. clin Invest. **47**, 595 (1968).
308. — Burrows, B. A., Hollander, W.: Body cholesterol metabolism in man. II. Measurement of the body cholesterol miscible pool and turnover rate. J. clin Invest. **41**, 1738 (1962).
309. — Hollander, W.: Body cholesterol metabolism in man. I. The equilibration of serum and tissue cholesterol. J. clin. Invest. **41**, 1732 (1962).
310. — — Studies on fatty acid metabolism in human blood vessels. Clin. Res. **11**, 216 (1963).
311. — — Phospholipid synthesis in human arterial intima. J. clin. Invest. **45**, 932 (1966).
312. Christiansen, I., Deckert, T., Kjerulf, K., Midtgaard, K., Worning, H.: Glucose tolerance, plasma lipids and serum insulin in patients with ischaemic heart diseases. Acta med. scand. **184**, 283 (1968).
313. Clark, E., Graef, I., Chasis, H.: Thrombosis of the aorta and coronary arteries with special reference to "fibrinoid" lesions. Arch. Path. **22**, 183 (1936).
314. Clements, R. S., Jr., Morrison, A. D., Winegrad, A. I.: Polyol pathway in aorta: regulation by hormones. Science **166**, 1007 (1969).

315. Clements, R. S., Jr., Weaver, J. P., Winegrad, A. I.: The distribution of polyol:NADP oxido-reductase in mammalian tissues. Biochem. biophys. Res. Commun. **37**, 347 (1969).
316. — Winegrad, A. I.: Modulation of mammalian polyol:NADP oxidoreductase activity by ADP and ATP. Biochem. biophys. Res. Commun. **36**, 1006 (1969).
317. Cohen, L., Blaisdell, R. K., Djordjevich, J., Ormiste, V.: Xanthomatosis, familial hyperlipidemia and myelomatosis. Circulation **30**, Suppl. III, 5 (1964).
318. — — — — Dobrilovic, L.: Familial xanthomatosis and hyperlipidemia, and myelomatosis. Amer. J. Med. **40**, 299 (1966).
319. Cole, D. R., Singian, E.B., Katz, L. N.: The long term prognosis following myocardial infarction and some factors which affect it. Circulation **9**, 321 (1954).
320. Connor, W. E.: Dietary cholesterol and the pathogenesis of atherosclerosis. Geriatrics **16**, 407 (1961).
321. — Hoak, J. C., Warner, E. D.: The role of lipids in thrombosis. In: F. Koller, F. Duckert and F. Streuli (eds.), Pathogenesis and treatment of thromboembolic diseases including coronary, cerebral and peripheral thrombosis, p. 193. Thrombos. Diathes. haemorrh. (Stuttg.) Suppl. **21**, 1966.
322. — Hodges, R. E., Bleiler, R. E.: The serum lipids in men receiving high cholesterol and cholesterol-free diets. J. clin Invest. **40**, 894 (1961).
323. — Witiak, D. T., Brahmankar, D. M., Wartman, A., Parker, R.: Prevention of hypercholesterolemia and atherosclerosis by 3β, 5α, 6β-cholestane triol. Circulation **38**, VI-58 (1968).
324. — — Stone, D. B., Armstrong, M. L.: Cholesterol balance and fecal neutral steroid and bile acid excretion in normal men fed dietary fats of different fatty acid composition. J. clin. Invest. **48**, 1363 (1969).
325. Consolazia, C. F., Johnson, R. E., Pecora, L. J.: Physiological measurements of metabolic functions in man. New York: McGraw-Hill 1963.
326. Constantinides, P.: Experimental atherosclerosis, p. 40, 43. Amsterdam-London-New York: Elsevier Publishing Company 1965.
327. — Plaque fissures in human coronary thrombosis. J. Atheroscler. Res. **6**, 1 (1966).
328. Cook, R. P.: Cholesterol—chemistry, biochemistry and pathology, p. 145, **170** New York: Academic Press 1958.
329. Cookson, F. B., Altschul, R., Fedoroff, S.: The effect of alfalfa feeding on serum cholesterol and in modifying or preventing cholesterol induced atherosclerosis in rabbits. J. Atheroscler. Res. **7**, 69 (1967).
330. Cornfield, J.: Joint dependence of risk of coronary heart disease on serum cholesterol and systolic blood pressure: a discriminiant function analysis. Fed. Proc. **21**, Suppl. II, 58 (1962).
331. — The Bayesian outlook and its application. Biometrics, in press (1970).
332. — Mitchell, S.: Selected risk factors in coronary disease possible intervention effects. Arch. environm. Hlth **19**, 328 (1969).
333. Cotlier, E., Beaty, C.: The transport of ^{14}C α-aminoisobutyric acid in galactose cataracts in rat and rabbit lenses incubated in high galactose media. Invest. Ophthal. **7**, 77 (1968).
334. Coulter, A. W., Talalay, P.: Studies of the microbiological degradation of steroid ring A. J. biol. Chem. **243**, 3238 (1968).
335. Cox, G. E., Taylor, C. B., Patton, D., Davis, C., Jr., Blandin, N.: Origin of plasma cholesterol in man. Arch. Path. **76**, 60 (1963).
336. Cramer, K., Isaksson, B.: An evaluation of the Theorell method for the determination of total serum cholesterol. Scand. J. clin. Lab. Invest. **11**, 213 (1959).
337. Crawford, M. A.: Fatty-acid ratios in free-living and domestic animals. Possible implications for atheroma. Lancet **1968 I**, 1329.
338. Crawford, M. D., Crawford, T.: Lead content of bones in soft water area. Lancet **1969 I**, 699.
339. — Gardner, M. J., Morris, J. N.: Mortality and hardness of water supplies. Lancet **1968 I**, 747.

340. Crawford, T.: The healing of puncture wounds in arteries. J. Path. Bact. **72**, 547 (1956).
341. — Crawford, M. D.: Prevalence and pathological changes of ischaemic heart disease in a hard-water and in a soft-water area. Lancet **1967 I**, 229.
342. — — Lead content of bones in a soft and a hard water area. Lancet **1969 I**, 699.
343 — Levene, C. I.: Incorporation of fibrin in the aortic intima. J. Path. Bact. **64**, 523 (1952).
344. Cremer, M. D., Tiselius, A.: Elektrophorese von Eiweiß in Filterpapier. Biochem. J. **320**, 273 (1950).
345. Creyssel, R., Manuel, Y., Richard, G. B., Fine, G. M.: Sur les caractères hétérogènes des paraprotéines des myélomes beta. Rev. franç. Étud. clin. biol. **7**, 253 (1962).
346. Cristafalo, V. J., Howard, B. V., Kritchevsky, D.: The biochemistry of human cells in culture. In: U. Gallo and L. Santamaria (eds.), *Research progress in organic, biological and medicinal chemistry*, p. 1. Amsterdam: Noord Hollandsche Uitgevers-Mij. 1968.
347. Cronholm, T., Sjövall, J.: Bile acids in portal blood of rats fed different diets and cholestryramine. Europ. J. Biochem. **2**, 375 (1967).
348. Crout, J. R., Johnston, R. R., Webb, W. R., Shore, P. A.: The antihypertensive action of metaraminol in man. Clin. Res. **13**, 204 (1965).
349. Cunningham, V. J., Robinson, D. S.: Clearing-factor lipase in adipose tissue. Biochem. J. **112**, 203 (1969).
350. Curnow, D. H., Cullen, K. J., McCall, M. G., Stenhouse, N. S., Welborn, T. A.: Health and disease in a rural community. Aust. J. Sci. **31**, 281 (1969).
351. Curran, G. L., Brewster, K. C.: A cholesterol metabolizing escherichia coli. Bull. Johns Hopk. Hosp. **91**, 68 (1952).
352. Daly, M. M., Deming, Q. B., Raeff, V. M., Brun, L. M.: Cholesterol concentration and cholesterol synthesis in aortas of rats with renal hypertension. J. clin. Invest. **42**, 1606 (1963).
353. Damon, A., Page, L. B., Moellering, R. C., Jr.: Cardiovascular status of four Solomon Island populations. Report to New Orelans Conference on Cardiovascular Epidemiology **1969**.
354. Danhof, I. E.: The effect of cholestyramine on fecal excretion of ingested radioiodinated lipids. Amer. J. clin. Nutr. **18**, 343 (1966).
355. Danielsson, H.: Present status of research on catabolism and excretion of cholesterol. In: R. Paoletti and D. Kritchevsky (eds.), *Advances in lipid research* p. 335. London: Academic Press 1963.
356. — Einarsson, K.: On the conversion of cholesterol 7α, 12α-dihydroxycholest-4-en-3-one. J. biol. Chem. **241**, 1449 (1965).
357. — — Johansson, G.: Effect of biliary drainage on individual reactions in the conversion of cholesterol to taurocholic acid. Europ. J. Biochem. **2**, 44 (1967).
358. — Enroth, P., Hellström, K., Lindstedt, S., Sjövall, J.: On the turnover and excretory products of cholic acid and chenodeoxycholic acid in man. J. biol. Chem. **238**, 2299 (1963).
359. — Tschen, T. T.: Steroid metabolism. In: D. M. Greenberg (ed.), *Metabolic pathways*, vol. 2, p. 117. New York: Academic Press 1968.
360. Danowski, T. S., Aliey, R.: Thyroxine and hypolipidaemic effect of clofibrate. Lancet **1967 I**, 854.
361. Daoud, A. S., Goodale, F., Florentin, R., Beadenkoff, W. G.: Chemico-anatomic studies in geographic pathology. A practical quantitation of cornary arteriosclerosis. Arch. Path. **73**, 74 (1962).
362. — Jarmolych, J., Zumbo, A., Fani, K., Florentin, R.: "Pre-atheroma" phase of coronary atherosclerosis in men. Exp. molec. Path. **3**, 475 (1964).
363. — Jones, R. M., Scott, R. F.: Dietary-induced atherosclerosis in miniature swine. Part II. Electron microscopy observations; characteristics of endothelial and smooth muscle cells in proliferative lesions and elsewhere in the aorta. Exp. molec. Path. **8**, 263 (1968).

364. Datey, K. K., Nanda, N. C.: Hyperglycemia after acute myocardial infarction. New Engl. J. Med. **276**, 262 (1967).
365. Davey, M. G., Lüscher, E. F.: Release reactions of human platelets induced by thrombin and other agents. Biochim. biophys. Acta (Amst.) **165**, 490 (1968).
366. Davidson, P. C., Albrink, M. J.: Insulin resistance in hyperglyceridemia. Metabolism **14**, 1059 (1965).
367. — — Abnormal plasma insulin response with high plasma triglycerides independent of clinical diabetes or obesity. (Abs.) J. clin. Invest. **45**, 1000 (1966).
368. Davies, M. J., Woolf, N., Bradley, J. P. W.: Endothelialisation of experimentally produced mural thrombi in the pig aorta. J. Path. **97**, 589 (1969).
369. Davignon, J., Simmonds, W. J., Ahrens, E. H., Jr.: Usefulness of chromic oxide as an internal standard for balance studies in formula-fed patients and for assessment of colonic function. J. clin. Invest. **47**, 127 (1968).
370. Dawber, T. R., Kannel, W. B., McNamara, P. M.: The prediction of coronary heart disease. Trans. Ass. Life Insur. med. Dir. Amer. **47**, 70 (1964).
371. Day, A. J.: Lipid metabolism by macrophages and its relationship to atherosclerosis. In: R. Paoletti and D. Kritchevsky (eds.), *Advances in lipid research*, vol. 5, p. 185. New York: Academic Press 1967.
372. — Incorporation of oleic acid into combined lipid by foam cells from rabbit atheromatous lesions. J. Atheroscler. Res. **9**, 141 (1969).
373. — Fidge, N. H., Wilkinson, G. N.: Effect of cholesterol in suspension on the incorporation of phosphate into phospholipid by macrophages *in vitro*. J. Lipid Res. **7**, 132 (1966).
374. — Gould-Hurst, P. R. S.: Esterfication of ^{14}C-labeled cholesterol by reticuloendothelial cells. Quart. J. exp. Physiol. **46**, 376 (1961).
375. — — Cholesterol esterase activity of normal and atheromatous rabbit aorta. Biochim. biophys. Acta (Amst.) **116**, 169 (1966).
376. — Newman, H. A. I., Zilversmit, D. B.: Synthesis of phospholipid by foam cells isolated from rabbit atherosclerotic lesions. Circulat. Res. **19**, 122 (1966).
377. — Tume, R. K.: *In vitro* incorporation of ^{14}C-labeled oleic acid into combined lipid by foam cells isolated from rabbit atheromatous lesions. J. Atheroscler. Res. **9**, 141 (1969).
378. — Wahlqvist, M. L.: Uptake and metabolism of ^{14}C-labeled oleic acid by atherosclerotic lesions in rabbit aorta. A biochemical and radioautographic study. Circulat. Res. **23**, 779 (1968).
379. — — Localization by autoradiography of phospholipid synthesis in rabbit atherosclerotic aorta. Exp. molec. Path. **11**, 263 (1969).
380. — Wilkinson, G. K.: Incorporation of ^{14}C labeled acetate into lipid by isolated foam cells and by atherosclerotic arterial intima. Circulat. Res. **21**, 593 (1967).
381. Day, C. E., Levy, R. S.: Determination of the molecular weight of apoprotein subunits from low density lipoprotein by gel filtration. J. Lipid. Res. **9**, 789 (1968).
382. Dayton, S., Hashimoto, S.: Movement of labeled cholesterol between plasma lipoprotein and normal arterial wall across the intimal surface. Circulat. Res. **19**, 1041 (1966).
383. — Pearce, M. L.: Prevention of coronary heart disease and other complications of atherosclerosis by modified diet. Amer. J. Med. **46**, 751 (1969).
384. — — Hashimoto, S. D., Dixon, W. J., Tomiyasu, W.: A controlled clinical trial of a diet high in unsaturated fat in preventing complications of atherosclerosis. Circulation, **40**, Suppl. II, 1 (1969).
385. Dearborn, D. G., Wetlaufer, D. B.: Reversible thermal conformation changes in human serum low-density lipoprotein. Proc. nat. Acad. Sci. (Wash.) **62**, 179 (1969).
386. De Lalla, O., Gofman, J. W.: Ultracentrifugal analysis of serum lipoproteins. In: D. Glick (ed.), *Methods of biochemical analysis*, vol. 1, p. 459. New York: Interscience Publishers, Inc. 1954.

387. Dempsey, M. E.: Inhibition of lipid biosynthesis. Ann. N. Y. Acad. Sci. **148**, 631 (1968).
388. — Δ^7-sterol Δ^5-dehydrogenase and $\Delta^{5,7}$-sterol Δ^7-reductase of rat liver. In: R. B. Clayton (ed.), *Steroids and terpenoids*, vol. 15, Methods in enzymology, p. 501. New York: Academic Press 1969.
389. Denny-Brown, D., Meyer, J. S.: The cerebral collateral circulation. 2. Production of cerebral infarction by ischemic anoxia and its reversibility in early stages. Neurology (Minneap.) 7, 567 (1957).
390. Des Prez, R. M., Horowitz, H. I., Hook, E. W., Jr.: Effects of bacterial endotoxin on rabbit platelets. I. Platelet aggregation and release of platelet factors *in vitro*. J. exp. Med. **114**, 857 (1961).
391. Detzer, S., Stampfl, B., Wetzstein, R.: Gestaltwandel der Thrombozyten in experimentelen Thrombus. Verh. anat. Ges. **115**, 221 (1965).
392. Dietschy, J. M.: The role of bile salts in controlling the rate of intestinal cholesterologenesis. J. clin. Invest. **47**, 286 (1968).
393. — Wilson, J. D.: Cholesterol synthesis in the squirrel monkey: relative rates of synthesis in various tissues and mechanisms of control. J. clin. Invest. **47**, 166 (1968).
394. Dintenfass, L.: Rehological approach to thrombosis and atherosclerosis. Angiology **15**, 333 (1964).
395. — Rozenberg, M. C.: The influence of the velocity gradient on *in vitro* blood coagulation and artificial thrombosis. J. Atheroscler. Res. **5**, 276 (1965).
396. Doerr, W.: Perfusionstheorie der Arteriosklerose. In W. Bargmann and W. Doerr (eds.), Zwanglose Abhandlungen aus dem Gebiet der normalen und pathologischen Anatomie. H. 13. Stuttgart: Georg Thieme 1963.
397. Dole, V. P.: A relation between non-esterified fatty acids in plasma and the metabolism of glucose. J. clin. Invest. **35**, 150 (1956).
398. Donath, W. F. H., DeLangen, C. D.: Vitamin D sclerosis of the arteries and the danger of feeding extra vitamin D to older people with a view on the development of different forms of arteriosclerosis. Proc. kon. ned. Akad. Wet. C **60**, No. 1 (1957).
399. Douglas, W. W.: Stimulus-secretion coupling: the concept and clues from chromaffin and other cells. Brit. J. Pharmacol. **34**, 451 (1968).
400. Doyle, J. T.: Etiology of coronary disease: risk factors influencing coronary disease. Mod. conc. cardiov. Dis. **35**, 81 (1966).
401. — Dawber, T. R., Kannel, W. B., Kinch, S. H., Kahn, H. A.: The relationship of cigarette smoking to coronary heart disease. J. Amer. med. Ass. **190**, 108 (1964).
402. — Kinch, S. H., Coronary heart disease in the United States: some preliminary findings from the pooling project of the Council on Epidemiology of the American Heart Association. Circulation **40**, Suppl. III, 72 (1969).
403. Dreyfuß, F., Shanan, J., Sharon, M.: Some personality characteristics of middle-aged men with coronary artery disease. Psychosom. **14**, 1 (1966).
404. Dubber, A. H. C., Rifkind, B., Gale, M., McNicol, G. P., Douglas, A. S.: The effect of fat feeding on fibrinolysis, "Stypven" time and platelet aggregation. J. Atheroscler. Res. **7**, 225 (1967).
405. Duff, G. L., McMillan, G. C.: The effect of alloxan diabetes on experimental cholesterol atherosclerosis in the rabbit. I. The inhibition of experimental cholesterol atherosclerosis in alloxan diabetes. J. exp. Med. **89**, 611 (1949).
406. — — Pathology of atherosclerosis. Amer. J. Med. **11**, 92 (1951).
407. — Payne, T. P. B.: The effect of alloxan diabetes on experimental cholesterol atherosclerosis in the rabbit. III. The mechanism of the inhibition of experimental cholesterol atherosclerosis in alloxan-diabetic rabbits. J. exp. Med. **92**, 299 (1950).
408. Duguid, J. B.: Thrombosis as a factor in the pathogenesis of coronary atherosclerosis. J. Path. Bact. **58**, 207 (1946).

409. Duguid, J. B.: Thrombosis as a factor in the pathogenesis of aortic atherosclerosis. J. Path. bact. **60**, 57 (1948).
410. — Pathogenesis of atherosclerosis. Lancet **1949 II**, 925.
411. — The arterial lining. Lancet **1952 II**, 207.
412. Duncan, C. H., Best, M. M., Despopoulos, A.: Inhibition of hepatic secretion of triglyceride by chlorophenoxyisobutyrate (CPIB). (Abs.) Circulation **30**, Suppl. III, 7 (1964).
413. Duncan, L. E.: Mechanical factors in the localization of atheromata. In: R. J. Jones (ed.), *The evolution of the atherosclerotic plaque*, p. 171. Chicago: Chicago University Press 1963.
414. — Buck, K., Lynch, A.: The effect of pressure and stretching on the passage of labeled albumin into canine aortic wall. J. Atheroscler. Res. **5**, 69 (1965).
415. Dustan, H. P., Schneckloth, R. E., Corcoran, A. C., Page, I. H.: The effectiveness of long-term treatment of malignant hypertension. Circulation **18**, 644 (1958).
416. Eastwood, M. A., Girdwood, R. H.: Lignin, a bile-salt sequestrating agent. Lancet **1968 II**, 1170.
417. — Hamilton, D.: Studies on the absorption of bile salt to non absorbed components of the diet. Biochim. biophys. Acta (Amst.) **152**, 156 (1968).
418. Eaton, R. P., Berman, M., Steinberg, D.: Kinetic studies of plasma free fatty acid and triglyceride metabolism in man. J. clin. Invest. **48**, 1560 (1969).
419. Eber, L. M., Kemp, H. G., Gorlin, R.: Short term changes in coronary atherosclerosis determined by coronary arteriography. Circulation Suppl. VI, **38**, 7 (1968).
420. Eder, H. A., Russ, E. M., Pritchett, R. A. R., Wilber, M. M., Barr, D. P.: Protein-lipid relationships in human plasma: in biliary cirrhosis, obstructive jaundice, and acute hepatitis. J. clin. Invest. **34**, 1147 (1955).
421. Egeberg, O., Owren, P. A.: Oral contraception and blood coagulability. Brit. med. J. **1963 I**, 220.
422. Eggen, D. A., Solberg, L. A.: Variation of atherosclerosis with age. Lab. Invest. **18**, 571 (1968).
423. Ehrlich, J. C., Shinohara, Y.: Low incidence of coronary thrombosis in myocardial infarction. A restudy by serial block technique. Arch. Path. **78**, 432 (1964).
424. Eiken, O.: Thrombotic occlusion of experimental grafts as a function of the regional blood flow. Acta chir. scand. **121**, 410 (1961).
425. Einarsson, K.: On the properties of the 12α-hydroxylase in cholic acid biosynthesis. Europ. J. Biochem. **5**, 101 (1968).
426. — Studies on the biosynthesis of bile acids. Opusc. med. (Stockh.) Suppl. **19** (1968).
427. Eisen, M. N., Little, J. R., Osterland, C. K., Simms, E. S.: Cold Spr. Harb. Symp. quant. Biol. **32**, 75 (1967).
428. Emmons, P. R., Hampton, J. R., Harrison, M. J. G., Honour, A. J., Mitchell, J. R. A.: Effect of prostaglandin E_1 on platelet behaviour *in vitro* and *in vivo*. Brit. med. J. **1967 II**, 468.
429. — Harrison, M. J. G., Honour, A. J., Mitchell, J. R. A.: Effect of dipyridamole on human platelet behavior. Lancet **1965 II**, 603.
430. Eneroth, P., Gordon, B., Ryhage, R., Sjövall, J.: Identification of mono- and dihydroxy bile acids in human feces by gas-liquid chromatography. J. Lipid Res. **7**, 511 (1966).
431. — — Sjövall, J.: Characterization of trisubstituted cholanoic acids in human feces. J. Lipid. Res. **7**, 524 (1966).
432. — Hellstrom, K., Sjövall, J.: A method for quantitative determination of bile acids in human feces. Acta chem. scand. **22**, 1729 (1968).
433. Engelberg, H.: Cigarette smoking and *in vitro* thrombosis of human blood. J. Amer. Ass. **193**, 1033 (1965).
434. Enos, W. F., Jr, Beyer, J. C., Holmes, R. H.: Pathogenesis of coronary disease in American soldiers killed in Korea. J. Amer. med. Ass. **158**, 912 (1955).

435. Epstein, F. H.: The epidemiology of coronary artery disease. A review. J. chron. Dis. **18**, 735 (1965).
436. — Hyperglycemia, a risk factor in coronary heart disease. Circulation **36**, 609 (1967).
437. — Predicting coronary heart disease. J. Amer. med. Ass. **201**, 795 (1967).
438. — Some uses of prospective observations in the Tecumseh Community Study. Proc. roy. Soc. Med. **60**, 56 (1967).
439. — Ostrander, L. D., Johnson, B. C., Payne, M. W., Hayner, N. C., Keller, J. B., Francis, T.: Epidemiological studies of cardiovascular diseases in a total community—Tecumseh, Michigan. Ann. intern. Med. **62**, 1170 (1965).
440. Erichson, R. B., Citron, J. R.: Ultrastructural observations on platelet adhesion reactions: III. Platelet interaction with collagen and platelets. Thrombos. Diathes. haemorrh. (Stuttg.) **18**, 80 (1968).
441. Erickson, B. A., Coots, R. H., Mattson, F. H., Kligman, A. M.: The effect of partial hydrogenation of dietary fats, of the ratio of polyunsaturated to saturated fatty acids, and of dietary cholesterol upon plasma lipids in man. J. clin. Invest. **43**, 2017 (1964).
442. Evans, G., Mustard, J. F.: Platelet surface reaction and thrombosis. Surgery **64**, 273 (1968).
443. — Packham, M. A., Nishizawa, E. E., Mustard, J. F., Murphy, E. A.: The effect of acetylsalicylic acid on platelet function. J. exp. Med. **128**, 877 (1968).
444. Ewing, A. M., Freeman, N. K., Lindgren, F. T.: Analysis of human serum lipoprotein distributions. In: R. Paoletti and D. Kritchevsky (eds.), *Advances in lipid research*, vol III, p. 25. New York: London Academic Press 1965.
445. Eyssen, H., Sacquet, E., Evrard, E., Van den Bosch, J.: Effect of neomycin on cholesterol levels and bile acid excretion in germfree and conventional rats. Life Sci. **7**, 1155 (1968).
446. Fabry, P., Fodor, J., Hejl, Z., Geizerova, H., Balcarova, O., Zvolankova, K.: Meal frequency and ischaemic heart disease. Lancet **1968 II**, 190.
447. Fahey, J. L., McKelvey, E.: Quantitative determination of serum immunoglobulines in antibody-agar plates. J. Immunol. **94**, 84 (1965).
448. Faloona, G. R., Stewart, B. N., Fried, M.: The effects of actinomycin D on the biosynthesis of plasma lipoproteins. Biochem. **7**, 720 (1968).
449. Farquhar, J. W., Frank, A., Gross, R. C., Reaven, G. M.: Glucose, insulin, and triglyceride responses to high and low carbohydrate diets in man. J. clin. Invest. **45**, 1648 (1966).
450. — Gross, R. C., Wagner, R. M., Reaven, G. M.: Validation of an incompletely coupled two-compartment nonrecycling catenary model for turnover of liver and plasma triglyceride in man. J. Lipid Res. **6**, 119 (1965).
451. Farquhar, W., Hirsch, R. L., Ahrens, E. H.: Evidence that atheroma fatty acids are in flux. J. clin. Invest. **39**, 984 (1960).
452. Fauvert, R., Hartmann, R., Mallarme, J., Boivin, P.: Renseignements fournis par l'étude quantitative des protéines sériques au cours de 85 cas de maladie de Kahler. Rev. Prat. (Paris) **9**, 1749 (1959).
453. Feenstra, D. L., Wilkens, J. N.: Cholesterol on Vitamine D. Ned. T. Geneesk. **109**, 615 (1965).
454. Fejfar, Z.: Arterial hypertension, atherosclerosis and ischaemic heart disease. Med. Today (Karachi), **2**, 36 (1968).
455. Felts, J. M.: The metabolism of chylomicron triglyceride fatty acids by perfused rat livers and by intact rats. Ann. N. Y. Acad. Sci. **131**, 24 (1965).
456. Ferry, C. B.: The autonomic nervous system. Ann. Rev. Pharmacol. **7**, 185 (1967).
457. Filshie, I., Scott, G. B. D.: The organization of experimental venous thrombi. J. Path. Bact. **76**, 71 (1958).
458. Fimognari, G. M., Rodwell, V. W.: Cholesterol biosynthesis Mevalonate synthesis inhibited by bile salts. Science **147**, 1038 (1965).
459. Fischer, S.: Simple and atherogenic thrombosis in the coronary vessels. J. Atheroscler. Res. **4**, 230 (1964).

460. Fisher, H., Griminger, P.: Cholesterol lowering effect of certain grains and of oat fraction in the chick. Proc. Soc. exp. Biol. Med. (N. Y.) **126**, 108 (1967).
461. — — Siher, W. G.: Effect of pectin on atherosclerosis in the cholesterol fed rabbit. J. Atheroscler. Res. **7**, 381 (1967).
462. Fleischman, A. I., Hayton, T., Bierenbaum, M. L., Wildrick, E.: Serum lipid assay by automated methods: Analysis of variation in sample preparation and automated chemistry. In: *Analytical chemistry*. Proc. Technicon Symposium, vol. 1, p. 21. New York: Mediad 1958.
463. — Yacowitz, H., Hayton, T., Bierenbaum, M. L.: Long term studies on the hyperlipemic action of dietary calcium in mature male rats fed cocoa butter. J. Nutr. **91**, 151 (1967).
464. — — — — Effect of calcium and vitamin D3 upon the fecal excretion of some metals in the mature male rat fed a high fat cholesterol diet. J. Nutr. **95**, 19 (1968).
465. Flint, A., Jr.: Experimental researches into a new excretory function of the liver; consisting in the removal of cholesterine from the blood, and its discharge from the body in the form of stercorine. Amer. J. med. Sci. **44**, 305 (1962).
466. Florentin, R. A., Choi, B. H., Lee, K. T., Thomas, W. A.: Stimulation of DNA synthesis and cell division *in vitro* by serum from cholesterol-fed swine. Cell Biol. **41**, 641 (1969).
467. — Lee, K. T., Daoud, A. S., Davies, J. N. P., Hall, E. W., Goodale, F.: Geographic pathology of arteriosclerosis. A study of the age of onset of significant arteriosclerosis in adult Africans and New Yorkers. Exp. molec. Path. **2**, 103 (1963).
468. — Nam, S. C.: Dietary-induced atherosclerosis in miniature swine. I. Gross and light microscopy observations: Time of development and morphologic characteristics of lesions. Exp. molec. Path. **8**, 263 (1968).
469. — — Lee, K. T., Thomas, W. A.: Increased ^{3}H-thymidine incorporation into endothelial cells of swine fed cholesterol for three days. Exp. molec. Path. **10**, 250 (1969).
470 — — — — Increased mitotic activity in aortas of swine after 3 days of cholesterol feeding. Arch. Path. **88**, 463 (1969).
471. Florey, H. W.: Microscopical observations on the circulation of the blood in the cerebral cortex. Brain **48**, 43 (1925).
472. — Greer, S. J., Kiser, J., Poole, J. C. F., Telander, R., Werthessen, N. T.: The development of the pseudointima lining fabric grafts of the aorta. Brit. J. exp. Path. **43**, 655 (1962).
473. Fodor, I., Vazrik, M., Felt, V.: Investigations of coronary insufficiency in epidemiological aspect. In: Modern problems of cardiology, p. 275. Moscow 1960.
474. Fodor, J., Miall, W. E., Standard, K. L., Fejfar, Z., Stuart, K. L.: Myocardial disease in a rural population in Jamaica. Bull. Wd. Hlth. Org. **31**, 321 (1964).
475. Folch, J., Lees, M., Sloane, Stanley, G. H.: A simple method for the isolation and purification of total lipids from animal tissues. J. biol. Chem. **226**, 497 (1957).
476. Fontaine, R., Bollack, C., Ebel, A., Pantesco, V.: Les altérations structurales déclenchées par certains enzymes au cours de l'artériosclérose expérimentale du lapin et les répercussions biochimiques de cell-ci sur le collagène de la paroi aortique. In: Centre National de la Recherche Scientifique (eds.), Le rôle de la paroi artérielle dans l'athérogenèse, p. 913. Paris (1967).
477. Foote, J. L., Coles, E.: Cerebrosides of human aorta: isolation, identification of the hexose, and fatty acid distribution. J. Lipid Res. **9**, 482 (1968).
478. Ford, S., Jr., Bozian, R. C., Knowles, H. C., Jr.: Interactions of obesity, and glucose and insulin levels in hypertriglyceridemia. Am. J. clin. Nutr. **21**, 904 (1968).
479. Forman, D. T., Garvin, J. E., Forestner, J. E., Taylor, C. B.: Increased excretion of fecal bile acids by an oral hydrophilic colloid. Proc. Soc. exp. Biol. Med. (N.Y.) **127**, 1060 (1968).

480. Forte, G. M., Nichols, A. V., Glaeser, R. M.: Electron microscopy of human serum lipoproteins using negative staining. Chem. Phys. Lip. **2**, 396 (1968).
481. — — — Structure of high-density serum lipoproteins after partial or complete delipidation. Biophys. J. **9**, A-111 (1969).
482. Frame, B., Pachter, R. M., Nixon, R. K.: Myelomatosis with xanthomatosis. Ann. intern. Med. **54**, 134 (1961).
483. Frank, C. W., Weinblatt, E., Shapiro, S., Sager, R. V.: Myocardial infarction in men. Role of physical activity and smoking in incidence and mortality. J. Amer. Med. Ass. **198**, 1241 (1966).
484. — — — — Prognosis of coronary heart disease. Presented at 41st Scientific Sessions, Amer. Heart Assoc. (1968).
485. — — — — Prognosis of men with coronary heart disease as related to blood pressure. Circulation **38**, 432 (1968).
486. Frantz, I. D., Jr., Schroepfer, G. J., Jr.: Sterol biosynthesis. Ann. Rev. Biochem. **36**, 691 (1967).
487. Fredrickson, D. S., Lees, R. S.: System for phenotyping hyperlipoproteinemia. Circulation **31**, 321 (1965).
488. — — Familia hyperlipoproteinemia. In: J. B. Stanburg, J. B., Wyngaarden and D. S. Fredrickson (eds.), *The metabolic basis of inherited disease*, p. 430. New York: McGraw-Hill 1966.
489. — Levy, R. I., Lees, R. S.: Fat transport in lipoproteins—an integrated approach to mechanisms and disorders. New Engl. J. Med. **276**, 34, 94, 148, 215, 273 (1967).
490. — Ono, K., Davis, L. L.: Lipolytic activity of post-heparin plasma in hyperglyceridemia. J. Lipid Res. **4**, 24 (1963).
491. Freis, E. D.: Hypertension and atherosclerosis. Amer. J. Med. **46**, 735 (1969).
492. French, J. E.: Thrombosis as a factor in atherosclerosis. Angiology **17**, 590 (1966).
493. — Atherosclerosis in relation to the structure and function of the arterial intima. Int. Rev. exp. Path. **5**, 253 (1966).
494. — The fine structure of experimental thrombi. Proc. Conf. on Thrombosis. Nat. Acad. Sci., Washington, 1967, in press (1969).
495. — MacFarlane, R. G.: Haemostasis and thrombosis. In: Lord Florey (ed.), *General pathology*, 4th ed. London: Lloyd-Luke 1970.
496. — — Sanders, A. G.: The structure of haemostatic plug and experimental thrombi in small animals. Brit. J. exp. Path. **45**, 2167 (1964).
497. Frey, J.: Contribution à la connaisance du métabolisme physiologique du collagène fondée sur une étude de la biosynthèse de l'hydroxyproline protéinique. Thesis. Fac. Sciencies Lyon 1969.
498. Friedberg, C. K.: Diseases of the heart, second edit. Philadelphia: W. B. Saunders, Co. 1956.
499. Friedberg, S. J., Klein, R. F., Trout, D. L., Bogdonoff, M. D., Estes, E. H., Jr.: The incorporation of plasma free fatty acids into plasma triglycerides in man. J. clin. Invest. **40**, 1846 (1961).
500. Friedman, M., Byers, S. O.: Induction of thrombi upon prexisting arterial plaques Amer. J. Path. **46**, 567 (1965).
501. — Van den Bovenkamp, G. J.; The pathogenesis of a coronary thrombus. Amer. J. Path. **48**, 19 (1966).
502. Fritsch, H., Urbaschek, B.: Studies on small blood vessels during the early phase of endotoxin administration using the raster electron microscope. Proc. Gravenbrüch, Heidelberg Symposium on Platelets and the Vessel Wall, Fibrin Deposition. Stuttgart: Thieme 1969.
503. Frost, H., Hess, H.: Untersuchungen zur Pathogenese der arteriellen Verschlußkrankheiten. III. Ein Modell zum Studium der Pathogenese der Kälteangiitis. Klin. Wschr. **47**, 507 (1969).
504. — — Richter, J. E.: Untersuchungen zur Pathogenese der arteriellen Verschlußkrankheiten; eine neue methode zum Studium früher Veränderungen auf der Gefäßwand. Klin. Wschr. **46**, 1099 (1968).

505. Fulton, G. P., Akers, R. P., Lutz, B. R.: White thromboemboli and vascular fragility in hamster cheek pouch after anticoagulants. Blood **8**, 140 (1953).
506. Furchner, J. E., Richmond, C. R.: Effect of dietary zinc on the absorption of orally administered Zn^{65}. Hlth. Phys. **8**, 35 (1962).
507. Furman, R. H., Sanbar, S. S., Alaupovic, P., Bradford, R. M., Howard, R. P.: Studies on the metabolism of radio-iodinated human serum alpha lipoprotein in normal and hyperlipidemic subjects. J. Lab. clin. Med. **63**, 193 (1964).
508. Gaarder, A., Jonsen, J., Laland, S., Hellem, A., Owren, P. A.: Adenosine diphosphate in red cells as a factor in the adhesiveness of human blood platelets. Nature (Lond.) **192**, 531 (1961).
509. Gan, J. C., Narashimha Murthy, P. V., Nichols, C. W., Chaikoff, I. L.: Mucosubstances in the chicken aorta. Part 1. Changes with age in acid mucopolysaccharides, glycoproteins, collagen and elastin. J. Atheroscler. Res. **7**, 629 (1967).
510. Garcia Palmieri, M. R.: Epidemiological study of coronary heart disease in Puerto Rico. Proc. VIIIth Interamerican Congress of Cardiology. Lima, Peru 1968.
511. — Feliberti, M., Costas, R., Benson, H., Blanton, J. H., Aixala, R,; Coronary heart disease mortality — a death certificate study. J. chrn. Dis. **18**, 1317 (1965).
512. Gardais, A., Picard, J. Tarasse, C.: Micro-fractionnement et micro-dosage des glycosaminoglycanes par électrophorèse sur bandes d'acétate de cellulose gélatinisées. J. Chromatog. **42**, 396 (1969).
513. Garfinkel, A. S., Baker, N., Schotz, M. C.: Relationship of lipoprotein lipase activity to triglyceride uptake in adipose tissue. J. Lipid Res. **8**, 274 (1967).
514. Geer, J. C.: Fine structure of human aortic intimal thickening and fatty streaks. Lab. Invest. **14**, 1764 (1965).
515. — Catsulis, C., McGill, H. C., Strong, J. P.: Fine structure of the baboon aortic fatty streak. Amer. J. Path. **52**, 265 (1968).
516. — Guidry, M. A.: Cholesteryl ester composition and morphology of human normal intima and fatty streaks. Exp. molec. Path. **3**, 485 (1964).
517. — Malcom, G. T.: Cholesterol ester fatty acid composition of human aorta fatty streaks and normal intima. Exp. molec. Path. **4**, 500 (1965).
518. Geiringer, E.: Intimal vascularization and atherosclerosis. J. Path. Bact. **63**, 201 (1951).
519. Geissinger, H. D., Mustard, J. F., Rowsell, H. C.: The occurrence of microthrombi on the aortic endothelium of swine. Canad. med. Ass. J. **87**, 405 (1962).
520. Gelin, J., Elgrishi, I., Ducimetière, P., Richard, J. L.: L'électrocardiogramme dans une population à haut risque. In: Enquête épidémiologique sur les facteur de l'athérosclérose. Bull. Inst. nat. Santé Rech. Méd. **22**, No. 2 (1961).
521. Gelin, L. E.: The significance of intravascular aggregation following tissue injury. Bull. Soc. int. Chir. **18**, 4 (1959).
522. Gerber, G. V., Gerber, G., Altman, K. I.: Studies on the metabolism of tissue proteins. I. Turnover of collagen labeled with proline $U^{14}C$ in young rats. J. biol. Chem. **235**, 2653 (1960).
523. Germuth, F. G., Senterfit, L. B., Pollack, A. D.: Immune complex disease. I. Experimental acute and chronic glomerulonephritis. J. Hopk. med. J. **120**, 225 (1967).
524. Gerő, S., Gergely, J., Jakab, L., Székely, J., Virág, S.: Comparative immunoelectrophoretic studies on homogenates of aorta, pulmonary arteries and inferior vena cava of atherosclerotic individuals. J. Atheroscler. Res. **1**, 88 (1961).
525. Gertler, M. M., Garn, M. G., Bland, E. F.: Age, serum cholesterol and coronary artery disease. Circulation **2**, 517 (1950).
526. — White, P. D.: Coronary artery disease in young adults, p. 177. Cambridge, Mass: Harvard University Press 1954.
527. Getty, R.: The gross and microscopic occurrence and distribution of spontaneous atherosclerosis in the arteries of swine. In: J. C. Roberts, Jr., and R. Straus (eds.), *Comparative atherosclerosis*, p. 11. New York: Hoeber Medical Division, Harper and Row 1965.

528. Getz, G. S., Vesselinovitch, D., Wissler, R. W.: A dynamic pathology of atherosclerosis. Amer. J. Med. **46**, 657 (1969).
529. — Wissler, R. W., Hughes, R. H., Graber, C., Tantra, S.: Lipid composition and biosynthesis of lecithin in atherosclerotic aorta of Rhesus monkey fed three food fats. (Abs.) Circulation **36**, II-13 (1967).
530. — — — Miller, L.: Composition and synthesis of lipids of atherosclerotic Rhesus monkey aortas. (Abs.) Circulation **34**, III-11 (1966).
531. Gisler, R., Pillot, J.: Activité anticardiolipide liée à un complexe macroglobuline de Waldenstrom IgG cryoprécipitant. Immunochemistry **5**, 543 (1968).
532. Glaumann, H., Dallner, G.: Lipid composition and turnover of rough and smooth microsomal membranes in rat liver. J. Lipid Res. **9**, 720 (1968).
533. Glazunov, I. C.: On the level of blood cholesterol and increase of myocardial infarction in some cities of the USSR. Cardiologia (Basel) **3**, 130 (1961).
534. Glomset, J. A.: The plasma lecithin: cholesterol acyl-transferase reaction. J. Lipid Res. **9**, 155 (1968).
535. — Janssen, E. T., Kennedy, R., Dobbins, J.: Role of plasma lecithin: cholesterol acyltransferase in the metabolism of high density lipoproteins. J. Lipid Res. **7**, 638 (1966).
536. Glueck, C. J., Brown, W. V., Levy, R. I., Greten, H., Fredrickson, D. S.: Amelioration of hypertriglyceridemia by progestational drugs in familia Type V hyperlipoproteinemia. Lancet **1969 I**, 1290.
537. — Levy, R. I., Fredrickson, D. S.: Immunoreactive insulin, glucose tolerance and carbohydrate inducibility in familial endogenous hypertriglyceridemia. (Abs.) Clin. Res. **16**, 343 (1968).
538. — — Glueck, H. I., Gralnick, H. R., Kaplan, A. P., Barth, W. F., Fredrickson, D. S.: Low post-heparin lipolytic activity and exogenous fat intolerance associated with abnormal heparin resistance and heparin binding globulins. Circulation, **38**, Suppl. VI, 7 (1968).
539. Glueck, H. I., Hong, R.: A circulating anticoagulant in γ_{1A}-multiple myeloma: its modification by penicillin. J. clin. Invest. **44**, 1866 (1965).
540. Glynn, M. F., Mustard, J. F., Buchanan, M. R., Murphy, E. A.: Cigarette smoking and platelet aggregation. Canad. med. Ass. J. **95**, 549 (1966).
541. Gofman, J. W., Hanig, M., Jones, H. B., Lauffer, M. A., Lawry, E. Y., Lewis, L. A., Mann, G. V., Moore, F. E., Olmsted, F., Yeager, J. F., Andrus, E. C., Barach, J. H., Beams, J. W., Fertig, J. W., Page, I. H., Shannon, J. A., Stare, F. J., White, P. D.: Evaluation of serum lipoprotein and cholesterol measurements as predictors of clinical complications of atherosclerosis. Circulation **14**, 691 (1956).
542. — Ruhm, L., McGinley, J. P., Jones, H. B.: Hyperlipoproteinemia. Amer. J. Med. **17**, 514 (1954).
543. Goldsmith, G. A., Hamilton, J. G., Miller, O. N.: Investigation of mechanisms by which unsaturated fats, nicotinic acid and neomycin lower serum lipid concentrations: excretion of sterols and bile acids. Trans. Ass. Amer. Phycns. **72**, 207 (1959).
544. Golup, E. S., Spitznagel, J. K.: Dermal lesions induced by homologous PMN lysosomes. Fed. Proc. **23**, 509 (1964).
545. Goodman, D. S.: The *in vivo* turnover of individual cholesterol esters in human plasma lipoproteins. J. clin. Invest. **43**, 2026 (1964).
546. — Noble, R. P.: Turnover of plasma cholesterol in man. J. clin. Invest. **47**, 231 (1968).
547. Gorden, P., Roth, J.: Circulating insulins "big" and "little". Arch. intern. Med. **123**, 237 (1969).
548. Gordon, E. S.: Non-esterified fatty acids in the blood of obese and lean subjects. Amer. J. clin. Nutr. **8**, 740 (1960).
549. Gotte, L., Mamri, M., Pezzin, G.: Some structural aspects of elastin revealed by x-ray diffraction and other physical methods. In: W. G. Crewther (ed.), *Symposium on fibrous proteins*, p. 236. Australia: Butterworths 1968.

550. Gotto, A. M., Levy, R. I., Fredrickson, D. S.: Observations on the confirmation of human beta lipoprotein: evidence for the occurence of beta structure. Proc. nat. Acad. Sci. (Wash.) **60**, 1436 (1968).
551. — — — Preparation and properties of an apoprotein derivative of human serum β-lipoprotein. Lipids **3**, 463 (1968).
552. — Shore, B.: Conformation of human serum high-density lipoprotein and its peptide components. Nature (Lond.) **224**, 69 (1969).
553. Gould, B. S.: Collagen biosynthesis. In: BERNARD S. GOULD (ed.), *Biology of collagen*, vol. 2, p. 139. London-New York: Academic Press 1968.
554. Gould, R. G.: Absorbability of beta-sitosterol. Trans. N. Y. Acad. Sci. **18**, 129 (1955).
555. — Lotz, L. V., Lilly, E. M.: Absorption and metabolism of dihydrocholesterol and beta-sitosterol. In: G. J. POPJAK and E. LE BRETON (eds.), *Proceedings of the Second International Conference on biochemical problems of lipids*, Ghent, Belgium, 1955, p. 353. London: Butterworth & Co., Ltd. 1956.
556. — Swyrud, E. A.: Sites of control of hepatic cholesterol synthesis. J. Lipid Res. **7**, 698 (1966).
557. — — Avoy, D., Coan, B.: The effects of α-p-chlorophenoxyisobutyrate on the synthesis and release into plasma of lipoproteins in rats. Progr. Biochem. Pharmacol. **2**, 345 (1967).
558. — — Coan, B. J., Avoy, D. R.: Effects of chlorophenoxyisobutyrate (CPIB) on liver composition and triglyceride synthesis in rats. J. Atheroscler. Res. **6**, 555 (1966).
559. Graham, J. M., Green, C.: The binding of sterols in cellular membranes. Biochem. J. **103**, 16c (1967).
560. Granda, J. L., Scanu, A.: Solubilization and properties of the apoproteins of the very low- and low-density lipoproteins of human serum. Biochemistry **5**, 3301 (1966).
561. Grande, F.: Dietary carbohydrates and serum cholesterol. Amer. J. clin. Nutr. **20**, 176 (1967).
562. — Anderson, J. T., Keys, A.: The effect of carbohydrates of leguminous seeds, wheat and potatoes on serum cholesterol concentration in man. J. Nutr. **86**, 313 (1965).
563. Grant, L.: The sticking and emigration of white blood cells in inflammation. In: B. W. ZWEIFACH, L. GRANT and R. T. MCCLUSKEY (eds.), *The inflammatory process*. New York: Academic Press 1965.
564. Grant, M. E., Freeman, I. L., Schofield, J. D., Jackson, D. S.: Variations in the carbohydrate content of human and bovine polymeric collagens from various tissues. Biochem. biophys. Acta (Amst.) **177**, 682 (1969).
565. Green, J. G., Brown, H. B., Meredith, A. P., Page, I. H.: Use of fat-modified foods for serum cholesterol reduction. J. Amer. med. Ass. **183**, 5 (1963).
566. Green, K., Samuelsson, B.: Mechanism of bile acid biosynthesis studied with 3α-^{3}H- and 4β-^{3}H-cholesterol. J. biol. Chem. **239**, 2804 (1964).
567. Greenough, W. B., III. Crespin, S. R., Steinberg, D.: Hypoglycaemia and hyperinsulinaemia in response to raised free-fatty acid levels. Lancet **1967 II**, 1334.
568. Gresham, G. A., Howard, A. N.: The independent production of thrombosis and atherosclerosis in rats. Brit. J. exp. Path. **41**, 633 (1960).
569. Greten, H., Levy, R. I., Fredrickson, D. S.: A further characterization of lipoprotein lipase. Biochim. biophys. Acta (Amst.) **164**, 185 (1968).
570. — — — Evidence for separate monoglyceride hydrolase and triglyceride lipase in post-heparin human plasma. J. Lipid Res. **10**, 326 (1969).
571. Grette, K.: Studies on the mechanism of thrombin-catalyzed hemostatic reactions in blood platelets. Acta physiol. scand. **495**, Suppl. 56, 1 (1962).
572. Groden, B. M.: Return to work after myocardial infarction. Scot. med. J. **12**, 297 (1967).
573. Groen, J. J.: Effect of bread in the diet on serum cholesterol. Amer. J. clin. Nutr. **20**, 191 (1967).

574. Groen, J. J., Balogh, M., Yaron, E.: Effect of the Yeminite diet on the serum cholesterol of healthy non-Yemenite volunteers. Israel J. med. Sci. **2**, 196 (1966).
575. — Dreyfuss, F., Futtman, L.: Epidemiological, nutritional and sociological studies of atherosclerotic (coronary) heart disease among different ethnic groups in Israel. Progr. Biochem. Pharmacol. **4**, 20 (1968).
576. Grosgogeat, Y., Anguera, G., Lellouch, J., Jacotot, B., Beaumont, J. L.: L'intoxication chronique par la nicotine chez le lapin nourri au cholesterol. J. Atheroscler. Res. **5**, 291 (1965).
577. Gross, P., Weicker, H.: Die Bedeutung des Lipoidelektrophoresediagrammes. Klin. Wschr. **32**, 509 (1954).
578. Grundy, S. M., Ahrens, E. H., Jr.: An evaluation of the relative merits of two methods for measuring the balance of sterols in man: isotopic balance versus chromatographic analysis. J. clin. Invest. **45**, 1503 (1966).
579. — — Measurements of cholesterol turnover, synthesis and absorption in man, carried out by isotope kinetic and sterol balance methods. J. Lipid Res. **10**, 91 (1969).
580. — — Davignon, J.: The interaction of cholesterol absorption and cholesterol synthesis in man. J. Lipid Res. **10**, 304 (1969).
581. — — Miettinen, T. A.: Quantitative isolation and gas-liquid chromatographic analysis of total fecal bile acids. J. Lipid Res. **6**, 397 (1965).
582. — — Salen, G.: Dietary sitosterol as an internal standard to correct for cholesterol losses in sterol balance studies. J. Lipid Res. **9**, 374 (1968).
583. — — — Quintao, E.: Mode of action of Atromid-S on cholesterol metabolism in man. J. clin. Invest. **48**, 33a (1969).
584. — Hofman, A. F., Davignon, J., Ahrens, E. H., Jr.: Human cholesterol synthesis is regulated by bile acids. J. clin. Invest. **45**, 1018 (1966).
585. Grusin, H.: Peculiarities of the African's electrocardiogram and the changes observed in serial studies. Circulation **9**, 860 (1954).
586. Gunn, C. G., Friedman, M., Byers, S., O.: Effect of chronic hypothalamic stimulation upon cholesterol-induced atherosclerosis in the rabbit. J. clin. Invest. **39**, 1963 (1960).
587. Gunning, A. J., Pickering, G. W., Robb-Smith, A. H. T., Ross-Russell, R. W.: Mural thrombosis of the internal carotid artery and subsequent embolism. Quart. J. Med. **33**, 155 (1964).
588. Gurpide, E., Mann, Jr., Sandberg, E.: Determination of kinetic parameters in a two-pool system by administration of one or more tracers. Biochemistry **3**, 1250 (1964).
589. Gustafson, A.: Studies on human serum very low density lipoproteins. Acta med. scand. **179**, Suppl. 446 (1966).
590. — Alaupovic, P., Furman, R. H.: Studies of the composition and structure of serum lipoproteins. Separation and characterization of phospholipid-protein residues obtained by partial delipidization of very low-density lipoproteins of human serum. Biochemistry **5**, 632 (1966).
591. Guzmán, M. A., McMahan, C. A., McGill, H. C., Jr., Strong, J. P., Tejada, C., Restrepo, C., Eggen, D. A., Robertson, Wm. B., Solberg, L. A.: Selected methodologic aspects of the International Atherosclerosis Project. Lab. Invest. **18**, 479 (1968).
592. Haft, D. E., Roheim, P. S., White, A., Eder, H. A.: Plasma lipoprotein metabolism in perfused rat livers. I. Protein synthesis and entry into the plasma. J. clin. Invest. **41**, 842 (1962).
593. Hagerman, J. S., Gould, R. G.: The *in vitro* interchange of cholesterol between plasma and red cells. Proc. Soc. exp. Biol. Med. (N. Y.) **78**, 329 (1956).
594. Hales, C. N., Randle, P. J.: Immunoassay of insulin with insulin antibody precipitate. Lancet **1963 I**, 200.
595. Hall, A. D.: The identification and estimation of elastase in serum and plasma Biochem. J. **101**, 29 (1966).

596. Hallberg, D.: Cross-transfusion of lipoprotein lipase activity in dogs. Acta chir. scand. **134**, 327 (1968).
597. Halperin, M., Rogot, E., Gurian, J., Ederer, F.: Sample sizes for medical trials with special reference to long-term therapy. J. chron. Dis. **21**, 13 (1968).
598. Ham, A. W. (ed.): Histology, fifth edit. London: Pitman Medical Publ. Co., Ltd. 1965.
599. Hamilton, M., Thompson, E. N., Wisniewski, T. K. M.: The role of blood pressure control in preventing complications of hypertension. Lancet **1964 I**, 235.
600. Hamilton, R. L., Regen, D. M., Gray, M. E., LeQuire, V. S.: Lipid transport in liver. I. Electron microscopic identification of very low density lipoproteins in perfused rat liver. Lab. Invest. **16**, 305 (1967).
601. Hampton, J. R., Harrison, M. J. G., Honour, A. J., Mitchell, J. R. A.: Platelet behavior and drugs used in cardiovascular disease. Cardiovasc. Res. **1**, 101 (1967).
602. — Mitchell, J. R. A.: An estimate of the number of binding sites on human platelets. Nature (Lond.) **211**, 245 (1966).
603. Hand, R. A., Chandler, A. B.: Atherosclerotic metamorphosis of autologous pulmonary thromboemboli in the rabbit. Amer. J. Path. **40**, 469 (1962).
604. Hanig, M., Shainoff, J. R., Lowy, A. D.: Flotational lipoproteins extracted from human atherosclerotic aortas. Science **124**, 176 (1956).
605. Hansen, P. F., Geill, T., Lund, E.: Dietary fats and thrombosis. Lancet **1962 II**, 1193.
606. Harders, H.: Intravascular agglutination of erythrocytes. Schweiz. med. Wschr. **87**, 11 (1957).
607. Harkness, M. L. R., Harkness, R. D., McDonald, D. A.: The collagen and elastin content of the arterial wall in the dog. Proc. roy. Soc. **146**B, 541 (1957).
608. Harlan, W. R., Jr., Oberman, A., Mitchell, R. E., Graybiel, A.: Constitutional and environmental factors related to serum lipid and lipoprotein levels. Ann. intern. Med. **66**, 540 (1967).
609. — Winsett, P. S., Wasserman, A. J.: Tissue lipoprotein lipase in normal individuals and in individuals with exogenous hypertriglyceridemia and the relationship of this enzyme to assimilation of fat. J. clin. Invest. **46**, 239 (1967).
610. Harland, W. A., Holburn, A. M.: Coronary thrombosis and myocardial infarction. Lancet **1966 II**, 1158.
611. Harman, D.: Atherosclerosis: hypothesis concerning the initiating steps in pathogenesis. J. Geront. **12**, 199 (1957).
612. — Atherosclerosis: possible ill-effects of the use of highly unsaturated fats to lower serum cholesterol levels. Lancet **1957 II**, 1116.
613. — Atherosclerosis: effect of rate of growth. Circulat. Res. **10**, 851 (1962).
614. — Role of serum copper in coronary atherosclerosis. Circulation **28**, 658 (1963).
615. — Effect of dietary copper on rabbit atherosclerosis. Circulation **30**, III-12 (1964).
616. Harrington, M.., Kincaid-Smith, P., McMichael, J.: Results of treatment in malignant hypertension. Brit. med. J. **1959 II**, 969.
617. Harrison, C. V.: Experimental pulmonary atherosclerosis. J. Path. Bact. **60**, 289 (1948).
618. Harrison, J. H., Davalos, P. A.: Influence of porosity on synthetic grafts. Fate in animals. Arch. Surg. **82**, 8 (1961).
619. Harrison, M. J. G., Mitchell, J. R. A.: The influence of red blood-cells on platelet adhesiveness. Lancet **1966 II**, 1163.
620. Harrison, M. T., Harden, R. M.: Some effects of clofibrate in hypothyroidims and on the metabolism of thyroxine. Scot. med. J. **11**, 213 (1966).
621. Hartman, L., Boivin, P., Fauvert, R.: Macroglobulines et macroglobulinemies Exp. Ann. Biochem. Med. **19**, 13 (1957).
622. — Filitti-Wurmser, S., Leloevre-Ardaillow, N. Boivin, P.: Etude biologique des macroglobulines serqiues. Sang **31**, 491 (1960).
623. — — Ollier, M. P., Laudat, P.: Lipides, lipoproteines et immunoglobulines IgM. Ann. Biol. clin. **26**, 881 (1968).

624. Hartman, L., Ollier, M. P., Laudat, P., Ambert, J. P., Fillittei-Wurmses, S.: Etude des lipides et lipoproteines seriques dans la maladie de Waldenström. Ann. Biol. clin. **26**, 865 (1968).
625. Hashim, S. A., Arteaga, A., Van Itallie, T. B.: Effect of a saturated medium-chain triglyceride on serum-lipids in man. Lancet **1960 I**, 1105.
626. — Bergen, S. S., Jr., Van Itallie, T. B.: Experimental steatorrhea induced in man by bile salt sequestrant. Proc. Soc. exp. Biol. Med. (N.Y.) **106**, 173 (1961).
627. — Van Itallie, T. B.: Cholestyramine resin therapy for hypercholesterolemia. J. Amer. med. Ass. **192**, 289 (1965).
628. Hashimoto, S., Dayton, S.: Transfer of cholesterol and cholesterol esters into wall of rat aorta *in vitro*. J. Atheroscler. Res. **6**, 580 (1966).
629. Haslam, R. J.: Role of adenosine diphosphate in the aggregation of human blood platelets by thrombin and by fatty acids. Nature (Lond.) **202**, 765 (1964).
630. — Mechanism of blood platelet aggregation. In: S. A. Johnson and W. H. Seegers (eds), *Physiology of hemostasis and thrombosis*, p. 88. Springfield, Ill.: C. C. Thomas 1967.
631. Haslewood, G. A. D.: Comparative studies of "bile salts". 5. Bile salts of crocodylidae. Biochem. J. **52**, 583 (1952).
632. Hass, G. M.: Observations on vascular structure in relation to human and experimental arteriosclerosis. In: Symposium on Atherosclerosis, p. 24. National Academy of Sciences, National Research Council, Publ. 338, Washington, D. C. (1955).
633. Hatch, F. T. Lees, R. S. Practical methods for plasma lipoprotein analysis.Adv. Lipid Res. **6**, 1. (1968).
634. — Reissell, P. K., Poon-King, T. M. W., Canellos, G. P., Lees, R. S., Hagopian, L. M.: A study of coronary heart disease in young men — characteristics and metabolic studies of the patients and comparison with age-matched healthy men. Circulation **33**, 679 (1966).
635. Hauss, W. H., Berlach, U., Junge-Hulsing, G., Themann, H., Wirth, W.: Studies on the "nonspecific mesenchymal reaction" and the "transit zone" in myocardial lesions and atherosclerosis. Ann. N. Y. Acad. Sci. **156**, 207 (1969).
636. Haust, M. D.: Electron microscopic and immunohistochemical studies of fatty streaks in human aorta. In: C. J. Miras, A. Y. Howard and R. Paoletti (eds.), *Progr. Biochem. Pharmacol.*, vol. 4, p. 249. Basel-New York: S. Karger 1968.
637. — Balis, J. U., More, R. H.: Electron microscopy study of intimal lipid accumulations in human aorta and their pathogenesis. Circulation **26**, 656 (1962).
638. — More, R. H.: Significance of the smooth muscle cell in atherogenesis. In R. J. Jones (ed.), *Evolution of the atherosclerotic plaque*, p. 51. Chicago: Chicago University Press 1963.
639. — — Bencosme, S. A., Balis, J. U.: Electron microscopic studies in human atherosclerosis. Extracellular elements in aortic dots and streaks. Exp. molec. Path. **6**, 300 (1967).
640. — — Movat, H. Z.: The mechanism of fibrosis in arteriosclerosis. Amer. J. Path. **35**, 265 (1959).
641. — — — The role of smooth muscle cells in the fibrogenesis of arteriosclerosis. Amer. J. Path. **37**, 377 (1960).
642. — Wyllie, J. C., More, R. H.: Atherogenesis and plasma constituents. Amer. J. Path. **44**, 255 (1964).
643. — — — Electron-microscopy of fibrin in human atherosclerotic lesions. Immunohistochemical and morphologic identification. Exp. molec. Path. **4**, 205 (1965).
644. Havel, R. J.: Conversion of plasma free fatty acids into triglycerides of plasma lipoprotein fractions in man. Metabolism **10**, 1031 (1961).
645. — Metabolism of lipids in chylomicrons and very low-density lipoproteins. In: A. E. Renold and G. F. Cahill (eds.), *Handbook of physiology*, p. 499. Baltimore: The Williams & Wilkins Company 1965.

646. Havel, R. J.: Triglyceride and very low density lipoprotein turnover. In: G. Cowgill, D. L. Estrich, and P. D. Wood (eds.), *Proceedings of the 1968 Deul Conference on Lipids*, p. 115. Washington, D. C.: U. S. Government Printing Office 1968.
647. — Pathogenesis, differentiation and management of hypertriglyceridemia. In: G. Stollerman (ed.), *Advances in internal medicine*, vol. XV, p. 117. Chicago: Year Book Publishers 1969.
648. — Balasse, E. O., Williams, H. E., Kane, J. P., Segel, N.: Splanchnic metabolism in Von Gierke's disease (Glycogenosis Type I). Trans. Ass. Amer. Phycns, **82**, 305 (1969).
649. — Eder, H. A., Bragdon, J. H.: The distribution and chemical composition of ultracentrifugally separated lipoproteins in human serum. J. clin. Invest. **34**, 1345 (1955).
650. — Felts, J. M., Van Duyne, C. M.: Formation and fate of endogenous triglycerides in blood plasma of rabbits. J. Lipid Res. **3**, 297 (1962).
651. — Gordon, R. S., Jr.: Idiopathic hyperlipemia: metabolic studies in an affected family. J. clin. Invest. **39**, 1777 (1960).
652. Hayner, N. S., Kjelsberg, M. O., Epstein, F. H., Francis, T., Jr.: Carbohydrate tolerance and diabetes in a total community, Tecumseh, Michigan. I. Effects of age, sex and test conditions on one-hour glucose tolerance in adults. Diabetes **14**, 413 (1965).
653. Hazzard, W. R., Spiger, M. J., Bagdade, J. D., Bierman, E. L.: Studies on the mechanism of increased plasma triglyceride levels induced by oral contraceptives. New Engl. J. Med. **280**, 471 (1969).
654. Heard, B. E.: Mural thrombosis in the renal artery and its relation to atherosclerosis. J. Path. Bact. **61**, 635 (1949).
655. — An experimental study of thickening of pulmonary arteries of rabbits produced by organization of fibrin. J. Path. Bact. **64**, 13 (1952).
656. Hegsted, D. M., McGandy, R. B., Myers, M. L., Stare, F. J.: Quantitative effects of dietary fat on serum cholesterol in man. Amer. J. clin. Nutr. **17**, 281 (1965).
657. Hellem, A. J.: The adhesiveness of human blood platelets *in vitro*. Scand. J. clin. Lab. Invest. **12** (Suppl. 51), 63 (1960).
658. — Platelet adhesiveness. Ser. Haemat. **1**, 99 (1968).
659. Hellman, L., Rosenfeld, R. S., Eidinoff, M. L., Fukushima, D. K., Gallagher, T. F., Wang, C. I., Adlersberg, D.: Isotopic studies of plasma cholesterol of endogenous and exogenous origins. J. clin. Invest. **34**, 48 (1955) .
660. — — Insull, W., Jr., Ahrens, E. H., Jr.: Intestinal excretion of cholesterol: a mechanism for regulation of plasma levels. (Abs.) J. clin. Invest. **36**, 898 (1957).
661. — Zumoff, B., Kessler, G., Kara, E., Rubin, I. L., Rosenfeld, R. S.: Reduction of cholesterol and lipids in man by ethyl p-chlorophenoxyisobutyrate. Ann. intern. Med. **59**, 477 (1963).
662. — — — — — — Reduction of serum cholesterol and lipids by ethyl chlorophenosyisobutyrate. J. Atheroscler. Res. **3**, 454 (1963).
663. Hellström, K., Lindstedt, S.: Cholic acid turnover and biliary bile acid composition in humans with abnormal thyroid formation. J. Lab. clin. Med. **63**, 666 (1964).
664. — — Studies on the formation of cholic acid in subjects given standardized diet with butter or corn oil as dietary fat. Amer. J. clin. Nutr. **18**, 185 (1966).
665. Hemker, H. C., Esnouf, M. P., Hemker, P. W., Swart, A. C. W., MacFarlane, R. G. Formation of prothrombin converting activity. Nature (Lond.) **215**, 248 (1967).
666. — Kahn, M. J. P.: Reaction sequence of blood coagulation. Nature (Lond.) **215**, 1201 (1967).
667. Henschel, A., Mickelsen, O., Taylor, H. L., Keys, A.: Plasma volume and thiocyanate space in famine edema and recovery. Amer. J. Physiol. **150**, 170 (1947).
668. Henson, P. M., Cochrane, C. G.: Immunological induction of increased vascular permeability. II. Two mechanisms of histamine release from rabbit platelets involving complement. J. exp. Med. **129**, 167 (1969).

669. Henzel, J. A., Holtman, B., Keitzer, F., DeWeese, M., Lichti, E.: Trace elements in atherosclerosis; efficacy of zinc medication as a therapeutic modality. Second Annual Trace Metal Conference, Univ. of Mo. (1968).
670. Heptinstall, R. H.: The effects of high blood cholesterol on the pulmonary arterial changes produced in rabbits by the injection of blood clot. Brit. J. exp. Path. **38**, 438 (1957).
671. Heremans, J.: Les globulines sériques du système gamma. Leur nature et leur pathologie, p. 227. Bruxelles: Arscia S. A. 1960.
672. Herman, J. B., Keynan, A.: Hyperglycemia and uric acid. Israel J. med. Sci. **5**, 1048 (1969).
673. — Mount, F. W., Medalie, J. H., Groen, J. J., Dublin, T. D., Neufeld, H. N., Riss, E.: Diabetes prevalence and serum uric acid. Diabetes **16**, 858 (1967).
674. Hers, H. G.: Le metabolisme du fructose. Bruxelles: Editions Arsica 1957.
675. Hess, R., Bencze, W. L.: Hypolipidemic properties of a new tetralin derivative (CIBA 13,437-Su). Experientia (Basel) **24**, 418 (1968).
676. — Maier, R., Stäubli, W.: Evaluation of phenolic ethers as hypolipidemic agents. Abstracts 3rd International Symposium on Drugs Affecting Lipid Metabolism, in Milan, p. 47 (1968).
677. — Stäubli, W., Reiss, W.: Nature of the hepatomegalic effect produced by ethyl-chlorophenoxyisobutyrate in the rat. Nature (Lond.) **208**, 856 (1965).
678. Higgins, A. C., Pooler, W. S.: Myocardial infarction and subsequent re-employment in Syracuse, New York. Amer. J. Publ. Hlth **58**, 312 (1968).
679. Higgins, I. T. T., Cochrane, A. L., Thomas, A. J.: Epidemiological studies of coronary disease. Brit. J. prev. soc. Med. **17**, 153 (1963).
680. — Kannel, W. B., Dawber, T. R.: The electrocardiogram in epidemiological studies. Brit. J. prev. soc. Med. **19**, 53 (1965).
681. Hill, R. M., Mulligan, R. M., Dunlop, S. G.: Plasma cell myeloma associated with high concentration of plasma lipoproteins. Amer. J. Path. **24**, 688 (1948).
682. Hinkle, L. E., Jr, Carver, S. T., Stevens, M.: The frequency of asymptomatic disturbances of cardiac rhythm and conduction in middle aged men. Amer. J. Cardiol. **24**, 629 (1969).
683. — — — Plakun, E.: Asymptomatic dysrhythmias and subsequent coronary (Abs.) Circulation, Suppl. III to Vols. **39** and **40**, 107 (1969).
684. Hirsch, J., Ahrens, E. H., Jr.: The separation of complex lipide mixtures by the use of silicic acid chromatography. J. biol. Chem. **233**, 311 (1958).
685. — Gallian, E.: Methods for the determination of adipose cell size in man and animals. J. Lipid Res. **9**, 110 (1968).
686. — Goldrick, R. B.: Serial studies on the metabolism of human adipose tissue. I. Lipogenesis and free fatty acid uptake and release in small aspirated samples of subcutaneous fat. J. clin. Invest. **43**, 1776 (1964).
687. — Knittle, J. L., Salans, L. B.: Cell lipid content and cell number in obese and nonobese human adipose tissue. J. clin. Invest. **45**, 1023 (1966).
688. Hirsch, J. G.: Cinematographic observations on granule lysis in polymorphonuclear leukocytes during phagocytosis. Degranulation and release of granule-associated enzymes into soluble cell fractions during phagocytosis of microorganisms by rabbit polymorphonuclear leukocytes. J. exp. Med. **166**, 827 (1962).
689. Hirsh, J., Buchanan, M., Glynn, M. F., Mustard, J. F.: Effect of streptokinase on haemostasis. Blood **32**, 726 (1968).
690. Ho, K. J., Taylor, C. B.: Comparative studies on tissue cholesterol. Arch. Path. **86**, 585 (1968).
691. — — Biss, K., Mikkelson, B.: Studies on cholesterol metabolism in the Masai. (Abs.) Fed. Proc. **27**, 440 (1968).
692. Holland, W. W., Elliott, A.: Cigarette smoking, respiratory symptoms, and anti-smoking propaganda. Lancet **1968 I**, 41.
693. Hollander, W.: Recent advances in experimental and molecular pathology. Influx, synthesis and transport of arterial lipoproteins in atherosclerosis. Exp. molec. Path. **7**, 248 (1967).

694. Hållander, W., Chobanian, A. V.: Comparative effects of d-thyroxin and ethyl-p-chloro-phenoxyisobutyrate on body cholesterol metabolism in man. Circulation **33**, 18 (1965).
695. — Kramsch, D. M.: The distribution of intravenously administered ^{3}H-cholesterol in arteries and other tissues. Part I. J. Atheroscler. Res. **7**, 491 (1967).
696. — — Inoune, G.: The metabolism of cholesterol, lipoproteins and acid mucopolysaccharides in normal and atherosclerotic vessels. Progr. Biochem. Pharmacol. **4**, 270 (1968).
697. Hollister, L. E., Overall, J. E., Snow, H. L.: Relationship of obesity to serum triglyceride, cholesterol, and uric acid, and to plasma glucose levels. Amer. J. clin. Nutr. **20**, 777 (1967).
698. Holman, R. L., McGill, H. C., Strong, J. P., Geer, J. C.: Technics for studying atherosclerotic lesions. Lab. Invest. **7**, 42 (1958).
699. — Essential fatty acid deficiency. Progr. Chem. Fats and other Lipids **9**, 279 (1968).
700. Holmes, W. L.: Drugs affecting lipid synthesis. In: R. Paoletti (ed.), *Lipid pharmacology*, p. 132. New York-London: Academic Press 1964.
701. Holmsen, H.: Adenin nucleotide metabolism in platelets and plasma. In: E. Kowalski and S. Niewiarowski (eds.), *Biochemistry of blood platelets*, p. 81. London: Academic Press 1967.
702. — Day, A. J.: Release of beta-glucuronidase from platelets induced by thrombin. Nature (Lond.) **219**, 760 (1968).
703. — Day, H. J., Stormorken, H.: The blood platelet release reaction. Scand. J. Haemat., Suppl. 2 (1969).
704. Honour, A. J., Mitchell, J. R. A.: Platelet clumping in injured vessels. Brit. J. exp. Path. **45**, 75 (1964).
705. — Ross-Russell, R. W.: Experimental platelet embolism. Brit. J. exp. Path. **43**, 350 (1962).
706. Hood, B., Persson, B., Bjorntorp, P.: Lipoprotein lipase activity in human adipose tissue. I. Conditions for release and relationship to triglycerides in serum. Metabolism **15**, 730 (1966).
707. Horecker, B. L.: In: G. E. W. Wolstenholme and M. O'Connor (eds.), *Thiamine deficiency*, p. 148. Boston: Little, Brown & Co. 1967.
708. — The role of pentitols and other polyols in evolutionary development. Proc. Internat. Symposium on metabolism, physical and chemical uses of pentoses and polyols, in press (1969).
709. Horlick, L.: Platelet adhesiveness in normal persons and subjects with atherosclerosis. Effect of high fat meals and anticoagulants on the adhesive index. Amer. J. Cardiol. **8**, 459 (1961).
710. Hovig, T.: The ultrastructure of rabbit blood platelet aggregates. Thrombos. Diathes. haemorrh. (Stuttg.) **8**, 455 (1962).
711. — Release of a platelet aggregating substance (adenosine diphosphate) from rabbit blood platelets induced by saline "extract" of tendons. Thrombos. Diathes. haemorrh. (Stuttg.) **9**, 264 (1963).
712. — The effects of various enzymes on the ultrastructure, aggregation and clot retraction ability of rabbit blood platelets. Thrombos. Diathes. haemorrh. (Stuttg.) **13**, 84 (1965).
713. — The role of formed elements in thrombosis. Proc. Conf. on Thrombosis. National Academy of Science, Washington, D. C., 1967, in press (1969).
714. — Jørgensen, L., Packham, M. A., Mustard, J. F.: Platelet adherence to fibrin and collagen. J. Lab. clin. Med. **71**, 29 (1968).
715. — Rowsell, H. C., Dodds, W. J., Jørgensen, L., Mustard, J. F.: Experimental hemostasis in normal dogs and dogs with congenital disorders of blood coagulation. Blood **30**, 636 (1967).
716. Howard, A. N., Bowyer, D. E., Gresham, G. A.: Cholesterol metabolism in normal and atherosclerotic aortas. Circulation **38**, Suppl. VI, 11 (1967).

717. Howard, A. N., Gresham, G. A.: The dietary induction of thrombosis and myocardial infarction. J. Atheroscler. Res. **4**, 40 (1964).
718. — — Dietary aspects of atherosclerosis and thrombosis. Int. J. Vit. Res. **38**, 545 (1968).
719. — — Jones, D., Jennings, I. W.: The prevention of rabbit atherosclerosis by soy bean meal. J. Atheroscler. Res. **5**, 330 (1965).
720. — Jennings, I. W., Gresham, G. A.: Atherosclerosis in pigs obtained from two centres differing in hardness of water supply. Path. Microbiol. **30**, 676 (1967).
721. Howard, C. F., Jr.: *De novo* synthesis and elongation of fatty acids by subcellular fractions of monkey aorta. J. Lipid Res. **9**, 254 (1968).
722. — Portman, O. W.: Hydrolysis of cholesteryl linoleate by a high speed supernate preparation of rat and monkey aorta. Biochim. biophys. Acta (Amst.) **125**, 623 (1966).
723. Howell, R. W., Wilson, D. G.: Dietary sugar and ischaemic heart disease. Brit. med. J. **1969 III**, 145.
724. Hueper, W. C.: Arteriosclerosis. Arch. Path. **38**, 162, 245, 350, **39**, 51, 117, 187 (1944—45).
725. Huff, J. W., Gillillan, J. L., Hunt, V. M.: Effect of cholestyramine, a bile acid binding polymer on plasma cholesterol and fecal bile acid excretion in the rat. Proc. Soc. exp. Biol. (N.Y.) **114**, 352 (1963).
726. Huff, R. L., Feller, D. D.: Relation of circulating red cell volume to body density and obesity. J. clin. Invest. **35**, 1 (1956).
727. Hughes, A., Tonks, R. S.: The role of micro-emboli in the production of carditis in hypersensitivity experiments. J. Path. Bact. **77**, 207 (1959).
728. — — Intravascular platelet clumping in rabbits. J. Path. Bact. **84**, 379 (1962).
729. Hugues, J.: Accolement des plaquettes au collagene. C. R. Soc. Biol. (Paris) **154**, 866 (1960).
730. Hutton, H. R. B., Boyd, G. S.: The metabolism of cholest-5-one-3β, 7α-diol by rat liver cell fractions. Biochim. biophys. Acta (Amst.) **116**, 336 (1969).
731. Hyun, S. A., Vahouny, G. V., Treadwell, C. R.: Effect of hypocholesterolemic agents on intestinal cholesterol absorption. Proc. Soc. exp. Biol. Med. (N.Y.) **112**, 496 (1963).
732. Hyvärinen, A., Nikkilä, E. A.: Specific determination of blood glucose with o-toluidine. Clin. chim. Acta **7**, 140 (1962).
733. Ignatowski, A.: Influence of albumins of various origins, animal, vegetable, lactic, upon the organism of the rabbit. Izv. Imp. Voyenno-Med. Akad. (S.-Peterb.) **24**, 20 (1912).
734. Ilyinsky, B. V.: Cited by S. F. Oleynik and R. F. Zubova: The effect of cholesterol load on the total level of blood cholesterol. Cardiologia (Basel) **1**, 87 (1966).
735. Imai, Y., Kikuchi, S., Matsuo, T., Suzuoki, Z., Nishikawa, K.: Biological studies of cholestane-3β, 5α, 6β-triol and its derivatives. Part 2. Effect of cholestane 3β, 5α, 6β-triol on the absorption, synthesis, excretion, distribution of cholesterol in rats. J. Atheroscler. Res. **7**, 671 (1967).
736. Imai, H., Thomas, W. A.: Cerebral atherosclerosis in swine: role of necrosis in progression of diet-induced lesions from proliferative to atheromatous stage. Exp. molec. Path. **8**, 330 (1968).
737. Inagaki, A.: An experimental study on the role of microthrombi in the formation of venous thrombosis. Jap. Circulat. J. **32**, 715 (1968).
738. Inman, W. H. W., Vessey, M. P.: Investigation of deaths from pulmonary, coronary, and cerebral thrombosis and embolism in women of child-bearing age. Brit. med. J. **1968 II**, 193.
739. Insull, W., Jr.: Pathogenesis of the fatty streak lesions in human atherosclerosis: alterations in fatty acids of neutral lipids. Circulation **30**, Suppl. III, 16 (1964).
740. — Bartsch, G. E.: Cholesterol, triglyceride, and phospholipid content of intima, media, and atherosclerotic fatty streak in human thoracic aorta. J. clin. Invest. **45**, 513 (1966).

741. Iverius, P. H.: Solubility of low-density beta-lipoproteins in the presence of dextran. Clin. chim. Acta **20**, 261 (1968).

742. Jacobson, E. D., Prior, J. T., Faloon, W. W.: Malabsorptive syndrome induced by neomycin; morphologic alterations in the jejunal mucosa. J. Lab. clin. Med. **56**, 245 (1960).

743. Janoff, A., Schaeffer, S., Scherer, J., Bean, M.: Mediators of inflammation in leukocyte lysosomes. II. Mechanism of action of lysosomal cationic protein upon vascular permeability in the rat. J. exp. Med. **122**, 841 (1965).

744. Jarand, J., Oliver, M. F.: The effects of ethyl chlorophenoxyisobutyrate on serum cholesteryl, triglyceride and phospholipid fatty acids. J. Atheroscler. Res. **3**, 547 (1963).

745. Jarmolych, J., Daoud, A. S., Landau, J., Fritz, K. D., McElvene, E.: Aortic medial explant, cell proliferation and production of mucopolysaccharide, collagen and elastic tissue. Exp. molec. Path. **9**, 171 (1968).

746. Jennings, M. A., Brock, L. G., Lord Florey: A comparison of connective tissue lining aortic grafts with connective tissue. Proc. roy. Soc. B **165**, 206 (1966).

747. Jensen, J.: On the relationship between metabolic activity and cholesterol uptake by intima media of the rabbit aorta. Biochim. biophys. Acta (Amst.) **183**, 204 (1969).

748. Jerushalmy, Z., Kohn, A., deVries, A.: Interaction of myxoviruses with human blood platelets *in vitro*. Proc. Soc. exp. Biol. Med. (N.Y.) **106**, 462 (1961).

749. Jick, H., Slone, D., Westerholm, B., Inman, W. H. W., Vessey, M. P., Shapiro, S., Lewis, G. P., Worcester, J.: Venous thromboembolic disease. Lancet **1969 I**, 539.

750. Johnson, B. C., Remington, R. D.: A sampling study of blood pressure levels in white and negro residents of Nassau, Bahamas. J. chron. Dis. **13**, 39 (1961).

751. Johnson, S. A.: Platelets in hemostasis. In W. Seegers (ed.); *Blood clotting enzymology*, p. 380. New York: Academic Press 1967.

752. Johnsson-Hegyeli, R. I. E., Hegyeli, A. F.: Interaction of blood and tissue cells with foreign surfaces. J. biomed. Mater. Res. **3**, 115 (1969).

753. Jolliffe, N., Archer, M.: Statistical associations between international coronary heart disease death rates and certain environmental factors. J. chron. Dis. **9**, 636 (1959).

754. Jones, A. L., Rudermann, N. B., Herrera, M. G.: Electron microscopic and biochemical study of lipoprotein synthesis in the isolated perfused rat liver. J. Lipid Res. **8**, 429 (1967).

755. Jørgensen, L.: Experimental platelet and coagulation thrombi. A histological study of arterial and venous thrombi of varying age in untreated and heparinized rabbits. Acta path. microbiol. scand. **62**, 189 (1964).

756. — Organforandringer ved hypertensjon under patologisk-anatomisk synsvinkel. Nyrene. T. Norske Laegeforen. **88**, 1430 and 1450 (1968).

757. — Hoerem, J. W., Chandler, A. B., Borchgrevink, C. F.: The pathology of acute coronary death. Acta anaesth. scand., Suppl. **29**, 193 (1968).

758. — The role of platelet embolism from crumbling thrombi and of platelet aggregates arising in flowing blood. In: S. Sherry, K. M. Brinkhous, E. Genton and J. M. Stengle (eds.), *Thrombosis*, p. 506. Washington, D. C.: National Academy of Sciences 1969.

759. — Rowsell, H. C., Hovig, T., Glynn, M. F., Mustard, J. F.: Adenosine diphosphate-induced platelet aggregation and myocardial infarction in swine. Lab. Invest. **17**, 616 (1967).

760. — — — Mustard, J. F.: Resolution and organization of platelet-rich mural thrombi in carotid arteries of swine. Amer. J. Path. **51**, 681 (1967).

761. — Torvik, A.: Ischaemic cerebrovascular diseases in an autopsy series. Part 1. Prevalence, location and predisposing factors in verified thromboembolic occlusions, and their significance in the pathogenesis of cerebral infarction. J. neurol. Sci. **3**, 490 (1966).

762. — — Ischaemic cerebrovascular diseases in an autopsy series. Part 2. Prevalence, location, pathogenesis, and clinical course of cerebral infarcts. J. neurol. Sci. **9**, 285 (1969).

763. Jurgens, J. L., Edwards, J. E., Achor, R. W. P., Burchell, H. B.: Prognosis of patients surviving first clinically diagnosed myocardial infarction. Arch. intern. Med. **105**, 444 (1960).
764. Kabat, E. A. (ed.): Structural concepts in immunology and immunochemistry. New York: Holt, Rinehart and Winston 1968.
765. — Mayer, M. M. (eds.): Experimental immunochemistry. Springfield: C. C. Thomas 1964.
766. Kagan, A., Dawber, T. R., Kannel, W. B., Revotskie, N.: Framingham study: prospective study of coronary heart disease. Fed. Proc. **21**, 52 (1962).
767. Kahn, H. A., Medalie, J. H., Neufeld, H. N., Riss, E., Balogh, M., Groen, J. J.: Serum cholesterol: its distribution and association with dietary and other variables in a survey of 10,000 men. Israel J. med. Sci., **5**, 1117 (1969).
768. Kallner, M., Groen, J. J.: Mortality and hospitalization in relation to coronary and cerebrovascular disease in Israel. J. Atheroscler. Res. **6**, 419 (1966).
769. Kane, J. P., Longcope, C., Pavlatos, F. C., Grodsky, G. M.: Studies of carbohydrate metabolism in idiopathic hypertriglyceridemia. Metabolism **14**, 471 (1965).
770. Kannel, W. B.: The Framingham heart study: habits and coronary heart disease. Public Health Service Publications No 1515, Department of Health, Education and Welfare, U.S. Public Health Service. Washington, D. C.: U. S. Government Printing Office 1966.
771. — Castelli, W. P., McNamara, P. M.: The coronary profile: 12 year follow-up in the Framingham study. J. occup. Med. **9**, 611 (1967).
772. — Dawber, T. R., Friedman, G. D., Glennon, W. E., McNamarra, P. M.: Risk factors in coronary heart disease. An evaluation of several serum lipids as predictors of coronary heart disease. The Framingham study. Ann. intern. Med. **61**, 888 (1964).
773. — Kagan, A., Revotskie, N., Stokes, J.: Factors of risk in the development of coronary heart disease—six-year follow-up experiences. Ann. intern. Med. **55**, 33 (1961).
774. Kanzow, U.: Untersuchungen über serumlipoide bei paraproteinämien. In: European society of Haematology, Transaction of the 6th Congress, Copenhagen, Part 2, p. 103. Basel: S. Karger 1957.
775. Kao, K. Y. T., Hilker, D. M., McGavack, T. H.: Connective tissue. IV. Synthesis and turnover of proteins in tissues of rats. Proc. Soc. exp. Biol. Med. (N.Y.) **106**, 121 (1961).
776. Kao, V. C. Y., Wissler, R. W.: A study of the immunohistochemical localization of serum lipoproteins and other plasma proteins in human atherosclerotic lesions. Exp. molec. Path. **4**, 457 (1965).
777. — — Dzoga, K.: The influence of hyperlipaemic serum on the growth of medial smooth cells of rhesus monkey aorta *in vitro*. Circulation **38**, VI-12 (1968).
778. Kaplan, J. A., Cox, G. E., Taylor, C. B.: Cholesterol metabolism in man. Studies on absorption. Arch. Path. **76**, 359 (1963).
779. Karam, J. H., Pavlatos, F. C., Grodsky, G. M., Forsham, P. H.: Critical factors in excessive serum insulin response to glucose. Lancet **1965 I**, 286.
780. Kates, M., Chan, T. H., Stanacev, N.: Aliphatic diether analogue of glycerid-derived lipids. I. Synthesis of D-α, β-dialkyl glyceryl ethers. Biochemistry **2**, 394 (1963).
781. Katz, L. N., Stamler, J.: Experimental atherosclerosis. Springfield: C. C. Thomas 1953.
782. — — Pick, R.: Nutrition and atherosclerosis. Philadelphia: Lea and Febiger 1958.
783. Kayden, H. J., Franklin, E. C., Rosenberg, B.: Interaction of myeloma gammaglobulin with human beta-lipoprotein. Circulation **26**, 659 (1962).
784. Keeley, F. W., Labella, F., Queen, G.: Dityrosine in a nonhydroxyproline, alkali-soluble protein isolated from chick aorta and bovine ligament. Biochem. biophys. Res. Commun. **34**, 156 (1969).

785. Keen, H., Jarrett, R. J.: Modern concepts in the diagnosis of diabetes. In Charles Weller (ed.); *The new management of stable adult diabetes*. Springfield: C. C. Thomas 1969.
786. — — Chlouverakis, C., Boyns, D. R.: The effect of treatment of moderate hyperglycaemia on the incidence of arterial disease. Postgrad. med. J. **44**, 960 (1968).
787. — Rose, G. A., Pyke, D. A., Boyns, D. R., Chlouverakis, C., Mistry, S.: Blood sugar and arterial disease. Lancet **1965 II**, 505.
788. Keller, S., Levi, M. M., Mandl, I.: Antigenicity and chemical composition of an enzymatic digest of elastin. Arch. Biochem. **13**, 565 (1969).
789. Kelly, F. B., Jr., Taylor, C. B., Hass, G. H.: Experimental atheroarteriosclerosis. Localization of lipids in experimental arterial lesions of rabbits with hypercholesterolemia. Arch. Path. **53**, 419 (1952).
790. Kershbaum, A., Bellet, S., Khorsandian, R. K.: Elevation of serum cholesterol after administration of nicotine. Amer. Heart J. **69**, 206 (1965).
791. Keys, A., Anderson, J. T., Grande, F.: Prediction of serum cholesterol responses of man to changes of fat in the diet. Lancet **1957 II**, 959.
792. — — — Serum cholesterol response to changes in the diet. Metabolism **14**, 747 (1965).
793. — Aravanis, C., Blackburn, H. W., van Buchem, F. S. P., Buzina, R., Djordjevic, B. S., Dontas, A. S., Fidanza, F., Karvonen, M. J., Kimura, N., Lekas, D., Monti, M., Puddu, V., Taylor, H. L.: Epidemiological studies related to coronary heart disease. Acta med. scand., Suppl. **460**, 1 (1966).
794. — Fidanza, F., Scardi, V., Vergami, G., Keys, M. H., Lorenzo, F.: Studies in serum cholesterol and the characteristics of clinically healthy men in Naples. Arch. intern. Med. **93**, 328 (1954).
795. — Grande, F., Anderson, J. T.: Fibre and pectin in the diet and serum cholesterol concentration inman. Proc. Soc. exp. Biol. Med. (N.Y.) **106**, 555 (1961).
796. — Taylor, H. L., Blackburn, H., Brozek, J., Anderson, J. J., Simonson, E.: Coronary heart disease among Minnesota business and professional men followed fifteen years. Circulation **27**, 381 (1963).
797. — Viranco, F., Rodriguez Miron, J. L., Keys, M. H., Castro-Mendoza, H.: Studies on the diet, body fatness and serum cholesterol in Madrid, Spain. Metabolism **3**, 195 (1954).
798. Khachadurian, A. K.: Cholestyramine therapy in patients homozygous for familial hypercholesterolemia (familial hypercholesterolemic xanthomatosis). J. Atheroscler. Res. **8**, 177 (1968).
799. Kinlough, R. L., Packham, M. A., Mustard, J. F.: Glucose and platelet aggregation. Fed. Proc. **28**, 509 (1969).
800. Kinoshita, J. H.: Cataracts in galactosemia. Invest. Ophthal. **4**, 786 (1965).
801. Kint, A.: Les manifestations cutanees de la maladie de Kahler. Arch. belges. Derm. **17**, 148 (1961).
802. Kipshidze, N. N.: Effect of oxygen deficiency on the development of experimental atherosclerosis of coronary arteries. Bull. exp. Biol. Med. **47**, 54 (1959).
803. Kirk, J. E.: Intermediary metabolism of human arterial tissue and its changes with age and atherosclerosis. In: M. Sandler and G. H. Bourne (eds.), *Atherosclerosis and its origin*, chapt. 3. New York: Academic Press 1963.
804. — Laursen, T. J. S.: Diffusion coefficients of various solutes for human aortic tissue. J. Gerontol. **10**, 288 (1955).
805. Kissane, J. M., Robins, E.: The fluorometric measurement of deoxyribonucleic acid in animal tissues with special reference to the central nervous system. J. biol. Chem. **233**, 184 (1958).
806. Kjeldsen, K.: Smoking and atherosclerosis. Thesis. Copenhagen: Munksgaard 1969.
807. — Astrup, P., Wanstrup, J.: Reversal of rabbit atherosclerosis by hyperoxia. J. Atheroscler. Res., **10**, 173 (1969).
808. — Mozes, M.: Investigations on carboxyhaemoglobin and serum cholesterol levels after smoking. Acta med. scand., in press (1970).

809. Kjeldsen, K., Wanstrup, J., Astrup, P.: Enchancing influence of arterial hypoxia on the development of atheromatosis in cholesterol-fed rabbits. J. Atheroscler. Res. **8**, 835 (1968).

810. Kloeze, J.: Influence of prostaglandins on platelet adhesiveness and platelet aggregation. In S. Bergstrom and B. Samuelsson (eds.), *Proc. 2nd Nobel Symposium*, Stockholm, 1966, p. 241. Stockholm: Almqvist & Wiksell; New York: Interscience 1967.

811. — Influence of prostaglandins on ADP-induced platelet aggregation. (Abs.) Acta physiol. pharmacol. neerl. **15**, 50 (1969).

812. Knieriem, H. J., Kao, V. Y., Wissler, R. W.: Actomyosin and myosin and the deposition of lipids and serum lipoproteins. Arch. Path. **84**, 118 (1967).

813. Knisely, M. H.: Intravascular erythrocyte aggregation. In: P. Dow (ed.), *Handbook of physiology*, sect. 2, vol. III, p. 2249. Washington, D. C.: Amer. Physiol. Soc. 1965.

814. Knittle, J. L., Ahrens, E. H., Jr.: Carbohydrate metabolism in two forms of hyperglyceridemia. J. clin. Invest. **43**, 485 (1964).

815. Kobayashi, J.: Geographical relationship between chemical nature of river water and death rate from apoplexy: preliminary report. Ber. d. Ohara Inst. Landwirksch. Biol. **11**, 12 (1957).

816. Kodicek, E.: Vitamin D and calcium homeostasis. In *Advances in fluorine research and dental caries prevention*, Proc. 11th Congr. European Organization for Research on Fluorine and Dental Caries Prevention, Sandefjord, Norway. New York: Pergamon Press 1965.

817. Kopin, I. J.: Storage and metabolism of catecholamines: the role of monoamine oxidase. Pharmacol. Rev. **16**, 179 (1964).

818. Korn, E. D.: The fatty acid and positional specificities of lipoprotein lipase. J. biol. Chem. **6**, 1638 (1961).

819. Kornfeld-Poullain, N., Robert, L.: Effet de différents solvants organiques sur la dégradation alcaline de l'élastin. Bull. Soc. chim. biol. (Paris) **50**, 759 (1968).

820. Kottke, B. A.: Differences in bile acid excretion, primary hypercholesteremia compared to combined hypercholesteremia and hypertriglyceridemia. Circulation **40**, 13 (1969).

821. Kramsch, D. M., Gore, I., Hollander, W.: The distribution of intravenously administered ^{3}H-cholesterol in the arteries and other tissues. Part 2. Radioautographic findings. J. Atheroscler. Res. **7**, 501 (1967).

822. — Hollander, W.: The interaction of serum and arterial lipoprotein with elastin of normal and atherosclerotic human arterial intima. Circulation **38**, Suppl. VI, 12 (1968).

823. Kreisberg, R. A., Boshell, B. R., DiPlacido, J., Roddam, R. F.: Insulin secretion in obesity. New Engl. J. Med. **276**, 314 (1967).

824. Krishna, G., Weiss, B., Brodie, B. B.: A simple, sensitive method for the assay of adenyl cyclase. J. Pharmacol. exp. Ther. **163**, 379 (1968).

825. Kritchevsky, D., Moynihan, J. L., Langan, J. Tepper, S. A., Sachs, M. L.: Effects of D- and L-thyroxine and of D- and L-3,5,3'-triiodothyronine on development and regression of experimental atherosclerosis in rabbits. J. Atheroscler. Res. **1**, 211 (1961).

826. — Sallata, P., Tepper, S. A.: Experimental atherosclerosis in rabbits fed cholesterol-free diet. Part 2. Influence of various carbohydrates. J. Atheroscler. Res. **8**, 697 (1968).

827. — Tepper, S. A.: Effect of ethyl p-chlorophenoxy-isobutyrate on oxidation of cholesterol by rat liver mitochondria. (Abs.) Fed. Proc. **27**, 822 (1968).

828. — — Experimental atherosclerosis in rabbits fed cholesterol free diets. Influence of chow components. J. Atheroscler. Res. **8**, 357 (1968).

829. Kritzman, J., Kunkel, H. G., McCarthy, J., Mellors, R. C.: Studies of a Waldenström type macroglobulin with rheumatoid factor properties. J. Lab. clin. Med. **57**, 905 (1961).

830. Kroman, H., Nodine, J., Bender, S., Brest, A.: Lipids in normals and patients. with coronary artery disease. Amer. J. med. Sci. **248**, 571 (1964).

831. Krut, L. H., Bronte-Stewart, B.: The fatty acids of human depot fat. J. Lipid Res. **5**, 343 (1964).

832. Kumar, V., Berenson, G. S., Ruiz, H., Dalferes, E. R., Jr., Strong, J. P.: Acid mucopolysaccharides of human aorta. Part 1. Variation with maturation. J. Atheroscler. Res. **7**, 573 (1967).

833. Kunkel, H. G., Ahrens, E. H., Jr.: The relationship between serum lipids and the electrophoretic pattern, with particular reference to patients with primary biliary cirrhosis. J. clin. Invest. **28**, 1575 (1949).

834. — Slater, R. J.: Lipoprotein patterns of serum obtained by zone electrophoresis. J. clin. Invest. **31**, 677 (1952).

835. Kuo, P. T.., Carson, J. C.: Dietary fats and the diurnal serum triglyceride levels in man. J. clin. Invest. **38**, 1384 (1959).

836. — Feng, L., Cohen, N. N., Fitts, W. T., Jr., Miller, L. D.: Dietary carbohydrates in hyperlipemia (hyperglyceridemia); hepatic and adipose tissue lipogenic activities. Amer. J. clin. Nutr. **20**, 116 (1967).

837. Laedlein, R.: Les anomalies lipoidiques de la macroglobulinémie de Waldenström. These de Medecine, Paris 1964.

838. Lambert, F. F., Miller, J. P., Olsen, R. T., Frost, D. V.: Hypercholesterolaemia and atherosclerosis induced in rabbit by purified high fat ration devoid of cholesterol. Proc. Soc. exp. Biol. Med. (N.Y.) **97**, 544 (1968).

839. Langer, T., Levy, R. I.: Acute muscular syndrome associated with administration of clofibrate. New Engl. J. Med. **279**, 856 (1968).

840. — Strober, W., Levy, R. I.: Familial type II hyperlipoproteinemia: a defect of beta lipoprotein apoprotein catabolism? (Abs.) J. clin. Invest. **48**, 49a (1969).

841. Lansing, A. I., Rosenthal, M. A., Dempsey, E. W.: The structure and chemical characterization of elastic fibers as revealed by elastase and by electron microscopy. Anat. Rec. **114**, 555 (1952).

842. Lapiccirella, V., Lapiccirella, R., Abboni, F., Liotta, S.: Enquête clinique, biological et cardiographique parmi les tribes nomades de la Somalie qui se nourissent seulement de lait. Bull. Wld. Hlth. Org. **27**, 681 (1962).

843. Laurell, S., Tibbling, G.: An enzymatic fluorometric micro-method for the determination of glycerol. Clin. chim. Acta **13**, 317 (1966).

844. Laurent, T. C.: In G. Quintarelli (ed.), The chemical physiology of mucopolysaccharides, p. 153. New York: Little, Brown & Co. 1967.

845. Laurie, W., Woods, J. D., Roach, G.: Coronary heart disease in the South African Bantu. Amer. J. Cardiol. **5**, 48 (1960).

846. Lavy, S., Carmon, A., Schwartz, A.: An angiographic survey of one hundred patients with "completed stroke" with reference to their demographic distribution. Israel J. med. Sci. **1**, 423 (1965).

847. — Stern, S., Herishianu, Y., Carmon, A.: Electrocardiographic changes in ischemic stroke. J. neurol. Sci. **7**, 409 (1968).

848. Lee, C. C., Herrmann, R. G.: Effect of vitamine D, sucrose, corn oil and endocrines on tissue cholesterol in rats. Circulation Res. **7**, 354 (1959).

849. Lee, K. T., Goodale, F., Scott, R. F., Snell, E. S.: Geographic pathology of myocardial infarction. Part III. Myocardial infarction in Africians in Africa and Negroes and whites in the United States. Amer. J. Cardiol. **13**, 30 (1964).

850. — Kim, D. N., Shaper, A. F., Thomas, W. A.: Coagulation and clot-lysis studies in groups eating high and low fat diets. 1. Comparison of East Africans with New Yorkers. Exp. mol. Path. **3**, 500 (1964).

851. — Shaper, A. G., Scott, R. F., Goodale, F., Thomas, W. A.: Geographical studies pertaining to atherosclerosis. Comparison of fatty acid patterns of adipose tissue and plasma lipids in East Africans with those of North American white and Negro groups. Arch. Path. **74**, 481 (1962).

852. Lee, Y. P., Lardy, H. A.: Influence of thyroid hormones on L-α-glycerophosphate dehydrogenase and other dehydrogenases in various organs of the rat. J. biol. Chem. **240**, 1427 (1965).
853. Lees, R. S., Hatch, F. T.: Sharper separation of lipoprotein species by paper electrophoresis in albumin-containing buffer. J. Lab. clin. Med. **61**, 518 (1963).
854. Leffler, H. H., McDougald, C. H.: Estimation of cholesterol in serum. Amer. J. clin. Path. **39**, 311 (1963).
855. Leigh, T., Platt, D. S., Thorp, J. M.: Abstracts 3rd International Symposium on Drugs Affecting Lipid Metabolism, Milan, p. 138, 1968.
856. Lennard-Jones, J. E.: Myelomatosis with lipaemia and xanthomata. Brit. med. J. **1960 I**, 781.
857. Leren, P.: The effect of plasma cholesterol lowering diet in male survivors of myocardial infarction. Acta med. scand., Suppl. **466**, 1 (1966).
858. Levene, C. I.: The electron-microscopy of atheroma. Lancet **2**, 1216 (1955).
859. Levin, K., Linde, S.: Determination of glucose in blood, cerebrospinal fluid and urine with a new glucose oxidase reagent. J. Swed. med. Ass. **59**, 3016 (1962).
860. Levin, W. C., Aboumrad, M. H., Ritzmann, S. E., Brantly, C.: Gammatype I myeloma and xanthomatosis. Arch. intern. Med. **114**, 688 (1964).
861. Levine, R. A.: Effect of dietary gluten upon neomycin-induced malabsorption. Gastroenterology **52**, 685 (1967).
862. Levy, L.: A form of immunological atherosclerosis. In N. R. DiLuzzio and R. Paoletti (eds.), *The reticuloendothelial system and atherosclerosis*, p. 426. New York: Plenum Press 1967.
863. Levy, R. I., Fredrickson, D. S.: Diagnosis and management of hyperlipoproteinemia. Amer. J. Cardiol. **22**, 576 (1968).
864. — Lees, R. S., Fredrickson, D. S.: A functional role for plasma alpha-l-lipoprotein. J. clin. Invest. **44**, 1068 (1965).
865. — — — The nature of prebeta (very low-density) lipoproteins. J. clin. Invest. **45**, 63 (1966).
866. Lewis, L. A., Brown, H. B., Page, I. H.: Ten years treatment of hyperlipidemia. Circulation **38**, Suppl. VI, 128 (1968).
867. — — — Ten years treatment of hyperlipidemia. Geriatrics, in press (1970).
868. — Page, I. H.: Serum proteins and lipoproteins in multiple myelomatosis. Amer. J. Med. **17**, 670 (1954).
869. — — An unusual serum lipoprotein-globulin complex in a patient with hyperlipemia. Amer. J. Med. **38**, 286 (1965).
870. — Van Ommen, R. A., Page, I. H.: Association of cold precipitability with β-lipoprotein and cryoglobulin. Amer. J. Med. **40**, 785 (1966).
871. Liebetseder, F., Hugentobler, F., Wunderly, C., Wuhrmann, F.: Untersuchungen über die serumlipoide und proteine. Wien. Z. inn. Med. **32**, 1 (1951).
872. Likar, I. N., Likar, L. J., Robinson, R. W., Gouvelis, A.: Microthrombi and intimal thickening in bovine coronary arteries. Arch. Path. **87**, 146 (1969).
873. Lille, R. D., Chobanian, A. V.: Glucose metabolism in human arterial intima. (Abs.) Clin. Res. **16**, 516 (1968).
874. Lin, T. M., Kim, K. S., Karvinen, E., Ivy, A. C.: Effect of dietary pectin, "protopectin" and gum arabic on cholesterol excretion in rats. Amer. J. Physiol. **188**, 66 (1957).
875. Lindeman, R. D., Assenzo, J. R.: Correlation between water hardness and cardiovascular death in Oklahoma counties. Amer. J. publ. Hlth **54**, 1071 (1964).
876. Lindholm, B.: Body cell mass during long-term cortisone treatment in asthmatic subjects. Acta endocr. (Kbh.) **55**, 202 (1967).
877. — Body cell mass during long-term treatment with cortisone and anabolic steroids in asthmatic subjects. Acta endocr. (Kbh.) **55**, 222 (1967).
878. Lindstedt, S.: The formation of bile acids from 7α-hydroxycholesterol in the rat. Acta chem. scand. **11**, 417 (1957).
879. — The turnover of cholic acid in man. Acta physiol. scand. **40**, 1 (1957).

880. Lindstedt, S., Avigan, J., Goodman, D. S., Sjövall, J., Steinberg, D.: The effect of dietary fat on the turnover of cholic acid and on the composition of the biliary bile acids in man. J. clin. Invest. **44**, 1754 (1965).

881. — Samuelsson, B.: On the interconversion of cholic and chenodeoxycholic acid in the rat. J. biol. Chem. **234**, 2026 (1959).

882. Lisovsky, V. A.: Effect of oxygen on the biosynthesis of cholesterol in experimental atherosclerosis. Bull. exp. Biol. Med. **61**, 68 (1963).

883. — Mikushkin, M. K.: Effect of oxygen on the experimental atherosclerosis of rabbits. Path. Physiol. exp. Ther. **6**, 33 (1962).

884. Little, J. A., Shanoff, H. M., Roe, R. D., Csima, A., Yano, R.: Studies of male survivors of myocardial infarction. IV. Serum lipids and five year survival. Circulation **31**, 854 (1965).

885. Littman, D.: Persistence of the juvenile pattern in praecordial leads of healthy adult negroes. Amer. Heart J. **32**, 370 (1946).

886. Loeven, W. A.: The identification of the enzymes elastolipoproteinase and elastomucase in human plasma. Acta physiol. pharmacol. neerl. **12**, 497 (1963).

887. — Elastolysis III: the release of carbohydrate moieties during the incubation of acid- and alkali-treated elastin with the enzymes of the elastase complex. Acta physiol. Pharmacol. neerl. **13**, 278 (1965).

888. Lofland, H. B., Jr., Moury, D. M., Hoffman, C. W., Clarkson, T. B.: Lipid metabolism in pigeon aorta during atherogenesis. J. Lipid Res. **6**, 112 (1965).

889. — St. Clair, R. W., Clarkson, T. B., Bullock, B. C., Lehner, D. M.: Atherosclerosis in cebus monkeys. II. Arterial metabolism. Exp. molec. Path. **9**, 57 (1968).

890. Lombardi, B., Pani, P., Schlunk, F. F., Chen Shi-Hua: Labeling of liver and plasma lecithins after injection of 1-2-^{14}C-2-dimethylaminoethanol and ^{14}C-L-methionine-methyl to choline deficient rats. Lipids **4**, 67 (1969).

891. Long, E. R.: The development of our knowledge of arteriosclerosis. In E. V. Cowdry (ed.), *Arteriosclerosis*, p. 19. New York: MacMillan Co. 1933.

892. Loomeijer, F. J., Van den Veen, K. J.: Incorporation of I^{14}C acetate into various lipids of the rat aorta *in vitro*. J. Atheroscler. Res. **2**, 478 (1962).

893. Lovell, R. R. H., Maddocks, I., Rogerson, G. W.: The casual arterial pressure of Fijians and Indians in Fiji. Aust. Ann. Med. **9**, 4 (1960).

894. Luft, J. H.: Fine structure of capillary and endocapillary layer as revealed by ruthenium red. Fed. Proc. **25**, 1773 (1966).

895. Lugibuhl, H.: Spontaneous atherosclerosis in swine. In: L. K. Bustad and R. O. McClellan (eds.), *Swine in biomedical research* p. 347., Seattle: Frayn Printing Company 1966.

896. Luyombya-Sengero, J. M.: Venous thrombosis and pulmonary embolism. Makerere med. J. **12**, 20 (1963).

897. MacDonald, L., Bray, C., Field, C., Love, F., Davies, B.: Homocystinuria, thrombosis and the blood-platelets. Lancet **1964 I**, 745.

898. MacFarlane, R. G.: The basis of cascade hypothesis blood clotting thrombosis. Diath. Haemorrh. **15**, 591 (1966).

899. MacMillan, D. C.: Secondary clumping effect in human citrated platelet-rich plasma produced by adenosine diphosphate and adrenaline. Nature (Lond.) **211**, 140 (1966).

900. Maguire, H., Michal, F.: Powerful new aggregator of blood platelets—2-chloroadenosine-5′-diphosphate. Nature (Lond.) **217**, 571 (1968).

901. Mahler, R.: Diabetes and arterial lipids. Quart. J. Med. **34**, 484 (1965).

902. Mahley, R. W., Gray, M. E., Hamilton, R. L., LeQuire, V. S.: Lipid transport in liver. II. Electron microscopic and biochemical studies of alterations in lipoprotein transport induced by cortisone in the rabbit. Lab. Invest. **19**, 358 (1968).

903. — Hamilton, R. L., LeQuire, V. S.: Characterization of lipoprotein particles isolated from the Golgi apparatus of rat liver. J. Lipid Res. **10**, 433 (1969).

904. Majno, G., Leventhal, M.: Pathogenesis of histamine-type vascular leakage. Lancet **1967 II**, 99.
905. — Palade, G. E.: Studies on inflammation. I. The effect of histamine and serotonin on vascular permeability. An electron microscopic study. J. biophys. biochem. Cytol. **11**, 571 (1961).
906. Malaisse, W. J., Malaisse-Lagae, F.: Stimulation of insulin secretion by non-carbohydrate metabolites. J. Lab. clin. Med. **72**, 438 (1968).
907. Malcom, G. T., Restrepo, C., McMurry, M. T., Richards, M. I., Strong, J. P.: Serum cholesterol and triglyceride levels in two human populations. (Abs.) Circulation **38**; Suppl. VI, 15 (1968).
908. Malhotra, S. L.: Serum lipids, dietary factors and ischaemic heart disease. Amer. J. clin. Nutr. **20**, 462 (1967).
909. Malins, J.: Clinical diabetes mellitus, p. 130 and 462. London: Pub. Eyre and Spottiswood 1968.
910. Mallarme, J., Hartmann, L., Boivin, P., Orcel, L., Fauvert, R.: La macroglobulinemie de Waldenström. Path. et Biol. **5**, 649 (1957).
911. Mallory, F. B.: The infectious lesions of blood vessels. In: *The Harvey lectures*, p. 150. Philadelphia: J. B. Lippincott Co. 1912—1913.
912. Malmros, H.: Occasional survey: dietary prevention of atherosclerosis. Lancet **1969 II**, 479.
913. Malmros, H., Wigand, G.: Atherosclerosis and deficiency of essential fatty acids. Lancet **1959 II**, 749.
914. Mancini, M., Keys, A.: Cholesterol concentration in human serum and blood cells. Proc. Soc. exp. Biol. Med. (N.Y.) **104**, 371 (1960).
915. Manelis, G., Esscchar, J., Altman, S., Modan, M., Brunner, D.: Physical activity at work, lipoproteins and the incidence of angina pectoris, myocardial infarction and death due to ischemic heart disease. Israel J. med. Sci. **5**, 786 (1969).
916. Manley, G., Kent, P. W.: Aortic mucopolysaccharides and metachromasia and dissecting aneurysm. Brit. J. exp. Path. **44**, 635 (1963).
917. Mann, G. V., Shaffer, R. D., Anderson, R. S., Sandstead, H. H.: Cardiovascular disease in the Masai. J. Atheroscler. Res. **4**, 289 (1964).
918. Maragoudakis, M. E.: Effect of clofibrate and Su-13437 on acetyl-CoA carboxylase. Abstracts 3rd Internat. Symposium on Drugs Affecting Lipid Metabolism, p. 142, 1968.
919. — Inhibition of hepatic acetyl-CoA carboxylase by hypolipidemic agents. J. biol. Chem., **244**, 5005 (1969).
920. — Hankin, H.: Inhibition of hepatic acetyl-CoA carboxylase by the lipid-lowering agents, clofibrate and Su-13437. (Abs.) Fed. Proc. **28**, 876 (1969).
921. — — On the mode of action of lipid lowering agents. III. Inhibition of rat liver acetyl-CoA carboxylase *in vivo* and *in vitro*. J. biol. Chem., in press (1969).
922. Marchand, F.: Über Arteriosklerose. Verh. Kongr. inn. Med. **21**, 23 (1904).
923. Marchesi, V. T., Barrnett, R. J.: The demonstration of enzymatic activity in pinocytic vesicles of blood capillaries with the electron microscope. J. Cell Biol. **17**, 547 (1963).
924. Marcus, A. J.: Platelet function. New Engl. J. Med. **280**, 213 (1969).
925. — Zucker-Franklin, D.: Enzyme and coagulation activity of subcellular platelet fractions. J. clin. Invest. **43**, 1241 (1964).
926. — Zucker, M. B.: The physiology of blood platelets. London: Grune und Stratton 1965.
927. Margolis, S.: Separation and size determination of human verum lipoproteins by agarose gel filtration. J. Lipid Res. **8**, 501 (1967).
928. — Langdon, R. G.: Studies on human serum $beta_1$ lipoproteins. II. Chemical modifications. J. biol. Chem. **241**, 477 (1966).
929. Marinetti, G. V., Pettit, D.: The interaction of γ-globulin with lipids. Chem. Phys. Lipids **2**, 17 (1968).

930. Marmorston, J., Moore, F. J., Hopkins, C. E., Kuzma, O. T., Weiner, J.: Clinical studies of long-term estrogen therapy in men with myocardial infarction. Proc. Soc. exp. Biol. Med. (N.Y.) **110**, 400 (1962).

931. Marquis, N. R., Vigdahl, R. L., Tavormina, P. A.: Platelet aggregation: I. Regulation by cyclic AMP and prostaglandin E_1. Biochem. biophys. Res. Commun. **36**, 965 (1969).

932. Marsh, J. B.: Incorporation of amino-acids into soluble lipoproteins by cell-free preparations from rat liver. J. biol. Chem. **238**, 1752 (1963).

933. Marten, R. H.: Xanthomatosis and myelomatosis. Proc. roy. Soc. Med. **55**, 318 (1963).

934. Marticorena, E., Ruiz, L., Severino, J., Galvez, J., Penaloza, D.: Systemic blood pressure changes observed in sea level white males after a long residence at high altitudes. Amer. J. Cardiol. **23**, 364 (1969).

935. Martin, D. B., Vagelos, P. R.: The mechanism of tricarboxylic acid cycle regulation on fatty acid synthesis. J. biol. Chem. **237**, 1787 (1962).

936. Martin, M., Staubesand, J.: Über die primäre Deckung vasaler Endothelläsion. Verh. anat. Ges. **121**, 109 (1968).

937. Masironi, R.: Trace elements and cardiovascular diseases. Bull. Wld. Hlth. Org. **40**, 305 (1969).

938. Mason, H. S.: Mechanisms of oxygen metabolism. Advanc. Enzymol. **19**, 79 (1957).

939. Mathur, K. S., Wahi, P. N., Gahlaut, D. S., Sharma, R. D., Srivastava, S. K.: Prevalence of coronary heart disease in general population at Agra. Indian J. med. Res. **49**, 605 (1961).

940. — — Malhotra, K. K., Sharma, R. D., Srivastava, S. K.: Dietary fats, serum cholesterol and serum lipid phosphorous in different socio-enconomic groups in Utter Pradesh. J. Indian. med. Ass. **33**, 303 (1959).

941. Matthews, C. M. E.: The theory of tracer experiments with ^{131}I-labelled plasma proteins. Phys. in Med. Biol. **2**, 36 (1957).

942. Mattson, F., Beck, L. W.: The specificity of pancreatic lipase for the primary hydroxyl groups of glycerides. J. biol. Chem. **219**, 735 (1956).

943. Maupin, B.: Les plaquettes sanguines de l'homme, p. 102. Paris: Masson & Cie 1954.

944. Maximova, I. V.: Effect of oxygen therapy of lipids, lipoproteins and protein blood fraction of patients affected by atherosclerosis and with hypertonic disease. Summary of the thesis for Master's Degree, Leningrad 1960.

945. Mayer, Jean: Obesity, cardiovascular dieseases, and the dietitian. J. Amer. diet. Ass. **52**, 1 (1968).

946. McCandless, E. L., Zilversmit, D. B.: The effect of cholesterol on the turnover of lecithin, cephalin and sphingomyelin in the rabbit. Arch. Biochem. **62**, 402 (1956).

947. McClure, P. D., Ingram, G. I. C., Jones, R. V.: Platelet changes after adrenaline infusions with and without adrenaline blockers. Thrombos. Diathes. haemorrh. (Stuttg.) **13**, 136 (1965).

948. McCullagh, K., Lewis, M. G.: Spontaneous arteriosclerosis in the wild African elephants. Lancet **1967 II**, 492.

949. McDonald, D. A.: Blood flow in arteries. London: Arnold 1960.

950. McDonough, J. R., Garrison, G. E., Hames, C. G.: Blood pressure and hypertensive disease among negroes and whites — a study in Evans County, Georgia. Ann. intern. Med. **61**, 208 (1964).

951. McGandy, R. B., Hegsted, D. M., Myers, M. L., Stare, F. J.: Dietary carbohydrate and serum cholesterol levels in man. Amer. J. Clin. Nutr. **18**, 237 (1966).

952. McGill, H. C., Jr.: Introduction to the geographic pathology of atherosclerosis. Lab. Invest. **18**, 465 (1968).

953. — Geer, J. C., Strong, J. P.: The natural history of human atherosclerosis. In: M. Sandler and G. H. Bourne (eds.), *Atherosclerosis and its origin*, chap. 2. New York: Academic Press 1963.

954. McGinley, J., Jones, H., Gofman, J.: Lipoproteins and xanthomatous diseases. J. invest. Derm. **19**, 71 (1952).
955. McKeown, T.: Medicine in modern society. London: Allen & Unwin Ltd. 1965.
956. McKerron, C. G., Scott, R. L., Asper, S. P., Levy, R. I.: Effects of clofibrate (Atromid-S) on the thyroxine-binding capacity of thyroxine-binding globulin and free thyroxine. J. clin. Endocrinol. **29**, 957 (1969).
957. McLaren, D. S., Read, W. W. C.: Fatty acids composition of adipose tissue. A study in three races in East Africa. Clin. Sci. **23**, 247 (1962).
958. McMahan, C. A.: Autopsied cases by age, sex and "race". Lab. Invest. **18**, 468 (1968).
959. McMillan, G. C., Duff, G. L.: Mitotic activity in the aortic lesions of experimental atherosclerosis in rabbits. Arch. Path. **46**, 179 (1948).
960. —, Stary, H. C.: Preliminary experience with mitotic activity of cellular elements in the atherosclerotic plaques of cholesterol fed rabbits studied by labeling with tritiated thymidine. Ann. N. Y. Acad. Sci. **149**, 699 (1968).
961. McNicol, G. P., Bain, W. H., Walker, F., Rifkin, B. M., Douglas, A. S.: Thrombolysis studied in an artificial circulation. Lancet **1965 I**, 838.
962. Medalie, J. H.: The classification of Israeli Jews for medical scientific purposes. Israel med. J. **21**, 118 (1962).
963. — Kahn, H. A., Groen, J. J., Neufeld, H. N., Riss, E.: The prevalence of ischemic heart disease in relation to selected variables. Israel J. med. Sci. **4**, 789 (1968).
964. — — Neufeld, H. N., Riss, E., Groen, J. J.: Physician's fact book: selected measurements on 10,000 Israeli males. Jerusalem: Central Press 1968.
965. — Neufeld, H. N., Riss, E., Groen, J. J., Kahn, H. A., Bachrach, C. A.: Variations in prevalence of ischemic heart disease in defined segments of the male population of Israel. Israel J. med. Sci. **4**, 775 (1968).
966. Medical Research Council: An assessment of long-term anticoagulant administration after cardiac infarction: Second report of the working party on anticoagulant therapy in coronary thrombosis. Brit. med. J. **1964 II**, 837.
967. — — — Report of a Research Committee to the: Controlled trial of soya-bean oil in myocardial infarction. Lancet **1968 II**, 693.
968. Medina, M. A., Giachetti, A., Shore, P. A.: On the physiological disposition and possible mechanism of the antihypertensive effect of debrisoquin. Biochem. Pharmacol. **18**, 891 (1969).
969. Meessen, M.: Über den plötzlichen Herztod bei Frühsklerose und Frühthrombose der Koronararterien bei Männern unter 45 Jahren. Z. Kreisl.-Forsch. **36**, 185 (1944).
970. Melville, K. I., Blum, B., Shister, H. E., Silver, M. D.: Cardiac ischemic changes and arrhythmia induced by hypothalamic stimulation. Amer. J. Cardiol. **12**, 781 (1963).
971. Mendelsohn, D., Mendelsohn, L., Staple, E.: The *in vitro* catabolism of cholesterol: formation of 5β-cholestane-3α, 7α-diol and 5β-cholestane-3α, 12α-diol from cholesterol in rat liver. Biochemistry **4**, 441 (1965).
972. Menghini, G.: One second needle biopsy of the liver. Gastroenterology **35**, 190 (1958).
973. Merskey, C., Lackner, H., Gordon, H.: Blood coagulation and fibrinolysis in relation to coronary heart disease. A comparative study of normal white men, white men with overt coronary heart disease and normal Bantu men. Brit. med. J. **1960 I**, 219.
974. Mestel, A. L., Spain, D. M., Turner, H. A.: Atheroma absence distal to subtotal aorta occlusion. Arch. Path. **78**, 186 (1964).
975. Metzger, M.: Characterization of a human macroglobulin. V. A. Waldenström macroglobulin with antibody activity. Proc. nat. Acad. Sci. (Wash.) **57**, 1490 (1967).
976. Meyer, B. J., Meyer, A. C., Pepler, W. J., Theron, J. J.: Chemical composition of the aorta, coronary arteries and cerebral arteries of Europeans and Bantu. Amer. Heart J. **71**, 68 (1966).

977. Meyer, B. J., Pepler, W. J., Meyer, A. C., Theron, J. J.: Atherosclerosis in Europeans and Bantu. Circulation **29**, 415 (1964).
978. Meyer, J. S., Gotoh, F., Tazaki, Y.: Circulation and metabolism following experimental cerebral embolism. J. Neuropath. Exp. Neurol. **21**, 4 (1962).
979. Miall, W. E.: E. C. G. abnormalities in Jamaican population samples. Proc. Vth International Scientific meeting of International Epidemiological Association. Primosten, Yugoslavia 1968.
980. Michaelson, I. C., Eliakim, M., Avshalom, A., Medalie, J. H., Ivry, M., Neumann, E.: An approach to the investigation of the vascular changes in the fundus of the eye in hypertension and arteriosclerosis. Proc. XX International Congress of Opthalmology, Excepta Medica Intern't, Congress Series No 146. Amsterdam: Excepta Medica 1966.
981. Michal, F., Firkin, B.: Physiological and pharmacological aspects of the platelet. Ann. Rev. Pharmacol. **9**, 95 (1969).
982. — Maguire, M. H., Gough, G.: 2-methylthioadenosine-5′-phosphate: a specific inhibitor of platelet aggregation. Nature (Lond.) **222**, 1073 (1969).
983. Michon, P., Strieff, F.: Macroglobulinemie de Waldenström. Paris: Masson & Cie 1959.
984. Miettinen, T. A.: Effect of dietary cholesterol and cholic acid on cholesterol synthesis in rat and man. Progr. Biochem. Pharmacol. **4**, 68 (1968).
985. — Effect of nicotinic acid on catabolism and synthesis of cholesterol in man. Clin. chim. Acta **20**, 43 (1968).
986. — Fecal steroid excretion during weight reduction in obese patients with hyperlipidemia. Clin. chim. Acta **19**, 341 (1968).
987. — Fecal steroid excretion, liver lipids, and conversion of acetate and mevalonate to serum cholesterol during starvation and nicotinic acid treatment. Scand. J. clin. Lab. Invest. **21**, Suppl. 101, 20 (1968).
988. — Lanosterol and other methyl sterols in serum of fed and fasted human subjects. Ann. Med. exp. Fenn. **46**, 172 (1968).
989. — Mechanism of serum cholesterol reduction by thyroid hormones in hypothyroidism. J. Lab. clin. Med. **71**, 537 (1968).
990. — Fecal steroid excretion and serum methyl sterols during cholestyramine treatment. Scand. J. clin. Lab. Invest. **23**, Suppl. 108, 56 (1969).
991. — Serum squalene and methyl sterols as indicators of cholesterol synthesis *in vivo*. Life Sci. **8**, 713 (1969).
992. — Sterol blance in hypercholesterolemia. Scand. J. clin. Lab. Invest. **24**, Suppl. 110, 48 (1969).
993. — Ahrens, E. H., Jr., Grundy, S. M.: Quantitative isolation and gas-liquid chromatographic analysis of total dietary and fecal neutral steroid. J. Lipid Res. **6**, 411 (1965).
994. — Pelkonen, R., Nikkilä, E. A., Heinonen, O.: Low excretion of fecal bile acids in a family with hypercholesterolemia. Acta med. scand. **182**, 645 (1967).
995. Mikhnev, A. L., Bezuglyi, V. P., Osadchaya, N. V.: The contribution of hypoxia in the development of atherosclerosis. Vrachebnoye Delo **7**, 3 (1961).
996. — Zanozdra, N. S.: On the mechanism of hypoxia compensation in atherosclerosis. Trudy Ukr. Nauchni-issl. Inst. Clin. Med. **8**, 223 (1963).
997. — — Nuzhny, D. A.: Hypoxia and oxygen debt in atherosclerosis. Vrachebnoye Delo **6**, 3 (1964).
998. Miller, B., Anderson, C. E., Piantadosi, C.: Plasmalogen and glycerol ether concentrations in normal and atherosclerotic aortic tissue. J. Geront. **19**, 430 (1964).
999. Miller, J. K., Miller, W. J.: Experimental zinc deficiency and recovery of calves. J. Nutr. **76**, 467 (1962).
1000. Miller, L. L.: Some direct actions of insulin, glucagon and hydrocortisone on the isolated, perfused rat liver. Recent Progr. Hormone Res. **17**, 539 (1961).
1001. Miller, O. N., Hamilton, J. G.: Nicotinic acid and derivatives. In: R. Paoletti (ed.), *Lipid pharmacology*, p. 132. New York: Academic Press 1964.

1002. Miller, W. J., Martin, Y. G., Gentry, R. P., Blockman, D. M.: Zn^{65} and stable zinc absorption, excretion and tissue concentrations as affected by type of diet and level of zinc in normal calves. J. Nutr. **94**, 391 (1968).
1003. Mills, D. C. B.: The breakdown of adenosine diphosphate and of adenosine triphosphate in plasma. Biochem. J. **98**, 32P (1966).
1004. — Robb, I. A., Roberts, G. C. K.: The release of nucleotides, 5-hydroxytryptamine and enzymes from human blood platelets during aggregation. J. Physiol. (Lond.) **195**, 715 (1968).
1005. — Roberts, G. C. K.: Effects of adrenaline on human blood platelets. J. Physiol. (Lond.) **193**, 443 (1967).
1006. — — Membrane active drugs and the aggregation of human blood platelets. Nature (Lond.) **213**, 35 (1967).
1007. Mills, G. L.: The distribution of lipoprotein patterns in healthy Englishmen and patients with ischaemic heart disease. Clin. chim. Acta in press (1970).
1008. Minick, C. B., Murphy, C. E., Campbell, W. C.: Experimental induction of atherosclerosis by the synergy of allergic injury to arteries and lipid rich diet. I. Effect of repeated injections of horse serum in rabbits fed dietary cholesterol supplement. J. exp. Med. **124**, 635 (1966).
1009. Mishkel, M. A., Webb, W. F.: The mechanisms underlying the hypolipidaemic effects of "Atromid-S", nicotinic acid and benzmalecene. I. The metabolism of free fatty acid-albumin complex by the isolated perfused liver. Biochem. Pharmacol. **16**, 897 (1967).
1010. Mitchell, J. R. A., Schwartz, C. J.: Arterial disease, p. 97. Oxford: Blackwell Sci. Publ. 1965.
1011. — Sharp, A. A.: Platelet clumping *in vitro*. Brit. J. Haemat. **10**, 78 (1964).
1012. Mitchell, W. D., Fyffe, T., Smith, D. A.: The effect of oral calcium on cholesterol metabolism. J. Atheroscler. Res. **8**, 913 (1968).
1013. — Truswell, A. S., Bronte-Stewart, B.: The effect of "Atromid-S" on faecal neutral steroids and bile acids. Progr. Biochem. Pharmacol. **2**, 365 (1967).
1014. Mitrani, I., Karplus, H., Brunner, D.: Arteriosclerosis of the coronary arteries in cases of traumatic death. Israel J. med. Sci. **3**, 339 (1967).
1015. Mitton, J. R., Boyd, G. S.: The enzymic hydroxylation of cholesterol by microsomal preparations of rat liver. Biochem. J. **103**, 17P (1967).
1016. Moczar, M., Moczar, E., Robert, L.: Composition of the glycopeptides isolated from the structural glycoproteins of aorta of different species. Biochem. biophys. Res. Commun. **28**, 380 (1967).
1017. — Robert, L.: Extraction and fractionation of the media of thoracic aorta. Isolation and characterisation of structural glycoproteins. J. Atheroscler. Res., in press (1970).
1018. Montenegro, M. R., Solberg, L. A.: Obesity, body weight, body length and atherosclerosis. Lab. Invest. **18**, 594 (1968).
1019. Mookerjea, S., Jeng, D., Black, J.: Studies on the synthesis of plasma glycolipoprotein and hepatic subcellular glycoprotein in early choline deficiency. Canad. J. Biochem. **45**, 825 (1967).
1020. Moore, F. D., Olesen, K. H., McMurray, J. D., Parker, H. V., Ball, M. R., Boyden, C. M.: The body cell mass and its supporting environment. Philadelphia-London: W. B. Saunders Co. 1963.
1021. Moore, F. E.: Some preliminary findings from the Pooling Project of the Council on Epidemiology, American Heart Association. Paper presented at the Conference on Cardiovascular Disease Epidemiology, Council on Epidemiology, American Heart Association, March, New Orleans, La. 1969.
1022. — Gordon, T.: Serum cholesterol levels of adults: United States 1960—1962. Vital and Health Statistics: National Center for Health Statistics. USPHS No 1000, Ser. 11, No 22 1967.
1023. Moore, J. H.: The effect of the type of roughage in the diet on plasma cholesterol and atherosis in rabbits. Brit. J. Nutr. **21**, 207 (1967).

1024. Moore, R. B., Anderson, J. T., Taylor, H. L., Keys, A., Frantz, I. D., Jr.: Effect of dietary fat on the fecal excretion of cholesterol and its degradation products in man. J. clin. Invest. **47**, 1517 (1968).
1025. — Crane, C. A., Frantz, I. D., Jr.: An apparatus and a method using phenetylamine for liquid scintillation counting of $C^{14}O_2$ obtained by wet oxidation of biological materials. Analyt. Biochem. **24**, 545 (1968).
1026. — — — Effect of cholestyramine on the fecal excretion of intravenously administered cholesterol-4-^{14}C and its degradation products in a hypercholesterolemia patient. J. clin. Invest. **47**, 1664 (1968).
1027. — Frantz, I. D., Jr., Buchwald, H.: Changes in cholesterol pool size, turnover rate, and fecal bile acid and sterol excretion after partial ileal bypass in hypercholesteremic patients. Surgery **65**, 98 (1969).
1028. Moore, S., Mersereau, W. A.: Microembolic renal ischaemia, hypertension, and nephrosclerosis. Arch. Path. **85**, 623 (1968).
1029. More, R. H., Haust, M. D.: Atherogenesis and plasma constituents. Amer. J. Path. **38**, 527 (1961).
1030. Moreland, A. F.: Experimental atherosclerosis of swine. In: J. C. Roberts, Jr. and R. Strauss (eds.), *Comparative atherosclerosis*, p. 21. Hoeber Medical Division. New York: Harper & Row 1965.
1031. Moret, V., Serafini-Fracassini, A., Gotte, L.: The carbohydrate composition of the NaCl-soluble fraction from autoclaved elastin. J. Atheroscler. Res. **4**, 184 (1964).
1032. Morgan, A. D.: The pathogenesis of coronary occlusion. Oxford: Blackwell Sci. Publ. 1956.
1033. Morgan, C. R., Lazarow, A.: Immunoassay of insulin: two antibody system. Plasma insulin levels of normal, subdiabetic and diabetic rats. Diabetes **12**, 115 (1963).
1034. Morin, R.: J. *In vitro* incorporation of I^{14}C-acetate and I^{14}C-palmitate into the aortic phospholipids of non-pregnant and pregnant rabbits. J. Atheroscler. Res. **8**, 579 (1968).
1035. Morris, J. N., Crawford, M. D.: Coronary heart disease and physical activity of work. Evidence of a national necropsy sample. Brit. med. J. **1958 II**, 1485.
1036. — — Heady, J. A.: Hardness of local water supplies and mortality from cardiovascular disease. Lancet **1961 II**, 506.
1037. — Gardner, M. J.: Epidemiology of ischaemic heart disease. Amer. J. Med. **46**, 674 (1969).
1038. Morris, M. D.: Measurement of tissue 3-beta-hydroxy sterols by tritiated digitonin. Analyt. Biochem. **11**, 402 (1965).
1039. — Chaikoff, I. L., Felts, J. M., Abraham, S., Farsah, N. O.: The origin of serum cholesterol in the rat: diet versus synthesis. J. biol. Chem. **224**, 1039 (1957).
1040. — Fitch, C. D.: Spontaneous hyperbetalipoproteinemia in the rhesus monkey. Biochem. Med. **2**, 209 (1968).
1041. — — Cross, E.: Abnormalities of lipid metabolism in the vitamin E-deficient monkey. J. Lipid Res. **7**, 210 (1966).
1042. Morrison, E. S., Scott, R. F., Imai, H., Kroms, M., Nour, B. A., Briggs, R. G.: Effect of thrombogenic atherogenic diets on aspects of hepatic energy metabolism in rats. J. Atheroscler. Res., in press (1970).
1043. Moses, C.: Atherosclerosis. Mechanisms as a guide to prevention. Philadelphia: Lea & Febiger 1963.
1044. Moskowitz, M. S., Moskowitz, A. A.: Lipase: localization in adipose tissue. Science **143**, 72 (1965).
1045. Moutafis, C. D., Myant, N. B.: The metabolism of cholesterol in two hypercholesterolemic patients treated with cholestyramine. Clin. Sci. **37**, 443 (1969).
1046. Movat, H. Z., Haust, M. D., More, R. H.: The morphologic elements in the early lesions of arteriosclerosis. Amer. J. Path. **35**, 93 (1959).
1047. — Macmorine, D. L., Burke, J. S.: A permeability factor released from leukocytes after phagocytosis of immune complexes and its possible role in the arthus reaction. Life Sci. **3**, 1025 (1964).

1048. Movat, H. Z., More, R. H., Haus, M. D.: The diffuse intimal thickening of the human aorta with aging. Amer. J. Path. **34**, 1023 (1958).
1049. — Mustard, J. F., Taichman, N. S., Uriuhara, T.: Platelet aggregation and release of ADP, serotonin and histamine associated with phagocytosis of antigen-antibody complexes. Proc. Soc. exp. Biol. Med. (N.Y.) **120**, 232 (1965).
1050. Muir, H.: The chemistry of mucopolysaccharides of arteries. In: D. G. Chalmers and G. A. Gresham (eds.), *Biological aspects of occlusive vascular disease*, p. 60. London: Cambridge University Press 1964.
1051. Muir, H, H., Mustard, J. F.: Enhancement of platelet aggregation by glycosaminoglycans (mucopolysaccharides). In: Le rôle de la paroi artérielle dans l'atherogénèse. Ed. du Centre National de la Recherche Scientifique No 169 (1968).
1052. Muir, J. R.: The regional production of lipoprotein lipase in man. Clin. Sci. **34**, 261 (1968).
1053. Mukherjee, A. B.: Precocious ischaemic heart disease. J. Indian med. Ass. **51**, 207 (1968).
1054. Mulcahy, R.: The influence of water hardness and rainfall on the incidence of cardiovascular and cerebrovascular mortality in Ireland. J Irish med. Ass. **55**, 17 (1964).
1055. Mulhausen, R., Astrup, P. and Kjeldsen, K.: Oxygen affinity of hemoglobin in patients with cardiovascular diseases, anemia, and cirrhosis of the liver. Scand. J. clin. Lab. Invest. **19**, 291 (1967).
1056. Müller, E., Otto, H.: Untersuchungen über Art und Bedeutung strömungsmechanischer Vorgänge bei der Coronarthrombose nach Coronarsklerose. Virchows Arch. path. Anat. **328**, 353 (1956).
1057. Müller-Eckhard, C., Lüscher, E. F.: Immune reactions of human blood platelets. Thrombos. Diathes. haemorrh. (Stuttg.) **20**, 336 (1968).
1058. Murphy, E. A., Rowsell, H. C., Downie, H. G., Robinson, G. A., Mustard, J. F.: Encrustation and atherosclerosis: the analogy between early *in vivo* lesions and deposits which occur in extracorporeal circulations. Canad. med. Ass. J. **87**, 259 (1962).
1059. Musa, B. U., Ogilvie, J. T., Dowling, J. T.: Effects of ethyl chlorophenoxyisobutyrate on thyroxine distribution, transport and metabolism in man. Metabolism **17**, 909 (1968).
1060. Muscholl, E.: Autonomic nervous system: newer mechanisms of adrenergic blockade. Ann. Rev. Pharmacol. **6**, 107 (1966).
1061. Mustard, J. F.: Platelets, thrombosis and vascular disease. Canad. med. Ass. J. **85**, 621 (1961).
1062. — Recent advances in molecular pathology. A review. Platelet aggregation, vascular injury and atherosclerosis. Exp. molec. Path. **7**, 366 (1967).
1063. — Evans, G., Packham, M. A., Nishizawa, E. E.: The platelet in intravascular immunological reactions. 3rd Int. Symposium Cellular and Humoral Mechanisms in Anaphylaxis and Allergy. Basel: S. Karger (in press).
1064. — Glynn, M. F., Nishizawa, E. E., Packham, M. A.: Platelet surface interactions: relationship to thrombosis and hemostasis. Fed. Proc. **26**, 106 (1967).
1065. — Jørgensen, L., Hovig, T., Glynn, M. F., Rowsell, H. C.: In: F. Duckert (ed.), *Pathogenesis and treatment of thromboembolic diseases*. Stuttgart: Schattauer-Verlag 1966.
1066. — Movat, H. Z., Macmorine, D. R. L., Senyi, A.: Release of permeability factors from the blood platelet. Proc. Soc. exp. Biol. Med. (N.Y.) **119**, 988 (1965).
1067. — Packham, M. A.: The biochemistry of primary hemostasis. Plenary Session Paper, XII Congr. Int. Soc. Hematol., New York, p. 306 (1968).
1068. — — Nishizawa, E. W., Rowsell, H. C.: The relationship between thrombosis and atherosclerosis. Presented at Colloques Intern. du Centre National de la Recherche Scientific. In: Le rôle de la paroi arterielle dans l'atherogenese. Ed. du Centre National de la Recherche Scientific, Paris 1967.
1069. — — Rowsell, H. C., Jørgensen, L.: The role of thrombogenic factors in atherosclerosis. Ann. N. Y. Acad. Sci. **149**, 859 (1968).

1070. Mustard, J. F., Rowsell, H. C., Lotz, F., Hegardt, B., Murphy, E. A.: Effect of adenine nucleotides on thrombus formation, platelet count and blood coagulation. Exp. molec. Path. **5**, 43 (1966).
1071. — — Murphy, E. A.: Platelet economy (platelet survival and turnover). Brit. J. Haemat. **12**, 1 (1966).
1072. — — — Downie, H. G.: Intimal thrombosis in atherosclerosis. In: R. J. Jones (ed.), *Evolution of the atherosclerotic plaque*, p. 183. Chicago: Chicago University Press 1963.
1073. Myant, N. B.: Hormonal control of cholesterol metabolism. In: E. E. Bittar and N. Bittar (eds.), *The biological basis of medicine*, vol. 2, p. 193. London and New York: Academic Press 1963.
1074. Myasnikov, A. L.: Atherosclerosis. Moscow: Medgiz 1960.
1075. — Hypertonic disease and atherosclerosis. Moscow: Medgiz 1965.
1076. Nachman, R. L.: Platelet proteins. Seminars Hemat. **5**, 18 (1968).
1077. Nakatani, M., Sasaki, T., Miyazaki, T., Nakamura, M.: Synthesis of phospholipids in arterial walls. Part 1. Incorporation of ^{32}P into phospholipids of aortas and coronary arteries of various animals. J. Atheroscler. Res. **7**, 747 (1967).
1078. Nathaniel, E. J. H., Chandler, A. B.: Electron microscope study of adenosine-induced platelet thrombi in the rat. J. Ultrastruct. Res. **22**, 348 (1968).
1079. National Diet-Heart Study Research Group: The national diet-heart study final report. American Heart Association, Monograph 18. Circulation **37**, Suppl. I, 1 (1968).
1080. Natvig, H., Borchgrevink, C. F., Dedichen, J., Owren, P. A., Schiøtz, E. H., Westlund, K.: A controlled trial of the effect of linolenic acid on incidence of coronary heart disease. Scand. J. clin. Lab. Invest. **22**, Suppl. 105, 1 (1968).
1081. Nékam, L., Jr., Ottenstein, B.: Zur Frage des Cholesterins bei Xanthomatose. Klin. Wschr. **14**, 641 (1935).
1082. Nelson, W. R., Werthessen, N. T., Holman, R. T., Hadaway, H., James, A. T.: Changes in fatty acid composition of human aorta associated with fatty streaking. Lancet **1961 I**, 36.
1083. Nestel, P. J.: Carbohydrate-induced hypertriglyceridemia and glucose utilization in ischemic heart disease. Metabolism **15**, 787 (1966).
1084. — Relationship between FFA flux and TGFA influx in plasma before and during the infusion of insulin. Metabolism **16**, 1123 (1967).
1085. — Austin, W.: The effect of ethyl chlorophenoxy-isobutyrate (CPIB) on the uptake of triglyceride fatty acids, activity of lipoprotein lipase and lipogenesis from glucose in fat tissue of rats. J. Atheroscler. Res. **8**, 827 (1968).
1086. — Couzens, E., Hirsch, E. Z.: Comparison of turnover of individual cholesterol esters in subjects with low and high plasma cholesterol concentrations. J. Lab. clin. Med. **66**, 582 (1965).
1087. — Hirsch, E. Z., Couzens, E. A.: The effect of chlorophenoxyisobutyric acid and ethinyl estradiol on cholesterol turnover. J. clin. Invest. **44**, 891 (1965).
1088. — Whyte, H. M., Goodman, D. S.: Distribution and turnover of cholesterol in humans. J. clin. Invest. **48**, 982 (1969).
1089. Nevaril, C. G., Lynch, E. C., Alfrey, C. P., Jr., Hellums, J. D.: Erythrocyte damage and destruction induced by shearing stress. J. Lab. clin. Med. **71**, 784 (1968).
1090. Nevin, N. C., Slack, J.: Hyperlipidaemic xanthomatosis. III. Mode of inheritance in 55 families with essential hyperlipidaemia and xanthomatosis. J. med. Genet. **5**, 9 (1968).
1091. Newman, H. A. I., Day, A. J., Zilversmit, D. B.: *In vitro* phospholipid synthesis in normal and atheromatous rabbit aortas. Circulation Res. **19**, 132 (1966).
1092. — Gray, G. W., Zilversmit, D. B.: Cholesteryl ester formation in aortas of cholesterol-fed rabbits. J. Atheroscler. Res. **8**, 745 (1968).
1093. — McCandless, E. L., Zilversmit, D. B.: The synthesis of C^{14}-lipids in rabbit atheromatous lesions. J. biol. Chem. **236**, 1264 (1961).

1094. Newman, H. A. I., Zilversmit, D. B.: Quantitative aspects of cholesterol flux in rabbit atheromatous lesions. J. biol. Chem. **237**, 2078 (1962).
1095. — — Accumulation of lipid and nonlipid constituents in rabbit atheroma. J. Atheroscler. Res. **4**, 261 (1964).
1096. — — Uptake and release of cholesterol by rabbit atheromatous lesions. Circulat. Res. **18**, 293 (1966).
1097. Nichols, A. V.: Human serum lipoproteins and their interrelationships. Advanc. biol. med. Phys. **11**, 109 (1967).
1098. Nikkilä, E. A.: Control of plasma and liver triglyceride kinetics by carbohydrate metabolism and insulin. Adv. Lipid Res. **7**, 63 (1969).
1099. — Miettinen, T. A., Pelkonen, R., Taskinen, M. R.: Plasma insulin response to glucose in endogenous and alimentary hyperglyceridemia. Progr. biochem. Pharmacol. **4**, 208 (1968).
1100. — — Vesenne, M. R., Pelkonen, R.: Plasma-insulin in coronary heart-disease. Response to oral and intravenous glucose and to tolbutamide. Lancet **1965 II**, 508.
1101. — Ojala, K.: Determination of liver L-α-glycerophosphate. Acta chem. scand. **17**, 554 (1963).
1102. — Pelkonen, R., Miettinen, T. A.: Relationship between glucose metabolism and serum triglyceride and cholesterol levels. (Abs.) Diabetologia **2**, 232 (1966).
1103. — Pykälistö, O.: Regulation of adipose tissue lipoprotein lipase synthesis by intracellular free fatty acids. Life Sci. **7**, 1303 (1968).
1104. — Taskinen, M. R.: Measurement of insulin secretion rate and its clinical applications. (Abs.) Scand. J. clin. Lab. Invest. **24**, Suppl. 110, 65 (1969).
1105. — — Miettinen, T. A., Pelkonen, R., Poppius, H.: Effect of muscular exercise on insulin secretion. Diabetes **17**, 209 (1968).
1106. Noble, R. P.: Electrophoretic separation of plasma lipoproteins in agarose gel. J. Lipid Res. **9**, 693 (1969).
1107. Nordöy, A.: The influence of saturated fats, cholesterol, corn oil and linseed oil on experimental venous thrombosis in rats. Thrombos. Diathes. haemorrh. (Stuttg.) **13**, 244 (1965).
1108. — Chandler, A. B.: Platelet thrombosis induced by adenosine diphosphate in the rat. Scand. J. Haemat. **1**, 25 (1964).
1109. — Hamlin, J. T., Chandler, A. B., Newland, H.: The influence of dietary fats on plasma and platelet lipids and ADP-induced platelet thrombosis in the rat. Scand. J. Haemat. **5**, 458 (1968).
1110. Norum, K. L., Gjone, E.: Familial plasma lecithin-cholesterol acyl-transferase deficiency. Biochemical study of a new inborn error of metabolism. Scand. J. clin. Lab. Invest. **20**, 231 (1967).
1111. Nuffield Provincial Hospitals Trust: Screening in medical care. Oxford: Oxford University Press 1968.
1112. Numa, S., Ringelmann, E., Lynen, F.: Zur Hemmung der Acetyl-CoA-Carboxylase durch Fettsäure-Coenzym A-Verbindungen. Biochem. Z. **343**, 243 (1965).
1113. O'Brien, J. R.: A comparison of platelet aggregation produced by seven compounds and a comparison of their inhibitors. J. clin. Path. **17**, 275 (1964).
1114. — Effect of anti-inflammatory agents on platelets. Lancet **1968 I**, 894.
1115. Ockner, R. K., Bloch, K. J., Isselbacher, K. J.: Very low-density lipoprotein in intestinal lymph: evidence for presence of the A protein. Science **162**, 1285 (1968).
1116. — Hughes, F. B., Isselbacher, K. J.: Very low-density lipoproteins in intestinal lymph—origin, composition and role in lipid transport in the fasting state. J. clin. Invest., in press (1970).
1117. Ogilvie, R. F.: The islands of Langerhans in nineteen cases of obesity. J. Path. Bact. **37**, 473 (1933).
1118. Oliver, M. F.: Reduction of serum lipid and uric-acid levels by an orally active androsterone. Lancet **1962 I**, 1321.
1119. — Further observations on the effects of "Atromid" and of ethyl chlorophenoxyisobutyrate on serum lipid levels. J. Atheroscler. Res. **3**, 427 (1963).

1120. Oliver, M. F.: The present status of clofibrate. Circulation **36**, 337 (1967).
1121. — The primary prevention of ischemic heart disease by means of Atromid-S (clofibrate). Bull. N.Y. Acad. Med. **44**, 8 (1968).
1122. — Boyd, G. S.: Influence of reduction of serum lipids on prognosis of coronary heart disease—a five year study using estrogen. Lancet **1961 II**, 499.
1123. — Geizerova, H., Cumming, L. A., Heady, J. A.: Serum cholesterol and ABO and Rhesus blood-groups. Lancet **1969 II**, 605.
1124. — Kurien, V. A., Greenwood, T. W.: Relation between serum free fatty acids and arrhythmias and death after acute myocardial infarction. Lancet **1968 I**, 710.
1125. Olmer, J., Mongen, M., Muratora, R., Denizet, D.: Myélomes, macroglobulinémies et dysglobulinémies voisines. Paris: Masson & Cie 1961.
1126. Olsen, R. E., Vester, J. W.: Nutrition-endocrine interrelationships in the control of fat transport in man. Physiol. Rev. **40**, 677 (1960).
1127. O'Neal, R. M., Still, W. J. F., Hartroft, W. S.: Experimental atherosclerosis in the rat. J. Path. Bact. **82**, 183 (1961).
1128. Ontko, J. A.: Chylomicron, free fatty acid and ketone body metabolism of isolated liver cells and liver homogenates. Biochim. biophys. Acta (Amst.) **137**, 13 (1967).
1129. Osborn, G. R.: The incubation period of coronary thrombosis. London: Butterworth 1963.
1130. Ostrander, L. D., Jr., Brandt, R. L., Kjelsberg, M. O., Epstein, F. H.: Electrocardiographic findings among the adult population of a total natural community, Tecumseh, Michigan. Circulation **31**, 888 (1965).
1131. — Francis, T., Jr., Hayner, N. S., Kjelsberg, M. O., Epstein, F. H.: The relationship of cardiovascular disease to hyperglycaemia. Ann. intern. Med. **62**, 1188 (1965).
1132. Ott, E. A., Smith, W. H., Stob, M., Beeson, W. M.: Zinc deficiency syndrome in the young lamb. J. Nutr. **82**, 41 (1964).
1133. Ott, H., Lohss, F., Gergely, J.: Der Nachweis von Serumlipoproteiden in der Aortenintima. Klin. Wschr. **36**, 383 (1958).
1134. Ouchterlony, O.: Antigen-antibody reactions in gels. IV. Types of reactions in coordinated system of diffusion. Acta path. microbiol. scand. **32**, 231 (1953).
1135. Özge, A. H., Rowsell, H. C., Downie, H. G., Mustard, J. F.: The effect of adrenaline infusions on blood coagulation in normal and haemophilia B dogs. Thrombos. Diathes. haemorrh. (Stuttg.) **15**, 349 (1966).
1136. Packham, M. A., Ardlie, N. G., Mustard, J. F.: The effect of adenine compounds on platelet aggregation. Amer. J. Physiol., **217**, 1009 (1969).
1137. — Evans, G., Glynn, M. F., Mustard, J. F.: The effect of plasma proteins on the interaction of platelets with glass surfaces. J. Lab. clin. Med.**73**, 686 (1969).
1138. — Jørgensen, L., Rowsell, H. C., Mustard, J. F.: Relationship among protein and ^{14}C-cholesterol accumulation, focal injury, and early atherosclerosis in pig and rabbit aortas. Circulation **36**, Suppl. II, 30 (1967).
1139. — Mustard, J. F.: The effect of pyrazole compounds on thrombin-induced platelet aggregation. Proc. Soc. exp. Biol. Med. (N.Y.) **130**, 72 (1969).
1140. — Nishizawa, E. E., Mustard, J. F.: Response of platelets to tissue injury. In: *Biochem. Pharmacol.*, Suppl., p. 171. Oxford and London: Pergamon Press 1968.
1141. — Rowsell, H. C., Jørgensen, L., Mustard, J. F.: Localized protein accumulation in the wall of the aorta. Exp. molec. Path. **7**, 214 (1967).
1142. — Warrior, E. S., Glynn, M. F., Senyi, A. S., Mustard, J. F.: Alteration of the response of platelets to surface stimuli by pyrazole compounds. J. exp. Med. **126**, 171 (1967).
1143. Padmavati, S., Gupta, S., Pantulu, G. V.: Dietary fat, serum cholesterol levels and the incidence of atherosclerosis in Delhi. Circulation **19**, 849 (1959).
1144. Page, I. H.: Atherosclerosis: an introduction. Circulation **10**, 1 (1954).
1145. — Stare, F. J., Corcoran, A. C., Pollack, H., Wilkinson, C. F., Jr.: Atherosclerosis and the fat content of the diet. Circulation **16**, 163 (1957).
1146. Palmer, G. H., Dixon, D. G.: Effect of pectin dose on serum cholesterol levels. Amer. J. clin. Nutr. **18**, 437 (1966).

1147. Palmer, R. S., Muench, H.: Course and prognosis of essential hypertension. Follow-up of 453 patients ten years after original series was closed. J. Amer. med. Ass. **153**, 1 (1953).

1148. Panganamala, R. V., Buntine, D. W., Geer, J. C., Cornwell, D. G.: Alk-l-enyl groups of glycerophosphatides from human aortic intima, plasma and erythrocytes. Chem. Phys. Lipids, in press (1969).

1149. — Geer, J. C., Cornwell, D. G.: Long-chain bases in the sphingolipids of atherosclerotic human aorta. J. Lipid Res. **10**, 445 (1969).

1150. Paoletti, P., Vandenheuvel, F. A., Fumagalli, R., Paoletti, R.: The sterol test for the diagnosis of human brain tumors. Neurology (Minneap.) **19**, 190 (1969).

1151. Parker, F., Ormsby, J. W., Peterson, N. F., Odland, G. F., Williams, R. H.: *In vitro* studies of phospholipid synthesis in experimental atherosclerosis: possible role of myointimal cells. Circulat. Res. **19**, 700 (1966).

1152. Parkinson T. M.: Hypolipidemic effects of orally administered dextran and cellulose anion exchangers in cockerels and dogs. J. Lipid Res. **8**, 24 (1967).

1153. Parks, H. F.: Electron microscopic investigation of the source and direction of movement of lipid granules appearing in the hepatic perisinusoidal space following partial hepatectomy. Amer. J. Anat. **124**, 513 (1969).

1154. Parrish, H. M.: Epidemiology of ischaemic heart disease among white males. J. chron. Dis. **14**, 311 (1961).

1155. Partridge, S. M.: Elastin, biosynthesis and structure. Gerontologia (Basel) **15**, 85 (1969).

1156. Patelski, J., Bowyer, D. E., Howard, A. N., Gresham, G. A.: Changes in phospholipase A. Lipase and cholesteryl esterase activity in the aorta in experimental atherosclerosis in the rabbit and rat. J. Atheroscler. Res. **8**, 221 (1968).

1157. Patterson, J.C.: Vascularization and hemorrhage of the intima of arteriosclerotic coronary arteries. Arch. Path. **22**, 313 (1936).

1158. Patil, V. S., Magar, N. G.: Effect of dietary fat intake and age on polyunsaturated fatty acids in human blood serum. Biochem. J. **76**, 417 (1960).

1159. Paul, O., Lepper, M. H., Phelan, W. H., Depertuin, G. W., MacMillan, A., McKean, H., Park, H.: A longitudinal study of coronary heart disease. Circulation **28**, 20 (1963).

1160. Payza, A. N., Eiber, H. B., Walter, S.: Studies with clearing factor. V. State of tissue lipases after injection of heparin. Proc. Soc. exp. Biol. Med. (N.Y.) **125**, 188 (1967).

1161. Peeters, H., Blaton, V.: Lipid fatty acid relationships in electrochromatographic lipoprotein fractions. Progr. biochem. Pharmacol. **4**, 144 (1968).

1162. — — Comparison of lipid and lipoprotein patterns in primates. Acta Zool. Path. Antverpiensia **48**, 221 (1969).

1163. Pelkonen, R., Miettinen, T. A., Taskinen, M. R., Nikkilä, E. A.: Effect of acute elevation of plasma glycerol, triglyceride and FFA levels on glucose utilization and plasma insulin. Diabetes **17**, 76 (1968).

1164. Perera, G. A.: Hypertensive vascular disease. Description and natural history. J. chron. Dis. **1**, 33 (1955).

1165. Perley, M., Kipnis, D. M.: Plasma insulin responses to glucose and tolbutamide of normal weight and obese diabetic and non-diabetic subjects. Diabetes **15**, 867 (1966).

1166. Perry, H. M., Jr., Schroeder, H. A.: The effect of treatment on mortality rates in severe hypertension. A comparison of medical and surgical regimens. Arch. intern. Med. **102**, 418 (1958).

1167. Peters, N., Hales, C. N.: Plasma insulin concentrations after myocardial infarction. Lancet **1965 I**, 1144.

1168. Peterson, D. W.: Some properties of a factor in alfalfa causing growth depression in chicks. J. biol. Chem. **183**, 647 (1950).

1169. Pfleiderer, E.: Tierexperimentelle Untersuchungen über Arteriosclerose unter besonderer Berücksichtigung der coronaren Atherosklerose. Virchows Arch. path. Anat. **284**, 154 (1932).

1170. Pfleiderer, T., Morgenstern, E., Weber, E.: Funktionelle, morphologische und biochemische Veränderungen in Blutplättchen während der Fettphagocytose *in vitro*. Klin. Wschr. **14**, 853 (1966).
1171. Picard, J.: Les mucopolysaccharides artériels et leurs variations dans l'athérosclérose. Arch. Mal. Coeur (Revue de l'Athérosclérose) **3**, 2 (1962).
1172. — Gardais, A., Lacord, M., Hermelin, B.: Le métabolisme des glycosaminoglycanes dans la paroi artérielle. In: 7th Int. Congr. Clin. Chem. Genève. Basle: S. Karger in press 1969.
1173. — Lacord-Bonneau, M., Gardais, A.: Incorporation du radio-sulfate (^{35}S) dans les mucopolysaccharides acides de l'aorte de rat. In: C.N.R.S. (ed.), Colloque International sur le rôle de la paroi artérielle dans l'athérogénèse, p. 721. Paris: Centre Nationale Recherche Scientifique 1967.
1174. Pierce, F. J., Jr.: The relationship of serum lipoproteins to atherosclerosis in the cholesterol fed alloxanized rabbit. Circulation **5**, 401 (1952).
1175. Pierce, F. T., Gofman, J. W.: Lipoproteins, liver disease, and atherosclerosis. Circulation **4**, 25 (1951).
1176. Pine, E. K., Holland, J. F.: Heterogeneity in the composition of human collagen. Arch. Biochem. Biophys. **115**, 95 (1966).
1177. Pinto, I. J., Colaco, F.: Risk factors in ischaemic heart disease in the lower socio-economic class in Bombay, India. Proceedings of the conference on cardiac rehabilitation. Dubrovnik (Yugoslavia), in press 1969.
1178. Pirie, A., van Heyningen, R.: The effect of diabetes on the cataract of sorbitol, glucose, fructose, and inositol in the human lens. Exp. Eye Res. **3**, 124 (1964).
1179. Plotz, M. B.: Coronary disease. Moscow: Inostrannaya Literatura 1961.
1180. Pokrajac, N., Lossow, W. J.: The effect of tube feeding of glucose or corn oil on adipose tissue lipoprotein lipase activity and uptake of C-labeled palmitic acid of chyle triglyceride *in vitro*. Biochim. biophys. Acta (Amst.) **137**, 291 (1967).
1181. Polasek, J.: Particulate nature of acid phosphatase released from thrombocytes. Thrombos. Diathes haemorrh. (Stuttg.) **19**, 466 (1968).
1182. Polonovski, J., Douste-Blazy, L., Valdiguie, P.: Lipides plasmatiques dans les dysprotéinémies. In: Les dysprotéinémies, p. 207. Paris: Expansion Scientifique 1963.
1183. Poole, J. C. F.: Phagocytosis of platelets by monocytes in organising arterial thrombi. An electron microscopical study. Quart. J. exp. Physiol. **51**, 54 (1966).
1184. — French, J. E.: Thrombosis. J. Atheroscler. Res. **1**, 251 (1961).
1185. — Sanders, A. G., Florey, H. W.: The regeneration of aortic endothelium. J. Path. Bact. **75**, 133 (1958).
1186. Poon King, T., Henry, M. V., Rampersad, F.: Prevalence and natural history of diabetes in Trinidad. Lancet **1968 I**, 155.
1187. Pories, W. J., Henzel, J. A., Lankau, C. A., Jr., Rob, C. G., Strain, W. H.: Zinc deficiency: a factor in atherosclerosis. In: A. S. Prasod (ed.), ***Zinc metabolism***, p. 371. Springfield: C. C. Thomas 1966.
1188. Porte, D., Jr., Bierman, E. L.: The effect of heparin infusion on plasma triglyceride *in vivo* and *in vitro* with a method for calculating triglyceride turnover. J. Lab. clin. Med. **73**, 631 (1969).
1189. — O'Hara, D. D., Williams, R. H.: The relation between postheparin lipolytic activity and plasma triglyceride and myxedema. Metabolism **15**, 107 (1966).
1190. Portman, O. W.: Incorporation of fatty acids into phospholipids by cell-free and subcellular fractions of squirrel monkey and rat aorta: importance of endogenous lysophosphatidylcholine. J. Atheroscler. Res. **7**, 617 (1967).
1191. — Alexander, M.: Lipid composition of aortic intima plus media and other tissue fractions from fetal and adult rhesus monkeys. Arch. Biochem. Biophys. **117**, 357 (1966).
1192. — — Maruffo, C. A.: Nutritional control of arterial lipid composition in squirrel monkeys. Major ester classes and types of phospholipids. J. Nutr. **91**, 35 (1967).
1193. — Stare, F. J.: Dietary regulation of serum cholesterol levels. Physiol. Rev. **39**, 407 (1959).

1194. Poullin, M. F., Vilain, C., Beaumont, J. L.: Une méthode de purification des β-lipoprotéines sériques. Ann. Biol. clin. **25**, 645 (1967).

1195. Powell, R. C., Nunes, W. T., Harding, R. S., Vacca, J. B.: Influence of non-absorbable antibiotics on serum lipids and the excretion of neutral sterols and bile acids. Amer. J. clin. Nutr. **11**, 156 (1962).

1196. Prior, I. A. M.: Health survey in a rural Maori community with particular emphasis on the cardiovascular, nutritional and metabolic findings. N. Z. med. J. **61**, 333 (1962).

1197. — Davidson, F.: Epidemiology of diabetes in Polynesians and Europeans in New Zealand and the Pacific. N. Z. med. J. **65**, 375 (1966).

1198. — Harvey, H. P. B., Neave, M. I., Davidson, F.: The health of two groups of Cook Island Maoris. New Zealand Dept. Health Spec. Report No. 26, 1964.

1199. Puchtler, H., Sweat, F., Terry, M. S., Conner, H. M.: Investigation of staining, polarization and fluorescence-microscopic properties of myoendothelial cells. J. Microscopy **89**, 95 (1969).

1200. Puddu, V.: Mortality from rheumatic heart disease and cardiovascular disease in Italy as compared to the U.S.A.. In: A. Keys and P. White (eds.), *Cardiovascular epidemiology, World Trends in Cardiology*, I, p. 77, 1956.

1201. Puffer, R. R., Griffith, G. W.: Patterns of urban mortality. Report of the Interamerican Investigation of Mortality. In: Scientific Publication No. 151, Pan American Health Organization. W.H.O., Washington, D.C. 1967.

1202. Pugatch, E. M. J., Poole, J. C. F.: Studies on the fibrinolytic activity of an extract from vascular endothelium. Quart. J. exp. Physiol. **54**, 80 (1969).

1203. Puigbo, J. J., Nava-Rhode, J. R., Garcia Barrios, H., Suarez, J. A., Gil Yepez, C.: Clinical and epidemiological study of chronic heart involvement in Chagas' Disease. Bull. Wld Hlth Org. **34**, 655 (1966).

1204. Puppione, D. L.: Physical and chemical characterization of the serum lipoproteins of marine mammals. Thesis. University of California, Berkeley, 1969.

1205. Pyke, D. A.: Arterial disease and diabetes. In: W. G. Oakley, D. A. Pyke and K. W. Taylor (eds.), *Clinical diabetes and its biochemical basis*. Oxford and Edinburgh: Blackwell Scientific Publications 1968.

1206. Quarfordt, S. H., Goodman, D. S.: Heterogeneity in the rate of plasma clearance of chylomicrons of different size. Biochim. biophys. Acta (Amst.) **116**, 382 (1966).

1207. Rachmilewitz, D., Eisenberg, S., Stein, Y., Stein, O.: Phospholipases in arterial tissue. 1. Sphingomyelin choline phosphohydrolase activity in human, dog, guinea pig, rat and rabbit arteries. Biochim. biophys. Acta (Amst.) **144**, 624 (1967).

1208. Radding, C. M., Steinberg, D.: Studies in the synthesis and secretion of serum lipoproteins by rat liver slices. J. clin. Invest. **39**, 1560 (1960).

1209. Randle, P. J.: Carbohydrate metabolism and lipid storage and breakdown in diabetes. Diabetologia **2**, 237 (1966).

1210. Randle, P., Jr., Hales, C. N., Garland, P. B., Newsholme, E. A.: The glucose fatty acid cycle. Lancet **1963 I**, 785.

1211. Rappoport, Y. L.: The spreading of atherosclerosis in different parts of the man's vascular system and its correlation with different factors. Arch. Path. Anat. Path. Physiol. **1**, 66 (1935).

1212. Ravenhill, J. R., James, A. T.: A simple sensitive radioactive scanner for thin-layer chromatograms. J. Chromatog. **26**, 89 (1967).

1213. Reaven, G., Calciano, A., Cody, R., Lucas, C., Miller, R.: Carbohydrate intolerance and hyperlipemia in patients with myocardial infarction without known diabetes mellitus. J. clin. Endocr. **23**, 1013 (1963).

1214. Reaven, G. M., Hill, D. B., Gross, R. C., Farquhar, J. W.: Kinetics of triglyceride turnover of very low-density lipoproteins of human plasma. J. clin. Invest. **44**, 1826 (1965).

1215. — Lerner, R. L., Stern, M. P., Farquhar, J. W.: Role of insulin in endogenous hypertriglyceridemia. J. clin. Invest. **46**, 1756 (1967).

1216. Redgrave, T. G.: Inhibition of protein synthesis and absorption of lipid into thoracic duct lymph of rats. Proc. Soc. exp. Biol. Med. (N.Y.) **130**, 776 (1969).

1217. Redman, C. M.: The synthesis of serum proteins on attached rather than free ribosomes of rat liver. Biochem. biophys. Res. Commun. **31**, 845 (1968).

1218. Reissell, P. K., Mandella, P. A., Poon-King, T. M. W., Hatch, F. T., Hagopian, L. M.: Treatment of hypertriglyceridemia. I. Total caloric restriction followed by refeeding a low carbohydrate, high-fat diet in the carbohydrate-induced type (eight cases). II. Low-fat diet plus medium-chain triglycerides in the fat-induced type (two cases). Amer. J. clin. Nutr. **19**, 84 (1966).

1219. Relman, A. S.: Editorial comments. In: F. J. INGELFINGER, A. S., RELMAN and M. FINLAND (eds.), *Controversy in internal medicine*, p. 101. Philadelphia: W. B. Saunders 1966.

1220. Renaud, S., Allard, C.: Thrombosis in connection with serum lipid changes in the rat. Circulat. Res. **11**, 388 (1962).

1221. Reneau, D. D., Fruley, D. F., Knisely, M. H.: A mathematical simulation of oxygen release, diffusion, and comsumption in the capillaries, and tissue of the human brain. In: D. HERSHEY (ed.), *Chemical engineering in medicine and biology*. New York: Plenum Press 1967.

1222. Research Committee of Four London Hospitals: Low-fat diet in myocardial infarction; a controlled trial. Lancet **1965 II**, 501.

1223. Reumuth, H.: Die Raster-Elektronenmikroskopie. Dtsch. med. Wschr. **36**, 1832 (1969).

1224. Reunanen, A., Miettinen, T. A., Nikkilä, E. A.: Quantitative lipid analysis of human liver needle biopsy specimens. Acta med. scand. **186**, 149 (1969).

1225. Riccardi, B. A., Fahrenbach, M. J.: Effect of Guar gum and pectin on serum and liver lipids of cholesterol-fed rats. Proc. Soc. exp. Biol. Med. (N.Y.) **124**, 749 (1967).

1226. Richards, D. W., Bland, E. F., White, P. D.: A complete twentyfive year-follow-up study of 200 patients with myocardial infarction. J. chron. Dis. **4**, 415 (1956).

1227. Rinzler, S. H.: Primary prevention of coronary heart disease by diet. Bull. N. Y. Acad. Med. **44**, 936 (1968).

1228. Ritter, M. C., Dempsey, M. E.: Partial purification and characterization of a naturally occurring activator of cholesterol biosynthesis from Δ5,7-cholestadienol. Biochem. biophys. Res. Commun., **38**, 921 (1970).

1229. Ritz, E.: Der Pentosezyklus im Arteriengewebe. J. Atheroscler. Res. **8**, 445 (1968).

1230. Robbins, S. L., Bentov, I.: The kinetics of viscous flow in a model vessel. Effect of stenoses of varying size, shape and length. Lab. Invest. **16**, 864 (1967).

1231. Robert, B., Legrand, Y., Pignaud, G., Caen, J., Robert, L.: Activite élastinolytique associée aux plaquettes sanguines. Path. et Biol. **17**, 615 (1969).

1232. — Robert, A. M.: Mécanismes immunologiques dans l'athérosclérose. Med. et Hyg. (Genéve) **878**, 822 (1970).

1233. — Robert, L.: Determination of leastolytic activity with ^{125}I and ^{131}I-labelled elastin. Europ. J. Biochem. in press (1970).

1234. — — Studies on the structure of elastin and the mechanism of action of elastolytic enzymes. In: G. R. TRISTRAM and E. A. BALAZS (eds.), NATO *Symposium, The chemistry and molecular biology of the intercellular matrix*. New York: Academic Press (in press).

1235. Robert, L., Poullain, N.: Structure de l'élastine. Rôle des forces hydrophobes. In: H. BRICAUD (ed.), *Enzymologie et immunologie dans l'athérosclérose*, Colloque International, Bordeaux, p. 121. Paris: Bailliere & Fils 1964.

1236. — Robert, B.: Structural glycoproteins of membranes and connective tissue: biochemical and immunopathological properties. In: H. PEETERS, (ed.), *Protides of biological fluids*, vol. 15, p. 143. Amsterdam: Elsevier 1967.

1237. — Robert, M., Moczar, M., Moczar, E.: Constituants macromoléculaires de la paroi artérielle, antigénicité et rôle dans l'athérogénèse. In: CNRS (ed.), Le róle de la paroi artérielle dans l'athérogénèse, p. 395. Paris: CNRS 1968.

1238. Roberts, J. C., Straus, R. (eds.): Comparative atherosclerosis. New York: Harper & Row 1965.

1239. Robertson, A. L.: Transport of plasma lipoproteins and ultrastructure of human arterial intimacytes in culture. Wistar Symp. Monograph No. 6, 116 (1967).

1240. — Oxygen requirements of human arterial intima in atherogenesis. Progr. biochem. Pharmacol. 4, 305 (1968).

1241. Robertson, J. S.: Mortality and hardness of water. Lancet **1968 II**, 348.

1242. — The water story. Lancet **1969 I**, 1160.

1243. Robertson, W. B., Strong, J. P.: Atherosclerosis in persons with hypertension and diabetes mellitus. Lab. Invest. **18**, 538 (1968).

1244. Robinson, D. S.: The clearing factor lipase activity of adipose tissue. In: A. E. Renold and G. F. Cahill, Jr. (eds.), *Handbook of physiology*, Sect. 5, p. 295. American Physiological Society, Washington, D. C., 1965.

1245. — The role of the clearing factor lipase in the removal of chylomicron triglycerides from the blood. In: G. Cowgill and L. W. Kinsell (eds.), *Proceedings of the 1967 Deuel conference on lipids on the fate of dietary lipids*, p. 166. U.S. Government Printing Office, Washington, D. C., 1967.

1246. Robison, G. A., Butcher, R. W., Sutherland, E. W.: Adenyl cyclase as an adrenergic receptor. Ann. N. Y. Acad. Sci. **139**, 703 (1967).

1247. Roden, L.: Linkage of acid mucopolysaccharides to protein. In: E. Rossi and E. Stoll (eds.), *Biochemistry of glycoproteins and related substances*. Proc. of the 4th International Conference on Cystic Fibrosis of the Pancreas, Part II, p. 185. Basel and New York: S. Karger 1968.

1248. Rodman, N. R., Mason, R. G., Brinkhous, K. M.: Some pathogenetic mechanisms of white thrombus formation: Agglutination and self-destruction of the platelet. Fed. Proc. **22**, 1356 (1963).

1249. Roheim, P. S., Gidez, L. I., Eder, H. A.: Extrahepatic synthesis of lipoproteins of plasma and chyle: role of the intestine. J. clin. Invest. **45**, 297 (1966).

1250. Rokitansky, C. von: Lehrbuch der pathologischen Anatomie, vol. 2, p. 306. Vienna: Braunmüller 1856.

1251. Rokitansky, C. A.: W. E.: Swaine, E. Sieveking, C. H. More and G. E. Day, (translators), Manual of pathological anatomy, vol. 4, p. 198. Philadelphia: Blanchard & Lea 1855.

1252. Rose, G.: Physical activity and coronary heart disease. Proc. roy. Soc. Med. **62**, 1183 (1969).

1253. Rose, G. A.: Variability of angina. Brit. J. prev. Soc. Med. **22**, 12 (1968).

1254. — Ahmeteli, M., Checcacci, L., Fidanza, F., Glazunov, I., DeHaas, J., Horstmann, P., Kornitzer, M. D., Meloni, C., Menotti, A., Van der Sande, D., DeSoto-Hartgrink, M. K., Piza, Z., Thomsen, B.: Ischaemic heart disease in middle aged men. Prevalence comparisons in Europe. Bull. Wld. Hlth. Org. **38**, 885 (1968).

1255. — Blackburn, H.: Cardiovascular survey methods. Wld. Hlth. Org. Monograph Series, No 56, 1968.

1256. — Thomson, W. B., Williams, R. T.: Corn oil in treatment of ischaemic heart disease. Brit. med. J. **1965 I**, 1531.

1257. Rosenman, R. H.: The role of personality and behavior patterns in the genesis of coronary heart disease. J. Amer. med. Wom. Ass. **20**, 161 (1965).

1258. — Friedman, M. A., Straus, R., Wurm, M., Jenkins, D., Messinger, H. B.: Coronary heart disease in the western collaborative group study. Follow-up experience of two years. J. Amer. med. Ass. **195**, 86 (1966).

1259. Ross, R., Bornstein, P.: The elastic fiber. I.: The separation and partial characterization of its macromolecular components. J. Cell Biol. **40**, 366 (1969).

1260. Rossi, E. C.: The effects of imidazole upon platelets incubated *in vitro*. Thrombos. Diathes. haemorrh. (Stuttg.) **19**, 53 (1968).

1261. Rössle, R.: Über die serösen Entzündungen der Organe. Virchows Arch. path. Anat. **311**, 252 (1944).

1262. Rothblat, G. H., Hartzell, R. W., Miahle, H., Kritchevsky, D.: The uptake of cholesterol by LS178γ tissue-culture cells: studies with free cholesterol. Biochim. biophys. Acta (Amst.) **116**, 133 (1966).
1263. — Kritchevsky, D.: The metabolism of free and esterified cholesterol in tissue culture cells: a review. Exp. molec. Path. **8**, 314 (1968).
1264. Rouser, G., Solomon, R. D.: Changes in phospholipid composition of human aorta with age. Lipids **4**, 232 (1969).
1265. Rowley, D. A.: Mast cell damage and vascular injury in the rat. An electron microscopic study of a reaction produced by thorotrast. Brit. J. exp. Path. **44**, 284 (1963).
1266. Rozenberg, M. C., Holmsen, H.: Adenine nucleotide metabolism of blood platelets. II. Uptake of adenosine and inhibition of ADP-induced platelet aggregation. Biochim. biophys. Acta (Amst.) **155**, 342 (1968).
1267. — — Adenine nucleotide metabolism of blood platelets. IV. Platelet aggregation response to exogenous ATP and ADP. Biochim. biophys. Acta (Amst.) **157**, 280 (1968).
1268. Ruderman, N. B., Richards, K. C., Valles de Bourges, V., Jones, A. L.: Regulation of production and release of lipoprotein by the perfused rat liver. J. Lipid Res. **9**, 613 (1968).
1269. Ruiz, L., Figuero, M., Horna, C., Penaloza, D.: Prevalencia de hipertension arterial y cardiopatia isquemica en la grandes alturas. Arch. Inst. Cardiol. Méx. in press (1969).
1270. Russ, E. M., Raymunt, J., Barr, D. P.: Lipoproteins in primary biliary cirrhosis. J. clin. Invest. **35**, 133 (1956).
1271. Ryan, W. G., Schwartz, T. B.: The dynamics of triglyceride turnover: effect of "Atromid-S". (Abs.) J. Lab. clin. Med. **64**, 1001 (1964).
1272. — — Dynamics of plasma triglyceride turnover in man. Metabolism **14**, 1243 (1965).
1273. Ryvkin, I. A.: Morbidity and lethality of myocardial infarction. Cardiologia (Basel) **4**, 42 (1965).
1274. Sachs, B. A., Cady, P., Ross, G.: An abnormal lipid-like material and carbohydrate in the sera of patients with multiple myeloma. Amer. J. Med. **17**, 662 (1954).
1275. Sackett, D. L., Gibson, R. W., Bross, I. D. J., Pickren, J. W.: Aortic atherosclerosis and smoking. Relation between aortic atherosclerosis and the use of cigarettes and alcohol. New Engl. J. Med. **279**, 1413 (1968).
1276. — Winkelstein, W., Jr.: The relationship between cigarette usage and aortic atherosclerosis. Amer. J. Epidemiol. **86**, 264 (1967).
1277. Sacks, M. I., Vlodaver, Z.: An autopsy study of myocardial infarction in Israel. Path. et Microbiol. (Basel) **30**, 570 (1967).
1278. Sailer, S., Bolzano, K., Sandhofer, F., Spath, P., Braunsteiner, H.: Triglyceridspiegel und Insulin-Konzentration im Plasma nach oraler Glukosegabe bei Patienten mit primärer kohlenhydratinduzierter Hypertriglyceridämie. Schweiz. med. Wschr. **98**, 1512 (1968).
1279. — Sandhofer, F., Braunsteiner, H.: Overweight and triglyceride level in normal persons and patients with diabetes mellitus. Metabolism **15**, 135 (1966).
1280. — — — Regulation of endogenous lipoprotein-lipase activity in the plasma of normal subjects and patients with essential hyperlipaemia. German Med. Monthly **11**, 41 (1966).
1281. St. Clair, R. W., Lofland, H. B., Jr., Clarkson, T. B.: Composition and synthesis of fatty acids in atherosclerotic aortas of the pigeon. J. Lipid Res. **9**, 739 (1968).
1282. — — Prichard, R. W., Clarkson, T. B.: Synthesis of squalene and sterols by isolated segments of human and pigeon arteries. Exp. molec. Path. **8**, 201 (1968).
1283. Salans, L. B., Knittle, J. L., Hirsch, J.: The role of adipose cell size and adipose tissue insulin sensitivity in the carbohydrate intolerance of human obesity. J. clin. Invest. **46**, 1112 (1967).

1284. Salen, G., Ahrens, E. H., Jr., Grundy, S. M.: The metabolism of β-sitosterol in man. J. clin. Invest. in press (1970).
1285. Salzman, E., Chambers, D. A., Neri, L. L.: Possible mechanism of aggregation of blood platelets by adenosine diphosphate. Nature (Lond.) **210**, 167 (1966).
1286. Samani, O. T.: Coronary heart disease in low income population in India. Indian Heart J. **8**, 104 (1956).
1287. Samuel, P., Holtzman, C. H., Goldstein, J.: Long-term reduction of serum cholesterol levels of patients with atherosclerosis by small doses of neomycin. Circulation **35**, 938 (1967).
1288. — — Meilman, E., Perl, W.: Effect of neomycin on exchangeable pools of cholesterol in the steady state. J. clin. Invest. **47**, 1806 (1968).
1289. — Steiner, A.: Effect of neomycin on serum cholesterol level in man. Proc. Soc. exp. Biol. Med. (N. Y.) **100**, 192 (1959).
1290. Samuels, P. B., Webster, D. R.: The role of venous endothelium in the inception of thrombosis. Ann. Surg. **136**, 422 (1952).
1291. Sandberg, L. B., Weissman, N., Smith, D. W.: The purification and partial characterization of a soluble elastin-like protein from copper deficient porcine aorta. Biochemistry **8**, 2940 (1969).
1292. Sandhofer, F., Bolzano, K., Sailer, S., Braunsteiner, H.: Die Verwendung von Plasmaglucose-Kohlenstoff zur Bildung von Plasmatriglycerid-Glycerol bei Patienten mit primärer, ,,kohlenhydratinduzierter" Hypertriglyceridämie. Klin. Wschr. **46**, 1034 (1968).
1293. — — — — Zur Bestimmung des Einbaues von Plasmaglucose-Kohlenstoff in Plasmatriglyceride beim Menschen. Klin. Wschr. **46**, 1139 (1968).
1294. — — — — Quantitative Untersuchungen über den Einbau von Plasmaglucose-Kohlenstoff in Plasmatriglyceride und die Veresterungsrate von freien Fettsäuren des Plasmas zu Plasmatriglyceriden während oraler Zufuhr von Glukose bei primärer kohlenhydratinduzierter Hypertriglyceridämie. Klin. Wschr. **47**, in press (1969).
1295. Saphir, O., Stryzak, D., Ohringer, L.: Hypersensitivity changes in coronary arteries of rabbits and their relationship to arteriosclerosis. J. Lab. Invest. **7**, 434 (1958).
1296. Sarvotham, S. G., Berry, J. N.: Prevalence of coronary heart disease in an urban population — Northern India. Circulation **37**, 939 (1968).
1297. Savin, R. C.: Hyperglobulinemic purpura terminating in myeloma, hyperlipemia and xanthomatosis. Arch. Derm. Syph. (Chic.) **92**, 679 (1965).
1298. Scanu, A.: Forms of human serum high-density lipoprotein proteins. J. Lipid Res. **7**, 295 (1966).
1299. — Lewis, L. A., Bumpus, F. M.: Separation and characterization of the protein moiety of human lipoproteins. Arch. Biochem. **74**, 390 (1958).
1300. — Pollard, H., Hirtz, R., Kothary, K.: On the conformational instability of human serum low-density lipoprotein: effect of temperature. Proc. nat. Acad. Sci. (Wash.) **62**, 171 (1969).
1301. — — Reader, W.: Properties of human serum low density lipoproteins after modification by succinic anhydride. J. Lipid Res. **9**, 342 (1968).
1302. — Toth, J., Edelstein, C., Koga, S., Stiller, E.: Fractionation of human serum high density lipoprotein in urea solutions. Evidence for polypeptide heterogeneity. Biochemistry **8**, 3309 (1969).
1303. Scarborough, D. E., Mason, R. G., Dalldorf, F. G., Brinkhouse, K. M.: Morphologic manifestations of blood-solid interfacial reactions. Lab. Invest. **20**, 164 (1969).
1304. Scebat, L., Renais, J., Groult, N., Lenegre, J.: Experimental arteriopathy induced in the rabbit through rat aorta homogenate injections: a study of the aortic tissue specificity. In: N. R. Di Luzzio and R. Paoletti (eds.); *The reticuloendothelial system and atherosclerosis*, p. 451. New York: Plenum Press 1967.
1305. — — Iris, L., Groult, N., Lenegre, J.: Athérosclérose expérimentale du rat. III. Rôle des lésions préalables de la paroi artérielle par un processus immunopathologique. Arch. Mal. Coeur Rev. Atheroscler. **1**, 242 (1967).

1306. Schalch, D. S., Kipnis, D. M.: Abnormalities in carbohydrate tolerance associated with elevated plasma nonesterified fatty acids. J. clin. Invest. **44**, 2010 (1965).

1307. Schettler, G.: Arteriosklerose. Stuttgart: Thieme 1961.

1308. — Krauland, W.: Arteriosklerose im Tierversuch und beim Menschen. Ciba Symposium **14**, 15 (1966).

1309. Schless, G.: Serum Cholesterol-Globulin Complex in Multiple Myeloma. Amer. J. med. Sci. **235**, 562 (1958).

1310. Schneckloth, R. E., Corcoran, A. C. Stuart, K. L., Moore, F. E.: Arterial pressure and hypertensive disease in a West Indian negro population. Report of a survey in St. Kitts, West Indies. Amer. Heart J. **63**, 611 (1962).

1311. Schoefl, G., French, J.: Vascular permeability to particulate fat: morphological observations on vessels of lactating mammary gland and of lung. Proc. royal Soc. **169**, 153 (1968).

1312. Scholan, N. A., Boyd, G. S.: Solubilization of cholesterol 7α-hydroxylase from the microsomal fraction of rat liver. Biochem. J. **108**, 27P (1968).

1313. — — The cholesterol 7α-hydroxylase enzyme system. Hoppe-Seylers Z. physiol. Chem. **349**, 1628 (1968).

1314. Schönheimer, R., Breusch, F.: Synthesis and destruction of cholesterol in the organism. J. biol. Chem. **103**, 439 (1933).

1315. Schork, M. A., Remington, R.: Determination of sample size in treatment-control comparisons for chronic disease studies in which dropout or non-adherence give a problem. J. chron. Dis. **20**, 233 (1967).

1316. Schotz, M. C., Arnesjö, B., Olivecrona, T.: The role of the liver in the uptake of plasma and chyle triglycerides in the rat. Biochim. biophys. Acta (Amst.) **125**, 485 (1966).

1317. Schroeder, H. A.: Relation between mortality from cardiovascular disease and treated water supplies. Variations in states and 163 largest municipalities of the United States. J. Amer. med. Ass. **172**, 1902 (1960).

1318. — The water factor. New Engl. J. Med. **280**, 836 (1969).

1319. Schuberth, O., Wretlind, A.: Fat emulsion for intravenous nutrition. Nord. Med. **69**, 13 (1963).

1320. Schumaker, V. N., Adams, G. H.: Circulating lipoproteins. Ann. Rev. Biochem. **38**, 113 (1969).

1321. Schwartz, D., Lellouch, J.: Explanatory and pragmatic attitudes in therapeutical trials. J. chron Dis. **20**, 637 (1967).

1322. Schweizer, W.: Die Epidemiologie des Myokardinfarktes. Z. Präv. Med. **4**, 424 (1959).

1323. Scott, G. B. D., Gracey, L. R. H.: Analysis of the factors concerned in the organization of occlusive thrombi. Arch. Path. **87**, 643 (1969).

1324. Scott, P. J., Hurley, P. J.: Effect of clofibrate on low-density lipoprotein turnover in essential hypercholesterolaemia. J. Atheroscler. Res. **9**, 25 (1969).

1325. — — Low density lipoprotein accumulation in human aortic tissue. J. Atheroscler. Res., in press (1970).

1326. Scott, R. F., Daoud, A. S., Florentin, R. A., Davies, J. N. P., Coles, R. M.: Comparison of the amount of coronary arteriosclerosis in autopsied East Africans and New Yorkers. Amer. J. Cardiol. **8**, 165 (1961).

1327. — Florentin, R. A., Daoud, A. S., Morrison, E. S., Jones, R. M., Hutt, M. S. R.: Coronary arteries of children and young adults. A comparison of lipids and anatomic features in New Yorkers and East Africans. Exp. molec. Path. **5**, 12 (1966).

1328. — Jones, R., Daoud, A. S., Zumbo, O., Coulston, F., Thomas, W. A.: Experimental atherosclerosis in rhesus monkeys. Cellular elements of proliferative lesions and possible role of cytoplasmic degeneration in pathogenesis as studied by electron microscopy. Exp. molec. Path. **7**, 34 (1967).

1329. — Likimani, J. C., Morrison, E. S., Thuku, J. J., Thomas, W. A.: Esterified serum fatty acids in subjects eating high and low cholesterol diets. A comparative study of serum lipid metabolism in New Yorkers, indigenous poor East Africans and upper class East Africans. Amer. J. clin. Nutr. **13**, 82 (1963).

1330. Scott, R. F., Morrison, E. S., Hall, E. W., Davies, J. N. P., Goodale, F., Daoud, A.: Chemico-anatomic studies in geographic pathology. A comparison of lipids in New Yorkers and African coronary arteries. Exp. molec. Path. **1**, 481 (1962).

1331. — — Jarmolych, J. Nam, S. C., Kroms, M., Coulson, F.: Experimental atherosclerosis in rhesus monkeys. Exp. molec. Path. **7**, 11 (1967).

1332. — — Kroms, M.: Aortic respiration and glycolysis in the pre-proliferative phase of diet-induced atherosclerosis in swine. J. Atheroscler. Res. **9**, 5 (1969).

1333. Scrimshaw, N. S., Guzman, M. A.: Diet and atherosclerosis. Lab. Invest. **18**, 623 (1968).

1334. Searcy, R. L., Bergquist, L. M.: The determination of cholesterol directly upon acetone-ethanol filtrates. Amer. J. med. Technol. **25**, 237 (1959).

1335. Seegers, W. H., Schroer, H., Marchiniak, E.: Blood clotting enzymology. In: W. H. Seegers (ed.), *Activation of prothrombin*, p. 103. New York: Academic Press 1967.

1336. Segal, P., Roheim, P. S., Eder, H. A.: Mechanism of action of chlorophenoxyisobutyrate in hyperlipemic rats. Circulation **40**, Suppl. III, 182 (1969).

1337. Seidel, D., Alaupovic, P., Furman, R. H.: A lipoprotein characterizing obstructive jaundice. I. Method for quantitative separation and identification of lipoproteins in jaundiced subjects. J. clin. Invest. **48**, 1211 (1969).

1338. Sekhar, N. C., Weeks, J. R., Kupiecki, F. P.: Antithrombotic activity of a new prostaglandin, 8-iso-PGE_1. Circulation **38**, Suppl. VI, 23 (1968).

1339. Seligmann, M., Danon, F., Basch, A., Bernard, J.: IgG myeloma cryoglobulin with antistreptolysin activity. Nature (Lond.) **220**, 711 (1968).

1340. Seyffert, W. A., Madison, L. L.: Physiologic effects of metabolic fuels on carbohydrate metabolism. I. Acute effect of elevation of plasma free fatty acids on hepatic glucose output, peripheral glucose utilization, serum insulin, and plasma glucagon levels. Diabetes **16**, 765 (1967).

1341. Shafer, A. J., Jones, K. W.: Serum cholesterol, diet and coronary heart diesase. Lancet **1959 II**, 534.

1342. Shah, V. V., Shah, S. R., Panse, V. N.: Nutritional and physical factors in coronary heart disease. Geriatrics **23**, 99 (1968).

1343. Shaper, A. G. (ed.): Symposium on blood pressure and hypertension in Africa. E. Afric. med. J. **46**, 220 (1969).

1344. — Jones, K. W., Jones, M., Kyobe, J.: Serum lipids in three nomadic tribes of northern Kenya. Amer. J. clin. Nutr. **13**, 135 (1963).

1345. — — Kyobe, J., Jones, M.: Fibrinolysis in relation to body fatness, serum lipids and coronary heart disease in African and Asian men in Uganda. J. Atheroscler. Res. **6**, 313 (1966).

1346. — Lee, K. T., Scott, R. F., Goodale, F., Thomas, W. A.: Comparison of adipose tissue fatty acids and plasma lipids in diabetics from East Africa and the United States with different frequencies of myocardial infarction. Amer. J. Cardiol. **10**, 390 (1962).

1347. Shapiro, H. L.: The Jewish people: a biological history. Liège (Belgium): UNESCO Gerages Thone 1963.

1348. Shapiro, S., Weinblatt, E., Frank, C. W., Sager, R. V.: Incidence of coronary heart disease in a population insured for medical care (HIP). Myocardial infarction, angina pectoris, and possible myocardial infarction. Amer. J. Publ. Health **59**, 1 (1969).

1349. Sharp, C. L. E. H., Butterfield, W. J. H., Keen, H.: Diabetes survey in Bedford. Proc. roy. Soc. Med. **57**, 193 (1964).

1350. Sheppard, B. L., French, J. E.: Observations by combined use of scanning and transmission electron microscopy on platelet adhesion in arteries. Nature (Lond.) in press (1969).

1351. Shimamoto, T.: Damages to "silicone-like property" of vascular endothelial cells and prevention by monoamine oxidase inhibitor, nialamide. Asian med. J. **3**, 479 (1960).

1352. Shore, B., Shore, V.: Heparin-released lipolytic and esterolytic activities of human and rabbit plasmas. Amer. J. Physiol. **201**, 915 (1961).
1353. — — The protein moiety of human serum β-lipoproteins. Biochem. biophys. Res. Commun. **28**, 1003 (1967).
1354. — — Heterogeneity in protein subunits of human serum high-density lipoproteins. Biochemistry **7**, 2773 (1968).
1355. — — Isolation and characterization of polypeptides of human serum lipoproteins. Biochemistry **8**, 4510 (1969).
1356. Shore, M. L., Zilversmit, D. B., Ackerman, R. F.: Plasma phospholipide deposition and aortic phospholipide synthesis in experimental atherosclerosis. Amer. J. Physiol. **181**, 527 (1955).
1357. Shore, P. A.: Release of serotonin and catecholamines by drugs. Pharmacol. Rev. **14**, 531 (1962).
1358. Shore, V., Shore, B.: Some physical and chemical studies on the protein moiety of a high-density (1.126—1.195 g/ml) lipoprotein fraction of human serum. Biochemistry **6**, 1962 (1967).
1359. — — Some physical and chemical studies on two polypeptide components of high-density lipoproteins of human serum. Biochemistry **7**, 3396 (1968).
1360. Shuhachi, K., Okazaki, Y., Yoshida, A.: Hypocholesterolemic effect of polysaccharides and polysaccharide-rich foodstuffs in cholesterol-fed rats. J. Nutr. **97**, 382 (1969).
1361. Siegal, I., Cohen, S.: Action of staphylococcal toxin on human platelets. J. infect. Dis. **114**, 488 (1964).
1362. Siggaard-Andersen, J., Bonde-Petersen, F., Hansen, T. I., Mellemgaard, K.: Plasma volume and vascular permeability during hypoxia and carbon monoxide exposure. Scand. J. clin. Lab. Invest. **22**, Suppl. 103, 39 (1968).
1363. Sih, C. J., Whitlock, H. W., Jr.: Biochemistry of steroids. Ann. Rev. Biochem. **37**, 661 (1968).
1364. Sinapius, D.: Häufigkeit und Morphologie der Coronarthrombose und ihre Beziehungen zur antithrombotischen und fibrinolytischen Behandlung. Klin. Wschr. **43**, 37 (1965).
1365. — Histological findings in coronary thrombosis. In: *Proc. Gravenbruch-Heidelberg symposium on platelets and the vessel wall-fibrin deposition*. Stuttgart: Thieme 1969 (in press).
1366. Sinclair, A. J., Collins, F. D.: Fatty livers in rats deficient in essential fatty acids. Biochem. biophys. Acta (Amst.) **152**, 498 (1968).
1367. Sinnett, P. F., Goldrick, R. B., Whyte, H. M.: Coronary heart disease in a New Guinea population. Proc. 4th Asian-Pacific Cong. Cardiol., Tel-Aviv 1968.
1368. Siperstein, M. D., Chaikoff, I. L.: Conversion of cholesterol to bile acids. Fed. Proc. **14**, 767 (1955).
1369. — Fagan, V. M.: Studies on the feedback regulation of cholesterol synthesis. In: G. Weber (ed.), *Advances in enzyme regulation*, vol. 2, p. 249. New York: Pergamon Press 1964.
1370. — — Feedback control of mevalonate synthesis by dietary cholesterol. J. biol. Chem. **241**, 602 (1966).
1371. — Guest, M. H.: Studies on the site of the feedback control of cholesterol synthesis. J. clin. Invest. **39**, 642 (1960).
1372. Skalhegg, B. A., Hellem, A. J., Odegaard, A. E.: Investigation on adenosine diphosphate (ADP) induced platelet adhesiveness *in vitro*. Part II. Studies on the mechanism. Thrombos. Diathes. haemorrh. (Stuttg.) **11**, 305 (1964).
1373. Skoza, L., Zucker, M. B., Jerushalmy, Z., Grant, R.: Kinetic studies of platelet aggregation induced by adenosine diphosphate and its inhibition by chelating agents, guanidino compounds and adenosine. Thrombos. Diathes. haemorrh. (Stuttg.) **18**, 713 (1967).
1374. Slack, J., Nevin, N. C.: Hyperlipidaemic xanthomatosis. I. Increased risk of death from ischaemic heart disease in first degree relatives of 53 patients with essential hyperlipidaemic xanthomatosis. J. med. Genet. **5**, 4 (1968).

1375. Slater, R. S., Smith, E. B.: The extraction and immunological assay of β-lipoprotein in the aortic intima. (Abs.) Biochem. J. **104**, 11P (1967).
1376. Smith, E. B.: Intimal and medial lipids in human aortas. Lancet **1960 I**, 799.
1377. — The influence of age and atherosclerosis on the chemistry of aortic intima. 1. The lipids. J. Atheroscler. Res. **5**, 241 (1965).
1378. — Evans, P. H., Downham, M. D.: Lipid in the aortic intima: the correlation of morphological and chemical characteristics. J. Atheroscler. Res. **7**, 171 (1967).
1379. — Slater, R. S., Chu, P. K.: The lipids in raised fatty and fibrous lesions in human aortas: a comparison of the changes at different stages of development. J. Atheroscler. Res. **8**, 399 (1968).
1380. Smith, R. H.: Lipid-protein isolates. In: *A.C.S. Advances in Chemistry Series*, No. 57, World Protein Resources, p. 133 (1966).
1381. Smythe, H. A., Orgyzlo, M. A., Murphy, E. A., Mustard, J. F.: The effect of sulfinpyrazone (Anturan) on platelet economy and blood coagulation in man. Canad. med. Ass. J. **92**, 818 (1965).
1382. Sodhi, H. S., Gould, R. G.: Combination of delipidized high density lipoprotein with lipids. J. biol. Chem. **242**, 1205 (1967).
1383. Sokolow, M., Perloff, D.: Five-year survival of consecutive patients with malignant hypertension treated with antihypertensive agents. Amer. J. Cardiol. **6**, 858 (1960).
1384. — — The prognosis of essential hypertension treated conservatively. Circulation **23**, 697 (1961).
1385. Somoza, C.: Serum cholesterol levels and aortic medial calcification in rabbits with lesions in the brain. Amer. J. Path. **47**, 271 (1965).
1386. Soppitt, G. D., Mitchell, J. R. A.: Periwinkle alkaloids and platelets (letters). Lancet **1969 II**, 539.
1387. — — The effect of colchicine on human platelet behavior. J. Atheroscler. Res. **10**, 247 (1969).
1388. Spaet, T. H., Erichson, R. B.: The vascular wall in the pathogenesis of thrombosis. In: F. Duckert (ed.), *Pathogenesis and treatment of thrombo-embolic diseases*. Stuttgart: Schattauer-Verlag 1966.
1389. — Zucker, M. B.: Mechanism of platelet aggregation by formation and role of ADP. Amer. J. Physiol. **206**, 1267 (1964).
1390. Spain, D. M., Aristizabal, N.: Rabbit local tissue response to triglycerides, cholesterol and its ester. Arch. Path. **73**, 82 (1962).
1391. — Bradess, V. A.: The relationship of coronary thrombosis to coronary atherosclerosis and ischemic heart disease. (A necropsy study covering a period of twentyfive years). Amer. J. med. Sci, **240**, 701 (1960).
1392. — Greenblatt, I. J., Snapper, I., Cohn, T.: Degree of coronary and aortic atherosclerosis in necropsied cases of multiple myeloma. Amer. J. med. Sci. **231**, 165 (1956).
1393. Sparagen, S. C., Bond, V. P., Dah, L. K.: Role of hyperplasia in vascular lesions of cholesterol-fed rabbits studied with thymidine-^{3}H autoradiography. Circulation Res. **11**, 329 (1962).
1394. — Giordano, A. R., Poon, T. P.: Autoradiographic evidence for participation of rabbit aortic cells in genesis of atheroma. (Abs.) Circulation **38**, Suppl VI, 24 (1968).
1395. Special Projects Review Committee, U. S. National Heart Institute: Organization, review and administration of cooperative studies report to National Advisory Heart Council. Washington, D. C.: U. S. Government Printing Office 1967.
1396. Spielvogel, A. R.: An ultrastructural study of the mechanisms of platelet-endotoxin interaction. J. exp. Med. **126**, 235 (1967).
1397. Spikes, J. L., Jr., Cohen, L., Djordjevich, J.: The identification of a myeloma serum factor which alters sera beta-lipoproteins. Clin. chim. Acta **20**, 413 (1968).

1398. Splitter, S. D., Michaels, G. D., Schlierf, G., Wood, P. D. S., Kinsell, L. W.: Evaluation of the effects of egg yolk lipids upon plasma lipids in human subjects. Metabolism **17**, 1129 (1968).

1399. Spritz, N., Ahrens, E. H., Jr., Grundy, S.: Sterol balance in man as plasma cholesterol concentrations are altered by exchanges of dietary fats. J. clin. Invest. **44**, 1482 (1965).

1400. — Lieber, C. S.: Decrease of ethanol-induced fatty liver by ethyl α-p-chlorophenoxyisobutyrate. Proc. Soc. exp. Biol. Med. (N.Y.) **121**, 147 (1966).

1401. — Mishkel, M. A.: Effects of dietary fats on plasma lipids and lipoproteins: an hypothesis for the lipid-lowering effects of unsaturated fatty acids. J. clin. Invest. **48**, 78 (1969).

1402. Srikantia, S. G., Jagannathan, S. N., Gopalan, S.: Serum cholesterol and blood pressure levels in some South Indian population groups. Indian J. med. Res. **49**, 99 (1961).

1403. Stamler, J.: The epidemiology of atherosclerotic coronary heart disease. Postgrad. Med. **25**, 610, 685 (1959).

1404. — Current status of the dietary prevention and treatment of atherosclerotic coronary heart disease. Progr. cardiovasc. Dis. **3**, 56 (1960).

1405. — The problem of elevated blood cholesterol. Amer. J. publ. Hlth. **50**, 14 (1960).

1406. — Lectures on preventive cardiology. New York: Grune & Stratton 1967.

1407. — Regional differences in mortality, prevalence and incidence of ischaemic heart disease. In: A. A. Snellen (ed.), *Voerhaave course on ischaemic heart disease*. Leiden, the Netherlands: 1969 (in press).

1408. — Berkson, D. M., Lindbergh, H. A., Hall, Y., Miller, W., Mojonnier, L., Levinson, M., Cohen, D. B., Young, Q. D.: Coronary risk factors; their impact, and their therapy in prevention of coronary heart disease. Med. Clin. N. Amer. **50**, 229 (1966).

1409. — — Lindberg, H. A., Whipple, I. T., Miller, W.: Mojonnier, L., Hall, Y. F., Soyugenc, R., Levinson, M. J.: Longterm epidemiologic studies on the possible role of physical activity and physical fitness in the prevention of premature clinical coronary heart disease. In: E. Jokl and D. Brunner (eds.), *Medicine and sport*, vol. 4. Basel, Switzerland: S. Karger 1969.

1410. — — Young, Q. D., Hall, Y., Miller, W.: Approaches to the primary prevention of clinical coronary heart disease in high risk, middle-aged men. Proc. N. Y. Acad. Sci. **97**, 932 (1963).

1411. — Lewis, L. A., Page, I. H., Berkson, D. M., Kaplan, B. M., Katz, L. N., Pick, R., Century, D.: Estrogens and androgens in the treatment of hyperlipidemia. In: J. H. Moyer and A. N. Brest (eds.), *Cardiovascular drug therapy*. p. 353. New York: Grune & Stratton 1965.

1412. — Lindberg, H. A., Berkson, D. M., Shaffer, A., Miller, W., Poindexter, A.: Prevalance and incidence of coronary heart disease in strata of the labor force of a Chicago industrial corporation. J. chron. Dis. **11**, 405 (1960).

1413. — Pick, R., Katz, L. N., Pick, A., Kaplan, B. M., Berkson, D. M., Century, D.: Effectiveness of estrogens for therapy of myocardial infarction in middle-aged men. J. Amer. Med. Ass. **183**, 632 (1963).

1414. Stary, H. C., McMillan, G. C.: Kinetics of cellular proliferation in the atherosclerotic lesion of cholesterol-fed rabbits. Arch. Path. **89**, 173 (1970).

1415. Stein, O., Selinger, Z., Stein, Y.: Incorporation of $I^{14}C$ linoleic acid into lipids of human umbilical arteries. J. Atheroscler. Res. **3**, 189 (1963).

1416. — Stein, Y.: Fine structure of the ethanol induced fatty liver in the rat. Israel J. med. Sci. **1**, 378 (1965).

1417. — — Lipid synthesis, intracellular transport, storage, and secretion. I. Electron microscopic radioautographic study of liver after injection of tritiated palmitate or glycerol in fasted and ethanol-treated rats. J. Cell Biol. **33**, 319 (1967).

1418. — — Lecithin synthesis, intracellular transport, and secretion in rat liver. IV. A radioautographic and biochemical study of choline-deficient rats injected with choline-^{3}H. J. Cell Biol. **40**, 461 (1969).

1419. Stein, Y., Stein, O.: Incorporation of fatty acids into lipids of aortic slices of rabbits, dogs, rats and baboons. J. Atheroscler. Res. **2**, 400 (1962).
1420. — — Shapiro, B.: Enzymic pathways of glyceride and phospholipid synthesis in aortic homogenates. Biochim. biophys. Acta (Amst.) **70**, 33 (1963).
1421. Steiner, G.: Lipoprotein lipase in fat-induced hyperlipemia. New Engl. J. Med. **279**, 70 (1968).
1422. Sternby, N. H.: Atherosclerosis in a defined population: an autopsy survey in Malmö, Sweden. Acta path. Microbiol. Scand., Suppl. 194 (1968).
1423. Stewart, J.: Cited from I. V. Ilyinsky. Atherosclerosis and other forms of arterial sclerosis. In: *Guidebook on internal diseases*, vol. 2, p. 155. Moscow 1964.
1424. Still, W. J. S.: An electron microscopic study of the organization of experimental thromboemboli in the rabbit. Lab. Invest. **15**, 1492 (1966).
1425. Stout, R. W.: Insulin-stimulated lipogenesis in arterial tissue in relation to diabetes and atheroma. Lancet **1968 II**, 702.
1426. Strisower, E. H.: The combined use of CPIB and thyroxine in treatment of hyperlipoproteinemias. Circulation **33**, 291 (1966).
1427. — Adamson, G., Strisower, B.: Treatment of hyperlipidemias. Amer. J. Med. **45**, 488 (1968).
1428. — Kradjian, R. M., Nichols, A. V., Coggiola, E., Tsai, J.: Effect of ileal bypass on serum lipoproteins in essential hypercholesterolemia. J. Atheroscler. Res. **8**, 525 (1968).
1429. — Strisower, B.: The separate hypolipoproteinemic effects of dextrothyroxine and ethyl chlorophenoxyisobutyrate. J. clin. Endocr. **24**, 139 (1964).
1430. Strong, J. P., Correa, P., Solberg, L. A.: Water hardness and atherosclerosis. Lab. Invest. **18**, 620 (1968).
1431. — McGill, H. C., Jr.: The pediatric aspects of atherosclerosis. J. Atheroscler. Res. **9**, 251 (1969).
1432. — Richard, M. L., McGill, H. C., Jr., Eggen, D. A., McMurry, M. T.: On the association of cigarette smoking with coronary and aortic atherosclerosis. J. Atheroscler. Res., **10**, 303 (1969).
1433. Stuart, K. L., Hayes, J. A.: A cardiac disorder of unknown aetiology in Jamaica. Quart. J. Med. N.S. **32**, 99 (1963).
1434. — Schneckloth, R. E., Lewis, L. A., Moore, F. E., Corcoran, A. C.: Diet, serum cholesterol, protein, blood haemoglobin and glycosuria in a West Indian community (St. Kitts). Brit. Med. J. **1962 II**, 1283.
1435. Studer, A.: Experimentelle Angipathien mit besonderer Berücksichtigung der Arteriosklerose. In: Verhandlungen der Deutschen Gesellschaft für Kreislaufforschung, 9. Tagung, p. 17. Darmstadt: Dietrich Steinkopff 1963.
1436. — Experimental platelet thrombus. In: F. Duckert (ed.), *Pathogenesis and treatment of thrombo-embolic diseases*. Stuttgart: Schattauer-Verlag 1966.
1437. — Lorez, H. P.: Experimentelle Untersuchungen über die Bedeutung vorbestehender Gefäßveränderungen für die Anlagerung von Fibrin. Path. et Microbiol. **29**, 406 (1966).
1438. — — Zum Mechanismus der Thrombininduzierten Fibrin-Bildung an der geschädigten kaninshenaorta. Path. et Microbiol. **29**, 285 (1966).
1439. — Reber, K., Lorez, H. P.: Experimentelle Untersuchungen zur Frage der Bedeutung intravasler Fibrinabscheidung für die Entstehung arteriosklerotischer Wandveränderungen. Path. et Microbiol. **27**, 287 (1964).
1440. Sugrue, M. F., Shore, P. A.: The mode of sodium-dependency of the adrenergic neuron amine carrier. Evidence for a second, sodium-dependent, optically specific and reserpine-sensitive system. J. Pharm. Pharmacol., in press (1970).
1441. Sullivan, J. M., Harken, D. E., Gorlin, R.: Pharmacologic control of thromboembolic complications of cardiac-valve replacement. A preliminary report. New Engl. J. Med. **279**, 576 (1968).
1442. Summerell, J. M., Hayes, J. A., Bras, G.: Autopsy data on heart disease in Jamaica. Trop. geogr. Med. **20**, 127 (1968).

1443. Sutherland, E. W., Robison, G. A., Butcher, R. W.: Some aspects of the biological role of adenosine 3',5'-monophosphate (cyclic AMP). Circulation **37**, 279 (1968).
1444. Svoboda, D., Grady, H., Azarnoff, D.: Microbodies in experimentally altered cells. J. Cell Biol. **35**, 127 (1967).
1445. Swan, D. M., McGowan, J. M.: Ileal bypass in hypercholesterolemia associated with coronary heart disease. Amer. J. Surg. **116**, 22 (1968).
1446. Swank, R. L.: Adhesiveness of platelets and leukocytes during acute exanguination. Amer. J. Physiol. **202**, 261 (1962).
1447. Swell, W., Law, M. D., Treadwell, C. R.: Dietary induction of atherosclerosis. J. Nutr. **76**, 429 (1962).
1448. Switzer, S.: Plasma lipoproteins in liver disease: I. Immunologically distinct low-density lipoproteins in patients with biliary obstruction. J. clin. Invest. **46**, 1855 (1967).
1449. Symposium on Atromid: Proceedings of a conference held in Buxton (England). J. Atheroscler. Res. **3**, 351 (1963).
1450. Tannhauser, S. J.: Lipidoses. Third edition, p. 360. New York: Grune & Stratton 1958.
1451. Taub, W., Cais, M.: The synthesis of δ-ketolactones with potential pharmacodynamic properties. Bull. Res. Coun. Israel **11A**, 18 (1962).
1452. Tayeau, F.: Sur la constitution et la stabilite des lipoproteines. In: *The blood lipids and the clearing factors*, p. 35. IIIe Cong. Internat. sur les problemes de la Biochimie des lipides, Bruxelles 1956.
1453. Taylor, C. B.: The reaction of arteries to injury by physical agents. With a discussion of arterial repair and its relationship to atherosclerosis. In: *Symposium on Atherosclerosis*. National Academy of Sciences, National Research Council, Publication **338**, p. 74. Washington, D. C. 1955.
1454. — Gould, R. G.: Effect of dietary cholesterol on rate of cholesterol synthesis of cholesterol. J. biol. Chem. **182**, 629 (1950).
1455. — Patton, D., Yogi, N., Cox, G. E.: Diet as source of serum cholesterol in man. Proc. Soc. Exp. Biol. (N.Y.) **103**, 768 (1960).
1456. Technical Group of the Comittee on Lipoproteins and Atherosclerosis. Report of the: Evaluation of serum lipoprotein and cholesterol measurements as predictors of clinical complications of atherosclerosis; report of a cooperative study of lipoproteins and atherosclerosis. Circulation **14**, 691 (1956).
1457. Tejada, C., Strong, J. P., Montenegro, M. A., Restrepo, C., Solberg, L. A.: Distribution of coronary and aortic atherosclerosis by geographic location, race and sex. Lab. Invest. **18**, 509 (1968).
1458. Tennent, D. M., Siegel, H., Zanetti, M. E., Kuron, O. W., Ott, W. H., Wolf, F. J.: Plasma cholesterol lowering action of bile acid binding polymers in experimental animals. J. Lipid Res. **1**, 469 (1959).
1459. Texon, M.: The haemodynamic concept of atherosclerosis. Bull. N. Y. Acad. Med. **36**, 263 (1960).
1460. Thienes, C. H.: Chronic nicotine poisoning. Ann. N. Y. Acad. Sci. **90**, 239 (1960).
1461. Thomas, W. A., Davies, J. N. P., O'Neal, R. M., Dimakulangan, A. A.: Incidence of myocardial infarction correlated with venous and pulmonary thrombosis and embolism. Amer. J. Cardiol. **5**, 41 (1960).
1462. Thomas, W. A., Florentin, R. A., Nam, S. C., Kim, D. N., Jones, R. M., Lee, K. T.: Pre-proliferative phase of atherosclerosis in swine fed cholesterol. Arch. Path. **86**, 621 (1968).
1463. — Hartroft, W. S.: Myocardial infarction in rats fed high fat and cholesterol diets containing thiouracil and sodium cholate. Circulation **19**, 65 (1959).
1464. — O'Neal, R. M., Kyu, T. L.: Thromboembolism, pulmonary arteriosclerosis, and fatty meals. Arch. Path. **61**, 380 (1956).
1465. Thomasson, H. J., de Boer, J., de Iongh, H.: Influence of dietary fats on plasma lipids. 9th Int. Soc. Geograph. Path., Leyden, 1966. Path. et Microbiol. **30**, 629 (1967).

1466. Thorp, J. M.: Experimental evaluation of an orally active combination of androsterone with ethyl chlorophenoxyisobutyrate. Lancet **1962 I**, 323.

1467. — An experimental approach to the problem of disordered lipid metabolism. J. Atheroscler. Res. **3**, 351 (1963).

1468. — Cotton, R. C., Oliver, M. F.: Role of the endocrine system in the regulation of plasma lipids and fibrinogen, with particular reference to the effects of "Atromid-S". Progr. biochem. Pharmacol. **4**, 611 (1968).

1469. — Waring, W. S.: Modification of metabolism and distribution of lipids by ethyl chlorophenoxyisobutyrate. Nature (Lond.) **194**, 948 (1962).

1470. Tibblin, G.: High blood pressure in men aged 50. A population study of men born in 1913. Acta med. scand., Suppl. **470** (1967).

1471. Tibbs, D. J.: Arterial replacement and reconstruction. A five-year review. Lancet **1960 II**, 1313.

1472. Todd, A. S.: Localization of fibrinolytic activity in tissues. Brit. med. Bull. **20**, 210 (1964).

1473. Tolman, E. L., Tepperman, H. M., Tepperman, J.: The effect of ethyl p-chlorophenoxyisobutyrate (CPIB) on adipose tissue lipoprotein lipase activity. Fed. Proc. **28**, 677 (1969).

1474. Torvik, A., Jorgensen, L.: Thrombotic and embolic occlusions of the carotid arteries in an autopsy series. Part 2. Cerebral lesions and clinical course. J. Neurol. Sci. **3**, 410 (1966).

1475. Tracy, R. E., Merchant, E. B., Kao, V. C.: On the antigenic identity of human serum β- and α_2-lipoproteins and their identification in the aortic intima. Circulat. Res. **9**, 472 (1961).

1476. Treadwell, C. R., Vahouny, G. V.: Cholesterol absorption. In: ***Handbook of physiology***, Sect. 6, vol. III, American Physiological Society, p. 1407. Washington, D. C. 1968.

1477. Truett, J., Cornfield, J., Kannel, W.: A multivariate analysis of the risk of coronary heart disease in Framingham. J. chron. Dis. **20**, 511 (1967).

1478. Ts'ao, C., Spaet, T. H.: Ultramicroscopic changes in the rabbit inferior vena cava following partial constriction. Amer. J. Path. **51**, 789 (1967).

1479. Turpeinen, O., Miettinen, M., Karvonen, M. J., Roine, P., Pekkarinen, M., Lehtosuo, E. J., Alivirta, P.: Dietary prevention of coronary heart disease: long term experiment. I. Observations on male subjects. Amer. J. clin. Nutr. **21**, 255 (1968).

1480. Tyavokin, V. V.: On the evaluation of ECG changes in cases of coronary insufficiency. Kazansky Med. J. **3**, 8 (1962).

1481. — Electrocardiographic dynamics of patients with coronary insufficiency as a response to the change in hospital regimen. Leningrad, Trudy Leningr. Paediatr. Med. Inst. **31**, 366 (1963).

1482. — The reproduction of atherosclerosis in rabbits by mobility restriction. Bull. Exp. Biol. Med. **2**, 19 (1967).

1483. — On the paper by Prof. I. V. Davydovsky, "Atherosclerosis as a problem of age". Cardiologia **8**, 143 (1967).

1484. — Experimental atherosclerosis in rabbits with mobility restriction. Cor et Vasa (Praha) **9**, 68 (1967).

1485. — Experimentelle Coronarsklerose durch Bewegungseinschränkung beim Kaninchen, ein neues Modell der Arteriosklerose. Virchows Arch. Abt. Path. Anat. **346**, 29 (1969).

1486. Tzagournis, M., Chiles, R., Ryan, J. M., Skillman, T. G.: Interrelationships of hyperinsulinaemia and hypertriglyceridaemia in young patients with coronary heart disease. Circulation **38**, 1156 (1968).

1487. Uri, N.: Physico-chemical aspects of autoxidation. In: W. O. Lundberg (ed.), ***Autoxidation and antioxidants***, p. 55. New York: Interscience Publishers 1961

1488. Vagelos, P. R.: Lipid metabolism. Ann. Rev. Biochem. **33**, 139 (1964).

1489. Vainstein, K. I.: Oxygen deficiency and oxygen therapy of atherosclerosis. Reports of the Scientific conference of the Chelyabinsk Medical Inst., p. 16. Chelyabinsk 1964.

1490. Vaishwanam, I., Nath, M. C.: Study of serum triglycerides in health and metabolic disorders. Indian Heart J. **15**, 114 (1963).

1491. Van den Bosch, J. F., Claes, P. J.: Correlation between the bile salt-precipitating capacity of derivatives of basic antibiotics and their cholesterol lowering effect *in vivo*. Progr. biochem. Pharmacol. **2**, 97 (1967).

1492. Van Handel, E., Zilversmit, D. B.: Micromethod for the direct determination of serum triglycerides. J. Lab. clin. Med. **50**, 152 (1957).

1493. Van Orden, D. E., Treffers, M. P.: A demonstration of the coprecipitation of β-lipoproteins with specific precipitates of chicken antibodies and human serum albumin. J. Immunol. **100**, 664 (1968).

1494. Van Reen, R.: Effect of excessive dietary zinc in rats and the interrelation with copper. Arch. Biochem. **46**, 337 (1953).

1495. Vasalli, P., Simon, G., Roullier, C.: Ultrastructural study of platelet changes initiated by thrombin. J. Ultrastruct. Res. **11**, 374 (1964).

1496. Velican, C., Velican, D.: Histochimie des glycoprotéines. Paris: Gauthiers Villars 1969.

1497. Vengsarkar, A. S., Misra, S. N., Rodrigues, P. F., Pinto, I. J.: Serum cholesterol, triglycerides and uric acid levels in ischaemic heart disease in the low-income population in Bombay. Indian J. med. Sci. **22**, 851 (1968).

1498. Veterans Administration Cooperative Study Group on Antihypertensive Agents: Effects of treatment on morbidity in hypertension. Results in patients with diastolic blood pressures averaging 115 through 129 mm. Hg. J. Amer. med. Ass. **202**, 1028 (1967).

1499. Virchow, R.: Aus dem pathologisch—anatomischen Curse. Wien. med. Wschr. **6**, 809 (1856).

1500. — Gesammelte Abhandlungen zur wissenschaftlichen Medizin, p. 219. Frankfurt: Medinger, Son & Co. 1856.

1501. Vital Statistics of U.S.: Deaths from arteriosclerotic heart disease, including coronary disease. U.S. Department of Health, Education and Welfare, Public Health Service, Superintendent of Documents, U.S. Government Printing Office, Washington, D. C., 1966.

1502. Vital Statistics of U.S. Special Reports: Death rates by age, race, and sex. United States, 1900—1953. All causes. U.S. Department of Health, Education and Welfare, Superintendent of Documents, U.S. Government Printing Office, Washington, D. C., **43**, 1 (1956).

1503. Vlodaver, Z., Kahn, H. A., Neufeld, H. N.: The coronary arteries in early life in three different ethnic groups. Circulation **39**, 541 (1969).

1504. — Medalie, J., Neufeld, H. N.: Coronary arteries in immature monkeys: Preliminary report of the relationships to activity and diet. J. Atheroscler. Res. **8**, 923 (1968).

1505. — Neufeld, H. N.: The musculo-elastic layer in the coronary arteries. Vascular Dis. **4**, 136 (1967).

1506. — — The coronary arteries in coarctation of the aorta. Circulation **37**, 449 (1968).

1507. Vogel, W. C., Bierman, E. L.: Post-heparin serum lecithinase in man and its positional specificity. J. Lipid Res. **8**, 46 (1967).

1508. — — Evidence for *in vivo* activity of postheparin plasma lecithinase in man. Proc. Soc. exp. Med. Biol. (N.Y.) **127**, 77 (1968).

1509. Volkov, N. F.: Cobalt, Manganese and zinc content in blood of atherosclerosis patients. Fed. Proc. trans. Suppl. **22**, T897 (1963).

1510. Wacker, W. E., Ulmer, D. D., Vallee, B. L.: Metalloenzymes and myocardial infarction. II. Malic and lactic dehydrogenase activities and zinc concentrations in serum. New Engl. J. Med. **255**, 449 (1956).

1511. Waddell, W. R., Geyer, R. P., Harley, N., Stare, F. J.: Abnormal carbohydrate metabolism in patients with hypercholesterolemia and hyperlipemia. Metabolism **7**, 707 (1958).
1512. Wahlberg, F.: Intravenous glucose tolerance in myocardial infarction, angina pectoris and intermittent claudication. Acta med. Scand., Suppl. **453**, 180 (1966).
1513. Wahlqvist, M. L., Day, A. J.: Phospholipid synthesis by foam cells in human atheroma. Exp. molec. Path. **11**, 275 (1969).
1514. — — Tume, R. K.: Incorporation of oleic acid into lipid by foam cells in human atherosclerotic lesions. Circulat. Res. **24**, 123 (1969).
1515. Wakil, S. J.: Lipid metabolism. Ann. Rev. Biochem. **31**, 369 (1962).
1516. Waldenstrom, J.: Abnormal proteins in myeloma. Advanc. intern. Med. **5**, 398 (1952).
1517. — Winblad, S., Hallen, J., Liumgman, S.: The occurrence of serological "antibody" reagins or similar γ-globulins in conditions with monoclonal hyperglobulinemia such as myeloma, macroglobulinemia. Acta med. scand. **176**, 619 (1964).
1518. Waldron, J. M.: Clot-accelerating property of *in vitro* epinephrine and norepinephrine on whole blood coagulation. J. appl. Physiol. **3**, 554 (1950–51).
1519. Walker, G., Doniach, D.: Antibodies and immunoglobulins in liver disease. Gut **9**, 266 (1968).
1520. — — Roitt, M., Sherlock, S.: Serological tests in the diagnosis of primary biliary cirrhosis. Lancet **1965 I**, 827.
1521. Walton, K. W., Williamson, N.: Histological and immunofluorescent studies on the evolution of the human atheromatous plaque. J. Atheroscler. Res. **8**, 599 (1968).
1522. Wanstrup, J., Kjeldsen, K., Astrup, P.: Acceleration of spontaneous intimal-subintimal changes in rabbit aorta by a prolonged moderate carbon monoxide exposure. Acta path. microbiol. scand. **75**, 353 (1969).
1523. Warren, R., Gomez, R. L., Marston, J. A. P., Cox, J. S. T.: Femoropopliteal arteriosclerosis obliterans—arteriographic patterns and rates of progression. Surgery **55**, 135 (1964).
1524. Warrier, C. B. C.: Venugopal, N. S., Ramchandran, C. K.: Incidence and pattern of cardiovascular disease in Kerala. J. Ass. Phys. India **15**, 229 (1967).
1525. Watts, H. F.: Role of lipoproteins in the formation of atherosclerotic lesions. In: R. J. Jones (ed.), *Evolution of the atherosclerotic plaque*, p. 117. Chicago: University of Chicago Press 1963.
1526. Weeks, J. R., Chandra Sekhar, N., Ducharme, D. W.: Relative activity of prostaglandins E_1, A_1, E_2 and A_2 on lipolysis, platelet aggregation, smooth muscle and the cardiovascular system. J. Pharm. Pharmacol. **21**, 103 (1969).
1527. Wegener, K.: Koronarverschluß. Histogenese der sklerotischen plaque und regressive Veränderungen. Arch. Kreisl.-Forsch. **58**, 102 (1969).
1528. Weinblatt, E., Frank, C. W., Shapiro, S., Sager, R. V.: Prognostic factors in angina pectoris—a prospective study. J. chron. Dis. **21**, 231 (1968).
1529. — Shapiro, S., Frank, C. W., Sager, R. V.: Prognosis of men after first myocardial infarction: mortality and first recurrence in relation to selected parameters. Amer. J. Publ. Hlth **58**, 1329 (1968).
1530. Weiss, H. J., Aledort, L. M., Kochwa, S.: The effect of salicylates on the hemostatic properties of platelets in man. J. clin. Invest. **47**, 2169 (1968).
1531. Weiss, M. M.: Ten years prognosis of acute myocardial infarction. Amer. J. med. Sci. **231**, 9 (1956).
1532. Welborn, T. A., Breckenridge, A., Rubenstein, A. H., Dollery, C. T., Fraser, T. R.: Serum insulin in essential hypertension and in peripheral vascular disease. Lancet **1966 I**, 1336.
1533. — Cumpston, G. N., Cullen, K. J., Curnow, D. M., McCall, M. G., Stenhouse, N. S.: The prevalence of coronary heart disease and associated factors in an Australian rural community. Amer. J. Epidemiol. **89**, 521 (1969).

1534. Welch, L. C., Twiehaus, M. J.: Nebraska miniature swine. In: L. K. Bustad and R. O. McClellan (eds.), *Swine in biomedical research*, p. 803. Seattle: Frayn Printing Company 1966.
1535. Wells, V. M., Bronte-Stewart, B.: Egg yolk and serum cholesterol levels: importance of dietary cholesterol intake. Brit. med. J. **1963 I**, 577.
1536. Wenzel, D. G., Turner, J. A., Jordan, S. W., Singh, J.: Cardiovascular interaction of nicotine, ergonovine, and hypercholesterolemia in the rabbit. Circulat. Res. **9**, 694 (1961).
1537. — — Kissil, D.: Effect of nicotine on cholesterol induced atherosclerosis in the rabbit. Circulat. Res. **7**, 256 (1959).
1538. Westerfeld, W. W., Richert, D. A., Ruegamer, W. R.: The role of the thyroid hormone in the effect of p-chlorophenoxyisobutyrate in rats. Biochem. Pharmacol. **17**, 100 (1968).
1539. Wexler, B. C.: Spontaneous arteriosclerosis in repeatedly bred male and female rats. J. Atheroscler. Res. **4**, 57 (1964).
1540. Whayne, T. F., Felts, J. M., Harris, P. A.: Effect of heparin on the inactivation of serum lipoprotein lipase by the liver in unanesthetized dogs. J. clin. Invest. **48**, 1246 (1969).
1541. Whereat, A. F.: Lipid biosynthesis in aortic intima from normal and cholesterol-fed rabbits. J. Atheroscler. Res. **4**, 272 (1964).
1542. — Fatty acid synthesis in cell-free system from rabbit aorta. J. Lipid Res. **7**. 671 (1966).
1543. — Recent advances in experimental and molecular pathology. Atherosclerosis and metabolic disorder in the arterial wall. Exp. molec. Path. **7**, 233 (1967),
1544. — Orishimo, M. W.: The effect of cholesterol administration on lipid biosynthesis by rabbit aortic mitochondria. Exp. molec. Path. **9**, 230 (1968).
1545. White, J. G.: Fine structural alterations induced in platelets by adenosine-diphosphate. Blood **31**, 604 (1968).
1546. Whyte, H. M., Nestel, P. J., Goodman, D. S.: Cholesterol distribution and turnover in obesity in man. Israel J. med. Sci. **5**, 644 (1969).
1547. Wieland, O., Neufeldt, I., Numa, S., Lynen, F.: Zur Störung der Fettsäuresynthese bei Hunger und Alloxandiabetes. Biochem. Z. **336**, 455 (1963).
1548. Wilcox, E. B., Galloway, L. S.: Serum and liver cholesterol, total lipids and lipid phosphorus levels of rats under various dietary regimes. Amer. J. clin. Nutr. **9**, 236 (1961).
1549. Wilson, D. E., Schreibman, P. H., Arky, R. A.: Post-heparin lipolytic activity in diabetic patients with a history of mixed hyperlipemia. Diabetes **18**, 562 (1969).
1550. Wilson, J. D.: Biosynthetic origin of serum cholesterol in squirrel monkey: evidence for a contribution by the intestinal wall. J. clin. Invest. **47**, 175 (1968).
1551. — The measurement of the exchangeable pools of cholesterol in the baboon. J. clin. Invest., in press (1970).
1552. — Dietschy, J. M.: The biosynthetic origin of serum cholesterol in the monkey. J. clin. Invest. **45**, 1086 (1966).
1553. — Lindsey, C. A., Jr.: Studies on the influence of dietary cholesterol on cholesterol metabolism in the isotopic steady state in man. J. clin. Invest. **44**, 1805 (1965).
1554. Wilson, R. B., Martin, J. M., Hartroft, W. S.: Failure of insulin therapy to prevent cardiovascular lesions in diabetic rats fed an atherogenic diet. Diabetes **18**, 225 (1969).
1555. Windmueller, H. G., Levy, R. I.: Total inhibition of hepatic β-lipoprotein production in the rat by orotic acid. J. biol. Chem. **242**, 2246 (1967).
1556. — — Production of beta-lipoprotein by intestine in the rat. J. biol. Chem. **243**, 4878 (1968).
1557. — Spaeth, A. E.: *De novo* synthesis of fatty acid in perfused rat liver as a determinant of plasma lipoprotein production. Arch. Biochem. **122**, 362 (1967).

1558. Winegrad, A. I., Yalcin, S., Mulcahy, P. D.: Alterations in aortic metabolism in diabetes. In: B. S. Leibel and G. A. Wrenshall (eds.), *On the nature and treatment of diabetes*, p. 452. Amsterdam: Excepta Medica Foundation 1965.
1559. Wing, D. R., Robinson, D. S.: Clearing-factor lipase in adipose tissue. Biochem. J. **109**, 841 (1968).
1560. Wirtz, K. W. A., Zilversmit, D. B.: Exchange of phospholipids between liver mitochondria and microsomes *in vitro*. J. biol. Chem. **243**, 3596 (1968).
1561. Wissler, R. W., Frazier, L. E., Hughes, R. H., Rasmussen, R. A.: Atherogenesis in the cebus monkey. 1. A comparison of three food fats under controlled dietary conditions. Arch. Path. **74**, 312 (1962).
1562. — Vesselinovitch, D.: Experimental models of human atherosclerosis. Ann. N. Y. Acad. Sci. **149**, 907 (1968).
1563. — — Getz, G. S., Hughes, R. H.: Aortic lesions and blood lipids in rhesus monkeys fed three different food fats. Fed. Proc. **26**, 371 (1967).
1564. — — Hughes, R., Roch, T.: Atherosclerosis and blood lipids in rhesus monkeys confined in widely varying space. (Abs.) Fed. Proc. **28**, 447 (1969).
1565. Witiak, D. T., Parker, R. A., Dempsey, M. E., Ritter, M. C., Connor, W. E.: Synthesis and *in vivo, in vitro* biological evaluation of cholestane-3β-5α-6β-triol analogues as hypocholesterolemic agents. J. med. Chem., in press (1970).
1566. Woerner, C. A.: Vasa vasorum of arteries, their demonstration and distribution. In: A. I. Lansing (ed.), *The arterial wall*, p. 1. Baltimore: Williams and Wilkins 1959.
1567. Wolinsky, H., Glagov, S.: Nature of species difference in the medial distribution of aortic *vasa vasorum* in mammals. Circulat. Res. **20**, 409 (1967).
1568. Wood, P. D. S., Shioda, R., Kinsell, L. W. W.: Dietary regulation of cholesterol metabolism. Lancet **1966 II**, 604.
1569. Woolf, N., Bradley, J. W. P., Crawford, T., Carstairs, K. C.: Experimental mural thrombi in the pig aorta. The early natural history. Brit. J. exp. Path. **49**, 257 (1968).
1570. — Carstairs, K. C.: Infiltration and thrombosis in atherogenesis. A study using immunofluorescent techniques. Amer. J. Path. **51**, 373 (1967).
1571. — — The survival time of platelets in experimental mural thrombi. J. Path. **97**, 595 (1969).
1572. — Crawford, T.: Fatty streaks in aortic intima studied by an immunohistochemical technique. J. Path. Bact. **80**, 405 (1960).
1573. — Pilkington, T. R. E.: The immunohistochemical demonstration of lipoproteins in vessel walls. J. Path. Bact. **90**, 459 (1965).
1574. — — Carstairs, K. C.: The occurrence of lipoproteins in thrombi. J. Path. Bact. **91**, 383 (1966).
1575. W. H. O.: Epidemiological and vital statistics report. Geneva: W. H. O. 1969.
1576. W. H. O. Health Organization Executive Board Report: International work in cardiovascular diseases. Geneva: W. H. O. 1969.
1577. W. H. O. Regional Office for Europe: Ischaemic heart disease registers: report of a working group. Document EURO 5010 (1). Geneva: W. H. O. 1968.
1578. W. H. O. Scientific Group on Paediatric Research: Report, W. H. O. Techn. Rep. Ser. No 400. Geneva: W. H. O. 1968.
1579. Wright, H. P.: The adhesiveness of blood platelets in normal subjects with varying concentrations of anticoagulants. J. Path. Bact. **53**, 255 (1941).
1580. Yacowitz, H., Fleischman, A. A., Beirenbaum, A. A.: Effect of oral calcium on serum lipids in man. Brit. Med. J. **1965 I**, 1352.
1581. Yalcin, S., Winegrad, A. I.: Defect in glucose metabolism in aortic tissue from alloxan diabetic rabbits. Amer. J. Physiol. **205**, 1253 (1963).
1582. Yalow, R. S., Berson, S. A.: Immunoassay of endogenous plasma insulin in man. J. clin. Invest. **39**, 1157 (1960).
1583. Yankeelov, J. A., Mitchell, C. D., Crawford, T. H.: A simple trimerization of 2,3-butanedione yielding a selective reagent for the modification of arginine in proteins. J. Amer. Chem. Soc. **90**, 1664 (1968).

1584. Yerushalmy, J., Hilleboe, H. E.: Fat in the diet and mortality from heart disease—a methodological note. N. Y. St. J. Med. 57, 2343 (1967).
1585. Young, W., Hotovec, R. L., Romero, A. G.: Tea and atherosclerosis. Nature (Lond.) **216**, 1015 (1967).
1586. Yudkin, J.: Diet and coronary thrombosis. Lancet **1957 II**, 155.
1587. Zahavi, J., Dryfuss, F.: An abnormal pattern of adenosine diphosphate—induced platelet aggregation in acute myocardial infarction. Thrombos. Diathes. haemorrh. (Stuttg.) **21**, 76 (1969).
1588. Zemplényi, T. (ed.): Vascular enzymes and atherosclerosis. J. Atheroscler. Res. **7**, 725 (1967).
1589. — Enzyme biochemistry of the arterial wall. London: Lloyd Luke 1968.
1590. — Grafnetter, D.: The lipolytic activity of the aorta; its relation to aging and atherosclerosis. Gerontologia (Basel) **3**, 55 (1959).
1591. Ziegler, E.: In: A. H. BUCK (ed.), *General pathology*, translated from the 8th German edition, p. 127, 290. New York: William Wood & Co. 1896.
1592. Zilversmit, D. B.: Phospholipid turnover in atheromatous lesions. In: G. PINCUS (ed.), *Hormones and atherosclerosis*, p. 145. New York: Academic Press 1959.
1593. — The design and analysis of isotope experiments. Amer. J. Med. **29**, 832 (1960).
1594. — Cholesterol flux in the atherosclerotic plaque. Ann. N. Y. Acad. Sci. **149**, 710 (1968).
1595. — Davis, A. K.: Microdetermination of plasma phospholipids by trichloroacetic acid precipitation. J. Lab. clin. Med. **35**, 155 (1950).
1596. — McCandless, E. L.: Independence of arterial phospholipid synthesis from atherotions in blood lipids. J. Lipid Res. **1**, 118 (1959).
1597. — — Jordan, P. H., Henly, W. S., Ackerman, R. F.: The synthesis of phospholipids in human atheromatous lesions. Circulation **23**, 370 (1961).
1598. — Shore, M. L., Ackerman, R. F.: The origin of aortic phospholipid in rabbit atheromatosis. Circulation **9**, 581 (1954).
1599. — Sweeley, C. C., Newman, H. A. I.: The fatty acid composition of rabbit aortic tissue. Circulat. Res. **9**, 235 (1961).
1600. Zucker, M. B., Borelli, J.: In: S. A. JOHNSON, R. W. MONTO, J., W. REBUCK, and R. C. HORN, JR. (eds.), *Blood platelets*. Boston: Little & Brown 1961.
1601. Zugibe, F. T.: Atherosclerosis in the miniature pig. In: J. C. ROBERTS, JR., and R. STRAUSS (eds.), *Comparative atherosclerosis*, p. 37. New York: Hoeber Medical Division, Harper & Row 1965.

SUBJECT INDEX